FOODS *that* HARM FOODS *that* HEAL

AN A-Z GUIDE TO SAFE AND HEALTHY EATING

Chief Consultants:
Joe Schwarcz, Ph.D., and Fran Berkoff, R.D.

The Reader's Digest Association, Inc.
Pleasantville, New York • Montreal

Library of Congress Cataloging-in-Publication Data

Foods that harm, foods that heal / Reader's Digest.—1st ed.
416 p. cm.
   Includes index.
   ISBN 978-0-7621-0505-2 (hardcover)
   1. Nutrition—Popular works. 2. Food—Composition—Popular works. I. Reader's Digest Association.
RA784.F639 2004
613.2—dc22

                                        2003027879

Address any comments about FOODS THAT HARM, FOODS THAT HEAL to:
The Reader's Digest Association, Inc.
Editor-in-Chief, Home & Health Books
Reader's Digest Road
Pleasantville, NY 10570-7000
or
Reader's Digest Association (Canada) Ltd.
1125 Stanley Street, Montreal, Quebec H3B 5H5

For information on this and other Reader's Digest products, visit our website:
www.rd.com (in the United States)
www.readersdigest.ca (in Canada)

7 9 10 8

US 4577/G

NOTE TO READERS:

**The information in this book should not be substituted for, or used
to alter, medical therapy without your doctor's advice.
For a specific health problem, consult your physician for guidance.**

READER'S DIGEST PROJECT STAFF

EDITORS: **Pamela Johnson,
Marianne Wait**
ART DIRECTORS: **John McGuffie,
Michele Laseau**
DESIGNERS: **Cécile Germain,
Andrée Payette**
ASSISTANT EDITORS: **Carolyn Jackson,
Robert Ronald**
COPY EDITOR: **Gilles Humbert**
PRODUCTION MANAGER: **Holger Lorenzen**
PRODUCTION COORDINATOR: **Susan Wong**

READER'S DIGEST HEALTH PUBLISHING

EDITOR-IN-CHIEF AND PUBLISHING DIRECTOR:
Neil Wertheimer
MANAGING EDITOR: **Suzanne G. Beason**
DESIGN DIRECTOR: **Michele Laseau**
PRODUCTION TECHNOLOGY MANAGER:
Douglas A. Croll
MANUFACTURING MANAGER: **John L. Cassidy**
MARKETING DIRECTOR: **Dawn Nelson**
VICE PRESIDENT AND GENERAL MANAGER:
Keira Krausz

READER'S DIGEST ASSOCIATION (CANADA) LTD.

VICE PRESIDENT AND EDITORIAL DIRECTOR,
BOOKS AND HOME ENTERTAINMENT:
Deirdre Gilbert
ART DIRECTOR: **John McGuffie**
ADMINISTRATOR: **Elizabeth Eastman**

READER'S DIGEST ASSOCIATION, INC.

PRESIDENT, NORTH AMERICA
GLOBAL EDITOR-IN-CHIEF: **Eric W. Schrier**

CONTRIBUTORS

2004 EDITION
CONSULTANTS: **Joseph A. Schwarcz, Ph.D.,
Fran Berkoff, R.D.**
WRITERS: **Sandra Brazel, Susan Fyshe,
Marilyn Linton**
PICTURE RESEARCHER: **Rachel Irwin**
IMAGE TREATMENT: **Yves Lachance**
INDEXER: **Patricia Buchanan**

1997 EDITION
EDITORIAL DIRECTOR:
Genell J. Subak-Sharpe, M.S.
MEDICAL CONSULTANTS:
**Morton D. Bogdonoff, M.D.,
Karen Levine, R.D.**
WRITERS/EDITORS: **Arlyn Apollo,
Diana Benzaia, Jean Callahan,
Mikola De Roo, Nicole Freeland,
Emily Paulsen, Rosemary Perkins,
Ann Forer Stockton**
TECHNICAL SUPPORT: **Debra Rabinowitz,
Dushan G. Lukic, Carl Li**
RESEARCHERS: **Helene MacLean,
Sarah Subak-Sharpe**
COPY EDITORS: **Gina Grant, Diana Marsh,
Joseph Marchetti, Judy Yelon**
PHOTOGRAPHERS: **Karl Adamson,
Colin Cooke, Gus Filgate, Vernon Morgan,
Carol Sharpe, Jon Stewart**
FOOD STYLISTS: **Nir Adar, Karen Temple**

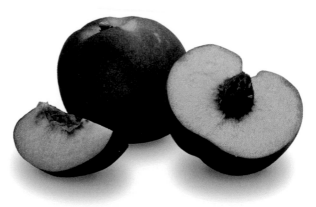

TABLE OF CONTENTS

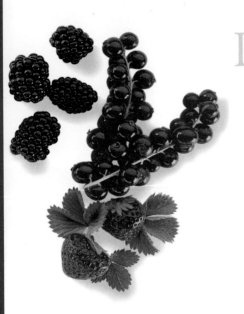

SPECIAL FEATURES

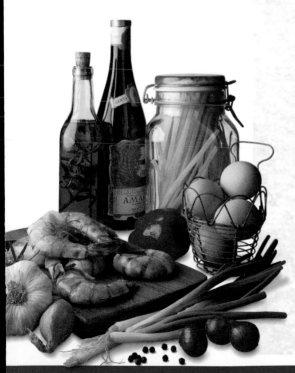

PREFACE

"Let thy food be thy medicine and thy medicine be thy food" advised Hippocrates more than 2,000 years ago. An alluring notion, to be sure. And certainly a sensible one given that food is the source of all of the components that make up the human body. But the famous Greek physician's dietary prescriptions were hampered by a lack of understanding of the chemical complexity of food and the intricacies of human physiology.

Throughout history, advances in nutrition came about more or less through chance discoveries. Jacques Cartier's second voyage to the New World in 1535 is a typical example. Many of Cartier's men came down with scurvy, a potentially deadly ailment for which the French explorers had no solution. But the Iroquois did! These people of the first nations of North America showed the sailors how to strip leaves from a white cedar tree and boil them into a tea that was rich in vitamin C. Today we know why drinking the tea had an almost miraculous effect. Scurvy is caused by a lack of vitamin C, which is present in cedar but was almost nonexistent in the explorers' diet while at sea.

By the 20th century researchers had discovered a number of links between diet and health. In addition to vitamin C, it became clear that 12 other vitamins, a host of minerals, and a proper blend of carbohydrates, fats, and proteins were required to prevent deficiency diseases. Then as such deficiency diseases were eliminated, at least in the developed world,

researchers began to shift their attention to tackling the modern plagues of heart disease, cancer, and obesity. Information accumulated quickly and the first edition of *Foods That Harm, Foods That Heal,* published in 1997, was able to make concrete recommendations about which foods to eat and which to avoid. Since then nutritional research has exploded, allowing us to fine-tune our recommendations and offer new advice.

North American waistlines have expanded dramatically in the last few years, necessitating a fresh look at various weight-loss programs. So, in this updated edition, we examine low-carb diets and investigate new findings about the glycemic index of foods. But of course, there is more to life than weight control. Recent research has used epidemiological studies, laboratory experiments, and clinical trials to tease out information about certain components of foods and help determine which ones fight disease. We discovered that lignans in flaxseed may reduce the risk of certain cancers, that beta glucan in oats lowers cholesterol, and that omega-3 fats in fish fight heart disease and maybe even depression, as well as ease allergies and inflammation-related arthritis pain. Lycopene, the red pigment in tomatoes, can reduce the risk of prostate cancer, and sulforaphane in broccoli has decided anticancer properties.

In the wake of new research findings, food itself is changing. Stanols, isolated from pine trees, are being added to some margarines to reduce blood cholesterol; inulin from chicory, which fosters the growth of beneficial bacteria in the digestive tract, is sometimes added to foods such as yogurt; and some eggs now contain omega-3 fats. On the other hand, we have also learned that hydrogenating fats introduces undesirable trans fatty acids into our food supply, and that many dietary supplements may not live up to the hype that surrounds them.

Numerous food and health questions arise everyday in our lives, and the information available is often confusing. Are artificial sweeteners safe? Can specific foods control the symptoms of menopause? Does sugar make children hyperactive? Is a glass of red wine a day good for us? In this book we address all of these issues, give you the most recent scientific findings, and make practical dietary recommendations that everyone can understand. As our population ages and medical and drug costs soar, it is becoming vitally important to learn how to avoid and treat various problems through the best food choices. Many experts have shared their views about such choices here and have ensured that the reader will be armed with the most up-to-date information about foods that harm and foods that heal.

Joe Schwarcz, Ph.D.
Director, McGill University
Office for Science and Society

ABOUT THIS BOOK

Does this sound familiar? You finally get it into your head that margarine is better for you than butter, and then you hear a news report that in fact, some margarine might be even worse than butter—unless you buy the right kind. Or maybe you're confused by the advice of health "experts," some of whom tell you to eat less meat, while others insist it should be front and center on your plate.

The story of food has as many twists and turns as a bowl of fusilli (pasta itself being one of the hottest subjects of debate). Yet you don't want to spend your time unraveling its mysteries. You just want to enjoy delicious food and know that what you're eating is good for you—maybe even good enough to keep the doctor away (or, since doctors no longer make house calls, to keep you away from the doctor). *Foods That Harm, Foods That Heal* will show you how.

More than 150 food entries, organized from A to Z, give you the lowdown on the nutritional value of everything from acorn squash to eggs to zucchini. Look up Chocolate and you'll find out why dark chocolate is better for you than milk chocolate. The Nuts and Seeds entry explains why peanut butter is now considered a good-for-you food. Tomatoes tells an anticancer tale so compelling you'll want to fire up a jar of sauce for that bowl of fusilli right away. Elsewhere, read about the surprising, newly discovered benefits of beer and coffee.

Food can do more than keep you healthy. Like the best modern medicines, it can also help heal what ails you. If you have a specific health concern, such as arthritis or diabetes, look it up here to learn what the right diet can do. More than 80 ailment entries reflect the latest, best thinking on which foods can tame inflammation, stop an asthma attack, clean your arteries, and even guard against Alzheimer's disease, stroke, and cancer. Turn to Depression and find inspiring reasons to eat more fish. And read Hay Fever to learn which plant foods can actually trigger symptoms.

Beyond the food and ailment entries are special features dedicated to key topics including Fast Food, Genetically Modified Organisms, Low-Carb Diets, Pesticides and Pollutants, and Probiotics. Use them to find answers to such questions as: Which fish have the lowest levels of mercury? Is organic produce worth the price? Do grilled foods cause cancer? Turn to Glycemic Index to find out how to choose foods that will give you more energy and improve your mood. Check Dieting to learn which mineral can help you lose weight. And in Omega-3s and Omega-6s, discover how these "good" fats can benefit people with arthritis, diabetes, and heart disease, and where to get them.

A team of medical and nutritional experts sifted through the latest scientific studies and reports in order to separate myths from facts and help us create the most authoritative, up-to-date food reference possible. Use it to clear up nagging confusion over carbohydrates, cholesterol, fats, and more. Follow its practical advice about the foods you eat every day and how to buy and prepare them. Trust it to help you make subtle changes to your diet that will pay off in big benefits over time.

There's no doubt that the right diet is the best prescription for better health. And now we know more than ever before about the power of food to prevent, treat, and even cure major ailments and minor annoyances. With *Foods That Harm, Foods That Heal* you can use that information to look better, function better, feel better—and enjoy more years of eating well.

—The Editors

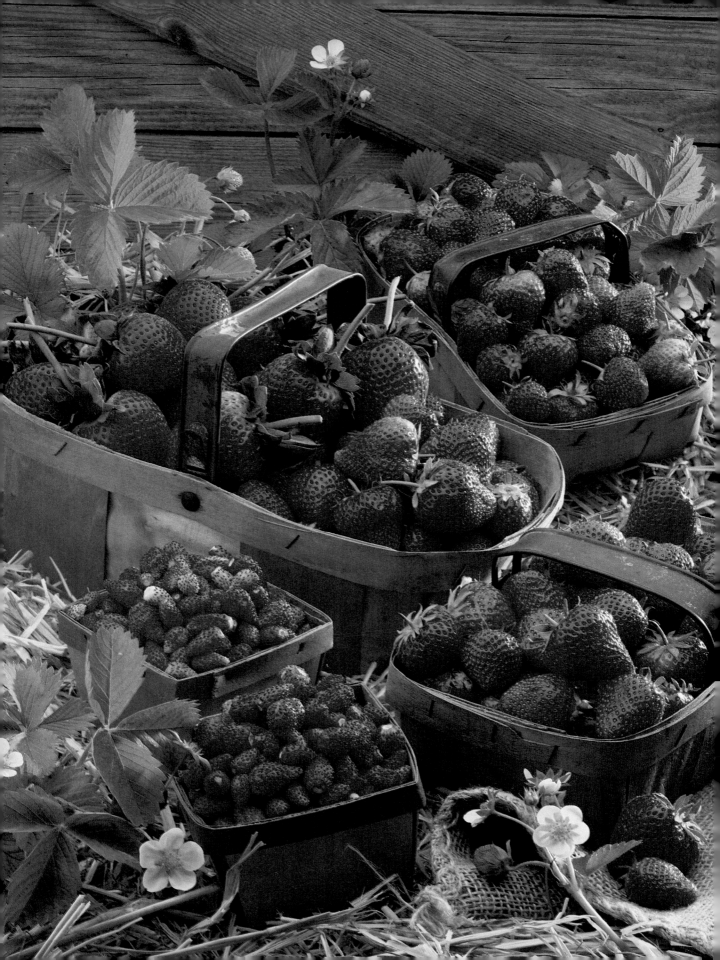

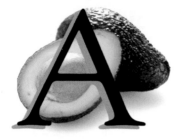

ACNE

EAT PLENTY OF
- Fresh fruits and vegetables for beta carotene and vitamin C.
- Seafood, lean meat, poultry, yogurt, and whole grains for zinc and vitamin B_6.

LIMIT
- Kelp supplements.
- Iodized salt.
- High doses of vitamins B_6 and B_{12}.

Almost everyone experiences an occasional flare-up of acne, but it is most prevalent during adolescence, afflicting 85 percent of teenagers to some degree. Hormones are responsible for most cases of acne. Diet and other lifestyle factors, including cleanliness and sexual activity, do not cause acne. In rare instances, sensitivity to a food may exacerbate existing acne, but food does not actually cause it. An exception is kelp, a seaweed that can cause severe cystic acne. Iodized salt can also provoke an acne flare-up. If you think your acne is a result of a food sensitivity, try eliminating suspect foods from your diet for several weeks. Then, add them back to see if your skin is affected.

Heredity is suspected in some cases of severe acne. A number of medications can also cause acne; major offenders include steroids and other hormonal agents, iodine preparations, lithium, and anticonvulsants. Stress often triggers a flare-up of acne, most likely by altering hormone levels. In turn, hormonal changes can stimulate food cravings. Consequently, the acne sufferer may erroneously attribute the acne to food, rather than stress, the real culprit.

HOW FOOD CAN HELP
Clear, glowing skin reflects overall good health. This requires regular exercise, adequate sleep, quitting smoking, and avoiding excessive exposure to the sun, as well as a diet rich in some important nutrients.

Eat vitamin A- and C-rich foods. They help build and maintain healthy skin. There is some evidence that beta carotene, which is converted by the body into vitamin A, may reduce sebum production. The best dietary sources of beta carotene are brightly colored fruits and dark green vegetables. Citrus fruits, berries, kiwi, melons, peppers, broccoli, cabbage, and potatoes are especially rich in vitamin C.

Include B_6. It's found in meat, fish, poultry, whole grains, beans, lentils, avocados, nuts, potatoes, bananas, and leafy greens. It may reduce acne by helping to regulate hormones implicated in the development of acne lesions.

Don't forget zinc. Some studies link this mineral to skin health and claim it may help to improve acne. Zinc promotes healthy hormone levels and advances healing. Seafood—especially oysters—red meat, poultry, yogurt, milk, and whole grains are rich in zinc.

Do not attempt to self-treat acne with high-dose vitamin and mineral supplements; this might worsen the condition. Some studies show that high doses of vitamins B_6 and B_{12} can aggravate acne symptoms, and high doses of vitamin A can cause dry, flaking skin and hair loss. Excessive intake of vitamin A has also been linked with the risk of osteoporosis.

Good nutrition is the first line of defense. Most persistent mild to moderate acne can be controlled with proper skin care, good nutrition, and nonprescription drugs, such as 2.5- to 10-percent strength benzoyl peroxide gel, lotion, or ointment.

A dermatologist may prescribe tretinoin, a topical medication derived from vitamin A; an antibiotic may also be tried. Isotretinoin (Accutane), a potent oral drug, is reserved for severe cystic acne. Since Accutane can cause severe birth defects, women taking this medication should be counseled to use multiple methods of birth control. ❖

MYTH BUSTER

Myth: Some people believe that eating foods like chocolate, French fries, and other high-fat favorites can lead to acne or make it worse.

Reality: Food does not cause acne, dermatologists stress, but eating a healthy, balanced diet is vitally important for great-looking skin.

CHEMICALS AND STREET DRUGS CAN ALSO CAUSE ACNE

"Chloracne" is a well-recognized clinical sign of exposure to certain chemicals, like dioxins—seen in Vietnam veterans who were exposed to the defoliant Agent Orange. Steroids, and the use of the drug Ecstasy, have also been linked with acnelike skin rashes.

ACORN SQUASH

See Squash

ADDITIVES
■ HELPFUL OR HARMFUL? ■

For centuries, people have enhanced their foods with various flavorings, preservatives, and dyes. But some ingredients on today's food labels can be downright scary.

Few foods reach today's supermarkets free of additives—substances that do not occur naturally in a food but are added for various reasons. These include preservatives to prevent spoilage; emulsifiers to prevent water and fat from separating; thickeners; vitamins and minerals (either to replace nutrients lost in processing or to increase nutritional value); sweeteners (both natural and artificial), salt, flavorings to improve taste; and dyes to make everything from candies to soft drinks more visually appealing.

In all, North American food processors may use any of about 2,800 additives. Although many people question the safety of these additives, the fact is that their use is governed by stringent regulations. Authorities require extensive studies before an additive is allowed on the market. In spite of this, rare reactions to certain additives are possible. The appropriate use of additives, though, allows us to enjoy history's safest and most abundant assortment of foods.

The most common food additives are sugar, corn syrup, other sweeteners, and salt; they are used both to enhance flavor and to retard spoilage. Other additives offer their own unique health benefits; these include calcium, as well as ascorbic acid (vitamin C), vitamin E, and other antioxidants that prevent fats from turning rancid and may also offer some protection against cancer, heart disease, and other ailments.

Additives can perform useful functions

Additives can be safe even though they sound distasteful. Shellac, for example, the resinous secretion of the female Indian "lac" bug, is often referred to in the trade as "confectioner's glaze." It can be used to give a protective, glossy coating to candies, jelly beans, and ice cream cones. Since it is insoluble in water, it can prevent the food product from drying out by forming a moisture impermeable layer. That's the reason citrus fruits and avocados are sometimes treated with shellac. This substance has long been used as a food additive without any problem, and animal tests have shown no adverse reactions.

Substances such as sodium stearyl fumarate, an additive to improve the texture and handling properties of baked goods, and dioctyl sodium sulfosuccinate, an emulsifier and flavor

Does Chinese restaurant syndrome really exist?

Used as a flavor enhancer, monosodium glutamate (MSG) is a common ingredient in Asian cooking. It does not actually change the flavor of food, it acts on the tongue to heighten the perception of certain tastes and minimize others. It masks any unpleasant tastes and brings out agreeable flavors. MSG occurs naturally in dried seaweed; more commonly, it is made from wheat or corn gluten or the liquid waste of sugar-beet refining.

In susceptible people, MSG may trigger headaches or idiosyncratic reactions. These problems, however, are more infrequent than is generally believed. Some people avoid MSG because they fear experiencing "Chinese restaurant syndrome." So much so that restaurants have taken to posting signs declaring "No MSG added."

Numerous studies around the world have failed to prove the existence of this condition. Perhaps the victims of this syndrome are reacting to other components in Chinese food. Histamine, tyramine, and phenylethylamine can all cause flushing, palpitations, and headaches, and are found in black beans, shrimps, and soy sauce, which are all common in Chinese cuisine.

COMMON FOOD ADDITIVES

Food additives play a vital role in today's food supply. Consumer concerns over food additives often stem from misinformation or confusion over long chemical names. All new additives receive federal government approval; older additives are presumed to be generally safe.

TYPE OF ADDITIVE	FOUND IN	FUNCTION
PRESERVATIVES		
Benzoic acid and benzoates	Soft drinks, beer, fruit products, margarine, and acidic foods.	Extend shelf life and protect food from fungi and bacteria.
Nitrites and nitrates	Processed meats, such as sausages, hot dogs, bacon, ham, and lunch meats. Smoked fish.	Extend shelf life and protect food from fungi and bacteria; preserve color in meats and dried fruits.
Sulfites	Dried fruits, shredded coconut, fruit-based pie fillings, and relishes.	Extend shelf life and protect food from fungi and bacteria.
ANTIOXIDANTS		
Ascorbic acid (vitamin C) and ascorbates	Fruit products (juices, jams, and canned fruits), acidic foods, and fatty foods that become rancid.	Ascorbates prevent fruit juices from turning brown and fatty foods from becoming rancid. They also improve baking quality in wheat.
BHA or BHT	Fatty foods that can turn rancid, such as baked products, cereals, potato chips, and fats and oil.	Extend shelf life and protect food from fungi and bacteria.
Tocopherols (vitamin E)	Oils and shortenings.	Prevent rancidity in fats and other damage to food due to exposure to oxygen.
COLORINGS		
Beta carotene Caramel Carrot oil Citrus red #1 　　Dehydrated beets 　　FD&C colors: Blue # 1, 2; 　　Red # 40; Yellow # 5, 6	Many processed foods, especially sweets and products marketed for children, soft drinks, baked goods, and confectionery items, such as frosting, jams, and margarine. Also used in bologna and other processed meats, as well as to color the skin of oranges and certain other fruits.	Make food look more appetizing by meeting people's food color expectations; for example, turning cherry Jell-O red.
FLAVOR ENHANCERS		
Disodium guanylate	Canned meats and meat-based foods.	Improve the flavor of many canned or processed foods.
Hydrolyzed vegetable protein	Mixes, stock, and processed meats.	Improve the flavor of many canned or processed foods.
Monosodium glutamate (MSG)	Chinese food, dry mixes, stock cubes, and canned, processed, and frozen meats.	Heightens taste perception so that foods seem to taste better.
EMULSIFIERS, STABILIZERS, AND THICKENERS		
Carageenan Cellulose Glycerol Guar gum Gum arabic Lecitin Pectins	Sauces, soups, breads, baked goods, frozen desserts, ice cream, low-fat and artificial cream cheese, condiments, jams, jellies, chocolate, puddings, and milk shakes.	Improve texture and consistency of processed foods by increasing smoothness, creaminess, and volume. Hold in moisture and prevent separation of oil and water. Excessive pectin can result in bloating.

enhancer, although harmless, make those of us without a degree in chemistry understandably wary.

The questionable few

The majority of food additives are safe, but there are exceptions, and every now and then, one is removed from the market. The fact that some dyes, such as Red # 2, are banned in the United States but allowed in Canada demonstrates that, in some cases, "safety" is open to interpretation. Red # 40, which was used in the United States to replace Red # 2 and is allowed in Canada, is banned in Austria, Belgium, Denmark, France, Germany, Norway, Sweden, and Switzerland.

Controversial actions by activist groups have fueled worries about complete groups of additives in some instances. The case of artificial sweeteners is a prime example (for further discussion, see Artificial Sweeteners).

Accidental additives

Some 10,000 substances make their way into food during growing, processing, and packaging; some of these accidental additives can pose more of a health threat than preservatives and other direct additives. Some foods, for example, contain traces of pesticides sprayed on crops or applied to the soil. Environmental pollutants in foods, such as PCBs, mercury, and lead, are harmful when ingested in large quantities.

Sometimes allergic reactions that are blamed on foods or intentional additives are actually triggered by an unintended one. For example, a person who has never had a food allergy may inexplicably develop a rash after drinking milk. Allergists have traced the symptoms in some cases to penicillin used to treat mastitis in cows. The resulting small amounts of penicillin in the milk would not be harmful for most people, only to those who are allergic to the drug.

A prudent approach

Even though the benefits of most food additives outweigh any potential risks, prudence and moderation should prevail in their use; some can be avoided entirely. Some additives pose problems for people with certain medical conditions. Anyone with high blood pressure or any condition that mandates a low-salt diet should check the labels on all processed foods for various forms of sodium. People trying to reduce sugar intake should look for lactose and other ingredients ending in "ose"; these are forms of sugar. Those with an inherited tendency to store excessive iron, a condition called hemochromatosis, should avoid iron-enriched breads, cereals, and other products. Sulfites used to preserve the color of dried fruits, frozen French fries, and sauerkraut can trigger an asthma attack in susceptible people. Some people may experience headaches after eating foods preserved with nitrites, and in rare cases children with attention deficit disorder may respond adversely to certain food colorants. Some additives amount to overkill; this is especially true of highly fortified breakfast cereals.

Preserved foods have more additives than their fresh counterparts. Fresh meat, poultry, and fish, for example, do not contain the nitrites and other preservatives found in smoked or processed meats. Highly processed foods tend to contain the most additives. These, though, should be avoided more on account of their poor nutritional value than simply because of their additives.

CAUTION

Watch out for yellow colorant # 5, or tartrazine. It has been linked with adverse reactions in sensitive people who are typically aspirin intolerant, allergic, or asthmatic. Symptoms may include hives, itching, runny nose, and asthma. This dye is the only dye that must be identified by name on food labels. Although it does not represent a major health risk to most people, its use in childrens' medications is clearly inappropriate.

AIDS and HIV Infection

CONSUME PLENTY OF

- Meat, poultry, liver, eggs, milk, nuts, and other high-calorie, high-protein foods to prevent weight and muscle loss.
- Pasta, rice, and other starchy foods, cooked vegetables, juices, and canned or stewed fruits for essential vitamins and minerals.
- Small meals/snacks through the day.

LIMIT

- Fatty foods and whole-grain products if they cause diarrhea.
- Coffee, tea, and other caffeinated drinks that can cause diarrhea and reduce absorption of some nutrients.

AVOID

- Raw or undercooked foods, especially shellfish, eggs, and meats.
- Alcohol, which can worsen diarrhea and interact with AIDS medications.

There is still no cure for AIDS (acquired immune deficiency syndrome), nor is there a special diet for people infected with HIV, the human immunodeficiency virus that causes the disease. But good nutrition can prevent or delay weight loss and other complications.

Asymptomatic HIV-infected individuals should follow the same dietary practices recommended for healthy people, but with added precautions. Because the HIV organism attacks the immune system, it makes a person more vulnerable to infections, including food poisoning from salmonella, shigella, campylobacter, and other bacteria. Such food-borne infections occur more frequently and are more severe in people with reduced immunity.

Keep up your food intake. AIDS is a wasting disease, and death is often due to starvation rather than to other HIV complications. A patient should eat as much as possible and, unless markedly obese, not worry about gaining weight. The extra weight can be critical in seeing a patient through a crisis when he can't eat.

Unfortunately, maintaining good nutrition is complicated by the ways in which AIDS affects the digestive system. It reduces absorption of nutrients, especially folate, riboflavin, thiamine, and vitamins B_6 and B_{12}; it often causes intractable diarrhea, which causes further nutritional loss; and it increases the risk of intestinal infections. Many AIDS patients also suffer appetite loss and bouts of nausea, either from the disease or from medications.

If rapid weight loss occurs, the patient may require artificial (hyperalimentation) feeding; this is generally administered through a gastric feeding tube inserted into the stomach or an intravenous line that pumps predigested nutrients into the bloodstream. Some AIDS specialists advise artificial feeding if nutrients are not being absorbed properly.

FOOD SAFETY

Anyone who is HIV-positive, or a person who prepares food for an AIDS patient, must pay special attention to food safety. Wash hands before handling food, during its preparation and after. Keep hot foods hot and cold foods cold. Avoid contact between raw and cooked foods. Eggs should be boiled for at least 7 minutes; meat and fish should be well cooked, with an internal temperature of 165°F to 212°F (74°C–100°C). Raw shellfish, sushi, steak tartare, rare hamburgers, as well as homemade mayonnaise and ice cream made with raw eggs must be avoided. Commercial mayonnaise and hard ice cream are safe.

Wash fruits and vegetables well. They are not as likely to cause problems as animal products, but they should be washed thoroughly. Many doctors advise following the same precautions as when traveling abroad; eat only cooked vegetables, and eat fruits that are peeled, stewed, or canned. Some feel salads and raw fruits and vegetables are safe but may be difficult to digest.

USE OF SUPPLEMENTS

Nutritionists often recommend that HIV-positive people take a multiple vitamin

---

PRACTICAL HINTS AND TIPS FOR HIV-INFECTED PEOPLE

When mouth or throat infections, such as thrush or ulcers, make eating uncomfortable: Try soft, moist foods that are easy to swallow, like mashed potatoes and gravy. Use a straw for liquids. Keep food at room temperature as hot foods can add to discomfort. Drink low-acid beverages such as milk or apple juice. Avoid foods and juices with high acid content.

When you suffer from nausea or diarrhea—common side effects of many HIV medications: Drink plenty of fluids to replace what you've lost, such as water, broth, or flat ginger ale, or eat popsicles. When you are ready to eat, start with bland foods such as toast or crackers. Try small snacks through the day. Eat slowly and chew food well. If the smell of food bothers you, let someone else prepare it and stay away from the kitchen. As the diarrhea improves, try nonirritating foods such as chicken, eggs, fish, applesauce, and peanut butter.

When you suffer from frequent bouts of diarrhea: Avoid raw fruits and vegetables and high-fiber foods such as whole-grain breads and cereals. Also avoid gassy foods such as onions, beans, cabbage, spicy foods, and carbonated beverages. Stay away from rich, fatty foods, caffeine, alcohol, and chocolate.

INFECTION-FIGHTING
MUSHROOMS COULD
HELP PEOPLE
WITH AIDS

Many nutritionists
consider fungi
to be champions in
the fight against
disease and, shiitake
mushrooms in
particular, are known
to stave off infection.
Lentinan, a compound
found in shiitakes, is
thought to have
immune-enhancing
properties and
therefore beneficial
to AIDS sufferers.

and mineral pill to prevent nutritional deficiencies; however, supplements with more than 100 percent of the Recommended Dietary Allowance (RDA) should be used only if prescribed by a doctor. Many patients self-treat with high-dose supplements, a course that can lead to serious problems. High doses of vitamin C, for example, can worsen diarrhea.

Avoid harmful dietary approaches. Some self-help groups advocate taking high doses of zinc and selenium to bolster the immune system. There is no proof that supplements of these nutrients protect against AIDS-related infections; in fact, studies show that taking 200 mg to 300 mg of zinc a day for 6 weeks actually lowers immunity. Excessive selenium can also cause vomiting and diarrhea.

Another dangerous dietary approach entails following a macrobiotic regimen, especially one restricted to brown rice and a few vegetables. Such a diet can actually worsen AIDS, because it fails to provide adequate nutrition; additionally, the excessive fiber can exacerbate diarrhea.

Herbal medicine is a popular self-care approach, though there is no evidence for its efficacy. Caution is needed as some herbal preparations contain substances that can cause serious side effects or interact with medications. Check with a doctor before taking any herbal or other preparation or engaging in self-treatment or alternative medicine. ❖

ALCOHOL

BENEFITS
- Moderate consumption cuts heart-attack risk by raising HDL cholesterol and reducing the risk of blood clot formation.
- May protect the brain against age-related dementia.
- In small amounts, it can improve appetite and aid digestion.
- May foster a happy mood.

DRAWBACKS
- Can provoke mood swings, aggression, and hangovers. Can be addictive.
- Interacts with many medications.
- Over time, moderate to high intake increases the risk of cancers, as well as heart and liver disease.

People have used alcohol in one form or another since prehistoric times. While alcohol is primarily drunk for its mood-altering effects, the results of recent studies suggest that there are benefits to moderate drinking. (Moderate drinking is defined as one or two drinks containing either 1½ oz/45 ml of alcohol, 5 oz/150 ml of wine, or 12 oz/355 ml of beer, each.)

WHAT IS ALCOHOL?
Ethyl alcohol (ethanol), the main active ingredient of alcoholic beverages, is made by yeast fermentation of starch or sugar. Almost any sweet or starchy food—potatoes, grains, honey, grapes and other fruits, even dandelions—can be turned into alcohol.

Unlike most foods, alcohol is not digested; 95 percent of it is absorbed into the bloodstream from the stomach and small intestine within an hour. (The other 5 percent is eliminated through the kidneys, lungs, or skin.) The liver breaks down, or metabolizes, alcohol; the time this takes depends upon whether the alcohol is ingested with food and upon the person's sex, weight, body type, and tolerance level, which increases with time and use. On average, however, it takes the liver 3 to 5 hours to completely metabolize 1 oz (30 ml) of alcohol.

LATEST MEDICAL RESEARCH ON ALCOHOL
Recent medical studies have found that drinking small amounts of alcohol, especially red wine, lowers the risk of a heart attack. This is good news for anyone who enjoys a little Chianti with their chicken. But the news also raises other questions: Does alcohol provide other protective health benefits? And can protection come with red wine only?

Another study revealed that having two alcoholic drinks a day offers more than double the protection from cardiovascular disease than one drink provides. In the long term, having one drink a day lowers your risk by 5 percent, but having two cuts it by 10 to 13 percent.

The risk of a heart attack lowers because alcohol reduces the detrimental effects of elevated blood cholesterol while also preventing clot formation. In this study levels of bad cholesterol (low-density lipoprotein, or LDL) lowered, as did triglyceride levels: High levels of either raise the risk of heart disease. Other studies show that moderate drinking may increase the levels of protective (high-density lipoprotein, or HDL) cholesterol.

The results are especially significant for women over 50 since a woman's risk of heart disease rises sharply after menopause.

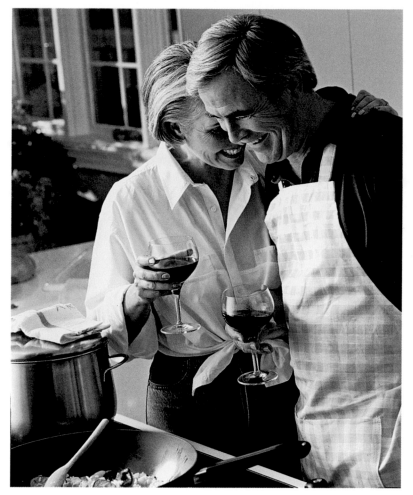

CHEERS! *Moderate drinking has been proven to improve appetite and aid digestion.*

than nondrinkers to develop dementia, an age-related decline in mental ability; they were also more than 30 percent less likely to develop Alzheimer's disease. Alcohol appears to offer a number of brain-related benefits. It thins the blood and helps prevent clots from jamming tiny blood vessels in the brain; and it appears to stimulate the release of acetylcholine, a brain chemical involved in learning and memory.

Consume no more than two drinks daily. Alcohol's protective effects are indeed impressive, but studies also show that overconsumption may significantly raise the risk of developing a number of health problems, including high blood pressure, cardiac arrhythmias,

WHAT DOES "PROOF" MEAN?

The term proof indicates alcohol concentrations; in the United States and Canada, proof is twice the alcohol content. Thus, a 90-proof liquor is 45 percent alcohol.

The mechanisms by which alcohol protects are still unclear, but some researchers note that because red wines in particular contain certain polyphenols, which can act as antioxidants—resveratrol being the prime example—they can be expected to protect cells from damage that normally occurs when the body uses oxygen. It's believed that oxidation of LDLs is what causes blood vessels to clog. The polyphenols may also fortify LDL cholesterol against oxidation.

It is not just red wine that's protective. The results of several studies have linked the moderate consumption of alcohol with a 32 percent lower risk of heart attack, and a decrease in stroke of 20 to 28 percent. Results from other studies also suggest that people who drink light to moderate amounts of alcohol daily significantly lower their risk of diabetes.

ALCOHOL PROTECTS THE BRAIN

A 2002 study reports that people who imbibe moderately daily were 70 percent less likely

WHAT CAUSES A HANGOVER?

Overconsumption of alcohol invariably results in a hangover; just how much alcohol is necessary to produce one depends on the biochemical individuality of the consumer, and the type of drink consumed. Distilled liquors, such as whiskey and gin, have a more immediate impact than wines or beers, and all alcohol is absorbed more quickly when mixed with a carbonated beverage. Once in the bloodstream, alcohol reaches the brain in minutes. At first it acts as a stimulant, producing euphoria. This soon gives way to central nervous system depression and feelings of numbness, and finally to sleep or unconsciousness. Rapid ingestion of a large amount of alcohol can be fatal. The severity of a hangover is partially influenced by congeners, by-products of the fermentation process that contribute to the taste and aroma of an alcoholic beverage. The more congeners in a drink, the more severe a hangover may be. Brandy has the greatest number of congeners, followed by red wine, rum, whiskey, white wine, gin, and vodka.

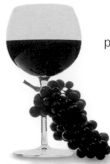

What's in a Drink?

Alcohol contains 7 calories per gram, compared with 4 calories per gram of protein or carbohydrate and 9 calories per gram of fat. Some wines provide small amounts of iron and potassium, and beer contains niacin, vitamin B$_6$, chromium, and phosphorus. To benefit from the nutrients in these beverages, you would have to consume much more than the recommended limit of two drinks per day for a man or one for a woman. Each beverage listed below provides about $\frac{1}{2}$ oz (15 ml) of ethanol, the usual definition of a drink.

ITEM	ALCOHOL VOLUME	SERVING SIZE	CALORIES
MIXED DRINKS WITH DISTILLED SPIRITS			
Bloody Mary	12%	5 oz (150 ml)	116
Daiquiri	28%	2 oz (60 ml)	111
Gin and tonic	9%	7$\frac{1}{2}$ oz (220 ml)	171
Manhattan	37%	2 oz (60 ml)	128
Martini	38%	2$\frac{1}{2}$ oz (75 ml)	156
Piña colada	12%	4$\frac{1}{2}$ oz (130 ml)	262
Screwdriver	8%	7 oz (200 ml)	174
Tequila sunrise	14%	5$\frac{1}{2}$ oz (160 ml)	189
Tom Collins	9%	7$\frac{1}{2}$ oz (220 ml)	121
Whiskey sour (using bottled mix)	17%	3$\frac{1}{2}$ oz (100 ml)	160
WINE AND WINE-RELATED PRODUCTS			
Regular wines	10%–14%	4 oz (120 ml)	85
Sweet white wine	10%–14%	4 oz (120 ml)	100
Light wines	6%–10%	5 oz (150 ml)	65
Wine coolers (fruit juice, carbonated water, white wine, sugar)	3.5%–6%	12 oz (355 ml)	220
Port	19%	4 oz (120 ml)	158
Sherry	19%	3 oz (90 ml)	125
ORDINARY BEER			
Regular	3%–5%	12 oz (355 ml)	150
Light	3%–5%	12 oz (355 ml)	100
STRONGER BREWED BEVERAGES			
Ales, porters, stouts, and malt liquors	5%–8%	12 oz (355 ml)	150

COMPARISON OF UNIT MEASURES

$\frac{1}{2}$ oz (15 ml) ethanol = 1$\frac{1}{2}$ oz (45 ml) of 80-proof liquor = 4 oz (120 ml) or 5 oz (150 ml) of wine = 12 oz (355 ml) of beer

liver disease, stroke, dementia, and several kinds of cancer, including cancer of the liver, pancreas, esophagus, and mouth. Also, alcohol is addictive. Overindulgence quickly erases any benefits. Even a weekend of heavy drinking causes a buildup of fatty cells in the liver. While this organ has remarkable recuperative powers, continued use of alcohol can lead to permanent liver damage and problems with glucose metabolism, and eventually scarring, or cirrhosis.

Alcohol also interferes with the body's metabolism of various vitamins and minerals. Women at risk for breast cancer should moderate their consumption. It has been shown that those who consume alcohol daily have a higher risk of breast cancer than those who do not. The risk increases with amount of alcohol consumed.

Alcohol's heart benefits stop after that second drink. A third does more harm than good, actually raising triglyceride levels without reducing LDL cholesterol. The key, as with everything else in life, is moderation. ❖

ALCOHOLISM

CONSUME PLENTY OF

- Seafood, lean pork, and enriched cereals and breads for extra thiamine.
- Dark green leafy vegetables, orange juice, liver, lentils, enriched cereals and breads for folate.
- Legumes, pasta, rice, and other starchy foods for carbohydrate.

AVOID

- Alcohol in any form.

Alcoholism is defined as chronic drinking that interferes with one's personal, family, or professional life. While an occasional drink is not likely to be harmful, it's important to recognize that alcohol is easily abused.

Various factors can foster alcoholism. Genetic predisposition, learned behavior, and childhood experiences, including abuse, are all thought to foster alcoholism. Progression of the disease varies from one person to another. For some, it develops as soon as they begin to drink; for most people, however, it progresses slowly from periodic social drinking to more frequent indulgence until finally the person is addicted.

Some alcoholics are binge drinkers and can go for weeks or even months without alcohol. But once they have a drink, they are unable to stop until they are incapacitated or pass out. Although these drinkers have difficulty maintaining sobriety, they are unlikely to suffer severe withdrawal symptoms when they abstain. In other cases, abstinence of 12 to 24 hours will produce withdrawal symptoms, such as sweating, irritability, nausea, vomiting, and weakness. More severe symptoms develop in 2 to 4 days and may include delirium tremens (DTs), a condition marked by fever and delirium.

Chronic overuse of alcohol takes a heavy psychological and physical toll. Alcoholics often do not appear to be intoxicated, but their ability to work and go about daily activities becomes increasingly impaired. They are very susceptible to depression, mood changes, and even violent behavior. Their suicide rate is higher than that of the general population. On average, alcoholism shortens life expectancy, not only from suicide but also because it raises the risk of other life-threatening diseases, including cancer of the pancreas, liver, and esophagus. Women who drink heavily while pregnant may have a baby with fetal alcohol syndrome, a constellation of birth defects, including mental retardation.

NUTRITIONAL EFFECTS OF ALCOHOLISM

Alcoholism can lead to malnutrition, not only because chronic drinkers tend to have poor diets, but also because alcohol alters digestion and metabolism of most nutrients. Severe thiamine deficiency (marked by muscle cramps and wasting, nausea, appetite loss, nerve disorders, and depression) is extremely common, as are deficiencies of folate, riboflavin, vitamin B_6, and selenium. Because many alcoholics suffer deficiency of vitamin D, which helps the body absorb calcium, they are at risk of bone fractures and osteoporosis. Impaired liver and pancreatic function may result in faulty fat digestion. Since alcohol stimulates insulin production, glucose metabolism speeds up and can result in low blood sugar. And alcoholics are often overweight, due to the calories in alcohol.

Diet and supplements help. Once an alcoholic stops drinking, the nutritional problems are tackled one by one. Supplements are prescribed to treat deficiencies. A diet addresses underlying problems; for example, an overweight person needs a diet that reverses nutritional deficiencies without additional weight gain. If there is liver damage, protein intake must be monitored to prevent further liver problems. ❖

FACTS ABOUT ALCOHOL

- The hops that give beer its distinctive taste and aroma come from a vine that is a relative of cannabis.
- A cold shower, strong coffee, and similar remedies are of no value in helping a person sober up.
- Large amounts of alcohol lower sexual performance in men. Alcohol reduces levels of testosterone, the male sex hormone, while increasing estrogen levels, which can lead to impotence, shrunken testicles, and male breast growth.
- Women absorb alcohol into the bloodstream more efficiently than men.

ALLERGIES
▪ REACTIONS TO FOOD ▪

It is estimated that almost one-third of people say they, or a family member, have a food allergy. But in fact, only 2 to 8 percent of children, and 1 to 2 percent of adults have clinically proven allergic reactions to food. The reason for this discrepancy is that we often fail to discriminate between food allergies and food intolerances. True food allergies involve the body's immune system, whereas a food intolerance originates in the gastrointestinal system and involves an inability to digest or absorb certain substances.

Doctors do not completely understand why so many people have allergies, though heredity is an important consideration. If both parents have allergies, their children will almost always have them as well, although the symptoms and allergens may be quite different. Food allergies in infants and children, however, tend to lessen as they grow, and the problem may disappear by adulthood. There is no doubt that breastfeeding and the delayed introduction of solid foods reduces a child's chances of developing food allergies.

Allergies develop in stages. When the immune system first encounters an allergen (or antigen)—a substance that it mistakenly sees as a harmful foreign invader—it signals specialized cells to make antibodies, or immunoglobulins, against it. There is no allergic reaction in that first exposure; however, if the substance again enters the body, the antibodies programmed to mount an attack against it will go into action. In some instances, the response will not produce symptoms; but the stage will have been set for a future antigen-antibody reaction and an allergic response.

Common symptoms

There are many symptoms of food allergies, including nausea, vomiting, diarrhea, constipation, indigestion, headaches, skin rashes or hives, itching, shortness of breath (including asthma attacks), and, in severe cases, widespread swelling of the skin and mucous membranes. Swelling in the mouth or throat is potentially fatal because it can block the airways to the lungs. In the most severe cases, anaphylactic shock—a life-threatening collapse of the respiratory and circulatory system—may develop.

Allergens usually provoke the same symptoms each time, but many factors affect intensity, including how much of the offending food was eaten, and how it was prepared. Some people can tolerate small amounts of an offending food; others are so hypersensitive that they react to even a minute trace.

Pinpointing allergens

Some allergens are easily identified because symptoms will develop immediately after eating the offending food. The most allergenic foods in infancy are egg, milk, peanut, wheat, and soy (about 85 percent of children lose

The latest on peanut allergies

An allergy to peanuts is one of the most dangerous food allergies, both because peanut products are widely used in processed foods and because even minute amounts of peanut protein can be enough to trigger fatal anaphylactic shock.

Researchers have determined that diagnosis of a peanut allergy is not necessarily a life-long sentence. A blood test to measure peanut specific antibodies can identify children who may have outgrown their allergies. They can then be tested in a controlled situation with a small amount of peanut protein to see if they are still allergic. Children with a peanut allergy should be retested every few years.

TWO CURRENT AREAS OF RESEARCH:
✔ development of a vaccine to help tone down the body's overreaction to peanuts
✔ the use of activated charcoal to bind the allergy-causing proteins when an allergic person realizes they have accidentally eaten peanuts.

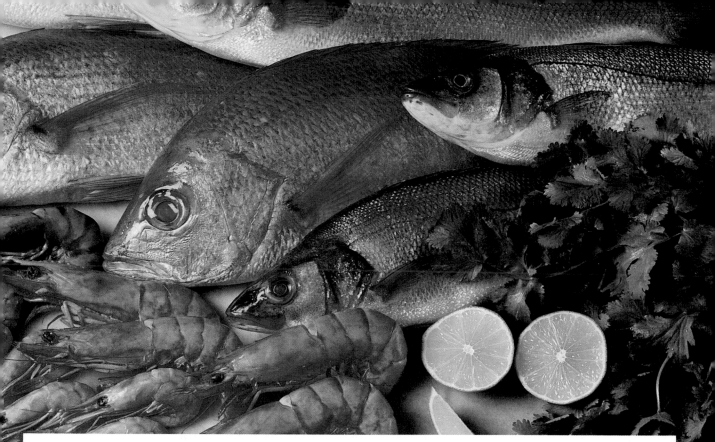

COMMON FOOD ALLERGENS

Almost any food can provoke an allergic reaction.
The following is a list of eight foods that account for 90 percent of allergic reactions.

FOOD TYPES	MAIN FOODS	HIDDEN SOURCES
Milk and milk products	Dairy products, such as milk, cheeses, yogurt, cream, ice cream, cream soups, and certain baked goods and desserts.	Deli meats cut on same slicer as cheese, some canned tuna, nondairy products, and prepared meats.
Eggs (especially egg whites)	Cakes, mousses, ice cream, sherbets, and other desserts; mayonnaise, salad dressings, French toast, waffles, and pancakes.	Toppings on specialty desserts, some egg substitutes, processed cooked pasta (e.g., in soup).
Soy and soy products	Soy, soybeans, tofu, textured vegetable protein, hydrolyzed protein, miso, soy sauce, tamari, tempeh, natural and artificial flavors, vegetable broth, and vegetable starch.	Major ingredient in processed foods.
Wheat and wheat products	Cereals, bread or bread-related products, dry soup mixes, cakes, pasta, gravies, dumplings, products containing flour; beer and ale.	Some hot dogs, ice cream, imitation crab, and imitation meats.
Peanuts	Peanuts and peanut oil, peanut butter, peanut flour, baked goods and candy with nuts, natural flavoring. Wise to avoid all nuts.	Many candies, sunflower seeds, African, Chinese, Mexican, Thai, and Vietnamese food.
Tree nuts	Candy and baked goods with pecans, walnuts, almonds, cashews, hazelnuts, and pistachios; oils from nuts.	Natural and artificial flavors, barbeque sauce, some cereals, crackers, and ice cream.
Fish	Fresh, canned, smoked or pickled fish, fish-liver oils, caviar, foods containing fish, such as bisques, broths, and stews.	Caesar salad dressings and imitation crab.
Shellfish	Crustaceans, such as shrimp, crab, lobster, and crayfish; mollusks, such as clams, oysters, and scallops; and seafood dishes.	Caesar salad dressings and imitation crab.

Avoiding hidden allergens

People with food allergies may experience allergic reactions to "safe" foods because of the following:
✔ contamination of foods through improper handling
✔ misleading labels, for example, when eggs are listed as an emulsifier
✔ ingredient switching, for example, when a shortage of vegetable oil results in substitution with a tropical oil such as coconut oil.

SO, WHAT SHOULD YOU DO?
✔ Read labels religiously.
✔ Use extreme caution when eating in restaurants or as a guest in someone's home. Don't be afraid to ask about a recipe's ingredients.
✔ Avoid processed foods.
✔ Carry an epinephrine self-injector (Epi-Pen) in case of accidental exposure.

Nutrition Facts

Serving Size 8 Crackers (29g)
Servings Per Container about 7

Amount Per Serving

Calories 130   Calories from Fat 30

	% Daily Value*
Total Fat 3g	5%
Saturated Fat 1g	5%
Cholesterol 0mg	0%
Sodium 310mg	13%
Total Carbohydrate 22g	7%
Dietary Fiber Less than 1g	3%
Sugars 3g	
Protein 3g	

Vitamin A	2%	Vitamin C	0%
Calcium	0%	Iron	4%

*Percent Daily Values are based on a 2,000 calorie diet. Your daily values may be higher or lower depending on your calorie needs:

	Calories:	2,000	2,500
Total Fat	Less than	65g	80g
Sat Fat	Less than	20g	25g
Cholesterol	Less than	300mg	300mg
Sodium	Less than	2,400mg	2,400mg
Total Carbohydrate		300g	375g
Dietary Fiber		25g	30g

What is anaphylactic shock?

Severe allergic reactions to foods can result in anaphylactic shock, a life-threatening collapse of the respiratory and circulatory system. If you have had, or believe you may be susceptible to, an anaphylactic reaction, you should wear medical identification, and carry emergency medical information in your wallet. Your doctor may also recommend that you carry an epinephrine self-injector (Epi-Pen).

their sensitivity within the first 3 to 5 years of life), whereas in older children and adults tree nuts, peanuts, and seafood are the most likely to cause severe reactions. Many people have mild allergies to various fruits and vegetables. Cooking can often reduce the allergenic potential of foods as proteins responsible for allergies are degraded by heat. This, however, is not always the case. Roasting peanuts makes them more allergenic.

Allergens are not always readily identified. It may be necessary to keep a carefully documented diary of the time and content of all meals and the appearance and timing of subsequent symptoms. After a week or two, a pattern may emerge. If so, eliminate the suspected food from the diet for at least a week, and then try it again. If symptoms develop, chances are you have identified the offending food.

In more complicated cases, allergy tests may be required. One or more of the following may be used:

Skin test: The most common test, where food extracts are placed on the skin, which is then scratched or pricked, allowing the penetration of a small amount of the extract. Development of a hive or itchy swelling usually indicates an allergic response.

RAST (radioallergosorbent test) blood study: Small amounts of the patient's blood are mixed with food extracts and then analyzed for signs of antibody action. This test may be safer for hypersensitive people, who may have a severe reaction to the skin test.

Medically supervised elimination diet and challenge tests: The patient is put on a hypoallergenic diet of foods that are unlikely to cause allergies for 7 to 10 days, at which time all allergic symptoms should completely disappear. (If they do not, a reaction to something other than food should be suspected.) The doctor then administers small amounts of food or food extracts to see if an allergic response occurs.

Living with food allergies

Once allergens have been identified, eliminating those foods from the diet should solve the problem. But this can be more complicated than it sounds. Some of the most common food allergens are hidden ingredients in many processed foods (see "Common Food Allergens," page 23). Also, many foods are chemically related; thus, a person allergic to lemons may also be allergic to oranges and other citrus fruits. In some cases, the real culprit may be a contaminant or an accidental additive in food. For example, some people who are allergic to orange juice and other citrus juices may actually be able to tolerate the peeled fruits themselves, since it is limonene, the oil in citrus peels, that often produces the allergic reaction.

Allergies and genetically modified foods

Genetic modification involves the introduction of novel proteins into foods and raises the question of increased allergenicity. Researchers, for example, have examined the possibility of introducing a gene from the arctic flounder into a tomato to prevent the tomato from freezing. This raises the question of someone with a fish allergy having a reaction to a tomato. No such tomatoes have been introduced and none will be until the question of transferred allergens is resolved. Traditional crossbreeding can also introduce novel proteins for which there are no allergy testing requirements. Also, in the case of genetically modified foods, the new proteins are not necessarily consumed. Canola oil, for example, contains none of the proteins that were introduced into the plant for improved agricultural performance.

ALMONDS

See Nuts

ALZHEIMER'S DISEASE

CONSUME PLENTY OF

- Leafy green vegetables, orange juice, liver, cooked beans and lentils, corn, asparagus, peas, nuts, enriched breads and cereals for folate.
- Lean meat, fish, poultry, or dairy products for vitamin B_{12}.
- Meat, fish, poultry, whole grains, beans, lentils, avocados, nuts, potatoes, bananas, and leafy greens for vitamin B_6.
- Fatty fish such as salmon, mackerel, herring, and sardines for the omega-3 fatty acids.
- Eggs, liver, soybeans and soy products, whole grains, brewer's yeast, and wheat germ—all reasonably good sources of lecithin and choline.

AVOID

- Antacids with aluminum.
- Using cooking utensils made of aluminum.

Alzheimer's disease is the leading cause of dementia in people over the age of 65, affecting over 4 million North Americans. The disease is characterized by abnormal deposits of a protein called beta-amyloid (plaque) in the brain as well as by twisted fibers caused by changes in a protein called "tau" (tangles). Before arriving at a diagnosis, tests are needed to rule out a stroke, a brain tumor, and other possible causes of dementia.

Blood tests can uncover genetic markers for the disease. The cause of Alzheimer's disease remains unknown, but researchers theorize that chromosomal and genetic factors are responsible for some cases. The increased incidence of Alzheimer's among those with Down's syndrome, which is caused by a chromosomal abnormality, seems to support this theory. Researchers have discovered a genetic marker, apolipoprotein E, which can be detected by blood tests, that identifies those likely to develop the disease. About 40 percent of sufferers have the gene that produces this protein.

In addition, hormonal factors are under study. Women are afflicted more often than men; studies suggest that estrogen replacement may be protective. A study published in 2003 in the *Journal of the American Medical Association*, however, has thrown cold water on this hypothesis. Women over the age of 65 who were taking combined estrogen-progestin therapy had a higher incidence of Alzheimer's disease than those not taking hormones. Thyroid disorders are also linked to the disease, while the long-term use of nonsteroidal anti-inflammatory drugs (NSAIDs) has been linked with a reduced Alzheimer's risk. These drugs may reduce inflammation in the brain linked with the disease. There is insufficient evidence for physicians to recommend taking anti-inflammatory drugs to ward off Alzheimer's.

DANGER: ALUMINUM?

There have been other intriguing leads, but researchers have been unable to pinpoint any specific dietary factors that increase the risk of or help to prevent Alzheimer's disease. Some research has implicated aluminum, which has been found in the abnormal tangles of brain cells in some Alzheimer's patients. However, extensive studies have failed to prove that aluminum actually causes the disease, and it now seems more likely that aluminum is found in Alzheimer's brains because the diseased brain retains it.

Avoid taking antacids containing aluminum. Although most researchers discount the aluminum factor, some argue that while the metal may not cause the disease, its increased concentration in the Alzheimer's brain worsens the condition. They suggest that patients avoid taking antacids with large amounts of aluminum or using cookware that allows the metal to leach into food. Concern has also been raised about the aluminum content of drinking water in areas where aluminum compounds are used as flocculating agents in city water treatment.

DIET AND ALZHEIMER'S

Researchers are studying the role of the B-vitamin folate in lowering risk of Alzheimer's. This vitamin helps regulate blood levels of homocysteine, an amino acid, high levels of which may play a part in the development of the disease. Studies have shown that people with Alzheimer's have high homocysteine levels and there is evidence that high concentrations of homocysteine in healthy adults may lead to Alzheimer's. In addition to folate, vitamins B_6 and B_{12}

FOODS THAT FIGHT ALZHEIMER'S

Researchers are finding many links between diet and dementia, and there is evidence that some foods are powerful allies in the battle against Alzheimer's

FISH, especially oily fish like salmon, mackerel, herring, and sardines, are rich in omega-3 fatty acids and should be eaten at least three times per week.

EGGS are a good dietary source of choline—a component of lecithin. They are also a good source of iron, vitamin B_{12} and other B vitamins, an excellent source of protein, and very easy to eat and digest.

MEDICAL PROOF THAT RISK CAN BE CUT BY 50 PERCENT THROUGH DIET ALONE

Researchers at Chicago's St. Luke's Medical Center found that people 65 and older who had fish once a week had a 60 percent lower risk of Alzheimer's than those who did not eat fish.

WHEAT GERM AND WHOLE GRAINS high in lecithin and choline, carbohydrate, vitamin E, B vitamins, and numerous minerals help forestall Alzheimer's. Whole-grain breads are a popular and readily available item to add to anyone's diet.

SOY products are rich in choline and provide protein, carbohydrate, calcium, and fiber. They are a good source of folic acid—also known as folate—and are known to lower blood levels of homocysteine.

help regulate homocysteine levels. People with high blood cholesterol and high blood pressure are also at increased risk and taking cholesterol-lowering drugs, particularly the "statins," has been shown to reduce the risk. Basically, it appears that what is good for the heart is good for the brain.

The brain is rich in DHA (docosahexaenoic acid), an omega-3 fatty acid that is plentiful in fatty fish such as salmon, mackerel, halibut, herring, and sardines. Low levels of this fat have been associated with age-related dementia, including Alzheimer's disease.

Antioxidants may be preventives. They mop up free radicals and have been touted as possible preventives for Alzheimer's since the body's ability to neutralize these rogue substances declines with age. The most recent studies, however, may end the hype. In a large trial published in 2003 in the *Archives of Neurology*, researchers at Columbia University found that people who had high intakes of vitamins C, E, and beta carotene did not have a reduced risk of Alzheimer's disease. Trials with ginkgo biloba, another antioxidant, have also been less than encouraging.

People with Alzheimer's disease have abnormally low levels of choline acetyltransferase, an enzyme necessary to make acetylcholine, a brain chemical believed to be instrumental in learning and memory. Also, the brain cells most affected by Alzheimer's are those that normally respond to acetylcholine. In addition, tacrine (Cognex), a drug that appears to improve the memory of some Alzheimer's patients, increases levels of acetylcholine. Some nutrition researchers theorize that supplements or foods high in lecithin or choline (the major component of acetylcholine) can also slow the progression of Alzheimer's by raising acetylcholine production. So far, studies have failed to document its value, but some nutritionists feel that foods high in lecithin and choline may help forestall symptoms and will certainly do no harm; these include egg yolks, organ meats, soy products, peanuts, wheat germ, and whole grains.

Monitor nutrition carefully. As the disease progresses, its victims may forget to eat or eat only sweets or other favorite foods. Patients should be persuaded to eat nutritionally balanced meals. They may need to be spoon-fed if they have difficulty feeding themselves. A multivitamin may also be advisable; high-dose supplements should not be administered unless specifically recommended by a physician.

Even in small amounts, alcohol destroys brain cells, a loss that a healthy person can tolerate but one that can accelerate the progression of Alzheimer's disease. Alcohol interacts with antidepressants, sedatives, and other medications prescribed for Alzheimer's patients. It's a good idea to avoid all alcohol.

Evidence is accumulating for the "use it or lose it" theory of reducing Alzheimer's risk. People who exercise their brains with education, puzzles, games, and museum visits seem to be less sensitive to brain damage. ❖

ANEMIA

CONSUME PLENTY OF
- Organ meats, beef and other meats, poultry, fish, and egg yolks for iron and vitamin B_{12}.
- Dried beans and peas, dates, raisins, dried apricots, nuts, seeds, and blackstrap molasses—all good nonheme sources of iron.
- Iron-enriched breads and cereals.
- Citrus fruits and other good sources of vitamin C—including orange juice—which increase the body's iron absorption.
- Green leafy vegetables, lentils and beans, asparagus, corn, and enriched grains for folate.

LIMIT
- Bran, spinach, rhubarb, Swiss chard, chocolate, and tea, which hinder iron absorption.

AVOID
- Iron supplements, unless prescribed by a physician.

Anemia is the umbrella term for a variety of disorders characterized by the inability of red blood cells to carry sufficient oxygen. This may be due to an abnormality of a low level of hemoglobin, the iron- and protein-based red pigment in blood that carries oxygen from the lungs to all body cells. Symptoms of anemia, therefore, reflect oxygen starvation. In mild anemia, this may include general weakness, pallor, fatigue, and brittle nails. More severe cases are marked by shortness of breath, fainting, and cardiac arrhythmias.

IRON-DEFICIENCY ANEMIA
In North America the most common type of anemia is due to iron deficiency, which is

---

DO ONE SIMPLE THING

COOK IN IRON POTS
Cook tomatoes and other acidic foods in iron pots that add large amounts of iron to food. Four ounces (120 ml) of tomato sauce cooked in a regular pot provides 0.7 mg of iron; cooking it in an iron pot adds 5 mg—ironware may discolor food, but taste is unaffected.

---

usually caused by blood loss of some type. Surgery patients, accident victims, people with a bleeding ulcer or certain cancers, or those with chronic or repeated bleeding such as nosebleeds often have iron-deficiency anemia. In fact, a blood test that shows iron deficiency often prompts a physician to investigate the possibility of colon cancer. Women with heavy menstrual periods, especially adolescents, are at risk as are young children, chronic dieters, female athletes, distance runners, or people on very restricted vegetarian diets. Pregnant women are predisposed to anemia because of the demands of the growing baby and placenta.

OTHER TYPES OF ANEMIA
Hemolytic anemia occurs when red blood cells are destroyed more rapidly than normal. The cause may be hereditary or one of a variety of diseases, including leukemia and other cancers, abnormal spleen function, autoimmune disorders, and severe hypertension.

Pernicious, or megaloblastic, anemia is caused by a deficiency of vitamin B_{12}, which is necessary to make red blood cells. Stomach acid releases B_{12} from protein in food. The vitamin then binds to a substance called intrinsic factor that enables B_{12} to be absorbed in the bloodstream. This means that you can develop a B_{12} deficiency if your stomach produces an insufficient amount of acid.

Older adults may need supplements. Up to one-third of older adults produce inadequate amounts of stomach acid and can no longer properly absorb B_{12} from food. People over 50 may have to meet their B_{12} need by consuming food fortified with B_{12} or by taking a supplement containing B_{12}. Vitamin B_{12} is found only in animal products and strict vegetarians are at risk and should consume fortified foods and/or take a supplement. Nitrous oxide (laughing gas) interferes with B_{12} metabolism and people who abuse this substance in search of a "high" have shown signs of B_{12} deficiency, which were reversed when supplements were administered.

CAUTION

Do not take iron supplements unless you have had a blood test to confirm an iron deficiency. Excess iron can be dangerous. It is estimated that as much as 10 percent of the population suffers from undiagnosed hemochromatosis, or "iron overload" disease. For these people, iron supplements can have catastrophic results.

Deficiency of folate, another B vitamin, can also cause anemia in pregnant women (who need extra folate for the developing fetus), in alcoholics, and in elderly people.

Relatively rare types of anemia include thalassemia, an inherited disorder, and aplastic anemia, which may be caused by infection, exposure to toxic chemicals or radiation, or a genetic disorder.

HOW MUCH IRON DO YOU NEED?

The human body recycles iron to make new red blood cells. Even so, the body loses an average of 1 mg for men and 1.5 mg for women during reproductive years. The body absorbs only a small percentage of dietary iron, so the Recommended Dietary Allowance (RDA) calls for consuming more than what is lost: 8 mg a day for men and postmenopausal women; 18 mg for women under 50; 27 mg for pregnant women.

Those who have nutrition-related anemias can benefit from a session with a registered dietitian or a qualified nutritionist to help structure a more healthful diet. The best sources of iron are animal products—meat, fish, poultry, and egg yolks. The body absorbs much more of the heme iron found in these foods than the nonheme iron from plant sources, such as green leafy vegetables, dried fruits, soy and other legumes, nuts, seeds, and iron-enriched breads and cereals. Strict vegetarians or people who rely heavily on plant food to get iron must increase their intake of these foods since they are poorly absorbed by the body. Adding a vitamin C-rich food to a plant-based meal can enhance the body's absorption of nonheme iron. Heme iron also promotes the absorption of nonheme iron from other foods when eaten at the same meal.

Watch out for natural compounds in tea, called tannins. They can bind with iron and make it unavailable for absorption. It is best to drink your tea between meals rather than during. Oxalates found in spinach, rhubarb, Swiss chard, and chocolate as well as phytates found in nuts, some greens, and bran cereal also can bind with iron and prevent the body from using it. ❖

RUNNERS BEWARE. *Female athletes and distance runners should include extra iron in their diet.*

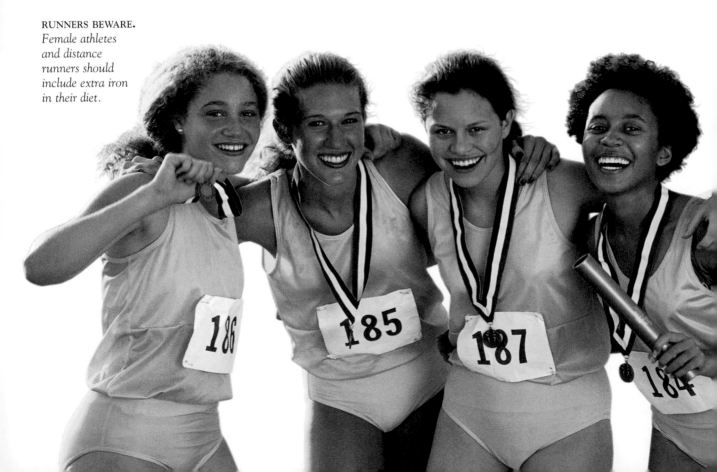

ANOREXIA NERVOSA

CONSUME

- A variety of nutritious foods in small amounts.
- Calorie-enriched liquid supplements and possibly multivitamin supplements, if approved by a doctor.

LIMIT

- Diet soft drinks and low-calorie diet foods.
- Appetite suppressants, diuretics, and laxatives.

The self-starvation that is a hallmark of anorexia nervosa is caused by a complex psychiatric disorder that afflicts between 2 and 6 percent of North Americans, mostly adolescent girls or, less commonly, young women. (Only about 5 percent of anorexics are males; they are often weight-conscious adolescent boys who are dancers or athletes.)

The cause of anorexia—a medical term for appetite loss—is unknown. Researchers believe that a combination of hormonal, social, and psychological factors are responsible. The disease often begins in adolescence, a time of tremendous hormonal and psychological change. Convinced that she is too fat, regardless of how much she weighs, a girl begins obsessive dieting. Some girls adopt a very restricted diet. Others become overly preoccupied with food, often planning and preparing elaborate meals that they then refuse to eat. And when the anorexic does eat, she may resort to self-induced vomiting or laxative abuse to avoid gaining weight. Many anorexics also exercise obsessively.

Take note of tell-tale signs. As the disease progresses, menstruation ceases and nutritional deficiencies develop. Many anorexics try to hide their thinness by wearing oversized clothes; physical indications of anorexia include fatigue, nervousness or hyperactivity, dry skin, hair loss, and intolerance to cold. More serious consequences include cardiac arrhythmias, loss of bone mass, kidney failure, and in about 6 percent of cases, death.

TREATMENT STRATEGIES

Anorexia often requires intensive long-term treatment, preferably by a team experienced with eating disorders: a doctor to treat starvation-induced medical problems, a psychiatrist, and a dietitian. Family members can also benefit from counseling.

CAUTION

Younger women are particularly vulnerable to eating disorders like anorexia nervosa, a serious, often chronic, and life-threatening condition. Although the term *anorexia* literally means loss of appetite, people with anorexia nervosa actually ignore hunger and deliberately control their desire to not eat.

Constant obsessive dieting may result in severe anorexia and sufferers may be at risk of death from starvation.

Should someone you know exhibit the following warning signs, contact a doctor knowledgeable about eating disorders immediately.
- Preoccupation with food
- Distorted body image, thinking they are fat when they are actually bone-thin
- Intense fear of gaining weight
- Refusal to eat
- Deliberate self-starvation
- Denial of hunger
- Obsessive exercise
- Loss of scalp hair
- Brittle nails and hair
- Constant complaining about feeling cold (due to low body temperature)
- A fine layer of hair on the body or face (like on a new born)
- Depression
- Irregular or absent periods.

Anorexics tend to defend their eating habits and resist treatment. Most are treated as outpatients; in severe cases, hospitalization and nutritional therapy are necessary.

The biggest hurdle is to help the anorexic overcome her abnormal fear of food and distorted self-image of being fat. Counseling is directed to uncovering the source of these fears.

In the beginning, the patient is offered small portions of nutritious and easily digestible foods, perhaps eggs, custards, soups, and milk shakes. Portion sizes and the variety of foods are increased gradually to achieve a steady weight gain. This does not require huge amounts of food; instead, doctors strive for a varied diet that provides adequate protein for rebuilding lost lean tissue, carbohydrate for energy, and a moderate amount of fat for extra calories. Extra calcium and multivitamins may also be given.

Monitor food intake closely. Anorexics are skilled at deceiving others about their eating. Relapses are common and close monitoring may be necessary to ensure that the anorexic is really eating. But avoid making food a constant source of attention and conflict; group therapy can be more helpful than parental nagging. ❖

ANTIAGING DIET
■ EAT RIGHT TO AGE WELL ■

As you get older, your body's energy needs drop; at the same time, demands for some nutrients increase. New studies indicate some of these can slow the aging process.

While aging is inevitable, many of the degenerative changes that prevail past middle age are not if preventive steps are taken. Recent medical research confirms that good nutrition can prevent, or at least slow, such debilitating conditions as osteoporosis, diabetes, and heart disease. In fact, one report estimates that one-third to one-half of the health problems of people over the age of 65 are related to diet.

Proper nutrition is an important part of any "aging-well" strategy. Yet, on the whole, seniors are the most poorly nourished group of all North Americans. There are many reasons for this: A person's appetite and the senses of taste and smell decline with age, making food considerably less appealing. Many older people experience difficulty chewing; in addition, heartburn, constipation, lactose intolerance, and other digestive problems increase with age and contribute to poor nutrition. Stomach acidity also declines with age, impairing absorption of nutrients. The loss of a partner, or difficulty in shopping or preparing meals, may result in a person subsisting on tea, toast, sweets, canned soups, and other convenience foods that provide little nutrition. Also, a number of older people living on a fixed income usually cannot afford such nutritious foods as fresh fruits, vegetables, fish, and meat.

Interesting facts about longevity

- Japan has the longest life expectancy in the world. Yet people in the Okinawan Islands in southern Japan enjoy even longer and healthier lives than the average Japanese. Their diet secret? Lots of grains, vegetables, soy, and fish; less meat, poultry, and dairy. There is, however, no scientific basis to the suggestion by some supplement manufacturers that "coral calcium" is the secret of the Okinawans' longevity.
- Various studies of Mormons, Seventh-Day Adventists, and Trappist monks— all people who follow a vegetarian diet and engage in a prudent lifestyle—also show that they enjoy increased life expectancy.
- North Americans also seem to be doing something right since they are healthier than they were two decades ago. People over age 85 are one of the fastest growing segments of the population, proving that today you can live longer and healthier if you practice good health habits.

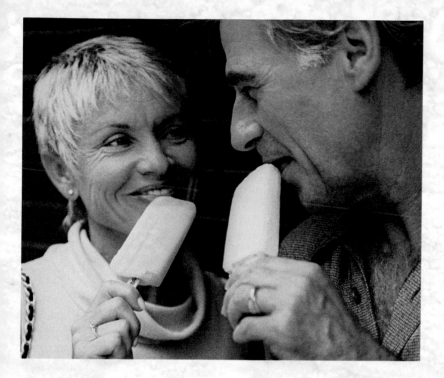

Changing needs

A person's body composition changes with age, as muscle mass decreases, often due to disuse, and fatty tissue increases. Because metabolism slows down, fewer calories are required; experts estimate that the average person should consume 10 percent fewer calories for every decade after the age of 50. Therefore, a 50-year-old who needs 1,800 calories a day will require 1,440 at age 70, and perhaps even fewer if he is sedentary. People who fail to cut back on food intake are likely to gain weight, increasing the risk of heart disease, diabetes, and osteoarthritis.

With increasing age, the body is less efficient in absorbing and using some nutrients; osteoporosis and other medical conditions common among older people also change nutritional needs. Consequently, an older person is likely to need extra amounts of the following essential nutrients:

- Calcium to prevent osteoporosis and maintain healthy bones.
- Vitamin D, which the body needs in order to absorb the calcium.
- Vitamin B_{12} to build red blood cells and maintain healthy nerves.
- Zinc to help compensate for lowered immunity due to aging.
- Potassium, especially in the presence of high blood pressure or the use of diuretic drugs.
- Folic acid, a B vitamin, which the body uses to make DNA and red blood cells, may also help to lower blood levels of homocysteine, a compound in the blood that has been associated with an increased risk of heart disease.
- Fiber to prevent constipation.

Supplements may be needed

A recent study in the *Journal of the American Medical Association* suggests that seniors may face the risk of vitamin

Medical proof that food is powerful medicine

According to a 2003 medical study there's nothing fishy about fish oil's ability to protect your heart. Omega-3 fatty acids from fish oils can prevent sudden cardiac death by blocking fatal heart rhythms, researchers say. Sudden cardiac death accounts for at least half of heart-related deaths. Eating fish, particularly fatty fish such as salmon, trout, mackerel, herring, and sardines, has long been associated with a reduced risk of heart disease. Omega-3 fats are credited with keeping arteries healthy and reducing the stickiness of platelets in the blood.

Elsewhere, researchers found that eating fish more than once a week was associated with a 50 percent reduced risk of macular degeneration in seniors: The chronic eye disease which accounts for one-third of all cases of vision loss that gradually destroys central vision.

Studies also indicate that fish oils may protect against Alzheimer's disease.

To increase your intake of protective fish oils, eat fish several times a week but be mindful of the fact that large fish such as swordfish and shark may be contaminated with mercury to the extent that frequent consumption presents a risk.

People who do not like fish or are allergic to it can look to flax or canola oils for omega-3 fats.

deficiencies, even if they are eating well. Some doctors recommend a daily vitamin and mineral supplement to ensure that an older person takes in 100 percent of the Recommended Dietary Allowances (RDAs). However, a multivitamin cannot take the place of healthy food because foods contain additional important components such as fiber, plant chemicals, and essential fatty acids. Also, high-dose supplements should be avoided unless recommended by a physician or dietitian, as they can lead to nutritional imbalances. For example, zinc supplements can interfere with the body's use of folic acid; iron can inhibit proper calcium and zinc absorption.

DO ONE SIMPLE THING

DRINK LOTS OF WATER EVERY DAY

Consume six to eight glasses each day. Water is an essential nutrient just like vitamins and minerals because your body cannot make enough of it to meet your daily requirements. It helps regulate body temperature, transports nutrients to your body's cells, and helps remove waste. Because sensitivity to thirst diminishes with age, older adults are susceptible to dehydration, which can cause confusion, fatigue, headache, and more.

Make the most of mealtimes

Although nutrition is all important for aging well, healthy eating isn't just about the nutrients. Sharing a meal with family and friends provides lots more benefits than just the food on your plate. If the thought of preparing and eating meals holds little pleasure, for whatever reason, try some of these practical tips to make dining more enjoyable.

✔ Strive to make meals pleasurable, even if you're eating alone. Set the table or prepare an attractive tray. Turn on your favorite music to improve your mood.

✔ If you dislike eating alone, organize regular potluck meals with friends and neighbors. Or consider joining an organization that provides an opportunity to dine with others.

✔ Select foods that supply contrasts in color, texture, and flavor. Avoid adding salt to improve flavor; instead, use herbs and spices. A sprinkling of nutmeg or cinnamon can compensate for a diminished sense of taste.

✔ Eat at least five servings a day of fruits and vegetables. Include a serving each time you eat. Many of these contain compounds that protect against diseases of aging such as heart disease and cancer. Choose brightly colored fruits and vegetables such as squash, carrots, peppers, melons, and berries.

✔ A small glass of wine or beer with a meal aids digestion and adds to eating pleasure. But don't substitute alcohol for food, and check with your doctor to make sure that it does not interact with any medications you might be taking.

✔ Make sure you drink six to eight glasses of water, juice, or other non-alcoholic fluids every day. Older people often experience decreased thirst or they reduce fluid intake because of bladder-control problems. This can contribute to constipation and kidney problems and increase the risk of dehydration in hot weather.

✔ If you have trouble chewing, there's no need to resort to a bland liquid diet, which can lead to constipation and perhaps even malnutrition. Instead, prepare fish or ground meat and purée vegetables, soups, and other nutritious foods.

✔ Take daily walks or engage in other exercise, but first consult your doctor for an appropriate routine. Exercise not only preserves muscle strength but also improves appetite and mood.

✔ If you're on a tight budget, organize a shopping co-op with others in a similar situation. Buying larger quantities is more economical; share with others, or divide the food into smaller portions and freeze them for future use.

✔ Read labels. Even if you have to take along a magnifying glass to see the small print, reading the breakdown of nutrients on a food package's label will help you to make healthier food choices.

Eat less to live longer?

Will cutting down on calories slow your aging clock as well as help cut extra weight off your waistline? Since the 1930s, scientists have known that restricting calories not only delays aging but even reverses some of its consequences in laboratory rats and mice. By feeding these animals a very low-calorie diet, a mere 30 to 50 percent of what they normally eat, scientists have been able to extend the lives of not only mice but also fruit flies.

One study was designed to see whether monkeys, fed a diet that included all required nutrients but two-thirds the usual calories, would live longer than normal. Data suggests that the primates who ingested a lean meal, as compared to their peers who ate all the food they wanted, had a lower incidence of heart disease, diabetes, and cancer. One theory as to why there's a link between eating less and living longer? Metabolism of food leads to the production of free radicals; the less food consumed, the fewer damaging free radicals produced.

Rats and monkeys, however, are not humans. Before caloric restriction is recommended as a potential antiaging strategy for people, carefully supervised studies on humans (such as those currently sponsored by the U.S. National Institute on Aging) need to be done. Caloric restriction is risky to try on your own: While it's generally known that seniors require fewer calories, the aging body is also less efficient in absorbing and using some nutrients. Knowing how to cut calories without compromising essential nutrients can be tricky; becoming undernourished would erase any benefits of such a diet—if indeed there are benefits to be had. Low-calorie diets are likely to be deficient in some nutrients, and leading proponents of such regimens, such as antiaging specialist Dr. Roy Walford, believe that supplementation with vitamins and minerals is essential.

CAUTION

If you live in a northern climate (that includes Boston, Seattle, Chicago, and much of Canada, as well as parts of Europe), your body may be seriously lacking in vitamin D, essential for the absorption of calcium. The majority of this vitamin is made in our skin upon exposure to sunlight. Not only do northern climates receive little sun in winter, but summer's bugs, poor air quality, and our desire to protect our skin against the sun's harmful rays lead many to shun it during summer months, too. Vitamin D is important in helping calcium to shore up bones to protect seniors against fractures. Seniors need between 400 IU and 600 IU of vitamin D daily. One cup of fluid milk contains 100 IU, as does one cup of fortified soy or rice beverage as well as some fortified orange juices.

DID YOU KNOW?

YOU MAY NEED A B_{12} SUPPLEMENT

If you're 50 or older, you should be taking a B_{12} supplement. B_{12} is essential for cell replication and red blood cell production. The acid in your stomach releases vitamin B_{12} from the meat you eat. The vitamin then binds to a substance called intrinsic factor that enables B_{12} to be absorbed into the bloodstream. Up to one-third of older adults produce inadequate amounts of stomach acid and therefore can no longer properly absorb B_{12} from food.

ANTIOXIDANTS
■ SORTING FACTS FROM HYPE ■

Recent research on antioxidant supplementation has yielded conflicting results. But there is no doubt about one thing—eating a diet high in antioxidant-rich foods is a smart choice. There are hundreds of studies linking antioxidant-rich fruits and vegetables to a lower risk of heart disease, cancer, and many other illnesses. But why is eating fruits and vegetables so healthy? Is it due to some specific compounds found in plant products or some special combination of nutrients? Or is it that people who eat lots of fruits and vegetables eat less meat, or that in general they consume fewer calories? In any case, the antioxidant theory merits investigation.

Just as a burning fire needs oxygen, every cell in our body needs a steady supply of oxygen to derive energy from digested food. But consuming oxygen comes with a price; it also generates free radicals, unstable molecules that can damage healthy cells. Free radicals are highly reactive because they contain an unpaired electron, and electrons prefer to pair up. So these free radicals search for a molecule from which they can steal an electron. The molecular victim then goes in search of an electron to satisfy its deficiency and sets off a chain reaction in the body that results in the creation of more free radicals. A molecule that has lost electrons in this manner is said to have been "oxidized."

Although all healthy cells produce small amounts of free radicals, there are a variety of other factors that can promote free-radical formation in the human body, such as radiation (including x-rays), cigarette smoke, alcohol, and environmental pollutants. Excessive free radicals can damage DNA and other genetic material. The body's immune system seeks out and destroys these mutated cells, in much the same way as it eliminates invading bacteria and other foreign organisms. This mechanism declines with age, however, and the body becomes more vulnerable to free-radical damage.

Antioxidants are molecules that interact with and stabilize free radicals, preventing the damage they might cause. Researchers have identified hundreds of antioxidants in our foods, including vitamins C and E; selenium and carotenoids such as beta carotene and lycopene. There are numerous other phytochemicals (chemicals derived from plants), such as the celebrated polyphenols in tea and wine that have antioxidant properties.

Over time, without the neutralizing action of antioxidants, the damage free radicals cause to cells can become irreversible, leading to cancer. Antioxidants also help prevent heart disease by hindering oxidation of LDL (low-density lipoprotein), the harmful cholesterol. It is actually oxidized cholesterol that damages arteries. There are hundreds of studies linking antioxidant-rich diets to a lower risk of both cancer and heart disease, as well as other degenerative diseases.

Possible detrimental effects

Less clear is the effect of antioxidant supplementation on health. Although research is ongoing, recent large-scale, randomized clinical trials have reached inconsistent conclusions. In five separate clinical

Top 10 antioxidant fruits and vegetables

Measured by their ORAC scores. ORAC refers to the Oxygen Radical Absorbance Capacity, an analysis that is used to measure the total antioxidant power of foods and other chemical substances. The higher the ORAC score, the greater its antioxidant capacity. This is a laboratory measurement and its relevance to the diet is unclear. Demonstrating that a substance neutralizes free radicals in a test tube and showing that it prevents some disease are quite different matters.

ORAC scores for 3½ oz (100 ml)

Prunes	5,770	Kale	1,770
Raisins	2,830	Spinach	1,260
Blueberries	2,400	Brussels sprouts	980
Strawberries	1,540	Broccoli florets	890
Raspberries	1,220	Beets	840
Plums	949	Red bell peppers	710
Oranges	750	Onions	450
Grapes	739	Corn	400
Cherries	670	Eggplant	390
Kiwi	602	Carrots	210

trials that studied the effects of antioxidants supplements on cancer in the last decade, results ranged from a reduced incidence of gastric cancer, to a possible increase in lung cancer rate associated with antioxidant intake.

Recently the U.S. Preventive Services Task Force scrutinized more than two dozen of the latest studies on the use of antioxidants to reduce the risk of cancer and heart disease and published its findings. The data led the lead researcher to conclude that people taking antioxidant supplements for the sole purpose of preventing heart disease or cancer "are basically creating expensive urine." Researchers at the Cleveland Clinic foundation carried out a study of studies that had examined the relationship between cardiovascular disease and antioxidant vitamins. They pooled the results and found that vitamin E provided no benefits to people suffering from cardiovascular disease and that beta carotene supplements actually increased the risk slightly.

Research is ongoing

Although results to date have been disappointing, research continues. It may be that the benefits of supplements only show up after many years. It is possible that while vitamin E is of no help once cardiovascular disease exists, it could help prevent the condition in the first place. There are many ongoing clinical trials investigating the effect of antioxidant supplementation on degenerative disease, and results are expected over the next few years. It is likely that antioxidants may have more dramatic effects with other diseases. Supplements of vitamin C (500 mg), vitamin E (400 IU), and beta carotene (25,000 IU), along with 80 mg of zinc and 2 mg of copper a day, may be of help in macular degeneration, a serious eye disease.

The value of getting antioxidants from food

For now, anyone taking supplements with amounts of nutrients higher than the RDAs should review their intake with their doctor, particularly if they are taking prescription drugs. High doses of vitamin E, for example, can interfere with blood clotting and increase the risk of a bleeding emergency. Some antioxidants may also reduce the effectiveness of the statin drugs, taken to reduce cholesterol levels.

The research results to date reinforce that foods rich in antioxidants remain the best source of these powerhouse nutrients.

CAUTION

Smokers who take high-dose beta carotene supplements actually increase their chances of developing lung cancer, say the results of two large medical trials. Ongoing studies continue to stress that everyone should get beneficial antioxidants the old-fashioned way—by eating their fruits and vegetables.

ANTIOXIDANT POWER

Researchers have investigated and identified literally hundreds of antioxidant phytochemicals in our food, from vitamins to pigments, that protect against disease, and the list continues to grow. Here are the main ones:

ANTIOXIDANT	FUNCTION	FOOD SOURCES
Vitamin C	Protects against heart disease, cataracts, macular degeneration, and some types of cancer.	Citrus fruit, tomatoes, melon, strawberries, kiwi, sweet peppers, broccoli.
Vitamin E	May help prevent heart disease and prostate cancer, and slow progression of Alzheimer's.	Nuts and seeds, oils, fruits and vegetables.
Carotenoids		
Beta carotene	Protective against cancer, particularly lung cancer, and heart disease.	Orange and dark green vegetables, including carrots, sweet potatoes, squash, broccoli, kale, spinach, apricots, peaches, and cantaloupe.
Lutein, zeaxathin	Protects against macular degeneration.	Dark green leafy vegetables, corn, sweet peppers, spinach, cabbage, oranges.
Lycopene	May protect against prostate cancer, lung cancer, and heart disease.	Tomatoes, pink grapefruit, watermelon.
Flavonoids		
Anthocyanidins	Protective against cancer.	Blueberries, cherries, cranberries, blackberries, black currents, plums, red grapes.
Hesperidin	Protective against heart disease and cancer.	Citrus fruits and juices.
Isoflavones	Protective against heart disease and cancer.	Soy, legumes, peanuts.
Quercetin	Protective against heart disease and cancer.	Onions, apples, berries, red grapes, kale, broccoli, red wine.
Selenium	May help prevent prostate cancer, colon cancer, and lung cancer.	Whole grains, nuts, Swiss chard, onions, garlic, poultry, seafood, meat.
Co-enzyme Q_{10}	May help reduce risk of heart disease. Works together with vitamin E.	All plants and animal foods.

APPETITE LOSS

EAT PLENTY OF

- Fresh fruits and vegetables for vitamin C.
- Lean meats, seafood, nuts, seeds, and whole grains for zinc and B vitamins.

AVOID

- Smoking and excessive alcohol, which dull the appetite.
- Liquids before meals.
- Bran and other high-fiber foods.

The pleasant anticipation of eating that we call appetite is controlled by two centers in the brain: one is the hypothalamus, which stimulates the release of hunger-producing hormones until hunger is satisfied; the other is the cerebral cortex, the center of intellectual and sensory function. Thus, a healthy appetite reflects both an unconscious response and learned behavior.

Many disorders and circumstances cause loss of appetite; most are temporary conditions, such as a cold, an upset stomach, dental problems, or stress. A persistent loss of appetite, however, can reflect a more serious illness; for example, clinical depression, anemia, kidney disease, AIDS, or cancer.

In unusual cases, appetite loss stems from nutritional deficiencies, usually of vitamin C, thiamine, niacin, biotin, and zinc. Excessive drinking of alcohol not only reduces appetite but may also cause nutritional deficiencies. Smoking is another activity that blunts appetite.

Eating large amounts of bran, whole-grain products, and other high-fiber foods interferes with the absorption of zinc and other minerals; such foods also diminish appetite because they are filling. Drinking large quantities of liquid before a meal reduces appetite too.

Loss of appetite related to illness usually corrects itself with recovery. There are several strategies, however, that may help trigger an appetite when it is lost inexplicably.

Eat small snacks through the day rather than three large meals. Keep snacks available to eat whenever you feel the urge.

Have a lemon drop. Before a meal, have a lemon drop; sucking something sour increases saliva flow, which in turn stimulates appetite.

Create a pleasant eating atmosphere. Put flowers on the table, play quiet music, use soft light—whatever makes you feel good. Surround yourself with appetizing odors, spices like cinnamon, or a favorite food.

Try a little exercise. Take a walk before meals; some people find that activity increases their appetite.

A little alcohol may help. Try drinking a glass of wine or beer—it may increase your appetite. ❖

APPLES

BENEFITS

- Low in calories and high in soluble fiber that helps lower cholesterol.
- Packed with numerous phytochemicals such as quercetin that may help prevent heart disease and cancer.
- Apples enhance dental hygiene.

DRAWBACKS

- Relatively low in nutrients.
- Skin may contain pesticide residues.

A fresh apple is an ideal snack. It's easy to carry, flavorful, filling, and low in calories; a 5-oz (140-g) piece of fruit has only 90 calories. Apples can be eaten fresh or cooked in myriad ways—baked into pies, crisps, and tarts; added to poultry stuffing; and made into jelly, apple butter, and sauce. Apple cider vinegar is an ingredient in many salad dressings. Pasteurized apple juice and fresh-pressed cider are popular drinks, while fermented apple cider, wine, and brandy are gaining in popularity.

Wash off the pesticide. Apple trees thrive in most temperate climates, but since they are vulnerable to worms, scale, and other insects, they are usually sprayed with pesticides several times. Apples should always be washed carefully before eating; some experts even suggest peeling them, especially if they have been waxed. The wax itself is not a problem but it may prevent pesticide residues from being rinsed off.

NUTRITIONAL VALUE

"An apple a day keeps the doctor away" is an old adage, but it may require more than one apple to do the job. The average apple provides only

CAUTION

Escherichia coli (*E. coli*) and *Cryptosporidium* have been identified as the cause of serious illness in people who consumed unpasteurized apple juice or apple cider. While the risk of becoming ill from these products is low, children, the elderly, and people with weakened immune systems are most susceptible and should take precautions by drinking pasteurized juice or cider. Most juices you buy in grocery stores are pasteurized (check the labels), but caution should be taken when buying drinks at roadside stands, country fairs, or visits to local orchards.

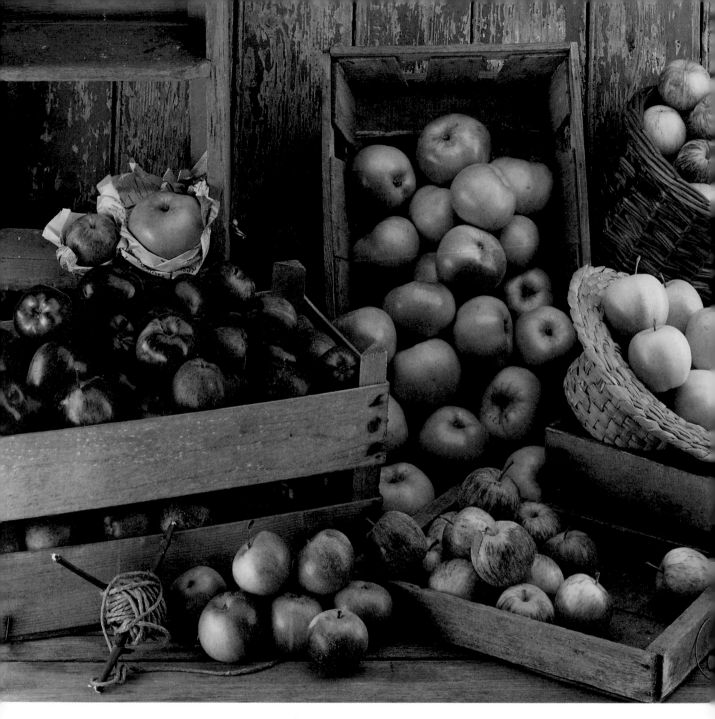

APPLE HARVEST. *More than 2,500 varieties of apples grow in North America; others are imported. Popular ones include (clockwise from far left) Red Delicious, Crispin, Royal Gala, Granny Smith, Empire, Golden Delicious, Royal Gala, and Cox.*

8 mg of vitamin C, which is not much. The nutritional value of an apple lies elsewhere. It contains a good dose of pectin, the soluble fiber that thickens jellies and helps lower artery-damaging LDL blood cholesterol levels. But the most positive nutritional aspect is the mix of antioxidants apples contain. Flavonoids, such as quercetin, prevent LDL cholesterol from being oxidized to a more dangerous form. Researchers have shown that as little as one and a half glasses of apple juice a day can significantly reduce the oxidation of LDL. Another study found that eating 3½ oz (100 g)

of a fresh apple with the skin provided the total antioxidant and anticancer activity equal to 1,500 mg of vitamin C.

Because applesauce is pleasant-tasting and easily digested, doctors recommend it as an early baby food. Apples have long been called nature's toothbrush; while they don't actually cleanse the teeth, they still enhance dental hygiene. Biting and chewing an apple stimulates the gums, and the sweetness of the apple prompts an increased flow of saliva, which reduces tooth decay by lowering the levels of bacteria in the mouth.

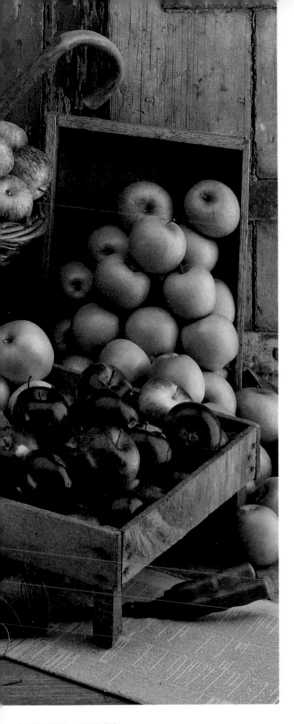

APRICOTS

BENEFITS

- A rich source of beta carotene, iron, and potassium.
- High in fiber, low in calories.
- Dried apricots are nutritious, fat-free foods.

DRAWBACKS

- Sulfite preservatives in some dried apricots can trigger an allergic reaction or asthma attack in people susceptible to these disorders.
- Dried apricots leave a sticky residue on teeth that can lead to cavities.
- A natural salicylate in apricots may trigger an allergic reaction in aspirin-sensitive people.

Apricots are ideal for both snacks and desserts. They are tasty, easy to digest, high in fiber, low in calories (about 50 calories in 3 fresh apricots and 85 in 10 dried halves), virtually fat-free, and highly nutritious.

Apricots' deep color indicates the presence of carotenoids, specifically beta carotene, an important antioxidant, linked with cancer prevention. Apricots are also a source of the soluble fiber pectin, which helps lower LDL cholesterol.

Although eating fresh apricots is a way to get the most vitamin C (which is depleted by heat and exposure to air when apricots are dried), other substances such as beta carotene and pectin are actually made more available to the body when the apricots are cooked. Regardless of form, apricots are high in iron and potassium, a mineral essential for proper nerve and muscle function that also helps maintain normal blood pressure and balance of body fluids. It is interesting to note dried apricots are a regular item in the diet of the inhabitants of Pakistan's Hunza Valley who profess to have legendary longevity (though they have no proof of such).

Apricots contain a natural salicylate, a compound similar to the active ingredient in aspirin. People sensitive to aspirin may experience allergic responses after eating apricots.

DRIED APRICOTS

Apricots are more nutritious when they are dried. The reason: Dried apricots are only 32 percent water, compared to 85 percent water in the fresh fruit. They are a more concentrated

IS LAETRILE AN EFFECTIVE CANCER TREATMENT?

Laetrile is a highly controversial substance derived from apricot pits. Legally, it cannot be sold as a medical treatment, but it is available, often called vitamin B_{17}, through the Internet. It is promoted as an alternative treatment for cancer, heart disease, and other ailments. However, numerous scientific studies have failed to find any benefit from laetrile. Indeed, laetrile from apricot pits can liberate cyanide and carries a risk of cyanide poisoning. Doctors warn that apricot pits in any form should not be ingested.

DRIED APPLES

Usually served as a snack or in pies, dried apples are a more concentrated source of energy than the fresh form. It takes about 5 lb (2.2 kg) of apples to make 1 lb (0.45 kg) of dried apple slices, which provide about 70 calories per ounce (30 g). Except for fiber and a small amount of iron, most nutrients are lost in the drying process. Dried apples are less likely to promote cavities than other dried fruits.

Sulfur dioxide is often added to dried apples to preserve moistness and color; it can provoke an allergic reaction in a susceptible person. ❖

source of calories—50 calories in 4 oz (115 g) of fresh apricots versus 260 in 4 oz (115 g) (about 30 halves) of the dried. When eaten in moderation, dried apricots are a compact and convenient source of nutrition.

Asthmatics should buy sulfite-free fruit. Apricots are often treated with sulfur dioxide before they are dried to preserve their color and certain nutrients. This sulfite treatment may trigger an asthma attack or allergic reaction in susceptible people. Unless dried apricots are labeled as sulfite-free, anyone with asthma should avoid them. ❖

ARTHRITIS

CHICKEN SOUP—
MORE THAN
JUST GOOD
FOR THE SOUL

Reports of the "chicken-bone cure" for rheumatoid arthritis were a bit premature, but results were promising. The goal of this treatment is to calm the overactive immune system by exposing it to large amounts of a substance similar to what it is attacking; in this instance, collagen made from chicken bones. In the study, all patients with severe RA saw an improvement after a few weeks of consuming chicken-bone collagen broth.

EAT PLENTY OF
- Salmon, sardines, and other fatty fish to counter inflammation.
- High-fiber, low-calorie foods to help control weight.

AVOID
- Any foods that provoke symptoms.

About one in seven North Americans suffers from some type of arthritis, any of more than 100 disorders characterized by joint inflammation, stiffness, swelling, and pain. The most common types are osteoarthritis, a painful condition in which joint cartilage gradually breaks down, and rheumatoid arthritis, a systemic disease that can cause severe pain and crippling.

Doctors do not understand why some individuals develop arthritis and others don't, but a combination of factors plays a role. People with osteoarthritis may have inherently defective

cartilage that makes it vulnerable to normal wear and tear. Rheumatoid arthritis (RA) develops when an overactive immune system attacks connective tissue in the joints and other organs, causing inflammation and pain.

ARTHRITIS AND FISH
Until recently, doctors generally dismissed dietary treatments for arthritis as quackery; new research shows, however, that for some patients, diet can make a difference. Studies have found that patients with RA can experience a marked reduction in swelling, pain, and redness of joints by adding omega-3 fatty acids to their diet. These are found in salmon, mackerel, and sardines, as well as in other cold-water fish. The omega-3 fats have anti-inflammatory properties, whereas the more common omega-6 fats found in soy, corn, safflower, and sunflower oils are proinflammatory.

Watch the levels of omega-6 in your diet. The best results with fish oils have been seen when the omega-6 fats in the diet have been reduced and the omega-3 fats increased so that they are consumed in roughly equal amounts.

Gamma linolenic acid (GLA) is another type of fat with anti-inflammatory properties. The best sources are borage oil (it contains up to 24 percent GLA), evening primrose oil (8 to 10 percent), and black current oil (15 to 17 percent). Benefits in rheumatoid arthritis can be seen with a dose of about 500 mg of GLA a day, but recent studies have indicated that 1 to 1.5 g a day may be more appropriate. Both fish oils and GLA may have to be taken for months before improvement occurs. There appears to be no risk in increasing GLA intake, but excessive fish oil consumption can increase the risk of bleeding problems.

Eat more vitamin C-rich foods. Since vitamin C is important for the manufacture of collagen, eating C-rich foods may help slow the progression of osteoarthritis. Best food sources are citrus fruits, berries, kiwi, melons, broccoli, peppers, potatoes, and cabbage. There is also evidence that antioxidants such as vitamin C, beta carotene, and vitamin E will fight the effects of free radicals, which are generated by inflammatory compounds and are thought to cause tissue damage in people with rheumatoid arthritis.

FOOD ALLERGIES
Some evidence indicates that a small percentage of people with arthritis have food allergies that exacerbate joint symptoms. Common offenders include shellfish, soy, wheat, corn,

TOP FOODS THAT FIGHT ARTHRITIS

FISH Eat lots of salmon, sardines, and other cold-water fish, rich in omega-3 oils, three or more times a week.

VEGETABLES Eat 5 to 10 servings every day of: dark green or bright orange vegetables to provide beta carotene; broccoli, peppers, cabbage, and brussels sprouts for vitamin C; and avocados for vitamin E.

FRUITS Eat daily: yellow-orange-colored fruits for beta carotene; citrus fruits, berries, melons, and kiwi for vitamin C.

NUTS AND WHOLE GRAINS Eat nuts, seeds, and whole grains regularly, for vitamin E, a potent antioxidant that helps relieve inflammation and stiffness.

MYTH BUSTER

Myth: Nightshade vegetables aggravate arthritis. The nightshades family includes eggplant, bell peppers, tomatoes, and potatoes.

Reality: No scientific studies support this belief. Arthritis sufferers should be encouraged to eat plenty of these nutritious vegetables.

alcohol, coffee, and possibly certain food additives. Researchers have found that, for these people, removing the allergy-causing foods from the diet has resulted in less pain. If you think a certain food is triggering your pain, remove it from your diet for two weeks and pay attention to any symptom changes. Then add it back, and see if your symptoms worsen.

THE WEIGHT FACTOR

Obesity greatly increases the risk and severity of osteoarthritis. Even a little extra weight strains the knees and hips. Losing weight and increasing exercise often improve symptoms.

Patients with rheumatoid arthritis often have the opposite problem; they may be too thin due to a lack of appetite, chronic pain, or depression. A doctor may recommend calorie- and nutrient-enriched liquid supplements.

VEGETARIAN DIET

Researchers have found that fasting followed by a strict vegetarian diet for at least three months can bring about significant symptom relief. They theorize that one benefit of this strict diet comes from fruits, vegetables, and grains, which contribute important antioxidants that can help counter some of the inflammation. The diet is also very low in or free of animal fats, which may promote the production of inflammatory immune compounds. A strict vegetarian diet requires professional supervision to ensure proper nutrition.

EXPERIMENTAL TREATMENTS

One promising approach entails rubbing painful joints with a cream containing capsaicin, a derivative of chilies. Capsaicin produces a stinging or burning feeling, but it appears to reduce inflammation.

Studies show a marked improvement in osteoarthritis when patients take glucosamine sulfate, a natural body compound vital in building and maintaining cartilage, in dosages of 500 mg three times a day.

Be wary of alternative treatments. Because arthritis has no cure, sufferers often turn to alternative therapies. Some may help, others are worthless, often costly, and sometimes dangerous. Bee venom injections do nothing for arthritis. Chelation, used to remove toxic metals from the body, has been touted in a series of 20 to 30 intravenous treatments as a remedy for RA, but there is no scientific evidence that it is effective. Herbal treatments, such as Chinese black balls sold under such names as Miracle Herb and Tung Shueh, have been found to contain the antianxiety drug diazepam. ❖

ARTICHOKES

BENEFITS

- A good source of folate, vitamin C, and potassium.
- Low in calories, high in fiber.

DRAWBACKS

- May provoke allergic reaction in people sensitive to ragweed.

Served either hot or cold, the globe artichoke is both a delicacy and a low-calorie, nutritious vegetable. Actually, a globe artichoke is the flower bud of a large, thistlelike plant, with only a few edible portions—the heart and the tender, fleshy part at the base of the tough outer leaves. Both the heart and the meaty leaves of the artichoke are edible, though it's the leaves that contain many of the vegetable's phytochemicals.

Use a light sauce. To prepare a fresh artichoke, the thorny top and leaf tips are trimmed away, and the vegetable is boiled, steamed, or baked. It can be served in many ways, but one of the most popular is to dip the edible portion of the leaves in a sauce. It's this sauce that dictates whether an artichoke is a healthful treat or a high-calorie indulgence. High-fat sauces like Hollandaise and melted butter are traditional favorites, but a much more healthful choice is lemon juice with a dash of olive oil.

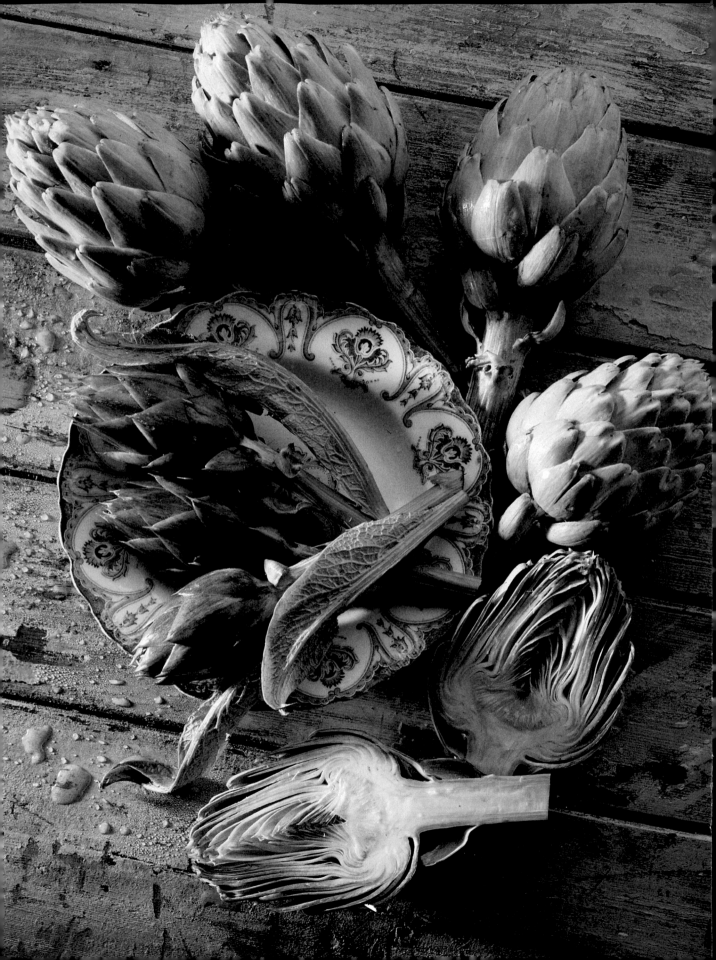

One artichoke provides 28 percent of the Recommended Daily Allowance (RDA) of folate, 16 percent of vitamin C, 300 mg of potassium, and about 3 g of fiber. Artichokes contain cynarin, an organic acid that stimulates the sweetness receptors in the taste buds of some people, causing the foods eaten afterward to taste sweeter. This chemical is thought to improve liver function and possibly lower blood cholesterol, but these claims are unproved. Also lacking proof are claims that artichokes lower blood sugar and stimulate bile flow.

Artichokes are members of the sunflower, or composite, plant family. People allergic to ragweed pollen may react to artichokes because of cross-reacting antigens that respond to both allergens. ❖

ARTIFICIAL SWEETENERS

BENEFITS

- Provide a sweet taste with fewer calories.
- Can be used as a sugar replacement for people with diabetes.
- They do not promote tooth decay.

DRAWBACKS

- Pregnant or lactating women should discuss the use of sweeteners with their physician.
- Aspartame should not be used by people with phenylketonuria (PKU).

Artificial sweeteners are popularly used to reduce both the total calorie intake and the amount of sugar consumed. They are many times sweeter than table sugar but, in measured amounts, add a taste to foods that is similar to that provided by regular sweeteners such as sugar, honey, molasses, or corn syrup. Because they do not contain any glucose, they can be effective sweeteners for people with diabetes. They come in a variety of forms and tastes. Each sweetener has a slightly different intensity or character to its taste.

Check your daily intake. Before any sweetener is approved for sale, it must meet rigorous guidelines and have been tested extensively. The Acceptable Daily Intake (ADI) is an average daily amount that can be used over a lifetime without causing harm. It is based on body weight and includes a very large safety margin (see "Acceptable Daily Intake" chart above).

ACCEPTABLE DAILY INTAKE (ADI) OF ARTIFICIAL SWEETENERS

Here's how to calculate your ADI. If, for example, you weigh 132 lb (60 kg), multiply your weight by the ADI figure of your sweetener in the chart. For Acesulfame K you would be allowed 924 mg per day (132 lb x 7 mg). One packet contains about 50 mg, so you could use up to 19 packets per day.

NAME	ADI mg/lb (mg/kg) body weight
Acesulfame K	7 (15)
Aspartame	18–23 (40–50)
Saccharin	2 (5)
Sucralose	2–7 (5–15)
Cyclamate (*Canada only*)	5 (11)

While sweeteners on the market are safe for consumption and do play a role, especially for people with diabetes, it is prudent to be moderate in your use of them. Here is a rundown of some of the most popular artificial sweeteners:

- Saccharin, sold as Sweet'n Low or Hermesetas, is the oldest of the sweeteners on the market. It is calorie-free, about 300 times sweeter than sugar, but has a slightly bitter aftertaste. It is allowed as an additive in the United States, but only as a tabletop sweetener in Canada. Although several studies have suggested that large quantities of saccharin can cause cancer in laboratory rats, no harmful effects have been shown in humans. The FDA in the United States has now dropped saccharin from its list of cancer-causing chemicals. It is heat stable and suitable for use in cooking and baking, and as an addition to beverages and foods.
- Aspartame, marketed under the brand name NutraSweet and also known as Equal, is made from two amino acids, phenylalanine and aspartic acid. It contains the same calories, weight for weight, as sugar, but since it is about 200 times sweeter, it can be used in minute quantities. Aspartame loses its sweetness when cooked or exposed to certain acids, so it is not used in baking. You'll find it in soft drinks, candies, and desserts. Studies suggest that in isolated cases aspartame can trigger seizures or headaches, but the vast majority use it without obvious problems. Because it contains phenylalanine, it is unsafe for people with phenylketonuria (PKU).

- Acesulfame potassium (acesulfame K) is 200 times sweeter than sugar and calorie-free. Marketed under the name Sunett, it is highly stable, withstands heat, and can be used for baking. It is not broken down by the body and is eliminated without providing any calories. It is found in spreads, beverages, candies, gum, and baked products. People on a potassium restricted diet or with sulfa-antibiotic allergies should discuss the use of Ace-K with their physician.
- Sucralose, made from sucrose, is about 600 times sweeter than sugar. Marketed as Splenda, it is highly stable and can be used in foods and beverages, cooking and baking. It is used as an additive in beverages and processed foods and as a tabletop sweetener. It is not broken down by the body and is eliminated without providing any calories.
- Cyclamates were banned in the United States in 1969, when a group of researchers reported an apparent increased incidence of cancer in rats fed large amounts of the sweetener. Canadian authorities were not convinced that this study showed a risk for humans, and Canada, and at least 40 other countries, allows the use of cyclamates. In Canada, cyclamates are sold in liquid, tablet, and powder forms. Cyclamate is marketed under the brand name Sucaryl and is used in Sugar Twin and Weight Watchers. You can cook and bake with this sweetener without it losing its sweet taste.
- Sugar alcohols are another category of sweeteners. They are derived from plant products such as fruit and are referred to as nutritive sweeteners because they provide calories and may affect blood sugar. They contain fewer calories than table sugar because they are not well absorbed. The most common include sorbitol, mannitol, xylitol, maltitol, and lactitol. One strong benefit of these sweeteners is their role in preventing dental cavities. You'll find them in candies, gum, jams and jellies, and some cough syrups. In excess, they can cause abdominal discomfort and bloating and have a laxative effect. They also can exacerbate the symptoms of irritable bowel syndrome (IBS) for some people. ❖

ASPARAGUS

BENEFITS
- A good low-calorie source of folate and potassium.
- Stalks are high in fiber.

DRAWBACKS
- Contains purines, which may precipitate an attack of gout.

Prized as a springtime delicacy for centuries, this edible member of the lily family is now so widely cultivated that it is available in every season. Lightly boiled or steamed, asparagus makes a tasty and nutritious appetizer, salad ingredient, or side dish.

The ancient Greeks and Romans thought that asparagus possessed medicinal qualities, curing everything from rheumatism to toothaches. None of these properties have been proven true, but asparagus does provide many essential nutrients: Six spears contain 100 mcg (micrograms) of folate, 25 percent of the adult Recommended Dietary Allowance (RDA), as well as 20 mg of vitamin C. Asparagus is low in calories (25 in six spears), contains fiber, important antioxidants such as glutathione, and is a useful source of vitamin B_6 and potassium.

Eat asparagus as soon as possible after picking. It spoils quickly, and if unrefrigerated, asparagus loses half its vitamin C and much of its flavor in just 2 or 3 days. If frozen quickly, asparagus retains most of its nutrients; canning destroys some flavor while adding large amounts of salt.

Gout sufferers may be advised to forgo asparagus because it contains purines, substances that can precipitate a painful attack of the disease. Some people notice that asparagus

> ## DID YOU KNOW?
>
> ### ASPARAGUS CAN CAUSE PAINFUL GOUT ATTACKS
>
> Asparagus contains purines, substances that promote the overproduction of uric acid that precipitates painful attacks of gout. Asparagus consumption should be kept to a minimum by gout sufferers.

gives their urine a pungent odor; this harmless reaction occurs when the body metabolizes the sulfur compounds in the food. Studies show, however, that only about 40 percent of people have this problem. ❖

ASTHMA

EAT PLENTY OF

- Fruits and vegetables (aim for 5 to 10 servings per day).
- Chicken soup, broth, and other fluids to help thin bronchial mucus.
- Foods high in omega-3 fatty acids such as salmon, mackerel, herring, and sardines to counter inflammation.

AVOID

- Any foods, including additives, that seem to bring on attacks.
- Mushrooms, cheese, soy sauce, and yeasty breads if molds trigger attacks.
- Salicylates, an ingredient in aspirin, tea, vinegar, salad dressings, many fruits, and a few vegetables.
- Any food preserved with sulfites.
- Foods containing tartrazine, or yellow food dye 5.

Asthma is a chronic lung condition that is a leading cause of childhood deaths, especially among city dwellers. The rising toll of asthma has puzzled doctors, but many attribute it to a combination of factors, such as the cost of asthma medications, which may be beyond the means of low-income families, improper use of asthma medications, and exposure to environmental pollutants.

Wheezing, chest tightness, labored breathing, and other asthma symptoms occur when the tiny muscles that control the airways to the lungs constrict, causing a bronchospasm. Normally, the airways narrow somewhat when exposed to smoke, pollutants, very cold air, or substances that are harmful if inhaled. In asthmatic people, however, the response is exaggerated and often triggered by otherwise harmless substances or activities, such as pollen and other allergens and exercise.

Heredity may be a factor. The reason some people have hyperreactive airways is unknown; heredity, however, is suspected of playing a role, because the disease runs in families. Many asthmatics also have hay fever and other allergies.

Although stress and emotional upsets can trigger or worsen an attack, experts emphasize that asthma is a lung disease, not a psychological disorder; as such, it should be treated as a serious and even debilitating physical condition.

Some asthma attacks are quickly reversed by taking a bronchodilator medication. These ease symptoms by opening the constricted airways. Other episodes are more prolonged, and, as the airways become more inflamed and clogged with mucus, breathing becomes increasingly difficult. In such cases, an injection of epinephrine (Adrenalin) and a corticosteroid drug may be needed to stop the attack.

Although asthma is a chronic disease, the changes that occur during an attack are temporary, and the lungs generally function normally at other times. When asthma starts during childhood, the frequency and severity of attacks tend to lessen as the youngster grows and may disappear by adulthood. Some adults, however, suffer a recurrence, often as an aftermath of a viral infection. In such cases, the asthma may be even more severe than it was in childhood.

ELIMINATING TRIGGERS

Doctors agree that the best treatment for asthma entails identifying and then avoiding its triggers. In some instances these are obvious— for example, exposure to tobacco smoke and other noxious fumes, cold air, exercise, or an allergy to animal dander. Seasonal asthma is usually due to various pollens, molds, and other environmental factors. Suspected allergens can usually be identified by blood and skin tests.

Food allergies can cause attacks. In many asthma sufferers, food allergies are a trigger; in these cases, identifying the culprits may require considerable detective work, especially in children. Because food allergies vary from person to person, there is no handy list of offenders. But sometimes a child unconsciously links a food with his asthma by fussing or refusing to eat it. Complaints such as "it makes my mouth feel funny" may point to an allergy. Often, foods that trigger asthma are

STAY AWAY FROM SULFITES

More prevalent—and potentially deadly— asthma triggers are sulfites, preservatives that are added to many foods to prevent spoilage and preserve color and texture. They are especially common in dried fruits, dehydrated or instant soup mixes, instant potatoes, dough conditioners, wine, beer, and white grape juice. Anyone sensitive to sulfites should carefully check food labels for any ingredient ending in sulfite—for example, potassium bisulfite—as well as sulfur dioxide. In addition to precipitating an asthma attack, sulfites sometimes lead to anaphylaxis in people hypersensitive to them.

DO ONE SIMPLE THING

DRINK ONE OR TWO CUPS OF COFFEE TO ABORT A MILD ASTHMA ATTACK

Coffee and tea are sources of theophylline, a bronchial muscle relaxant used to treat asthma in people who are not sensitive to salicylates. Anyone taking a theophylline drug, however, should avoid large amounts of tea to prevent an overdose.

identified by keeping a careful record of the time and ingestion of all foods and drinks, as well as any asthma symptoms. After a few weeks, a pattern of offending foods may emerge. A doctor can then do confirming skin or other allergy tests.

For some people, inadvertently ingested environmental allergens are the problem rather than the foods. People allergic to ragweed, for example, may also react to pyrethrum, a natural pesticide made from chrysanthemums, or to other allergens related to plants. Similarly, people allergic to mildew and other environmental molds may react to molds in foods; common offenders include cheese, mushrooms, hot dogs and other processed meats, as well as anything that is fermented, including soy sauce, beer, wine, and vinegar.

Salicylates—compounds in the same family as the active ingredient in aspirin and found naturally in many fruits—may trigger asthma. Yellow food dye 5 (tartrazine) is chemically similar to salicylate, although it is less potent.

HELPFUL FOODS

There are no specific foods that prevent asthma, but some may lessen its complications. Omega-3 fatty acids, found in salmon, mackerel, sardines, and other cold-water fish, have an anti-inflammatory effect and may counter bronchial inflammation. Evidence continues to grow on the protective effects of fruits and vegetables on lung function.

Eat at least 5 to 10 servings of fruits and vegetables daily and include one citrus fruit. These foods all provide a variety of vitamins, minerals, and antioxidants important for healthy lung function. Vitamin C helps promote a healthy immune system and may be helpful in reducing wheezing in children with asthma. Some studies have linked weight gain with adult-onset asthma. In addition, when obese people with asthma lose weight, there can be an improvement in asthma symptoms.

POTENTIAL PROBLEMS

Like everyone else, asthma patients need to consume a healthful, balanced diet, but this is sometimes difficult if allergies require eliminating entire food groups (for example, milk and other dairy products). A dietitian can recommend substitutes or supplements to ensure maintaining good nutrition.

Asthma drugs can create nutritional problems. Long-term steroid use, for example, causes bone loss; vitamin D and calcium supplements may be needed to strengthen bones. Potassium deficiency is another potential problem; it can be prevented by eating ample citrus fruits, bananas, dried fruits, berries, beets, tomatoes, and green leafy vegetables. Epinephrine and other bronchodilator drugs can cause feelings of nervousness, which are exacerbated by caffeine. It may be advisable to switch to decaffeinated coffee. ❖

ATHEROSCLEROSIS

EAT PLENTY OF
- Fresh fruits and vegetables for vitamin C, beta carotene, and folate.
- Wheat germ, nuts, seeds, and vegetable oils for vitamin E.
- Salmon, sardines, and other cold-water fish for omega-3 fatty acids.
- Apples, oatmeal, lentils, and legumes for soluble fiber.
- Soy proteins in foods such as soy beverages, tofu, or tempeh.

CUT DOWN ON
- Fats, especially saturated ones.
- Cookies, cakes, and snack foods rich in trans fatty acids.
- High-cholesterol foods.

AVOID
- Smoking, obesity, high alcohol intake, and physical inactivity.

As we become older, our arteries lose some of their elasticity and stiffen. This can lead to a progressive condition referred to as arteriosclerosis, the medical term for hardening (sclerosis) of the arteries. These stiffened blood vessels usually become clogged with fatty plaque, the hallmark of atherosclerosis (*athero* is the Greek term for porridge, which describes the thick, cheesy appearance of the deposits).

Some degree of atherosclerosis is a natural part of aging. It usually progresses slowly over years without producing noticeable symptoms. But serious problems develop when these stiffened blood vessels become severely narrowed with plaque. Complications include circulatory disorders, especially reduced blood flow to the lower legs and other extremities; angina, the chest pains caused by inadequate oxygen to the heart muscle; and heart disease and stroke.

TEN WAYS TO CUT SATURATED FAT

1. Choose leaner cuts of meat and remove fat whenever possible.
2. Downsize meat portions. Choose low-fat cheeses.
3. Cook with olive or vegetable oil instead of butter or margarine.
4. Use tofu or nuts in stir-fries instead of meat.
5. Try adding a slice of avocado instead of cheese to a sandwich.
6. Enjoy a baked potato instead of fries, and use low-fat yogurt instead of sour cream.
7. Switch to a lower-fat milk.
8. Substitute buttermilk instead of mayonnaise in salad dressings, or instead of butter in mashed potatoes.
9. Add more beans and vegetables to casseroles and chili—use less meat or veggie ground round.
10. Enjoy fruit served with frozen sherbet or low-fat frozen yogurt instead of ice cream for dessert.

By the time Western men have reached their late forties, most have some degree of atherosclerosis. In women the process is somewhat delayed, presumably due to the protective effects of estrogen during the reproductive years. After menopause, however, women quickly catch up with their male counterparts, and once in their sixties they are just as likely to develop severely clogged arteries as men are.

UNDERLYING CAUSES

Precisely what initiates atherosclerosis is unknown. Most experts agree, however, that a genetic susceptibility and a combination of lifestyle factors accelerate the process; these include a diet high in fats and cholesterol, cigarette use, excessive stress, and lack of exercise. Poorly controlled diabetes and high blood pressure also contribute to atherosclerosis.

Arteries can be narrowed by 85 percent (or more) without producing symptoms. Nevertheless, there is still a high risk of a heart attack or stroke because clots tend to form at the site of fatty deposits. Most heart attacks are caused by a clot blocking a coronary artery (a coronary thrombosis); similarly, a cerebral thrombosis, or a clot that blocks blood flow to the brain, is the most common type of stroke.

DIETARY APPROACHES

Researchers agree that diet plays a critical role in both the development and treatment of atherosclerosis. Cholesterol is the major component of atherosclerotic plaque, and numerous studies correlate high levels of blood cholesterol with atherosclerosis. Research indicates that atherosclerosis can be slowed and even reversed by lowering cholesterol in the blood—particularly the levels of low-density lipoproteins (LDLs), the bad type of cholesterol.

Elevated triglycerides, another type of lipid that circulates in the blood, also may contribute to atherosclerosis. People with diabetes tend to have high triglyceride and cholesterol levels, which may explain why diabetics are so vulnerable to heart disease.

Limit total fat intake. Dietary treatment for atherosclerosis entails limiting total fat intake to 20 to 30 percent of calories, with saturated fats (found mostly in animal products and palm, coconut, and palm kernel oils) comprising no more than 10 percent of calories. In addition to limiting saturated fats, experts suggest reducing intake of trans fatty acids and hydrogenated fats. These trans fats are the result of hydrogenation and are known to raise your LDL cholesterol. Trans fats come in packaged foods such as cookies and crackers and snack food such as chips. Some experts advocate even more stringent fat reduction; these include Dr. Dean Ornish, the cardiologist who has developed a comprehensive lifestyle approach to treating heart disease, which combines a healthy low-fat diet with exercise and methods for dealing with stress. His atherosclerosis-reversal regimen limits fat calories to 10 percent of the diet and virtually eliminates saturated fats.

Although consumption of high-cholesterol foods is not as instrumental as a high-fat diet, a high intake of dietary cholesterol can raise the levels of blood lipids. Experts recommend limiting dietary cholesterol to 300 mg a day—about the amount in 1½ egg yolks.

The omega-3 fatty acids in salmon, sardines, and other cold-water fish lower blood levels of triglycerides; they also

DO ONE SIMPLE THING

EAT MORE SOY

Add 25 g of soy protein to your daily diet. Try tofu or soy nuts. A variety of studies have shown that eating this amount daily should lower cholesterol in people with elevated levels by about 9 percent, and LDL cholesterol, by as much as 15 percent.

reduce the tendency to form blood clots. Oat bran, oatmeal, lentils and legumes, pectin-containing fruits such as pears, apples, and citrus fruits, barley, guar gum, psyllium all contain soluble fiber that lowers blood cholesterol, probably by interfering with the intestinal absorption of bile acids, which forces the liver to use circulating cholesterol to make more bile.

Antioxidants may help. Studies indicate that beta carotene and vitamins C and E may protect against atherosclerosis by preventing LDL cholesterol from collecting in atherosclerotic plaque. Regular intake of soy protein may raise HDL cholesterol (the "good" cholesterol) as well as provide antioxidant protection.

Many studies are looking at homocysteine, an amino acid (one of the building blocks of protein) that some scientists say is as risky or maybe even riskier than cholesterol. High levels have been shown to damage the lining of the artery walls, potentially leading to a buildup of plaque. Folate as well as vitamins B_{12} and B_6 appear to help lower homocysteine levels.

Diet is not the only factor that contributes. Maintaining an ideal weight, abstaining from smoking, increasing exercise, developing effective methods of coping with stress, and keeping blood pressure and blood sugar levels within normal limits are also important. ❖

AVOCADOS

BENEFITS

- A rich source of folate, vitamin A, and potassium.
- Useful amounts of protein, iron, magnesium, and vitamins C, E, and B_6.

DRAWBACKS

- Very high in calories, with 85 percent coming from fat.

Although it is often mistaken for a vegetable, the avocado is a fruit—the reproductive part of the plant. The rich, buttery flavor and smooth texture of an avocado make it a complementary addition to vegetable, meat, and pasta salads. When mashed and seasoned, it can also be served as a dip (as in guacamole), or a sandwich spread.

The avocado contains approximately 200 calories in a 4-oz (115-g) serving, and it has more fat and calories than any other fruit. However, because most of the fat in avocados is monounsaturated, it does not tend to elevate blood cholesterol levels, unlike the saturated oil that comes from palms and a number of other tropical plants.

When served as part of an otherwise low-fat meal or snack, an avocado contributes a number of important nutrients. Four ounces (115 g), about one-half of a medium-size fruit, provides 500 mg of potassium and more than 16 percent of the Recommended Dietary Allowance (RDA) of folate; it also supplies 10 percent or more of the RDAs for iron, vitamins C, E, and B_6. Avocados are also rich in two phytochemicals: beta-sitosterol, an important phytochemical linked with lower cholesterol levels; and glutathione, an antioxidant that may offer protection against several cancers.

Avocados should be served raw; they have a bitter taste when cooked. But they can be added to hot dishes that have already been cooked—for example, tossed with a spicy pasta sauce or sliced atop a broiled chicken breast. ❖

AN AVOCADO PRIMER

- Avocados are rich in monounsaturated oil, the same heart-friendly fat found in olive oil, and have more soluble fiber than any other fruit.

- Avocados are spilling over in a plant sterol called beta-sitosterol, which helps prevent cholesterol from being absorbed through the intestines.

- A medium-size (8-oz/230-g) California avocado contains about 30 g of fat—almost twice as much as its Florida cousin—and more calories than any other fruit.

- The avocado is popularly known as the alligator pear because of the shape and rough skin of its most common variety. Other types are larger in size, and range in color from dark green to crimson.

- Avocados start to ripen only after being cut from the tree. Mature fruit can be left on the tree for 6 months without spoiling. Once picked, it will ripen in a few days.

- Avocados have more protein than any other fruit—approximately 2 g in a 4-oz (115-g) serving.

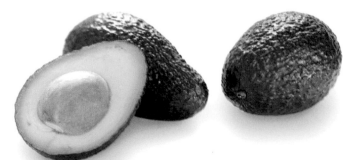

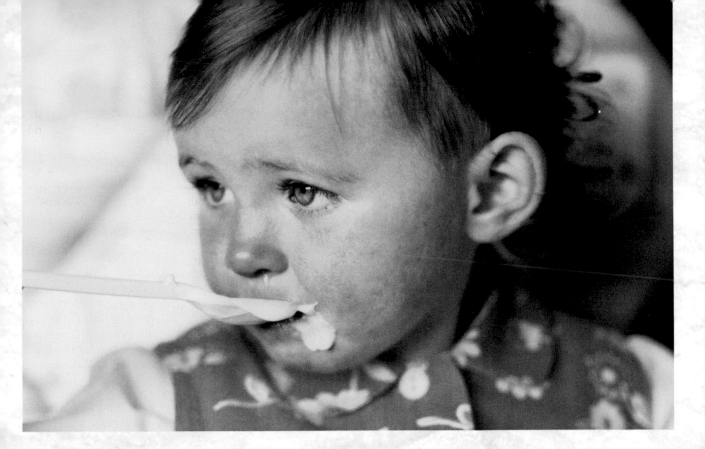

BABY FOOD
■ HEALTHY CHOICES FOR TODDLERS ■

Proper early nutrition is important. The eating patterns established in infancy determine how well a baby grows and also influence lifelong food habits and attitudes.

New parents probably worry more about feeding their baby than any other aspect of early child care. What if I can't breast-feed? How do I know if the baby is getting enough? Too much? Should I give the baby vitamins? When do I start solid food? Parents quickly learn that almost everyone is eager to answer such questions—grandparents, neighbors—even strangers in the supermarket. As might be expected, however, much of the advice is conflicting and adds to a parent's feelings of confusion and uncertainty. So let's begin with a few anxiety busters:

✔ Get to know your baby. No two infants are alike. Some enter the world ravenously hungry and demand to be fed every hour or two. Others seem to prefer sleeping, and may even need to be awakened to eat.

✔ Try to relax. It's natural for new parents to feel nervous and apprehensive, but raising a baby should be a joyful experience.

✔ Trust your own judgment and common sense. If a baby is growing and developing at a normal pace, he's getting enough to eat.

✔ Keep food in its proper perspective. It provides the essential energy and nourishment infants need to grow and develop. But food should not be a substitute for a reassuring hug or used as a bribe or reward for good behavior. Even an infant quickly learns how to use food as a manipulative tool, which can set the stage for later eating problems.

MYTH BUSTER

Myth: One glass of beer a day increases a mother's supply of breast milk.

Reality: There is no scientific evidence to support the claim that drinking beer boosts milk production or improves mother's milk, researchers say. However, studies have shown that beer can increase levels of a hormone necessary for milk production. In the late 1800s an American brewery marketed a new beer blend that was touted as a "tonic" for breast-feeding women.

Introducing New Foods in the First Year

During the first 3 months of life, breast milk or formula provides all the nutrients a newborn baby needs. The following chart summarizes the generally accepted guidelines for introducing new foods to babies under one year of age. It should be noted, however, that all babies are different; consequently, the timing varies considerably from one baby to another.

FIRST MONTH

If giving breast milk, enough for weight gain and to yield regular soft stools and 6 or more wet diapers a day. If giving formula, 2–4 oz (60–120 ml) per feeding (every 2 to 4 hours).

SECOND AND THIRD MONTHS

4–5 oz (120–150 ml) each feeding; six feeding a day.

Milk and dairy	Cereals and other starchy foods	Vegetables and fruits	Meat and meat alternatives	Occasional foods and foods to avoid
4 TO 6 MONTHS				
Total intake: About 30–40 oz (900–1,200 ml) of breast milk or formula per day, plus small amounts of new foods (starting 1–2 teaspoons and work up) at two or three feedings a day.				
5–6 oz (150–180 ml) breast milk or formula feeding five or six times a day.	Iron-fortified cereals— rice first, then barley, oat, and finally mixed cereal.	At 6 months: Plain, cooked pureed vegetables; plain, soft pureed fruits.		Avoid honey in the first year due to its link to botulism in infants, and egg white to reduce risk of egg allergy.
6 TO 9 MONTHS				
Total intake: 24–32 oz (720–960 ml) of breast milk or formula; 2–4 oz (60–120 ml) of cereal and/or pureed baby food should be given at each of the baby's three meals.				
For breast milk, continue or wean to bottle. Give five or six feedings per day. For formula, 6–8 oz (180–240 ml) per feeding four or five times each day.	Toast, dry unsweetened cereals, crackers. Daily intake: $1/4$ to $1/2$ cup starchy food over three meals.	Plain, cooked mashed vegetables; plain, soft, mashed fruits. Daily intake: Four $1/4$- to $1/2$-cup servings of fruits and vegetables.	Plain, pureed, minced, or finely chopped meat, poultry, fish; cooked egg yolk; mashed legumes, lentils, and tofu. Daily intake: Two $1/2$- to $3/4$-oz (14–21 g) portions.	Limited amount of unsweetened fruit juice in child-size cup. Citrus fruit juices tend to irritate the baby's skin and make stool acidic, so it is advisable to wait until at least 6 to 9 months.
9 TO 12 MONTHS				
Total intake: 24–32 oz (720–960 ml) of breast milk or formula; 750 to 900 total calories needed per day divided into three meals and two snacks.				
Yogurt; cheese; cottage cheese; pasteurized cow's milk.* *Pasteurized whole (homogenized) cow's milk can be offered around 12 months of age and continued until age 2.	Soft breads; plain muffins; other grains such as pasta and rice. Daily intake: $1/2$- to $3/4$-cup total a day.	Soft bite-size pieces of vegetables; mashed potatoes; soft, ripe, peeled fruit or canned fruits. Daily intake: Six $1/4$-cup servings a day.	Strips of lean tender meats; soft, whole legumes or lentils; diced tofu. Daily intake: Total of 2 oz (60 g) of meat a day.	May use moderate amounts of butter (unsalted) and small amounts of jam on bread, toast, and crackers. Do not give peanut butter, which can cause choking.

In the beginning, they are what *you* eat

Good infant nutrition actually begins before birth, because what the mother eats during pregnancy goes a long way toward determining her baby's initial nutritional health. A well-nourished mother provides plenty of nutrients her baby can use for proper growth and development in the uterus, as well as to store for later use. Skimping on food to avoid gaining excessive weight while pregnant can produce a low-birth-weight baby who has special nutritional needs or serious medical problems. An anemic woman is likely to have a baby with low iron reserves. A woman who does not consume adequate folate may have a baby with serious neurological problems. High doses of vitamin A before and during early pregnancy can cause birth defects. All pregnant women are strongly advised to have regular prenatal checkups and to eat a varied and balanced diet.

Breast milk—babies' first food

Physicians are in agreement that breast milk provides the best and most complete food to achieve optimal health, growth, and development for full-term infants. In fact, the recommendation of the World Health Organization is that a full-term, healthy infant should be exclusively breast-fed up to 6 month of age (premature and low-birth-weight babies may need specialized formula and breast milk). An adequate alternative to breast milk is commercial infant formula, which provides comparable nutrition but lacks some of the unique benefits of breast milk.

Although breast-feeding for 6 months may not be possible for every mother, a baby can benefit from any amount of breast milk—even a few feedings. Colostrum, the breast fluid that is secreted for the first few days after birth, is higher in protein and lower in sugar and fat than later breast milk. It has a laxative effect that activates the baby's bowels. Colostrum is also rich in antibodies, which increase the baby's resistance to infection. Hormones released in response to the baby's suckling increase the flow of breast milk, and within a few days women produce enough mature milk for their infants. Mature breast milk is easy to digest and provides just about all the nutrients a baby normally needs for the first 4 to 6 months. This milk has two parts—the beginning of the feed is foremilk, which is high in sugar and water and a real thirst quencher for the baby. As the baby continues to feed, the breast decreases in size and the milk becomes a fat and calorie-rich milk, known as hindmilk.

A breast-fed baby can remain on breast milk exclusively until the introduction of age-appropriate foods at 4 to 6 months of life. In addition, a daily supplement of vitamin D (400 IU) is recommended in the United States and Canada for breast-fed babies and should be continued until an adequate amount of vitamin D is consumed through diet. Beginning at 4 to 6 months of age, these babies usually require additional iron, which is typically provided by an iron-fortified cereal. Fluoride supplementation may be required for some infants after 6 months. Babies of vegan mothers may require a B_{12} supplement.

How to tell if your baby is getting enough to eat

Many new nursing mothers often worry that their babies are not getting enough to eat. Mothers should answer the following questions:
1. How many wet diapers and stools does my baby have each day?
2. Is my baby growing?
3. Does my baby appear hungry?

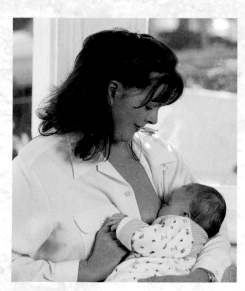

The advantages of breast-feeding

● Nursing stimulates uterine contractions that help prevent hemorrhaging and return the uterus to its normal size.
● Breast milk is convenient and economical; it is sterile, portable, and always the right temperature.
● Nursing promotes a special kind of mother-infant bonding.
● Breast-fed babies have fewer infections. The benefits extend beyond childhood; studies show that people who were breast-fed have a reduced incidence of obesity, diabetes, asthma, heart disease, and some types of cancer.
● Breast milk may protect infants with a strong family history of allergy from developing one.
● Women who breast-feed have a reduced risk of premenopausal breast cancer and postmenopausal osteoporosis (loss of bone mass).

DO ONE SIMPLE THING

DO ONE SIMPLE THING
TRY, TRY, AND TRY AGAIN WHEN INTRODUCING NEW FOODS TO BABY

Refusal to eat new foods is common among infants and may not reflect an actual dislike of the food. Reoffer the food from time to time. Persistence will help a child develop a varied diet in the long run.

Commercial baby food

Most babies' introduction to solid food comes in the form of small jars of pureed vegetables, fruits, and meats. For a young baby, the commercial foods offer several advantages—they are safe and most are salt- and sugar-free. For the mother, they offer convenience. If you use commercial baby foods, follow these precautions:

- Never feed the baby straight from the jar and then save the remaining food; saliva on the spoon can transmit bacteria to the food and result in spoilage.

- Commercial baby food typically tastes bland; resist the temptation to season it with salt. Excessive salt can cause future health problems.

A baby who has regular stools and produces six or more wet diapers a day is most likely getting plenty of food. Although this varies, breast-fed babies generally nurse every 2 to 4 hours for the first month or so. Experts promote "on demand" feeding; in other words, babies should be fed whenever they are hungry for the first 4 or 5 months. Some babies may be sleepy or disinterested in food; a baby who is not feeding at least six to eight times a day may need to be stimulated to consume more.

Growth is an important indicator of whether or not a baby is getting enough to eat. Remember, however, that babies tend to grow in spurts. During a growth spurt, an infant will want to nurse more often and longer than usual, which may empty the reserve of breast milk. This will signal the mother's body to increase milk production. But the mother should not be concerned if, a week or two later, her baby is less interested in eating.

Finally, hungry babies send out plenty of signals that they are hungry. Common cues are fussing, crying, and irritability as well as a variety of lip and tongue movements—such as lip smacking and fists in mouths.

Bottle-feeding

Although more than half of all North American women breast-feed for at least the first few weeks, many mothers elect to bottle-feed. They should be assured that commercial formulas provide all the essential nutrients and, when used according to the manufacturers' instructions, babies thrive on them. Choosing an iron-fortified formula is recommended. Babies under one year of age should not be given regular cow's milk because it is difficult for them to digest and may provoke an allergic reaction. The cow's milk in most infant formulas is modified to make it easier to digest. Despite this precaution, some babies may require a soy or rice formula.

Generally, bottle-fed babies consume more than breast-fed infants do; they may gain weight more rapidly, although the breast-fed babies will eventually catch up with them. On average, most babies double their birth weight in 4 to 5 months, and triple it by the time of their first birthday.

Bottle-feeding requires more work than nursing; bottles, nipples, and other equipment must be sterilized. Some formulas are premixed; others are concentrated or powdered, and must be mixed with sterile water. Formula mixed in advance should be refrigerated, but not longer than 24 hours; after that, it should be discarded. Any formula that is left in the baby's bottle after a feeding should be discarded; if not, there is a possibility of its being contaminated by microorganisms entering through the nipple opening.

Introducing foods

There is no specific age at which to start solid foods, but for most babies, 4 to 6 months is about right. Starting too early can be harmful because the digestive system may not be able to handle solid foods yet; also, the early introduction of solid foods may increase the risk of developing food allergies. An infant who is thriving solely on breast milk can generally wait until he is 5 or 6 months old; after that, nursing alone may not provide adequate calories and the nutrients that a baby needs for normal growth.

The first solid food must be easy to digest and unlikely to provoke an allergic reaction—infant rice cereal is a good choice. For the first few feedings, put a very small amount on the spoon, gently touch the baby's lips to encourage him to open his mouth, and place the cereal at the back of the tongue. Don't expect these feedings to go smoothly; a baby usually does a lot of spitting, sputtering, and protesting.

The baby should be hungry, but not ravenous. Some experts suggest starting the feeding with a few minutes of nursing or bottle-feeding, then offering a small amount of the moistened cereal—no more than a teaspoon or two—and finishing with the milk. After a few sessions, you can start with the cereal, then gradually increase the amount of solid foods as you reduce the amount of milk.

Beginning slowly, introducing only one or two new items a week. If you use home-cooked foods, make sure that they're thoroughly pureed. In addition to rice cereal, try oatmeal and barley cereals; strained vegetables and fruits; and pureed chicken and beef. At about 5 months, fruit juice can be added to the diet, starting with apple juice. Hold off on orange juice and other citrus products for at least 6 months; these may provoke an allergic reaction. Other potentially allergenic foods should be delayed until the baby is 6 to 9 months old, or even later if there is a family history of allergies. Withdraw any food that provokes a rash, runny nose, unusual fussiness, diarrhea, or any other sign of a possible allergic reaction or food intolerance.

Self-feeding

When they are about 7 or 8 months old, most babies have developed enough eye-hand coordination to pick up finger food and maneuver it into their mouths. The teeth are also beginning to come in at this age; giving a baby a teething biscuit, or cracker to chew on can ease gum soreness as well as provide practice in self-feeding. Other good starters are finger foods, which could include bite-size dry cereals, bananas, slices of apples and pears, peas, and cooked carrots, and small pieces of soft-cooked boiled or roasted chicken. The pieces should be large enough to hold but small enough so that they don't lodge in the throat and cause choking.

As soon as the baby can sit in a high chair, he should be included at family meals and start eating many of the same foods, even though they may need mashing or cutting into small pieces. Give the child a spoon, but don't be disappointed if he prefers using his hands. At this stage it's more important for the baby to become integrated into family activities and master self-feeding than to learn proper table manners. These will come eventually, especially if the parents and older siblings set a good example.

Weaning

Giving up the breast or bottle is a major milestone in a baby's development, but not one that should be rushed. When a woman stops nursing is largely a matter of personal preference. Some mothers wean their babies from the breast to a bottle after only a few weeks or months; others continue nursing for longer, even though the child is eating solid food. Similarly, some babies decide to give up their bottles themselves at 9 or 10 months; yet others will still want it—especially at nap or bedtime. If a baby under a year old drinks milk from a cup, it should still be a formula.

Dental hygiene

Many parents mistakenly assume that baby teeth aren't important because they are eventually replaced by permanent teeth. In fact, early dental decay not only threatens the underlying secondary teeth, it can cause severe toothaches. As soon as the first tooth comes in, parents should begin practicing preventive dental hygiene. Babies should not be permitted to fall asleep while nursing or sucking a bottle; this allows milk to pool in the mouth, and the sugar (lactose) in it can cause extensive tooth decay. Offering a little water at the end of a feeding rinses any remaining milk from the baby's mouth. The gums and emerging teeth can be wiped gently with a gauze-wrapped finger.

Sugar is the major cause of childhood tooth decay; avoid offering sugary soft drinks and sweet snacks. A chunk of cheese, or a piece of fruit are better alternatives that provide important nutrients without harming the teeth.

MYTH BUSTER

Myth: Vegetables should be introduced to baby's diet before fruits in order to increase the acceptance of vegetables.

Reality: This is not the case and fruits and vegetables should be introduced in an alternating manner.

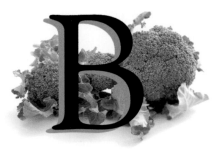

BACON

See Pork

BANANAS

BENEFITS

- An excellent source of potassium and vitamin B_6, as well as a source of folate and fiber.

Healthful, filling, and tasty, bananas are one of nature's ideal snacks. The fruit, which is grown in most of the world's tropical areas, is harvested while still green. When stored at room temperature, most bananas ripen in a few days; the process can be hastened by placing them in a plastic or paper bag along with an apple.

Try bananas for baby's first food. Because bananas are bland, easy to digest, and unlikely to produce allergies, they are an ideal early food for babies. Bananas, along with rice, applesauce, and toast, are one of the foods in the diet recommended after a bout of diarrhea. Some ulcer patients report that bananas alleviate some pain, but this is unproven. While allergies to bananas are rare, they are more common in people who are allergic to rubber products.

NUTRITIONAL VALUE

A medium banana contains close to 500 mg of potassium, a mineral that plays a role in lowering blood pressure. A study on 17,000 adults indicated that higher potassium levels are associated with lower blood pressure. Bananas also contain the amino acid tryptophan, which stimulates the production of serotonin, a neurotransmitter that has a calming effect on the body.

Bananas are an excellent source of vitamin B_6; a medium (4-oz/115-g) banana supplies 45 percent of the Recommended Dietary Allowance (RDA). It has 2 g of dietary fiber, some of which is soluble fiber, instrumental in lowering blood cholesterol levels. Bananas contain about 100 calories each, mostly in the form of fruit sugar and starch. A ripe banana can hold the equivalent of 5 teaspoons of sugar.

Plantains These resemble large green bananas, but they never become as sweet. Plantains can be baked or fried and served as a starchy side dish. They can also be a delicious addition to soups, stews, and meat dishes. Nutritionally, plantains are comparable to bananas, except that they contain about 10 times more beta carotene than a regular banana. ❖

BEANS

BENEFITS

- Contain folate and vitamins A and C.
- Mature (shelled) beans are high in protein and iron.

DRAWBACKS

- Shelled beans can cause flatulence.
- Fava beans are toxic to some people.

Green beans (which can also be yellow or purple) are harvested at an immature stage. Both the tender pods and small, soft seeds are eaten. These are sometimes called wax beans. In shelled varieties, only the seeds are eaten. Some, such as lima beans, are harvested while they are still tender; others are left to mature (see Legumes). Most pod beans—snap beans, Italian green beans, long Chinese beans, purple and yellow wax beans, and green beans—can be eaten raw. More commonly, they are steamed or boiled. Shelled beans should always be cooked; they can be served hot or cold.

NUTRITIONAL VALUE

Lima and fava beans are good sources of protein, providing about 7 g per half-cup serving. The same-size serving of baby or green lima beans contains 2 mg of iron, more than twice as much as in favas and four times the amount in a ½ cup of green snap beans. All these varieties hold folate and vitamins A and C. Shelled beans have more thiamine, vitamin B_6, potassium, and magnesium; the soluble fiber in shelled beans may lower cholesterol, but the presence of carbohydrates such as raffinose may also cause flatulence.

Warning: Some Mediterranean people lack an enzyme needed to protect red blood cells from damage by vicine, a toxic substance in fava beans that causes a type of anemia. Those taking monoamine oxidase (MAO) inhibitors to treat depression should avoid fava beans; the combination can raise blood pressure. ❖

BEAN SPROUTS

BENEFITS

- Some are high in folate; others are fair to good sources of protein, B vitamins, and iron.

DRAWBACKS

- Alfalfa sprouts may provoke a flare-up of symptoms in lupus patients.

Various types of sprouts are available in health-food stores, supermarkets, and restaurants. However, few live up to their reputation as the prototype of health foods. Some sprouts are much more nutritious than others. A cup of raw mung bean sprouts, for example, provides 16 percent of the Recommended Dietary Allowance (RDA) of folate and 18 percent of the RDA for vitamin C. In contrast, it takes approximately five cups of alfalfa sprouts to yield comparable amounts. Broccoli sprouts are receiving a lot of attention from researchers because they are a rich source of sulforaphane, one of the most potent anticancer compounds

CAUTION

Anyone who eats raw sprouts is at risk for exposure to *E. coli* 0157:H7 or salmonella bacteria. The risk is greatest for children, seniors, and people with weak immune systems. If you are at risk, you shouldn't eat raw sprouts of any kind, especially alfalfa sprouts. If you are a healthy adult, you can minimize the risk by taking the following precautions: Make sure the sprouts you buy are crisp and have buds attached. Avoid dark or musty smelling sprouts. Respect the "best before" date. Refrigerate them immediately after you get home. You can also reduce risk of illness by cooking them before consumption.

isolated from a natural source. Sprouts can contain 50 times more sulforaphane than mature broccoli.

Warning: Most sprouts, if free of bacterial contamination, can be eaten raw. An important exception is the sprouted soybean, which contains a potentially harmful toxin that is destroyed by cooking. People with lupus should avoid alfalfa sprouts; alfalfa in any form can prompt a flare-up of symptoms. ❖

BEEF AND VEAL

BENEFITS

- Major sources of high-quality protein.
- Contain a wide range of nutrients, especially vitamin B_{12}, iron, niacin, and zinc.

DRAWBACKS

- Beef fat contains saturated fat, which can increase blood cholesterol levels and the risk of cardiovascular disease.
- A high-meat diet may raise the risk of colon cancer and other cancers.
- Rare ground beef is a source of *E. coli*.

Although its consumption has decreased by more than 25 percent in recent decades, beef is still a popular red meat. One of the most versatile meats, beef may be prepared by roasting, stewing, broiling, frying, and grilling.

There is no question that beef is a highly nutritious food source; not only is it a leading source of high-quality protein, but a 4-oz (115-g) serving provides more than 100 percent of the Recommended Dietary Allowance (RDA) of vitamin B_{12}, an essential nutrient found only in animal products. Beef is also an excellent source of vitamin B_6, niacin, and riboflavin, as well as such essential minerals as iron and zinc.

A CASE OF LESS IS BEST

Beef's major nutritional drawback is the large amount of saturated fat in some cuts, especially in roasts and steaks. Studies link a diet with large amounts of meat to an increased risk of heart attacks and certain cancers.

The key factors concerning fat are the cut, portion size, and cooking method. Choose the leanest cuts—round or loin are good. Then, trim all visible fat from your meat. Reduce fat further by broiling, grilling, or roasting on a rack (so fat can drip away). Another approach is to cook stews and soups in advance, chill

BEEF FACTS

- The average North American buys more than 50 lb (23 kg) of beef a year.
- Fat content of today's beef is lower because of consumer demand and changes in breeding and feeding practices.
- While beef contains saturated fat, one-third of its fatty acids consist of stearic acid, which does not negatively effect blood cholesterol levels.

them so that the congealed fat can be removed easily, and then reheat the dishes before serving. Instead of gravy or sauce, serve your meat "au jus," after skimming off all the fat. A quick way to remove the fat is to drop an ice cube into the cooled liquid. The fat will harden around the ice cube and can be easily removed.

Trimming the fat can make a significant difference: By trimming the fat from 3½ oz (100 g) of beef, you can save 7 g of fat and 56 calories. Of course, controlling the size of the portion is also important. A 16-oz (450-g) T-bone steak, rack of beef ribs, or huge slab of prime rib roast each have 800 to 1,000 calories, with half or more of these coming from fat. A modest 4-oz (115-g) serving of eye of round provides about 200 calories, only 70 of which come from fat.

The liver, kidneys, and other organ meats are the most concentrated source of iron and vitamins A and B$_{12}$ in beef. At one time, women were urged to eat an occasional serving of liver to prevent iron-deficiency anemia. But enthusiasm for liver and other organ meats has been dampened in recent years for several reasons: They are very high in cholesterol, and they may increase the risk of heart disease. Another issue revolves around the fact that factory-reared animals are fed antibiotics and hormones, which concentrate in the animals' liver. Some experts contend that these drug and hormone residues pose a health risk to humans who ingest them; others, however, insist that they are safe.

HORMONES IN BEEF

If you are concerned about hormones in the meat you eat, recent research can help put your mind at ease. After extensive evaluation, the World Trade Organization has concluded that the use of growth-promoting hormones does not present a risk to those consuming beef or beef products. Hormones occur naturally in all animals. When you compare hormone levels in cattle that have been given hormones with those that have not, the difference is indistinguishable. In other words, giving hormones to animals does not alter the levels found in the meat of that animal. The greatest source of hormones for humans comes not from the food you eat but from that which your body produces naturally. In fact, every day your body naturally produces 100,000 to 100 million times more hormones than are found in a serving of beef.

E. COLI BACTERIA

Outbreaks of a deadly type of E. coli infection have been traced to contaminated beef. Many strains of E. coli bacteria are harmless ones that normally inhabit the human intestinal tract. But in 1982 researchers identified a different strain, later called 0157:H7, in the intestinal tract of cattle. This E. coli can invade meat during slaughter. Grinding the contaminated beef further spreads the bacteria through the meat. The organism can survive in hamburgers and other contaminated beef that is served rare. When the E. coli reaches the human intestinal tract, it can cause mild to severe diarrhea. More seriously, some people—especially children, the elderly, and individuals with weakened immune systems—can develop hemolytic uremic syndrome, a life-threatening disorder characterized by the rapid destruction of red blood cells and kidney failure. Although some infections have been traced to rare roast beef, and a few to unpasteurized milk, rare hamburgers are by far the most common source. Health officials stress that virtually all beef-borne E. coli infections can be prevented by cooking beef, especially hamburger, until it is well-done, 160°F (70°C).

DID YOU KNOW?

BEEF MAY NOT BE AS BAD FOR YOU AS YOU THINK

Beef may not affect your cholesterol level as much as you think. It contains a type of fatty acid called conjugated linoleic acid, or CLA, that has actually been shown to improve cholesterol ratios (the ratio of LDL, or "bad" cholesterol, to HDL, or "good" cholesterol), at least in animals. Studies on animals have also found that CLA can delay the development of atherosclerosis, and possibly even help with weight loss.

ABOUT VEAL

Very young calves produce the delicate pink, low-fat veal that has always been considered a luxury meat. It is an excellent source of high-quality protein and a source of iron, zinc, and vitamin B_{12}. On average, a trimmed, cooked 3-oz (85-g) serving of veal contains less than 200 calories and less than 8 g of fat. The leanest cuts include the cutlet, veal roast, arm steak, and loin chop.

Veal calves are Holstein or Holstein–cross intact bull calves. After consuming colostrum from their mothers, containing essential nutrients and antibodies, the calves are placed into individual pens or hutches for their first few weeks of life. This protects the calves from disease transfer from other calves and cows while their immune system develops. Veal producers do not restrict calf movement to promote meat tenderness—a common misconception. Veal calves are either weaned from milk at around 2 months of age and placed on a grain-based diet or they are maintained on a milk-based diet. The meat from milk-fed veal is pink. The meat from grain-fed veal is slightly darker and of similar quality.

MAD COW DISEASE

BSE (bovine spongiform encephalopathy), or "mad cow disease," is a fatal disease of the nervous system of cattle. It is also known as a transmissible spongiform encephalopathy, or TSE. Although the cause of BSE is unknown, it is associated with the presence of an abnormal protein called a prion. There is no treatment currently available for the disease.

BSE is not contagious. But the disease can be transmitted when rendered materials from an infected animal are fed to another animal. By banning the feeding of rendered materials, the major transmission method of BSE between animals can be eliminated.

A similar disease, Creutzfeldt-Jacob Disease (CJD), exists in humans. And people who ingest central nervous tissue (brain, spinal cord, and parts of the eye) of BSE-infected cattle may develop a variant of CJD called vCJD.

In December 2003, BSE was identified in the United States for the first time. The cattle originated from Canada, where several previous cases of BSE had been recorded. All cattle potentially affected were destroyed. Thanks to continuing vigilance on the part of both the United States and Canada, infected cattle are discovered rapidly, and contaminated tissues are unlikely to reach the food supply. In the United States, new regulatory measures have been introduced to further safeguard the population.

SOCIAL ISSUES

The process of producing 1 lb (0.45 kg) of beef requires more land and other resources than growing an equivalent amount of vegetable protein. Critics of our high beef consumption express concern over the increasing destruction of the Amazon rain forests and our own ecological systems in order to make room for more cattle ranching. There are also environmental worries about finding ways to dispose of animal waste without polluting our rivers and other natural resources. ❖

BEER

BENEFITS

- Is lower in alcohol concentrations than wine and hard liquor.
- Contains modest amounts of niacin, folate, vitamin B_6, and some minerals.

DRAWBACKS

- Overconsumption can cause unwanted weight gain and obesity.
- Heavy drinking can lead to inebriation and alcoholism.
- Causes feelings of aggression in some people.

Historians believe that humans began to brew beer some time around 5000 B.C. in what is now Iraq and Egypt. Barley, the grain that still dominates beer brewing, was abundant in that region. Nonetheless, almost every society worldwide has independently developed ways of making beer from local cereal grains: African tribes use sprouted corn, millet, and sorghum; Russians turn rye bread into a low-alcohol beer called kvass; the Chinese and Japanese use rice; and South and Central American Indians rely on corn to make their respective beers.

THE BREWING PROCESS

Although many societies around the world continue to use their traditional methods to make beer, modern brewing is a scientific process that begins with malting to convert grain starch into sugar that will ferment. To do this, the grain is sprouted in order to activate enzymes that will eventually turn the starch into sugar. The precise methods vary according to the type of beer being produced, but at some point the germination is stopped, the sprouts are removed, and the malted grain is then prepared for mashing.

The malt is heated slowly to allow the enzymes to continue converting starch into a sugary broth called wort. The grain is allowed to settle, and the wort is heated and filtered through it into the brewing kettles. (The grains are then rinsed and salvaged for livestock feed.)

Hops, which are dried flowers from the hop vine, are added to the wort, and the mixture is boiled and then strained. (The used hops are added to livestock feed.) The wort is allowed to settle so that the protein can be removed; the clear liquid is then fermented with yeast and aged. Eventually, yeast residue is skimmed off and used as a nutritional supplement (brewer's yeast) or added to livestock feed. The process may be varied and other ingredients added to give beer a distinctive flavor, color, or aroma. Adding extra hops produces the British draft beer known as bitters; ale, a more concentrated beer, uses a type of yeast that rises to the top; stout is a bitter ale brewed from a dark malt.

The specific brewing method influences the nutritional quality of beer. The cloudy German *weisse bier,* for example, retains many of the B vitamins found in brewer's yeast, but these are strained away to make clear beer.

Native African beers remain unfiltered; as a result, they retain many of the nutrients found in the grains and roots and tubers that are their main ingredients.

The type of yeast used by American and Canadian brewers contains selenium, an antioxidant mineral, and chromium, a mineral that aids carbohydrate metabolism.

NUTRITIONAL VALUE OF BEER

Beer's nutritional value is often overstated because most of the nutrients in grain are lost in the brewing process. About two-thirds of the 150 calories in 12 oz (355 ml) of ordinary beer come from the alcohol itself, with one-third coming from sugars; in contrast, only a trace of protein remains after brewing and straining. A 12-oz (355-ml) bottle of ordinary beer provides 5 to 10 percent or more of the RDAs of folate, niacin, vitamin B_6, and phosphorus, as well as significant amounts of chromium and selenium.

HOW MUCH IS ENOUGH?

Typically, the alcohol content of beer ranges from 3 to 8 percent, compared to an average of 12 percent in wine, and about 40 to 50 percent in hard liquor. Some people who are very sensitive to alcohol will react almost immediately to even this modest amount, often with feelings of aggression. Many people, however, can consume 1 qt (1 liter) or more of beer without obvious mental or physical effects. Since drinking more than 1 qt (1 liter) of fluid produces an uncomfortable feeling of fullness, most beer drinkers usually stop before they become inebriated. Even so, drinking 1 qt (1 liter) of beer may yield up to 600 calories, which can result in weight gain, and the excessive urination resulting from the diuretic effect of the alcohol can wash away important vitamins and minerals before the body can absorb them. Contrary to popular belief, chronic overconsumption of beer can very much lead to problem drinking and even alcoholism.

Watch what you eat with beer. Beer is frequently served with nuts, potato chips, pretzels, and other salty foods. Because these increase feelings of thirst, they actually promote consumption of excessive amounts of beer. Foods that are high in protein, vitamins, and minerals and moderate in fat are better alternatives; for example, eggs, meat, poultry, seafood, or whole-grain bread or crackers, pasta, and legumes. ❖

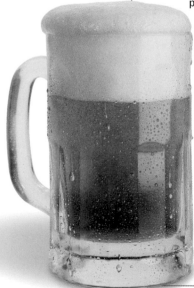

BEER AND HEALTH

A medical study examined the beer-drinking habits of a group of people who had had a heart attack, as well as of a group randomly selected from the Czech population. The Czech Republic is especially appropriate for such a study because it is a country of beer drinkers. Perhaps surprisingly, in both groups, the lowest risk for heart attack was found in men who drank about 11 to 24 pt (5.2–11.3 liters) of beer a week. Their risk was a third of that seen in the men who never drank beer. But if they drank more, the protection was lost and problems appeared! Dark beer seems to be especially protective. It was even found to reduce the potential harm caused by the notorious "heterocyclic aromatic amines" (HAAs) that form when food is heated to a high temperature. Serving dark beer at a barbecue is a good idea.

Beer's cardiovascular benefits are likely due to polyphenols, those pigmented antioxidants that are also found in fruits, tea, and wine. Researchers have found that drinking one beer a day alters the structure of fibrinogen, a protein in the blood responsible for clotting. In a study of men who had undergone bypass surgery, they found that those who drank 12 oz (355 ml) of beer a day were less likely to form blood clots, and at reduced risk for heart attacks and strokes.

Beets

BENEFITS

- A source of folate, fiber, and potassium.
- The greens are a rich source of potassium, calcium, iron, beta carotene, and vitamin C.
- Low in calories.
- Rich in phytochemicals such as anthocyanins and saponins, which may bind cholesterol in the digestive tract, lowering the risk for heart disease.

DRAWBACKS

- Turn urine and stools red, a harmless condition that nonetheless alarms people who mistake it for blood.
- If prone to kidney stones or gout, avoid beet greens as they are high in oxalates. Oxalates can form small crystals and contribute to the development of kidney stones.

Beets are a highly versatile vegetable. They can be cooked and served as a side dish, pickled and eaten as a salad or condiment, or used as the main ingredient in borscht, a popular Eastern European soup. Beet greens, the most nutritious part of the vegetable, can be cooked and served like spinach or Swiss chard.

According to folklore, beets were believed to possess curative powers for headaches and other painful conditions. Even today, some naturalist practitioners recommend beets to prevent cancer and bolster immunity; they also suggest using the juice of raw beets to speed convalescence. Although beets are a reasonably nutritious food source, there is no scientific proof that they confer any special medicinal benefits.

Don't forget the tops. A half-cup serving of cooked beets provides 45 mcg (micrograms) of folate, about 11 percent of the adult Recommended Dietary Allowance (RDA). The tops, if eaten while young and green, are more nutritious: 1 cup has 35 mg of vitamin C, almost 46 percent of what is advised for adult women; 720 RE of vitamin A; and 160 mg of calcium, 2.5 mg of iron, and 1,300 mg of potassium.

The most flavorful beets are small, with greens still attached. The best way to cook beet roots is to boil them unpeeled, which retains most of the nutrients, as well as the deep red color. After the beets have cooled, the skins slip off easily; the root can be sliced, chopped, or pureed, depending upon the method of serving. Beets may also be canned and pickled with

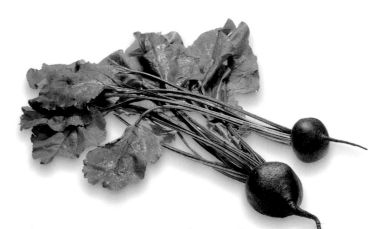

vinegar; some nutrients are lost in the processing, but the sweet flavor remains.

EFFECTS ON BODY WASTES

Many people notice that their urine and stools have turned pink or even red after eating beets. This is harmless and occurs in about 15 percent of people who lack the gut bacteria that normally degrade betalains, the bright red pigment in beets. The urine and stools usually return to their normal colors after a day or two. ❖

Bioflavonoids

BENEFITS

- Thought to function as antioxidants and also to enhance the antioxidant effects of vitamin C.
- Believed to be instrumental in proper capillary function.
- Some appear to be natural antibiotics and anticancer agents.

Bioflavonoids are a group of naturally occurring phytochemicals that act primarily as plant pigments and flavorants. Numerous compounds fall into this family of substances, linked by some common features in their molecular structure. Subcategories of bioflavonoids include isoflavones, anthocyanidins, flavans, flavonols, flavones, and flavanones.

WHERE ARE THEY?

Bioflavonoids are found in a wide range of foods, particularly fruits and vegetables. For example, flavanones are found in citrus fruits, isoflavones in soy products, anthocyanidins in wine, flavans in apples, and tea and rutin in the buckwheat plant. Other foods high in bioflavonoids include apricots, blackberries, black currants, broccoli, cantaloupe, cherries,

FACTS ABOUT BEETS

- Beets have one of the highest sugar content of any vegetable, yet are low in calories—about 50 per cup.
- Beets contain beta-cyanin, a type of plant pigment, which some preliminary research indicates might be helpful in defending cells against harmful carcinogens. It is also being studied for its potential as a tumor-fighting compound.
- Many cooks today discard the beet tops and use only the roots. In ancient times, however, only the tops were eaten as a vegetable; the roots were used as a medicine to treat painful disorders such as headaches and toothaches.
- Betalains, the bright red pigments in beets, are extracted and can be used as a natural food coloring or a dye.

SHOULD YOU TAKE BIOFLAVONOIDS SUPPLEMENTS?

There is no justification at this time for taking individual bioflavonoids in supplement form. These substances almost certainly act synergistically with other phytochemicals, vitamins, and minerals found in foods. Optimal doses, long-term adverse effects of high doses, and possible interactions with medicines are unknown.

Scientists at the University of Chicago Medical Center have expressed concern that certain bioflavonoids in supplement form, if taken during pregnancy, may result in childhood leukemias. They found that 10 out of 20 bioflavonoids tested caused DNA breaks in a gene known to be involved in infant leukemias. An earlier study had found that these rare leukemias were twice as common in large Asian cities where soy intake (soy contains a number of bioflavonoids) is two to five times as high as in North America.

The benefits of foods high in flavonoids is unquestioned but the benefits of supplements are not convincing. Pregnant women especially should be careful about taking bioflavonoid supplements. The best source of bioflavonoids is eating a wide variety of plant foods daily, especially fruits and vegetables.

grapefruit, grapes, green peppers, papayas, plums, tomatoes, as well as coffee and cocoa.

Ongoing studies of these compounds are focusing on their potential health-promoting effects:

- Capillaries are highly permeable blood vessels that allow oxygen, hormones, nutrients, and antibodies to pass from the bloodstream to individual cells. If the capillary walls are fragile, blood will seep out into the cells. This can result in bruising, brain and retinal hemorrhages, bleeding gums, and other abnormalities. Bioflavonoids improve capillary strength by helping to maintain the proper degree of permeability in the capillary wall.
- Recent research indicates that some bioflavonoids are inhibitors that prevent blood clot formation. These bioflavonoids may be useful in treating phlebitis and other clotting disorders.

- Bioflavonoids are also believed to protect against heart disease. Resveretrol and quercetin, bioflavonoids in grape skins, are thought to reduce the risk of heart disease among moderate wine drinkers.
- Many bioflavonoids prevent cellular damage caused by free radicals, unstable molecules that are formed when the body uses oxygen. Some bioflavonoids are used as food preservatives to prevent oxidation of fats. Others enhance the antioxidant action of nutrients.
- Bioflavonoids enhance the action of vitamin C. Bioflavonoids and vitamin C are present in the same foods, and the body metabolizes both in a similar way. This similarity has led researchers to theorize that some of the functions attributed to vitamin C are actually due to bioflavonoids instead; others feel that the two work together in a synergistic manner.
- Cancer-causing substances may be hampered by bioflavonoids. Laboratory studies indicate that some bioflavonoids stop or slow the growth of malignant cells; they may also help protect against cancer-causing substances.
- Some bioflavonoids destroy certain bacteria, retarding food spoilage, and protecting humans from food-borne infections.

POTENTIAL THERAPEUTIC USES

A number of bioflavonoids are currently being studied for potential therapeutic uses:

- **Hesperidin**, a bioflavonoid in the blossoms and peels of oranges, lemons, and a number of other citrus fruits, is being considered for

BENEFICIAL PIGMENTS. *These and many other brightly colored fresh fruits and vegetables are rich in bioflavonoids.*

treating easy bruising and other bleeding abnormalities.

- **Rutin,** found in buckwheat leaves and some other plants, is being studied for treating glaucoma and the retinal bleeding in diabetics, as well as for reducing tissue damage from frostbite, radiation exposure, and hemophilia.
- **Quercetin,** found in apples, onions, tea, red wine and grapes, raspberries, citrus fruits, cherries, and other foods, is being investigated to improve lung function and lower risk of certain respiratory diseases, such as asthma, bronchitis, and emphysema. It may also help treat or even prevent prostate cancer by blocking male hormones that encourage the growth of prostate cancer cells.

DIETARY REQUIREMENTS

No Recommended Dietary Allowance (RDA) has been established for bioflavonoids, but studies show that if a diet contains enough fruits and vegetables to supply 60 mg of vitamin C, it will provide adequate bioflavonoids. Good sources of vitamin C include oranges, lemons, cantaloupe, tomatoes, blackberries, broccoli, and green peppers. ❖

BLACKBERRIES

BENEFITS
- Low in calories and high in fiber.
- A good source of vitamin C and bioflavonoids; also contain folate, iron, and calcium.
- Contain anthocyanins, bioflavonoids with numerous health benefits including lowering risk of cancer and heart disease. Also contain ellagic acid, which has anticancer properties.

DRAWBACKS
- Contain salicylates, which can cause a reaction in aspirin-sensitive people.

When fully ripe, blackberries are sweet and juicy. Cultivated varieties include: boysenberries, which are maroon and slightly tart, and loganberries, which are dark red and very tart.

Their many seeds make blackberries high in fiber. A half-cup serving of raw berries has 40 calories and supplies 15 mg of vitamin C, or 20 percent of the Recommended Dietary Allowance (RDA) for adult women, as well as 20 mcg (micrograms) of folate and small amounts of iron and calcium.

Blackberries contain anthocyanins, which have numerous possible health benefits such as preventing cancer and heart disease and even combatting some of the effects of aging.

Blackberries contain ellagic acid, a substance that is believed to help prevent cancer. Cooking does not appear to destroy ellagic acid, so even jams may confer this health benefit.

People allergic to aspirin may find that they experience a similar reaction from eating blackberries. The reason for this is that blackberries are a natural source of salicylates, substances related to the active compound in aspirin. ❖

BLEEDING PROBLEMS

EAT PLENTY OF
- Spinach, broccoli and other leafy greens, and organ meats.
- Lean meat, poultry, seafood, and other foods high in iron and vitamin B_{12}.
- Citrus and other fresh fruits and vegetables for vitamin C.

LIMIT
- Supplemental sources of omega-3 fatty acids.

AVOID
- Alcohol, aspirin, and other drugs that suppress blood platelets and clotting.

Some bleeding disorders, such as hemophilia, are hereditary; others develop as a result of nutritional deficiencies, taking aspirin and other medications that suppress clotting, and as the consequence of certain diseases, including some cancers. Most of these bleeding disorders stem from some type of thrombocytopenia, the medical term for a reduced number of platelets, the blood cells instrumental in clotting. Symptoms vary, but they typically include easy bruising, frequent nosebleeds, and excessive bleeding from even minor cuts. Bleeding gums unrelated to dental problems are common. Affected women may experience very heavy menstrual periods. In some cases, there are no obvious symptoms, but blood tests reveal a low platelet count and reduced clotting time.

Check all medications. Treatment varies according to the underlying cause. Overuse of aspirin or other drugs that suppress normal platelet function or production is the most common cause of platelet abnormalities; stopping the offending medication usually solves

THE BLACKER THE BERRY, THE SWEETER THE FRUIT

Fresh blackberries are lush and delicious, an excellent source of vitamin C, and have more fiber than a serving of some bran cereals. Eat them while fresh, and lightly rinse just before serving.

the problem. In other cases, transfusions of platelets and blood cells may be necessary.

NUTRITIONAL INFLUENCES

Bleeding disorders due to nutritional deficiencies are uncommon in North America, but they do occur. For example, vitamin K—necessary for the blood to clot normally—is made by bacteria in the human intestinal tract; it is also found in green peas, broccoli, spinach and other green leafy vegetables, brussels sprouts, and organ meats. Sometimes prolonged antibiotic therapy destroys the bacteria that make vitamin K, resulting in bleeding. Increasing foods high in vitamin K may help, but often supplements of the vitamin are given.

Foods high in vitamin K should be limited by people taking anticoagulant medication such as coumadin. The vitamin can counteract the desired effect of the drug. Omega-3 fatty acids, found in salmon and other oily fish, can suppress platelet function. People taking high doses of fish oil supplements have an increased risk of developing bleeding problems; the risk is compounded if they are also taking aspirin.

Vitamin C deficiency can cause bleeding gums. This deficiency may occur in alcoholics or people who eat little fruits and vegetables.

Chronic blood loss can lead to anemia, a blood disorder that is characterized by inadequate levels of red blood cells. Dietary sources should supply extra iron, folate, and vitamins B_{12} and C. Supplements may be needed. ❖

BLOOD PRESSURE

CHECK IT OUT

All adults over age 40 should have their blood pressure checked annually. But just one blood pressure measurement is insufficient to diagnose hypertension unless the reading is in the severe range. Some people also have "white coat" hypertension, in which their blood pressure rises when they are in a doctor's office but is normal at other times. In order to properly diagnose hypertension, several measurements are needed—taken at different times and perhaps in different places.

EAT PLENTY OF

- Fresh vegetables, fresh and dried fruits, legumes, and dairy products for potassium.
- Recommended foods as part of the DASH diet (see page 63).

LIMIT

- Canned and other processed foods with added salt.
- Fatty foods.

AVOID

- Pickled and very salty foods.
- Excessive alcohol and caffeine.

As blood circulates through the body, it exerts varying degrees of force on artery walls; doctors refer to this as blood pressure. Over 60 million North Americans have blood pressure that is too high, or hypertension. In its early stages, high blood pressure is symptomless, so many people don't realize they have a potentially life-threatening disease. If the condition goes unchecked, high blood pressure damages the heart and blood vessels and can lead to a stroke, heart attack, and other serious consequences.

In about 5 percent of cases, there's an underlying cause for high blood pressure; for example, a narrowed kidney artery, pregnancy, an adrenal gland disorder, or a drug side effect. Most often there is no identifiable cause; this is referred to as primary, or essential, hypertension.

Blood pressure rises when the arterioles, the body's smallest arteries, narrow or constrict, requiring the heart to beat more forcefully in order to pump blood through them. Increased blood volume, often due to the body's tendency to retain excessive salt and fluids, raises blood pressure; so do high levels of adrenaline and other hormones that constrict blood vessels.

Monitor underlying factors. With age, blood pressure rises somewhat, but no one fully understands precisely what leads to hypertension, although a combination of factors seems to be involved. Because it tends to run in families, an inherited susceptibility is suspected. Diabetes, obesity, and certain other disorders increase risk. Stress prompts a surge in adrenal hormones and a temporary rise in blood pressure; some researchers believe that constant stress may play a role in developing hypertension. Other contributors include smoking, excessive alcohol, and a sedentary lifestyle.

There is little doubt that keeping blood pressure at normal levels makes a difference in the quality and length of life. Cardiovascular disease death rates, which had been steadily declining since the 1960s, thanks largely to lifestyle changes and improvements in hypertension treatment, are now on the increase again.

DIET AND HYPERTENSION

Diet plays a role in both prevention and treatment of high blood pressure, experts now agree. Simple things can help keep your blood pressure in check.

Limit your salt intake. A high-salt diet also contributes to the condition in people who have a genetic tendency to retain sodium; in these individuals, restriction of salt beginning at an early age reduces the risk of developing hypertension. A portion of the population, including older people and people with diabetes, appears to be particularly sensitive to sodium and may benefit significantly from

CONTROL BLOOD PRESSURE WITH THE DASH DIET

The most compelling evidence in support of diet as a means of controlling blood pressure comes from two trials sponsored by the National Institutes of Health. Together the studies are known as the DASH diet.

The first study, carried out in 1997, was called "DASH," for Dietary Approaches to Stop Hypertension. It found that blood pressure levels could fall significantly with an eating plan low in total fat, saturated fat, and cholesterol, and rich in fruits, vegetables, and low-fat dairy products. The diet was shown to prevent hypertension and in some cases reduce blood pressure as much as an antihypertensive drug. Results were seen within two weeks, and benefits remained eight weeks later regardless of a person's gender, ethnicity, or starting blood pressure.

The DASH diet provides foods that are high in fiber, calcium, magnesium, and potassium, all of which have been associated with lower blood pressure. It is also low in saturated fat. The diet calls for eating 8 to 10 servings of fruits and vegetables and 2 to 3 cups of low-fat dairy foods daily. Here are the broad DASH guidelines you can follow in menu planning:

- Grains and grain products: 7 to 8 servings daily
- Fruits and vegetables: 4 to 5 servings of each daily
- Low-fat or nonfat dairy foods: 2 to 3 servings daily
- Meats, poultry, and fish: 2 or fewer 3-oz (85-g) servings daily
- Nuts, seeds, or legumes: 4 to 5 servings per week
- Fats: 2 to 3 servings daily; avoid saturated fat
- Sweets: 5 per week

DASH-sodium trial

A follow-up trial, held in 2000, examined whether reducing salt could enhance results even more. Sodium in table salt and in other foods can raise blood pressure by causing the body to retain water thereby increasing blood volume and thus blood pressure. Sodium also causes small blood vessels to constrict. This study showed that the DASH diet combined with salt reduction was superior to either strategy alone. All the participants benefited from limiting their salt intake.

eating low-sodium foods. Experts disagree as to how much salt is too much; many recommend no more than 2,400 mg of sodium each day for healthy individuals. The best way to reduce sodium intake is to avoid adding salt, and to avoid most processed foods, which are usually loaded with sodium. Check labels carefully—look for the term "sodium" to find hidden salt. In addition to avoiding salty and pickled foods, use herbs and spices in cooking.

Keep your weight down. Being even slightly overweight contributes to hypertension; losing excess weight is often all that is needed to return blood pressure to normal. Even a modest weight loss will cause a drop in blood pressure.

Eat less fat. A high-fat diet not only leads to weight gain but may also contribute to high blood pressure. Limit fat intake to 30 percent or less of total calories, with 10 percent or less coming from saturated animal fats. This means cutting back on butter and margarine; switching to low-fat milk and other low-fat dairy products; choosing lean cuts of meat; and shifting to low-fat cooking methods, such as broiling instead of frying.

Reduce alcohol and caffeine consumption. Although a glass of wine or other alcoholic drink daily seems to reduce the chance of a heart attack, consuming more than this will negate any benefit and may increase the risk of hypertension. Too much caffeine can also raise blood pressure. Older adults with hypertension may be more sensitive to the effects of caffeine and should limit their intake.

Mind your minerals. Some nutrients may protect against high blood pressure. Potassium, an electrolyte that helps maintain the body's balance of salt and fluids, helps ensure normal blood pressure. Potassium can be found in fruits and vegetables, dairy products, and legumes.

Some studies have linked calcium deficiency to hypertension; the diet should provide two to three servings of low-fat milk products a day.

Get more garlic. Other research appears to validate the claims that garlic may lower blood pressure. The amount of garlic necessary to lower blood pressure, however, can cause other problems, especially unpleasant breath and body odor. Although garlic is available in odorless pills, it is not known if these pills produce the same benefits as eating garlic fresh or lightly cooked. A further problem

UNDERSTANDING BLOOD PRESSURE MEASUREMENTS

Blood does not flow through the body in a steady stream; instead, it courses in spurts. Thus, blood pressure is expressed in two numbers, such as 120/80. The higher number indicates the systolic pressure, the peak force when the heart contracts and pumps a small amount of blood into the circulation. The lower number, the diastolic reading, measures pressure exerted when the heart is resting momentarily between beats. The units of blood pressure measurement are millimeters of mercury; basically this measures how high the pressure of the blood can push a column of mercury in an evacuated tube.

A doctor usually uses a stethoscope and a sphygmomanometer to measure blood pressure. The cuff is tightened to stop blood flow, and as pressure is released, he listens for the sounds that indicate systolic and diastolic pressures. If your resting blood pressure is consistently 140/90 or higher, you have high blood pressure. Normal adult blood pressure is defined as below 120/80; hypertension is classified as follows:

	Systolic	Diastolic
• Normal:	Less than 120	Less than 80
• Prehypertension:	120–139	80–89
• Stage 1 hypertension:	140–159	90–99
• Stage 2 hypertension:	Greater than 160	Greater than 100

Note: Some people have a normal systolic reading but a high diastolic pressure; they are classified as hypertensive. Other people have isolated systolic hypertension.

with garlic supplements is that the lack of government regulations means there is no assurance that the product in the bottle matches the contents on the label.

OTHER LIFESTYLE CHANGES

While a proper diet is instrumental in maintaining normal blood pressure, it should be combined with other lifestyle changes. One of the most important is regular aerobic exercise, which lowers blood pressure by conditioning the heart to work more efficiently. If you smoke, give up the habit. Nicotine raises blood pressure. Quitting can drop blood pressure by 10 points or more.

Use medications with caution. Over-the-counter cold, allergy, and diet pills can raise blood pressure. In some women, birth control pills, or estrogen replacement therapy, can cause high blood pressure.

Reduce stress. Experts continue to debate the role of stress in hypertension. There is no doubt that stress temporarily raises blood pressure, and some experts think that it may have a long-term effect.

Meditation, yoga, biofeedback training, self-hypnosis, and other relaxation techniques may help lower blood pressure. Studies have found that people with pets have lower blood pressure than non-pet owners.

DRUG THERAPY

Doctors usually recommend 6 months of lifestyle changes to see if mild to moderate hypertension returns to normal levels. If not, drug therapy is often instituted. There are dozens of antihypertensive drugs and doctors can usually find one or a combination that lowers blood pressure with minimal adverse side effects. The most widely used drugs are diuretics, which reduce salt and fluid volume by increasing the flow of urine. Some classes of drugs reduce the heart's workload by helping to widen, or dilate, the arterioles to increase blood flow; others regulate nerve impulses to slow the pulse.

It is also important to treat disorders that contribute to high blood pressure; these include diabetes and elevated blood cholesterol, both of which compound the risk of developing heart problems. Dietary and other lifestyle changes that lower high blood pressure also help to control diabetes and blood cholesterol levels. ❖

BLUEBERRIES

BENEFITS

- A good source of dietary fiber.
- A excellent source of antioxidants.
- Provide some vitamin C and iron.
- May protect against some intestinal upsets.
- May help prevent urinary tract infections.
- Anthocyanins may help prevent heart disease and cancer and may help with memory loss.

DRAWBACKS

- Can make stool dark and tarry, which may be mistaken for intestinal bleeding.
- May cause allergic reactions in some people.

Blueberries are naturally sweet. Because cooking destroys vitamin C, eating blueberries raw preserves this antioxidant nutrient.

"Natural healers" also advocate eating one cup of raw berries or drinking one to two cups of unsweetened blueberry juice a day to treat and prevent urinary tract infections. Research appears to support this advice. Blueberries are in the same plant family as cranberries, and

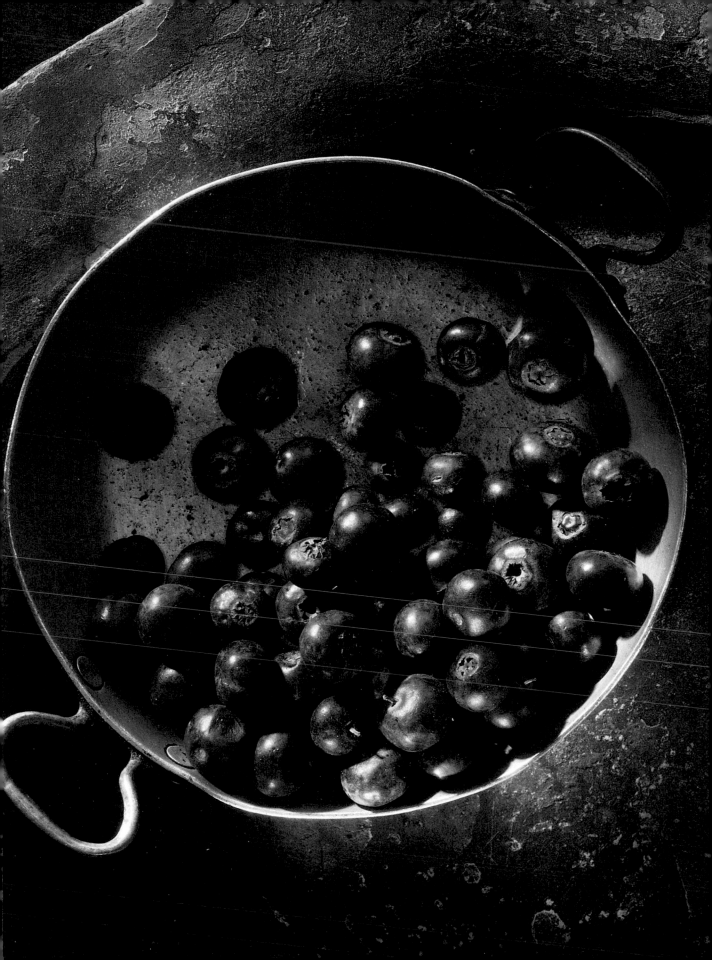

both contain a substance that prevents bacteria from adhering to the bladder walls, where they can multiply. These berries also make urine more acidic, which helps destroy bacteria that invade the bladder and urethra. Eating large amounts of blueberries, however, can make stools appear dark and tarry; this is a harmless situation but can be alarming, because it resembles intestinal bleeding.

Blueberries provide antioxidant power. They contain anthocyanins, flavonoids that give the fruit their distinctive blue color. These compounds are associated with numerous health benefits such as prevention of heart disease and cancer and may even combat aging. Studies on animals show that blueberries help to prevent and also reverse age-related memory loss. The specific substance has not been identified, but scientists speculate that the antioxidant power of blueberries protects brain cells from free-radical harm.

Like many fruits, blueberries are potential allergens in susceptible people. Common symptoms are itchy hives and swollen lips.

NUTRITIONAL VALUE

Although they are sweet and tasty, blueberries are not especially high in nutrients; one-half cup provides 10 mg of vitamin C, 0.7 mg of iron, and small amounts of potassium, folate, and beta carotene. A half-cup of raw blueberries has almost 2 mg of fiber, only 40 calories, and important disease-fighting anthocyanins, so they're an ideal low-calorie dessert. ❖

BRAN

BENEFITS

- Helps prevent constipation.
- Oat and rice brans help lower blood cholesterol levels.
- Promotes a feeling of fullness, which can lead to weight loss.
- May reduce the risk of some cancers.

DRAWBACKS

- Excessive bran consumption reduces the absorption of calcium, iron, and zinc.
- Can cause intestinal irritation, bloating, and gas.

Bran, one of the richest sources of dietary fiber, is the indigestible outer husk of wheat, rice, oats, and other cereal grains. At one time most bran was discarded when grains were milled. Then in the 1960s Dr. Dennis P. Burkitt, a British medical officer in Africa, published several scientific reports in which he theorized that bran and other types of fiber could prevent heart attacks, diverticulitis and other intestinal disorders, and cancers of the breast, colon, prostate, and uterus. He developed this theory after observing that these diseases are rare among rural Africans, who consume large amounts of whole grains. Prompted by a number of best-selling books, bran became the fad food of the 1970s, and raw miller's bran was added to everything from bread to such unlikely dishes as meat loaf and baked apples.

Since then, much of the enthusiasm for using raw bran has dissipated as researchers have learned more about its health benefits and possible hazards. We also know now that various types of bran have different properties and functions. Wheat bran, for example, is mostly insoluble fiber; although it absorbs large amounts of water, it makes its way through the intestinal tract intact. When used in moderation, insoluble fiber helps prevent constipation by producing a soft, bulky stool that moves quickly and easily through the colon. Excessive amounts, however, should not be taken as they can cause bloating and intestinal gas.

DOES BRAN PREVENT COLON CANCER?

Dr. Burkitt had theorized that bran prevented colon cancer by reducing the amount of time required for the stool to travel through the bowel. But studies to document this protective effect have produced mixed results. An Australian study found that women taking large amounts of wheat bran actually had a slightly increased incidence of colon cancer. In contrast, a 4-year study involving 58 high-risk adults with precancerous colon polyps found that those taking wheat bran achieved a reduction in the size and number of these growths.

Two 2003 medical studies—one on Americans and one on Europeans—showed that high intake of dietary fiber is associated with a lower risk of colorectal cancer. In the American study, investigators compared the daily fiber intake of more than 3,500 people who had precancerous colon polyps to the fiber intake of about 34,000 people who did not have these growths. They found that the people who ate the most fiber, about 35 g daily, had a 27 percent lower risk of precancerous growths than those who ate the least, about 12 g per day. The association was strongest for fibers from grains, cereals, and fruits. In the European study, researchers examined the link in more than 500,000 people in 10 countries. Those who ate the most fiber, about 35 g daily, had about a 40 percent lower risk of colorectal cancer compared to those who ate the least, about 15 g a day. An editorial accompanying publication of the studies concludes, "Eating a diet rich in plant foods, in the form of fruits, vegetables, and whole-grain cereals probably remains the best option for reducing the risk of colon cancer and for general health protection."

It also appears that including wheat bran in a high-fiber diet can help prevent diverticulitis, an intestinal disorder in which small pockets bulging from the colon wall become impacted and inflamed. And because it helps prevent constipation, bran may also be beneficial for persons suffering from hemorrhoids.

Diabetics may benefit from oat bran. Oat bran is high in soluble fiber, which is sticky and combines with water to form a thick gel. Some researchers have reported that this type of fiber reduces blood cholesterol levels. It also appears to improve glucose metabolism in diabetics. This benefit, in turn, reduces their need for insulin and other diabetes medications.

More recently, there have been reports that rice bran also reduces cholesterol levels. Researchers are not sure, however, whether this benefit comes from the insoluble fiber found in the bran or from the highly unsaturated oil in the rice germ—which is not separated from the grain husks during the milling process.

All types of bran, as well as other high-fiber foods, play an important role in weight control by promoting a feeling of fullness without overeating. This may provide an explanation for the lowered incidence of some obesity-related cancers and heart attacks among populations whose diets are high in fiber.

POSSIBLE HAZARDS

When the benefits of bran were first announced, many people started adding three, four, or even more tablespoons of raw miller's bran to their daily diet. It soon became apparent that this practice could cause bloating and discomfort and also aggravate irritable bowel syndrome. In addition, the phytic acid in raw

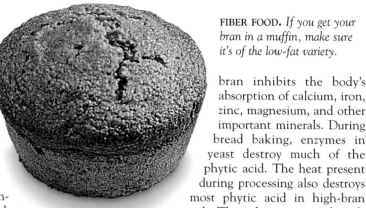

FIBER FOOD. *If you get your bran in a muffin, make sure it's of the low-fat variety.*

bran inhibits the body's absorption of calcium, iron, zinc, magnesium, and other important minerals. During bread baking, enzymes in yeast destroy much of the phytic acid. The heat present during processing also destroys most phytic acid in high-bran cereals. Thus, these processed products are safer than raw miller's bran.

There have been several reports of severe bowel obstruction in people who consumed large amounts of bran, especially if they don't drink enough water. Many nutritionists now advise people to eat whole-grain wheat bread, cereals, and other products that contain bran. Have oatmeal and cereals made with whole oats; substitute brown rice for the white. These foods are more palatable than raw bran, which tastes like sawdust, and are more beneficial. ❖

BREAD

BENEFITS
- A good source of complex carbohydrates.
- High in niacin, riboflavin, and other B complex vitamins.
- Some kinds provide good amounts of iron.
- Whole-grain breads are high in fiber.

DRAWBACKS
- People with celiac disease cannot tolerate the gluten found in many breads.
- May trigger an adverse reaction in people allergic to molds.
- Often high in salt.
- Some breads made from refined flour may have a high glycemic index.

Since prehistoric times, bread has been a staple food in virtually every society. As early hunter-gatherers settled into agricultural societies, they learned how to transform various grains into bread. This simple food required only stones to grind grain into flour or meal, water or another liquid to mix it into dough, and a means of baking or cooking it.

Over the centuries, each society developed its own unique types of bread. The huge variety

DO ONE SIMPLE THING

BUY BREAD WITH THE WORD "WHOLE" IN IT

Twenty grams of additional dietary fiber per day, such as found in whole-grain breads, is associated with an approximate 26 percent reduction in the risk of coronary heart disease.

of baked goods available to us at our supermarkets and bakeries today—different-shaped loaves of white, wheat, rye, pumpernickel, sourdough, and multigrain breads, croissants and matzos, bagels and muffins, tortillas, pita, and chapatis, among many others—represent a dietary melding of dozens of diverse cultures.

GIVING DOUGH A LIFT

The simplest and oldest breads are flat, or unleavened; they are made by mixing flour or meal with water and then baking, frying, or steaming it. Examples include matzo, tortillas, chapatis, and some types of crackers. The addition of yeast, baking soda, or other leavening agent to the flour-and-water mixture allows the dough to expand, or rise, and gives the bread a lighter, finer texture than unleavened types.

The type of flour used and the manner in which it and the other ingredients interact give the various kinds of breads their unique textures and flavors. In many industrialized countries the most popular breads are made from wheat flour, which produces a product with a light texture. When wheat flour is kneaded with liquid, the gluten proteins absorb water to form an elastic dough that traps gas from the fermenting yeast; bubbles of carbon dioxide are formed, resulting in the light texture. Rye and some other flours contain varying amounts of gluten, but none come close to that of wheat—which is why breads made from other grains tend to be heavy and coarse. To make a lighter-textured bread from rye, barley, or other grains, some wheat flour is usually added to the dough.

Flavor and texture are also influenced by the type of liquid mixed into the dough—plain water, milk, beer, and fruit juice are common choices. Sugar or honey may be added to "feed" the yeast and make the bread rise at a faster

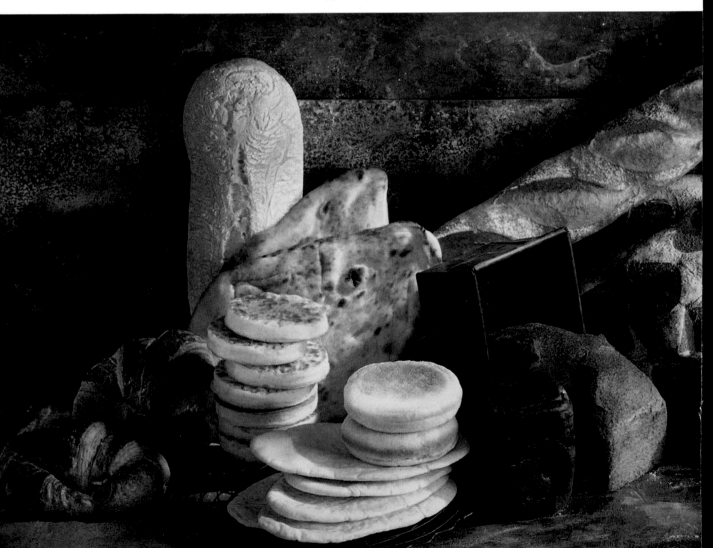

rate; it also results in a moister product. A small amount of salt is needed to strengthen the gluten and to temper the rate at which the yeast multiplies. Butter or other fat is often added to flavor commercial breads; it also makes pastry-like breads, such as croissants, rich and flaky.

Check the ingredients. Bread sold in North America is often mass-produced; such products contain various preservatives, emulsifiers, and bleaches or coloring agents to extend their shelf life and improve their appearance. These additives do not alter nutritional value, but most commercial bread may be too high in salt for people on low-sodium diets. Also, people who have celiac disease cannot tolerate the gluten in most bread. People with food allergies may react to specific ingredients; for example, people allergic to molds may react to sourdough or very yeasty breads. Some health food stores and specialty shops offer breads that are gluten-free; people with food allergies should always check labels for any offending ingredients.

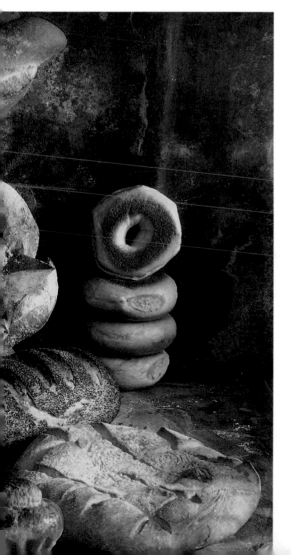

NUTRITIONAL VALUE

Traditionally, bread has been called the staff of life, implying that it alone is all that is required for total nutrition. This is inaccurate. While bread does provide starch, protein, and some vitamins and minerals, it is far from being nutritionally complete. It lacks such essentials as vitamins A, B_{12}, C, and D. Many of the nutrients in the grain are destroyed by milling and processing, but some (typically folate, iron, thiamine, riboflavin, and niacin) are added later to restore the nutrients to their original levels or, in some cases, even increase them; consequently, enriched white flour often has more of the B complex vitamins than are found in whole-wheat flour. In general, however, whole-grain flours are more nutritious than their highly processed counterparts; they also provide more dietary fiber.

Look for added nutrients. The addition of other ingredients also increases the nutritional value of bread. Depending upon the type, these may include soy, flax, eggs, molasses, raisins and other dried fruits, whole grains, seeds, and various types of cheese.

Contrary to popular belief, bread is not especially fattening; a typical slice of white or whole-wheat bread contains just 65 to 80 calories. But slathering bread with butter, margarine, or other fatty spreads does make it higher in calories; a low-sugar jam or an all-fruit preserve is a more healthful spread.

THE WORLD'S BREADBASKET

The growing popularity of international breads is reflected in the many types sold in supermarkets, delis, and bakeries. Some common breads include the following:

Bagel. This doughnut-shaped roll, identified with Eastern European and Jewish communities, is boiled and then baked. Traditionally, bagels are made from a high-gluten white flour, but whole wheat, rye, flax, pumpernickel, sourdough, and other versions are also commonly

CHOOSING YOUR LOAF. *Breads from around the world include: croissant, pita, English muffin, crumpet, Italian, naan, raisin, whole wheat, baguette, crusty whole wheat, bagel, poppy seed, pain de campagne, and brioche.*

available. Bagels may be topped with caraway, sesame seeds, poppy seeds, chopped onions, or coarse salt. Cinnamon and raisin bagels are also popular.

Brioche. A light yeast roll that originated in France, brioche falls somewhere between bread and cake in terms of texture and taste. It is usually made with refined white flour and enriched with butter and eggs.

Chapati. A flat Indian bread that is made with whole wheat or white flour and may be leavened or unleavened. Some are brushed with butter or oil, adding extra calories.

Ciabatta. Olive oil is added to this Italian raised bread, making it moist and chewy; oregano, basil, and various other herbs may also be added.

Cornbread. This bread is made from wheat flour, ground yellow cornmeal, eggs, milk, and sometimes sugar.

English muffin. High-protein white flour is used to make this round, honey-combed roll; it is cooked in a skillet or on a griddle.

Focaccia. An Italian yeast bread that is made from a dough similar to that of pizza, it is usually baked in a large disc and flavored with olive oil, onions, garlic, and herbs. The added oil in this recipe contributes extra calories.

Matzo. Made from wheat flour, water, and salt, this crackerlike unleavened Jewish bread is traditionally served at Passover meals.

Multigrain. Often promoted as a health food, this bread is usually made with a combination of flours and added ingredients, such as sprouts, various seeds, and raisins. Some multigrain breads are more nutritious than others, but a

check of their labels will often show that many are comparable to ordinary breads.

Naan. Baked on the hot side of a tandoori oven, this flat yeast bread originated in India.

Pita. This flat, leavened Middle Eastern bread puffs up during baking and then flattens out to leave a hollow middle, or pocket.

Pumpernickel. This heavy rye German bread derives its dark color from molasses or caramel. One dense type is steamed and baked for hours, then cut into thin slices.

Quick bread. Made from a variety of flours, it is leavened with baking powder or baking soda and rises as it bakes. Biscuits, muffins, scones, coffee cakes, and loaf breads are all quick breads.

Rye. All-rye bread is heavy and dense; most of the softer, deli-type rye breads are made mostly of wheat flour.

Sourdough. This bread is leavened with a "starter" and is usually made with white flour. True sourdough bread has a heavier, denser texture than yeast-leavened breads.

Tortillas. This unleavened Mexican bread is made of corn or wheat flour, salt, and water. Finely ground limestone is often added. ❖

BROCCOLI

BENEFITS

● An excellent source of vitamin C.

● A good source of beta carotene and folate.

● Significant amounts of protein, calcium, iron, potassium, and other minerals.

● Rich in glucosinolates, effective natural cancer fighters.

● Low in calories and high in fiber.

DRAWBACKS

● Overcooking releases unpleasant-smelling sulfur compounds and may cause gas.

One of our most nutritious and studied vegetables, broccoli's powerful disease-fighting properties give it the ability to protect against many common cancers. Over the last 20 years, numerous studies have found that people who eat an abundance of broccoli have a significantly reduced incidence of cancers of the colon, breast, cervix, lungs, prostate, esophagus, larynx, and bladder.

While other cruciferous vegetables (members of the cabbage family, whose flowers resemble crosses) are protective, broccoli seems to have more cancer-fighting compounds. Some

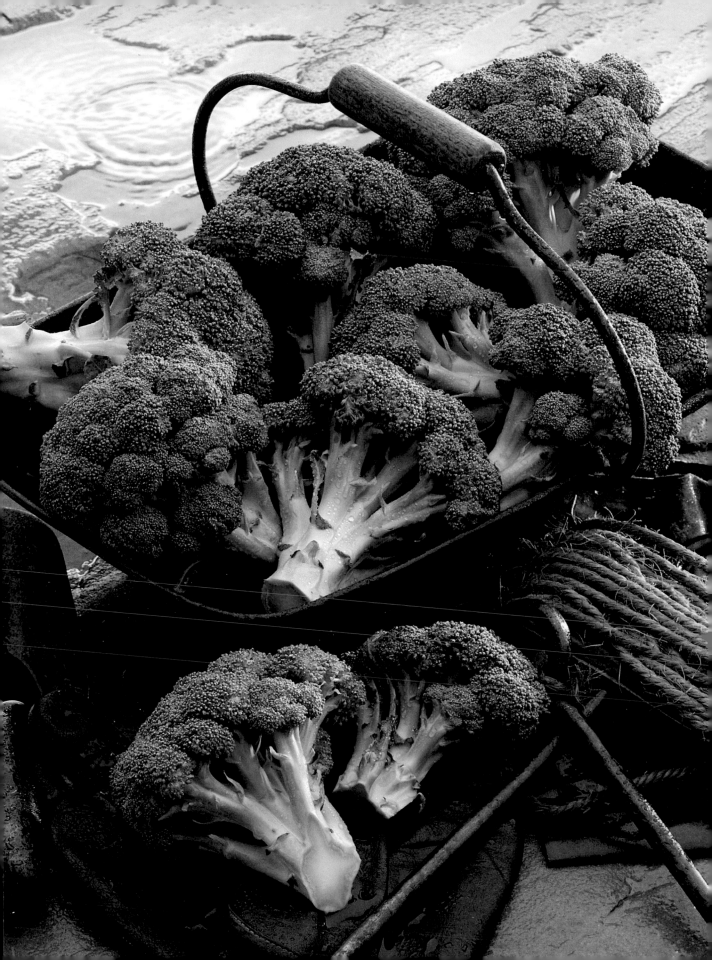

of these block the action of hormones that stimulate tumors; others work by inhibiting tumor growth or by boosting the action of protective enzymes. Broccoli contains glucosinolates, which, once ingested, break down into healthful compounds, including indoles, sulforaphane, and isothiocyanates, all of which may be cancer fighters. The most interesting compound is sulforaphane, which shows decided anticancer activity in both cultured rat and human cells. Broccoli sprouts are roughly fifty times richer in sulforaphane than mature broccoli. Broccoli is also high in bioflavonoids, including quercetin and other phytochemicals that protect cells against mutation and damage from unstable molecules.

Broccoli has an abundance of essential vitamins and minerals. A 1-cup serving of cooked broccoli contains only 44 calories, yet it provides more than 100 percent of the Recommended Dietary Allowance (RDA) of vitamin C, 20 percent of the RDA for folate, and a healthy amount of beta carotene. A cup of broccoli also provides 75 mg of calcium, 1.2 mg of iron, and 5 g of protein. Because 1 cup of cooked broccoli has 3.5 g of fiber and contains natural laxatives, it is often suggested to prevent constipation.

Fresh broccoli is available year-round; frozen broccoli is just as nutritious. Florets turning yellow are past their prime and less nutritious. Broccoli can be eaten raw, but most people prefer it cooked. Steaming or stir-frying it until crispy tender retains the most nutrients; boiling it in a large amount of water destroys many of the cancer-fighting compounds, vitamin C, and other nutrients. ❖

BRUSSELS SPROUTS

BENEFITS

- An excellent source of vitamin C.
- A good source of protein, folate, beta carotene, iron, and potassium.
- Contain bioflavonoids and other substances that protect against cancer.
- Low in calories and high in fiber.

DRAWBACKS

- Can cause bloating and flatulence.

Brussels sprouts resemble small cabbages and share many of the same health benefits. Like broccoli, cabbage, and other cruciferous vegetables, they contain chemicals that appear to protect against cancer. They are also very high in vitamin C; a cup of cooked brussels sprouts provides 99 mg, more than 100 percent of the adult Recommended Dietary Allowance (RDA); it also provides 20 percent or more of the folate, more than 10 percent of the daily needs of iron, and a healthy amount of beta carotene. A 1-cup serving has about 61 calories, almost a third of which come from protein. Serving brussels sprouts with a small amount of cheese, rice, or another grain adds complementary amino acids to make a complete protein.

THE CANCER FACTOR

Brussels sprouts have high amounts of bioflavonoids and indoles, plant chemicals that protect against cancer in several ways. Bioflavonoids have an antioxidant effect that helps prevent cellular damage and mutation caused by the unstable molecules released when the body uses oxygen. Bioflavonoids, along with indoles and perhaps other plant chemicals, inhibit hormones that promote tumor growth. Indoles are particularly active against estrogen, the hormone that stimulates the growth of some breast cancers.

Other studies indicate that bioflavonoids and indoles may protect against cancers of the prostate and uterus. Even if cancer does develop, these plant chemicals may slow tumor growth and spread of the disease.

SPROUTS AT THEIR BEST

When buying fresh brussels sprouts, select small, bright green ones with tightly packed leaves. Those past their prime will have patches of yellow, an unpleasant sulfurous smell, and a bitter taste. Frozen brussels sprouts retain most of their nutrients and flavor.

Sprouts can be boiled or steamed; to ensure that they are evenly cooked, cut a small cross into their base. When boiling, use a cup of water for each cup of sprouts. Bring it to a rapid boil, add the sprouts, and cook uncovered until they are crispy tender.

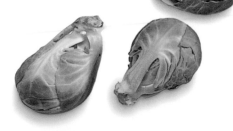

Overcooking destroys vitamin C and gives sprouts a bitter taste. When steaming sprouts, uncover the steamer for a few seconds every 2 or 3 minutes to prevent a buildup of the sulfurous gases. ❖

BUCKWHEAT

BENEFITS
- A good source of iron and magnesium.
- High in starches, protein, and fiber.

DRAWBACKS
- Whole kernels are prepared with mixed egg or egg white, which may cause an allergic reaction in those susceptible.

Although it's not a grain and is unrelated to wheat, buckwheat is generally used as if it were. North Americans are most familiar with buckwheat in pancakes, which are made from the flour of the plant's seeds. The hulled roasted seeds, commonly called groats or kasha, can be boiled to make cereal, pudding, or a side dish similar to bulgur wheat.

When cooked, the buckwheat groats have a nutty flavor that goes well with lamb and strong-tasting vegetables like cabbage. Typically, the dry groats are mixed with a beaten egg, sautéed briefly, then boiled in water. The protein in the egg white keeps the kernels from sticking together as the seeds expand and break their hulls. The amino acids from the egg combine with the amino acids in buckwheat to provide a complete protein dish. To avoid the fat and cholesterol in eggs, discard the yolk.

NUTRITIONAL CONTENT
A half-cup serving of buckwheat groats contains about 90 calories, 3 g of protein, and 51 mg of magnesium, a mineral needed for proper energy metabolism. It also contributes 0.8 mg of iron.

Sprouted buckwheat seeds are a nutritious and tasty addition to salads, stir-fried foods, and other dishes. Fresh unhulled seeds suitable for sprouting are available from health food stores. ❖

DID YOU KNOW?

RUTIN, FOUND IN BUCKWHEAT, IS A KNOWN CANCER FIGHTER

It also helps to lower cholesterol levels, strengthen blood vessels, and lower blood pressure.

BULIMIA

EAT PLENTY OF
- Fresh vegetables, fruits, and high-fiber foods to promote a feeling of fullness.
- Bananas, dried fruits, and a variety of fresh vegetables and fruits for potassium.

AVOID
- "Trigger" foods that are associated with binges.

Medically, bulimia is defined as recurrent episodes of binge eating—the rapid intake of unusually large amounts of food—an average of twice a week for at least 3 months. Although bulimia literally means "the hunger of an ox," the majority of bulimics do not have excessive appetites. Instead, their tendency to overeat compulsively seems to arise from psychological problems, possibly complicated by abnormal brain chemistry or a hormonal imbalance.

Far more women than men are affected by bulimia. Despite their overeating, most bulimics are of normal weight, although many have a frequent gain or loss of 10 lb (4.5 kg) or more. Their ability to maintain normal weight is attributed to the other aspect of bulimia; namely, their ability to compensate for overeating by strict dieting and excessive exercise or by purging through self-induced vomiting or abuse of laxatives or enemas.

Some bulimics purge after eating any amount of food. About half of anorexics suffer from bulimia, and both disorders are characterized by a perfectionist focus on dieting and weight and a fear of being unable to control eating behavior. These disorders typically begin with a strict weight-loss diet. Driven by extreme hunger, the dieter may succumb to gorging, usually on sweet food that is high in calories, such as cake and ice cream. Then, feeling guilty and ashamed, the dieter may purge to compensate for the indiscretion. Before long, the dieter may be caught in a cycle of binging and purging, with binges often triggered by feelings of anxiety, stress, loneliness, or boredom. A binge may be brief, or it may last for several hours, with anywhere from 1,000 to 50,000 calories consumed.

NUTRITIONAL DEFICIENCIES
Repeated purging can have serious consequences, including nutritional deficiencies and an imbalance of sodium and potassium, leading to fatigue, fainting, and palpitations. Acids in

vomit can damage tooth enamel and the lining of the esophagus. Laxative abuse can irritate the large intestine and produce rectal bleeding. Overuse of laxatives disrupts normal bowel function, leading to chronic constipation when they are discontinued. Perhaps one of the most severe consequences, however, is depression and the high suicide rate that is common among bulimics.

TREATMENT

Like all eating disorders, bulimia can be difficult to treat and usually requires a team approach involving nutrition education, medications, and psychotherapy. If the patient appears to be suicidal or the intractable binge-purge behavior does not respond to outpatient therapy, hospitalization may be necessary. Don't expect instant success, however; treatment often takes 3 years or more, and even then, relapses are common.

Treat nutritional deficiencies early. This is especially important if the body's potassium reserves have been depleted by vomiting or laxative abuse. Eating high-potassium foods, such as dried fruits, bananas, and fresh fruits and vegetables, usually restores the mineral; if not, a supplement may be needed.

Keep a diary. Nutrition education typically begins with asking the person with bulimia to keep a diary to help pinpoint circumstances that contribute to binging. A nutrition counselor may also give the patient an eating plan that minimizes the number of decisions she must make about what and when to eat. This diet should emphasize foods high in protein and starches while excluding favorite binge foods until the bulimia is under control; they can then be reintroduced in small quantities. At this stage of treatment, the person with bulimia learns how to give herself permission to eat desirable foods in reasonable quantities, in order to reduce the feelings of deprivation and intense hunger that often lead to loss of control in eating.

Bulimics who abuse laxatives may need a high-fiber diet to overcome constipation. Whole-grain cereals and breads, fresh fruits and vegetables, and adequate fluids should help restore normal bowel function.

DRUG THERAPY

Because chronic clinical depression often accompanies bulimia, treatment usually includes giving selective antidepressant drugs that restore normal levels of serotonin, a brain chemical instrumental in mood control and appetite. The most commonly prescribed drugs for bulimia are the serotonin-reuptake inhibitors like fluoxetine (Prozac), which also suppresses appetite, and sertraline (Zoloft). As patients recover from their depression, they are better able to control their compulsive eating. Two drugs that were originally developed for epilepsy, Topamax and Zonegran, also show promise for eating disorders.

Psychotherapy may be an option. It can take several forms, including family and group therapy, as well as cognitive behavioral therapy to help the patient shift the central focus of her life away from food. Bulimics also learn to recognize the warning signs of a binge and how to deal with stress or situations that make them vulnerable to binges.

Participation in self-help groups can also be useful. In addition, alternative therapies, such as meditation, guided imagery, and progressive relaxation routines, can help patients become less obsessive about weight and their eating habits. ❖

BURNS

CONSUME PLENTY OF

- Foods high in protein and zinc, such as lean meat, poultry, fish and shellfish, eggs, and legumes, to promote healing and tissue repair.
- Water, broth, fruit juices, and other non-alcoholic beverages to replace fluid loss.
- Fresh fruits and vegetables rich in vitamin C to foster healing.

In order to promote healing and tissue repair, it is essential for victims of extensive burns to have a well-balanced diet that provides extra calories, protein, vitamins, and minerals. Burn victims also require extra fluids, sodium, and potassium to replace those substances that seep out through damaged skin; if this is not done, there is a danger of dehydration and an imbalanced body chemistry. Second- and third-degree burns that cause blistering and tissue damage are very serious; they have a high risk of becoming infected by germs that enter the body through the damaged skin.

Patients hospitalized with extensive burns are usually given intravenous fluids and antibiotics. If they are unable to eat, they will also be fed intravenously. A diet that provides extra calories, protein, and zinc is needed for tissue repair. Zinc, found in seafood, meat, poultry and in slightly lesser amounts in eggs, milk, beans, nuts, and whole grains is essential for wound healing; it also bolsters the body's immune defenses to fight infection.

Include vitamin C in the diet to build and maintain healthy skin and ward off infection. Often liquid supplements are necessary to maintain a high-calorie intake during the day.

Tea, coffee, and other caffeinated beverages should be avoided; they have a diuretic effect that accelerates fluid loss. Alcohol should also be avoided because it, too, dehydrates the body; it also lowers immunity. ❖

BUTTER AND MARGARINE

BENEFITS

- Improve flavor, moistness, and texture of baked goods.
- Good sources of vitamins A and D.
- Margarine made with polyunsaturated oil contains essential fatty acids and vitamin E.
- Some margarines contain the additives sitostanol or sitosterol which can reduce cholesterol.

DRAWBACKS

- High in calories, all of which come from fats, which increase the risk of obesity, cancers, and other diseases.
- Butter is high in saturated fats, which increase the risk of heart disease.
- Stick margarine or margarines that are made from hydrogenated oils contain trans fatty acids, which also raise blood cholesterol levels.
- Both butter and margarine may be high in salt.

North American eating habits have changed over the last few decades, and nowhere is this more obvious than in the supermarket dairy case. Where butter once reigned, we now have a puzzling array of margarines and other substitutes from which to choose.

More and more people than ever use margarine instead of butter because they believe it is the more healthful of the two spreads. Although most people agree that butter is more flavorful than margarine, they also know that it is relatively high in dietary cholesterol and that

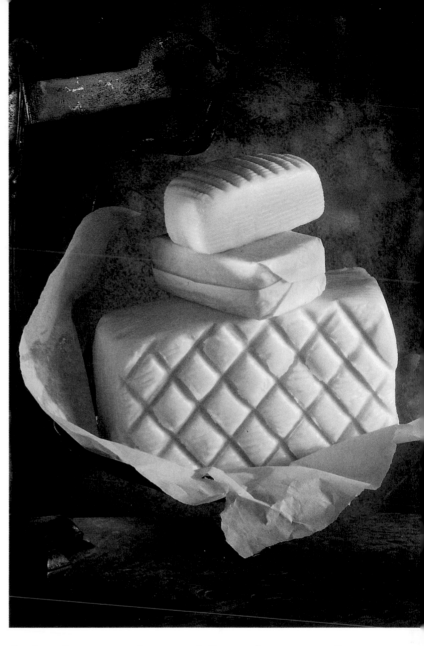

the fat in butter is mostly saturated. Saturated fats are presumed to raise blood cholesterol levels more than other types of fat.

Is margarine more healthful than butter? Doubts were raised in 1993, when Harvard researchers concluded that some types of margarine may actually increase the risk of heart disease more than butter. Understandably, this added fuel—and confusion—to the "butter versus margarine" debate. Not all margarines are created equal. The controversy lies in the level of trans fatty acids. (See "What Are Trans Fatty Acids?" page 76.) In general, the more solid the margarine is at room temperature, the more trans fat it contains. These days, many margarine manufacturers are changing their formulations to make products that do not contain any trans fats.

FAT STATS. *Butter, on average, has 108 calories per tablespoon, and 11 g of total fat (7.1 g saturated fat, 3.3 g mono-unsaturated fat, 0.4 g polyunsaturated fat) and 33 mg cholesterol.*

BUTTER OR MARGARINE?

The United States Department of Agriculture (USDA) studied 46 men and women who ate varying, but controlled, amounts of butter, tub margarine, or trans-free tub margarine over a period of several months. The results confirmed what cardiologists have been telling their patients. Subjects who consumed both types of margarine significantly improved cholesterol levels; subjects who consumed butter did not.

WHAT ARE TRANS FATTY ACIDS?

Trans fatty acids are produced when a vegetable oil is hydrogenated. Hydrogenation is a process used by many manufacturers to make liquid oil more solid (as in the manufacturing of spreads). This process improves shelf life and the stability of many baked goods and processed foods. Unfortunately, the process of hydrogenation creates trans fatty acids. Studies suggest that trans fats raise LDL cholesterol and also lower our HDL cholesterol, increasing risk of heart disease. Some experts say that eating too much trans fats may be as bad or even worse than eating too much saturated fat.

The primary sources of trans fats in the North American diet are partially hydrogenated vegetable oils used in the production of shortenings and hydrogenated margarine. These are used extensively in food preparation. The foods most likely to contain trans fats are processed foods like chips, breakfast waffles, doughnuts, pastries, cookies, crackers, fast food products like deep-fried sandwiches and French fries. They are also in some margarine and spreads.

Having a trans-free diet is pretty difficult and probably not necessary, but reducing your intake of trans fats is very important. Read labels and look for the listing of trans fats on packaged foods. You can also find trans fats in foods by looking for the words "hydrogenated vegetable oils" or "partially hydrogenated vegetable oils" in the ingredient list.

The best advice regarding these fats is to limit your intake of deep-fried, processed fatty foods, and snack foods. Look for "nonhydrogenated" on the label and for processed foods made with nonhydrogenated oils. Use a margarine that is nonhydrogenated. It's also a good idea to go easy on the trans fats that kids eat, which means cutting back on a lot of high-fat snack foods. Many manufacturers are now cutting trans fats from their products. It's almost impossible and probably unnecessary to avoid trans fats altogether but in this case, moderation is very important.

CHOOSING A MARGARINE

Choose soft-tub margarine made with non-hydrogenated fats. Check labels and select a product with high levels of monounsaturated and polyunsaturated fats; margarines made from canola, safflower, sunflower, olive, and corn oils are all good choices. Avoid products with hydrogenated or partially hydrogenated oils; they have more trans fatty acids than the other types do.

Margarines that have added sitostanol or sitosterol that reduce blood cholesterol can be sold in the United States, but not in Canada.

Scientists theorize that due to chemical similarity to cholesterol, these compounds compete with cholesterol for absorption into the bloodstream from the intestine. This interferes with the uptake of cholesterol from the diet, but more importantly, also lowers the amount of cholesterol that works its way into the blood from cholesterol synthesis in the liver. Cholesterol is an essential biochemical that our liver can supply. Much of it though arrives in the bloodstream in an indirect fashion. It is first secreted into the intestine via the bile, where it plays a role in fat absorption, and then is absorbed into the blood. Sitostanol or sitosterol block this absorption. Two tablespoons of margarine featuring these compounds are needed per day for the cholesterol-lowering effect.

A MATTER OF CALORIES

Butter and margarine are a major source of fat calories in the North American diet. Many people think that butter has more calories than margarine, but butter and margarine have about the same calories; both are also 16 to 20 percent water. Their calorie content can be reduced by adding extra water, air, or both, so anyone striving to cut fat intake should read product labels and select low-calorie items.

A QUESTION OF FLAVOR

It's no secret that butter tastes better than margarine, but it's also increasingly difficult to tell the difference. Whipped or light butter often loses some of its natural flavor; conversely, mixing a little butter with margarine gives it a more buttery taste. Butter-substitute powders or sprinkles are virtually fat-free, deriving their flavor from the essence of butter. These products won't spread, but they melt when sprinkled on vegetables or other hot dishes.

Salt is used to flavor both butter and margarine; anyone on a low-sodium diet should look for unsalted varieties.

MODERATION IS THE KEY

Used sparingly, both butter and margarine can be incorporated into a healthful diet. A little butter goes a long way; a teaspoon imparts as much flavor as a tablespoon, with one-third the fat. Further reduce butter or margarine by combining it with herbs, spices, or low-fat ingredients; for example, top baked potatoes with chives and blended nonfat cottage cheese. When making cakes, cut the amount of butter or margarine by one-third to one-half; top whole-grain breads with fruit preserves. ❖

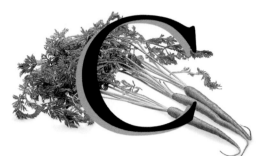

CABBAGE

BENEFITS
- An excellent source of vitamin C.
- Low in calories and high in fiber.
- May help prevent colon cancer and malignancies stimulated by estrogen.

DRAWBACKS
- Can cause bloating and flatulence.
- Gives off strong, somewhat unpleasant sulfurous odor when cooked.
- Coleslaw can be high in calories; sauerkraut is loaded with salt.

Although cabbage is not quite as nutritious as broccoli, brussels sprouts, and cauliflower, it does outrank these plant relatives in consumption. In fact, in some parts of the world, cabbage consumption is on a par with that of potatoes. Very high in fiber and very low in calories (a cup of chopped, raw green cabbage contains a meager 20 calories), the lowly cabbage is a rich source of vitamin C (with 33 mg per cup). Red cabbage contains almost twice as much vitamin C as the green cabbage, while the green variety contains twice as much folate as the red; both red and green cabbages contribute potassium and fiber. Savoy cabbage is a good source of beta carotene.

MYTH BUSTER

Myth: Prevailing folk wisdom states that cabbage juice is a miracle cure for ulcers.

Reality: There is little scientific evidence to prove that cabbage juice works. Nevertheless, there is probably no harm in trying cabbage juice along with conventional medical treatment for ulcers.

CABBAGE IS RICH IN CANCER-FIGHTING COMPOUNDS

Cabbages are members of the cruciferous family of vegetables, a family associated with numerous health benefits. It has long been known that people who eat large amounts of cabbage enjoy a low rate of colon cancer. This protective effect is assumed to come from bioflavonoids, indoles, monoterpenes, and other plant chemicals that inhibit tumor growth and protect cells against damage from free radicals, those unstable molecules released when the body uses oxygen. Some of these chemicals also speed up the body's metabolism of estrogen, which may explain why women whose diets provide ample amounts of cabbage and related vegetables have a reduced incidence of breast cancer. This chemical action may also protect against cancers of the uterus and ovaries. Of particular interest is indole-3-carbinol, a cabbage component that in animal studies had reduced the risk of cancer. Still, advice to take this compound in pill form, as advocated by some supplement manufacturers, would appear to be premature.

PREPARATION METHODS

Cabbage can be served raw—as coleslaw, cooked, or pickled into sauerkraut. Commercial coleslaw is high in calories (about 200 per cup) because it has large amounts of mayonnaise. You can reduce calories by using low-fat yogurt, vinegar, and oil. Sauerkraut is soaked in salt brine and then fermented; to lower the sodium content, rinse it before heating. Sulfites are often used to preserve cabbage color; asthma sufferers or anyone allergic to sulfites should check package labels.

Steaming and stir-frying preserves most nutrients. Don't use aluminum cookware, which causes a chemical reaction that discolors the vegetable and alters its flavor. ❖

TYPES OF CABBAGE

There are hundreds of different kinds of cabbage; the following are the most popular varieties in Canada and the United States:

- Green, the most common cabbage, has a mild flavor that can be enjoyed raw or cooked.
- Red cabbage is similar to the green varieties, but it is much higher in vitamin C than other types.
- Savoy cabbage has ruffled yellow-green outer leaves and is higher in beta carotene than other varieties.
- Bok choy, or Chinese cabbage, forms a celerylike stalk of white leaves; it is higher in calcium.

CAFFEINE

BENEFITS

- Temporarily enhances mental alertness and concentration.
- Can improve athletic performance by temporarily increasing endurance.
- May abort an asthma attack by relaxing constricted bronchial muscles.

DRAWBACKS

- Is mildly addictive and can result in withdrawal symptoms.
- Can cause insomnia.
- Excessive amounts can produce tremors, palpitations, and feelings of anxiety.
- Diuretic effect increases urination.
- Lowers the body's absorption of calcium by increasing the amount lost in urine and stools.
- Can increase blood pressure.

By far our most popular (and least harmful) addictive drug, caffeine is the stimulant in coffee, tea, chocolate, and soft drinks; it is also added to some painkillers, cold medications, weight-loss supplements, and drugs used to promote mental alertness. Within a few minutes after caffeine is ingested, it is absorbed from the small intestine into the bloodstream and carried to all the body's organs. It speeds the heart rate, stimulates the central nervous system, increases the flow of urine and the production of digestive acids, and relaxes smooth muscles, such as those that control the blood vessels and the airways.

Although caffeine in moderation is generally harmless, sudden withdrawal can often cause headaches, irritability, and other symptoms that vary in severity from one person to another. For example, in some people who are sensitive to caffeine, the substance can trigger migraine headaches, while in others it might actually abort a migraine by relaxing the constricted blood vessels that are causing the throbbing head pain. People with some types of heart-valve disease are very often advised to forgo caffeine altogether because it can provoke heart palpitations or other cardiac arrhythmias.

DID YOU KNOW?

COFFEE MAY KEEP ALZHEIMER'S AT BAY

It is possible that drinking coffee could help stave off Alzheimer's disease. In one small study, drinking three cups a day reduced the risk of developing Alzheimer's by as much as 60 percent.

CAFFEINE: A KNOWN PERFORMANCE ENHANCER

The stimulant in caffeine enhances mental performance by increasing alertness and the ability to concentrate. For many people a cup of coffee helps them "get going" in the morning, and coffee or tea breaks during the day give them a boost when energy lags.

Athletes have long observed that one or two caffeine drinks an hour before competition can improve performance, especially in endurance sports like distance running. Studies confirm that 250 mg of caffeine—the amount in two cups of strong coffee—increases endurance, presumably because caffeine increases the body's ability to burn fat for fuel. However, while high doses may improve performance, they can also cause side effects and any athlete must be aware of his individual tolerance.

POTENTIAL SIDE EFFECTS

Ingestion of caffeine late in the day can result in a sleepless night, and excessive intake can lead to caffeinism, a syndrome marked by insomnia, feelings of anxiety and irritability, a rapid heartbeat, tremors, and excessive urination. These symptoms abate with the gradual withdrawal of caffeine. Otherwise, caffeine is relatively nontoxic; a fatal adult dose of the stimulant would require rapidly consuming the amount found in 80 to 100 cups of coffee.

Because caffeine, especially that in coffee, increases the production of stomach acid, ulcer patients are often advised to limit coffee (including decaffeinated) consumption to one cup after a meal. Many ulcer patients can tolerate tea, however.

Caffeine can prompt a modest temporary rise in blood pressure; it also speeds up the heart rate. There's no need for most heart patients to eliminate coffee or tea from their diets, but they should use it in moderation—cardiologists generally advise no more than 400 to 450 mg of caffeine per day. Older people with hypertension may be more sensitive to caffeine and should limit their intake to one cup per day.

The safety of caffeine consumption during pregnancy is controversial. Some studies suggest that drinking one or two cups of coffee each day is associated with a very small increase in risk of miscarriage and low-birth-weight babies but others do not. There is stronger evidence that drinking large amounts of caffeine daily during pregnancy may increase risk of a miscarriage, preterm delivery or having a low-

SOURCES OF CAFFEINE

Coffee is our most prevalent caffeinated drink; however, many other products also contain caffeine. The following chart shows how much caffeine can be found in some of the most common sources.

AVERAGE CAFFEINE CONTENT

COFFEE (5 oz/150 ml)	Milligrams
Decaffeinated	1–5
Espresso (2 oz/60 ml)	90–100
Ground:	
Drip method	100–180
Percolated	75–170
Instant	65–120

TEA (5 oz/150 ml)	
Brewed, 1 min.	9–33
Brewed, 3 min.	20–46
Brewed, 5 min.	20–50
Decaffeinated	1–5
Iced tea (from mix)	22–36
Instant	12–28

SOFT DRINKS (12 oz/355 ml)	
Coca-Cola (Cherry, Classic, or diet)	46
Diet Pepsi	36
Dr. Pepper (regular and diet)	40
Pepsi-Cola	38
RC Cola (regular and diet)	48
Sunkist Orange	40

CHOCOLATE	
Baking chocolate (2 oz/60 g)	70
Cold chocolate milk (8 oz/240 ml)	2–7
Hot cocoa (6 oz/180 ml)	5
Milk chocolate candy (2 oz/60 g)	12
Sweet or dark chocolate (2 oz/60 g)	40

PAINKILLERS	
Anacin, 400 mg aspirin	32
Bayer Select, 500 mg acetaminophen	65
Excedrin, 500 mg aspirin/acetaminophen	65

birth-weight baby. Some experts suggest that women avoid coffee during pregnancy while others recommend that pregnant women limit their daily caffeine consumption to about 150 mg—the amount found in one-and-a-half cups of coffee—spread over the entire day. Because caffeine enters breast milk, nursing mothers should either skip caffeinated beverages altogether or consume them at least 3 hours before breast-feeding.

Caffeine reduces calcium absorption, which can increase the risk of osteoporosis, especially in older women. Those who are heavy coffee drinkers should either consume more milk, low-fat yogurt, and other high-calcium foods or consider taking calcium supplements.

Some people prefer decaffeinated coffee but worry that the decaffeination process introduces some undesirable substances into the coffee. While the process may be harmful to the flavor of the coffee, it is not harmful to its drinker. Basically green coffee beans are soaked in water to extract the caffeine. This solution is then treated with a solvent in which caffeine is highly soluble. The solvents that are used never come into contact with the beans themselves and in any case are readily removed. ❖

DO ONE SIMPLE THING

WASH YOUR ASPIRIN DOWN WITH COLA

If you are taking aspirin for a headache, wash it down with a glass of cola. The caffeine will help the pain medication work faster. It may also fight the headache directly by relaxing the constricted blood vessels in the head. Just don't go overboard: Too much caffeine can trigger a rebound headache.

POTENT POTABLES. *One source of caffeine is the kola nut, from which cola is made.*

CAKES, COOKIES, AND PASTRIES

BENEFITS

- In small amounts, a good source of quick energy.
- Delicious occasional snacks or desserts.

DRAWBACKS

- Most are high in fat and calories.
- Generally contain low amounts of most vitamins and minerals.
- Often contain trans fatty acids.

Although high on most people's list of favorite foods, cakes, cookies, pies, and other pastries are low on the scale of nutritious choices. Most are high in fats, sugar and other sweeteners, and calories—but relatively low in vitamins, minerals, protein, and starches. Worst of all, most packaged crackers and baked goods are loaded with trans fats, man-made fats that contribute to heart disease (see Atherosclerosis). If you see the word "hydrogenated" on the nutrition label, the food contains trans fats. Anyone who wants to avoid gaining weight should minimize consumption of these foods. Unfortunately, many people find it hard to resist overindulging in such foods, often at the expense of more nutritious items.

Refined flour, sugar, fat, eggs, and milk or cream are the basic ingredients in most cakes, cookies, and pastries. Solid and highly saturated fats, such as vegetable shortening, lard, butter, and palm and coconut oils, are generally more suitable for baking than liquid vegetable oils and reduced-fat margarines. Thus, the fats found in most baked goods are the types that are most likely to raise the blood levels of the detrimental low-density lipoprotein (LDL) cholesterol.

MYTH BUSTER

Myth: Low-fat cookies are better for you than regular cookies.

Reality: According to the latest thinking, it doesn't do any good to replace the fat in your diet with sugar. And low-fat cookies usually contain more sugar.

EIGHT TIPS FOR HEALTHIER BAKING

In recent years commercial and home bakers alike have developed low-sugar, low-fat versions of many cakes, cookies, and pies. Some of these lack the flavor and texture of their traditional counterparts, but others are quite acceptable alternatives. Don't be afraid to experiment with your favorite recipes; in general, fat can be cut by one-third or more and sugar by up to one-half without substantially jeopardizing texture and flavor. Here are a few tips for cutting fat and sugar.

1. Try using applesauce, strained prunes, mashed bananas, and other pureed fruits as substitutes for at least some of the fat in cookie and cake recipes. The fruit adds the moisture and texture generally contributed by fat; it also imparts sweetness and extra flavor.

2. Reduce or even eliminate sugar in fruit pies; use extra cinnamon and other spices to perk up flavor.

3. Cut the fat content in pies by using one crust; reduce it even further with a low-fat graham cracker crust or make a deep-dish crustless pie or cobbler. A low-fat graham cracker crust is a nutritious and flavorful alternative to the traditional butter crust used to make a fruit tart.

4. Discard half the egg yolks and increase the number of whites when baking a cake or cookies; this increases the protein and at the same time cuts down on fat and cholesterol.

5. Substitute condensed skim milk for cream in frostings and pie fillings. Similarly, try strained yogurt cheese instead of high-fat cream cheese for toppings and fillings. Fruit and fruit sauces are other options for low-calorie toppings.

6. Increase the nutritional content and cut the fat calories in cookies by sticking with old favorites like oatmeal cookies or fruit bars. These can be made even more healthful by substituting applesauce or strained prunes for part of the fat, using whole-wheat flour, and loading them with raisins and other dried fruits instead of nuts.

7. For a festive occasion, serve a chocolate angel food cake with fresh berries and strawberry or raspberry sauce; it has virtually no fat and a fraction of the calories contained in a comparable piece of devil's food cake with chocolate cream frosting.

8. Make a light lemon cheesecake by using a combination of nonfat cottage and ricotta cheeses and condensed skim milk, lemon zest, and egg whites. Top the cake with strained yogurt instead of sour cream.

The high sugar content can promote tooth decay and may pose a problem for some people with diabetes. Recent studies show, however, that most diabetics can tolerate moderate amounts of sweet foods.

Carrot cakes, zucchini and banana breads, and other such commercial baked goods are often promoted as healthy alternatives. In fact, most of these contain only negligible amounts of the fruit or vegetable, are still high in fat and sugar, and are often topped with butter frosting. However, these can be made healthier by using low-fat substitutes for some ingredients. ❖

CANCER

EAT PLENTY OF
- Citrus and other fruits and dark green or yellow vegetables for vitamin C, beta carotene, bioflavonoids, and the plant chemicals that protect against cancer.
- Whole-grain breads and cereals and other high-fiber foods to promote smooth colon function.

LIMIT
- Fatty foods, especially those high in saturated fats.
- Alcoholic beverages.
- Salt-cured, smoked, fermented, and charcoal-broiled foods.

AVOID
- Foods that may contain pesticide residues and environmental pollutants.

Recent research has dramatically changed our thinking about the role of diet in both the prevention and treatment of cancer. It's increasingly clear that certain dietary elements may help promote the development and spread of malignancies, while others slow or block tumor growth. Researchers estimate that at least 35 percent of all cancers may be related to diet, especially one high in fat and processed foods; they also believe that many of these cancers could be prevented by dietary changes.

THE ANTICANCER DIET

Eat more fruits and vegetables. Compelling data associate a diet that provides ample fruits and vegetables with a reduced risk of many of our most deadly cancers. These foods are rich in bioflavonoids and other plant chemicals (see Antioxidants; Bioflavonoids); dietary fiber; folate, and antioxidants beta carotene and vitamin C. All of these substances may slow, stop, or reverse the processes that can lead to cancer. They do so through several protective mechanisms: by neutralizing or detoxifying cancer-causing agents (carcinogens); by preventing precancerous changes in cellular genetic material due to carcinogens, radiation, and other environmental factors; by inducing the formation of protective enzymes; and by reducing the hormonal action that can stimulate tumor growth. Folate is crucial for normal DNA synthesis and repair and low levels are thought to make cells vulnerable to carcinogenesis.

Reduce your fat intake. Equally important is a reduced intake of fats. Numerous studies link a high-fat diet and obesity with an increased risk of cancers of the colon, uterus, prostate, and skin (including melanoma, the most deadly form of skin cancer). The link between fat consumption and breast cancer is more controversial. Experts stress that no more than 30 percent of total calories should come from fats, and many advocate a 20 percent limit on fat calories. Often, it takes only a few simple dietary changes to lower fat intake; for example, choosing lean cuts of meat, trimming away all visible fat, eating vegetarian dishes several times a week, adopting low-fat cooking methods, such as baking and steaming, and limiting the use of added fats such as butter, margarine, mayonnaise, shortening, and oils.

Eat more fiber. Increased intake of fiber may protect against cancer in several ways. It speeds the transit of waste through the colon, which some researchers think cuts the risk of bowel cancer. A high-fiber, low-calorie diet also protects against obesity and the increased risk of cancers linked to excessive body fat (see Bran).

EAT YOUR VEGETABLES AND FRUITS!

The pigments and other chemicals that give plant foods their bright colors also seem to contribute to their cancer-fighting properties. Nutritionists now agree with the age-old urging of mothers and advise people to eat at least three different-colored vegetables and two different fruits daily. Choose from among the dark green leafy vegetables and the dark yellow, orange, and red fruits and vegetables. Include one serving of citrus a day, and strive to have a cruciferous vegetable. The members of the cruciferous (or cabbage) family include bok choy, broccoli, brussels sprouts, cabbage, cauliflower, collards, kale, kohlrabi, mustard greens, rutabagas, and turnips.

Most fruits and vegetables have more than one cancer-fighting benefit. Broccoli, for example, contains beta carotene, vitamin C, fiber, as well as the phytochemicals found in the vegetables of the cruciferous family. This is why nutritionists recommend a variety of foods instead of supplements as your first line of defense. Here are some of the fruits and vegetables superstars:

Best vitamin C: citrus fruits, strawberries, cantaloupe, kiwi, mango, broccoli, brussels sprouts, cauliflower, peppers, and potatoes.

Best beta carotene: sweet potatoes, carrots, squash, cantaloupe, pumpkin, broccoli, red peppers, apricots, mangoes, papaya, and kale.

Best fiber: corn, pears, broccoli, brussels sprouts, potatoes (with skin on), carrots, apples, berries, figs, prunes, peas, and Swiss chard.

Best folate: green leafy vegetables, spinach, orange juice, broccoli, avocado, asparagus, and brussels sprouts.

TOP CANCER-FIGHTING FOODS

Apples, berries, broccoli and other cruciferous vegetables, and citrus fruits contain flavonoids, which act as antioxidants. Flavonoids are also thought to prevent DNA damage to cells.

Tomatoes and tomato products contain lycopene, which has been found to have protective effects against prostate cancer.

Onions and garlic contain sulfur compounds that may stimulate the immune system's natural defenses against cancer, and they may have the potential to reduce tumor growth. Studies suggest that garlic can reduce the incidence of stomach cancer by a factor of 12.

Green tea contains EGCG, a catechin that may help fight cancer in three ways: it may reduce the formation of carcinogens in the body, increase the body's natural defenses, and supress cancer promotion. Some scientists believe that EGCG may be one of the most powerful anticancer compounds ever discovered.

Brazil nuts, seafood, some meats and fish, bread, wheat bran, wheat germ, oats, and brown rice are the best sources of selenium, a trace mineral that is another powerful cancer-fighter. In one major study, selenium significantly reduced the incidence of lung, prostate, and colorectal cancers in participants who received 200 mcg selenium for 4.5 years. This has led to follow-up studies investigating whether selenium in combination with vitamin E has a protective effect against prostate cancer. Plant foods, especially wheat, provide much of the selenium in the North American diet although their selenium content will vary according to the selenium content of the soil in which they are grown.

CANCER-FIGHTING FOODS. *A variety of fresh fruits and vegetables, high-fiber legumes, and whole-grain breads are not only high in vitamins and minerals, but may also protect against cancer.*

BREAK HIGH-RISK HABITS

Limit your alcohol intake. Doctors warn against heavy use of alcohol, which is associated with an increased risk of cancers of the mouth, larynx, esophagus, and liver. Excessive alcohol consumption hinders the body's ability to use beta carotene, which appears to protect against these cancers. Alcohol can also deplete reserves of folate, thiamine, and other B vitamins, as well as selenium. Folate is known to reduce proliferation of cancer cells; low levels of folate are also associated with an increased risk of cervical cancer. Researchers have found that giving folate supplements slows the proliferation of other precancerous cells.

Stop smoking. Smoking, more than any other lifestyle factor, increases the risk of cancer; stopping the habit is the most important step that a smoker can take to avoid cancer. In addition to lung cancer, smoking is strongly associated with cancers of the esophagus, mouth, larynx, pancreas, and bladder; recent studies also link it to an increased risk of breast cancer. For people who find it impossible to stop smoking, there are some dietary measures that can somewhat lower their cancer risk. One is to consume broccoli or related cruciferous vegetables several times a week. These members of the cabbage family are known to be appreciably high in certain cancer-fighting compounds, including bioflavonoids, indoles, monoterpenes, phenolic acids, and plant sterols, precursors to vitamin D. Sulforaphane, a chemical particularly abundant in broccoli, is one of the most potent anticancer compounds identified to date; various studies show that eating broccoli several times a week lowers the incidence of lung cancer among smokers compared to those whose diet does not include the vegetable.

Low levels of vitamin C are linked to an increased risk of many of the cancers related to smoking. Because smoking works to deplete the body's reserves of vitamin C, it's a good idea for smokers to increase their intake of citrus fruits and other good sources of this nutrient. Similarly, smoking can deplete the body's stores of folate and other B-complex vitamins; increased consumption of lean meat, grains, fortified cereals, legumes, and green leafy vegetables may help counter this adverse effect.

Limit your consumption of processed foods. People who eat large amounts of smoked, pickled, cured, fried, charcoal-broiled, and processed meats have a higher incidence of stomach and esophageal tumors. Smoked foods contain polyaromatic hydrocarbons that are known carcinogens. The salt in pickled foods can injure the stomach wall and facilitate tumor formation. Nitrites, commonly found in bacon and hot dogs, as well as in processed meats, can form nitrosamines, established carcinogens. However, consuming these foods along with good sources of vitamins C and E reduces the formation of nitrosamines.

WHEN CANCER STRIKES

A qualified nutritionist should be part of any cancer treatment team, because both the disease and its treatment demand good nutrition as an aid to recovery. Surgery, which still remains the major treatment for cancer, also requires a highly nutritious diet for healing and recuperation. The cancer itself can cause nutritional problems that will require treatment along with the underlying disease; for example, colon cancer will often cause iron-deficiency anemia because of chronic intestinal bleeding.

Weight loss is common among most cancer patients. Most experience a loss of appetite as a result of the cancer itself; depression brought on by a diagnosis of a potentially fatal disease, as well as pain, understandably lessens any desire to eat. Cancer treatments, especially radiation and chemotherapy, curb appetite and produce nausea and other side effects. Surgery, too, can affect appetite and make eating undesirable, especially if it involves the digestive system. A qualified nutritionist can devise a diet or recommend supplements to provide the calories, protein, and other nutrients needed to maintain weight and promote healing.

Dietary guidelines for cancer patients must take into account the stage and type of malignancy. In most cases of early or localized cancer, patients are generally advised to follow a diet that is low in fat; high in whole-grain products and other starches; and high in fruits and vegetables. Fats, especially from animal sources, are discouraged because they are believed to support tumor growth. In contrast, fruits and vegetables contain an assortment of natural plant chemicals that are thought to retard the growth and spread of cancers.

Protein is essential because it helps the body repair tissue that has been damaged during treatment of the disease. Protein is also important for wound healing. Therefore, surgery patients should eat at least two—and more if possible—daily servings of lean meat, low-fat dairy products, eggs, fish and shellfish, or meat alternates such as tofu and other soy products. Many cancer patients find it difficult to tolerate red meat, however, because for some it takes on an unpleasant metallic taste; in such instances, substitute egg whites, poultry, and a combination of legumes and grains. They will provide the much-needed protein and zinc. In some cases, a prescription for supplements may be required.

EATING WHEN YOU HAVE CANCER

In many instances, loss of appetite, nausea, and other eating problems of cancer patients can be dealt with by changing daily habits and routines. The following tips have worked for many people.

- Plan your major meal for the time of day when you are least likely to experience nausea and vomiting. For many cancer patients, this is in the early morning. Otherwise, eat small, frequent meals and snacks throughout the day.

- Let someone else prepare the food; cooking odors often provoke nausea. Food that is served cold or at room temperature gives off less odor than hot food.

- If mouth sores are a problem, eat bland, pureed foods—for example, custards, rice and other puddings made with milk, and eggs, porridge, and blended soups. Avoid salty, spicy, or acidic foods. Sucking on zinc lozenges may speed the healing of mouth sores.

- Try to eat with others in a pleasant social atmosphere. Ask family members to bring home-cooked food to the hospital (but have them check with the dietitian first).

- Get dressed to eat, if possible, and strive to make meals visually attractive. A few slices of a colorful fruit give visual appeal to a bowl of oatmeal; a colorful napkin and bud vase perk up a tray of food.

- To overcome nausea, try chewing on ice chips or sucking on a ginger candy or sour lemon drop before eating. Sipping flat ginger ale or cola may also help.

- Rest for half an hour after eating, preferably in a sitting or upright position; reclining may trigger reflux, nausea, and vomiting.

- Pay extra attention to dental hygiene. If mouth sores hinder tooth brushing, make a baking soda paste and use your finger and a soft cloth to gently cleanse the teeth. Then rinse the mouth with a weak solution of hydrogen peroxide and baking soda. Diluted commercial mouthwashes freshen the breath, but avoid full-strength products that can further irritate sores.

- If a dry mouth makes swallowing difficult, liquefy foods in a blender or moisten them with low-fat milk, sauces, or gravies.

- If diarrhea is a problem (as is often the case during chemotherapy), avoid fatty foods, raw fruits, whole-grain products, and other foods that can make it worse. Instead, eat bland, binding foods, such as rice, bananas, cooked apples, and dry toast.

WISDOM OF THE BODY

Flying in the face of conventional wisdom, however, are recent recommendations from a growing number of cancer specialists who discourage urging some cancer patients to eat when they don't feel like it. In the past, forced feeding in the form of enriched dietary supplements, intravenous nutrition, or a gastric feeding tube was recommended to maintain nutrition, but these approaches usually did not result in weight gain or prolonged survival. Instead, many who were force-fed actually died sooner; experts now believe this may be because the feeding actually spurs tumor growth. Consequently, many medical scientists now believe that the anorexia and cachexia (a severe form of malnutrition and body wasting) that occurs in advanced cancer may be an example of the "wisdom of the body" as it attempts to starve the tumor. Although it may be difficult for family members and friends to watch loved ones stop eating and progressively lose weight, informed physicians now urge that, in some situations, cachectic patients be allowed to limit food intake while doctors undertake aggressive therapy to destroy the tumor. Once this is accomplished, appetite returns, and the lost weight is regained as recovery takes place.

THE LURE OF SUPPLEMENTS

Millions of North Americans take vitamin and mineral supplements, often in high doses. Most do so without consulting a doctor. Recent reports detailing the anticancer effects of antioxidants have resulted in greatly increased sales of high-dose supplements of beta carotene and vitamins A, C, and E. In theory, it is reasonable to assume that if a small amount of a nutrient protects against cancer, then a high dose should be even more protective. Unfortunately, this does not seem to be true. When consumed in the amounts that are generally found in foods, these nutrients do have an antioxidant effect, which prevents the potentially cancer-causing damage that occurs when the body uses oxygen. But when taken in the form of high-dose supplements, these substances may have an opposite effect; recent research indicates they may become pro-oxidants and may actually increase damage caused by free radicals, the unstable molecules released when the body uses oxygen. In addition, high doses of vitamin A can lead to toxicity. (It is best to consult with qualified professionals, including your doctor and pharmacist, before deciding to pursue high-dose supplement therapy.)

The situation may be quite different, however, for patients who are undergoing cancer treatment. Some may need high-dose supplements, while others may be advised to avoid certain nutrients. Since some forms of cancer treatment rely on the generation of free radicals to destroy cancer cells, the use of antioxidant supplements may be counterproductive. This is why it's important to consult a registered dietitian or nutritionist regarding any dietary change and supplementation. There is no scientific evidence to suggest that alternative therapies, which include Japanese maitake, Chinese herbs, blue-green algae, or shark cartilage extracts, have any added value in treating cancer. ❖

CANDIES

BENEFITS
- Flavorful source of quick energy.

DRAWBACKS
- High in calories and sometimes fat.
- Sugar candies can cause tooth decay.
- Licorice may raise blood pressure in susceptible people.

Candies offer little nutritional value, but they are enjoyed by people around the world. Occasional consumption of candy should not prove harmful to any healthy person who consumes an otherwise balanced diet.

Our preference for sweet tastes is evident at a very early age and is considered to be part of human evolution. For instance, edible berries and fruits tend to be sweet as opposed to the bitter taste of many poisonous plants.

Commercial candy production is generally believed to have begun when marzipan (a thick, creamy paste made of almonds and sugar) was brought to Italy and Spain through trade with the Arabs and Moors during the Middle Ages. In fact, the word candy is derived from the Arabic pronunciation of *khandakah*, the Sanskrit word for sugar.

European candies were first compounded by druggists who preserved herbs in sugar. Candies were rare treats, however, until the widespread cultivation of sugar cane and the development of large-scale refining processes in the 17th and 18th centuries. Modern candies are mostly variations on three basic forms: taffy, from the Creole French word for a mixture of sugar and molasses; nougat, from the Latin word for nutcake; and fondant, from the French for melting (which can be recognized in the texture of fudges and soft-centered chocolates and bars).

ENERGY HIGHS—AND LOWS

All candies are packed with simple sugars—sucrose, corn syrup, fructose—which supply about 375 calories in a 3½-oz (100-g) serving and provide quick energy because they rapidly convert to glucose, or blood sugar. Unfortunately a rapid rise in blood sugar causes insulin levels to spike, which encourages the liver to convert sugar into fat. And when your blood sugar crashes after its high, you're likely to feel hungry again—and tired.

ADDITIVES AND SENSITIVITIES

Practically all hard candies are made with artificial flavors and colorings. There is no scientific evidence that the rigorously tested food dyes allowed in candy cause allergies or adverse reactions. These additives are included in minute amounts. Some people may be hypersensitive to the ingredients in a candy, but since candy is not an essential part of the diet, it's easy enough to avoid the offending sweet.

Natural licorice is known to raise blood pressure in certain people. The effect takes place mainly through salt retention. If you know you're hypertensive, you may be better off avoiding licorice. Most "licorice" candies in North America are artificially flavored and did not originate from the licorice root.

SWEETS AND TOOTH DECAY

Sweets and sugary foods form an acid bath that is corrosive to tooth enamel and creates an environment where destructive, caries-causing bacteria flourish. The effect is less harmful if you brush your teeth regularly to remove dental

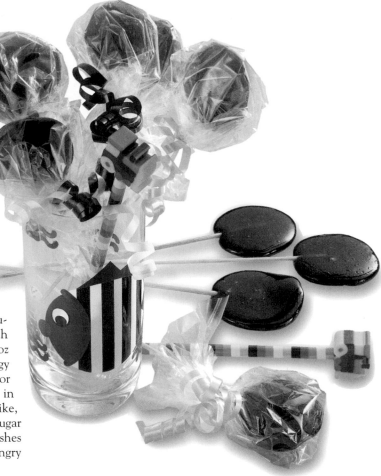

TRICK OR TREAT? *Babies respond positively to sugar the first time they taste it. Our affinity for sugar is probably in our genes.*

plaque. Candies that linger in the mouth are more damaging than those quickly swallowed.

When you can't brush after a meal, chewing sugarless gum may help to stimulate the saliva flow and flush food particles out of the mouth. "Sugarless" chewing gums fall into two categories. Some contain artificial sweeteners and therefore are very low in calories; others contain "sugar alcohols," such as xylitol. Although it does provide some calories, xylitol cannot be converted by bacteria in the mouth and on the teeth to acidic substances that erode tooth enamel. In rare cases sugar alcohols can cause diarrhea and gastric problems in those susceptible. ❖

MYTH BUSTER

Myth: Sweets make children hyperactive.

Reality: Many studies have shown that sugar does not cause hyperactivity, although some food dyes in candies may exacerbate existing hyperactivity.

CARBOHYDRATES
▪ A REASSESSMENT ▪

There is probably no greater debate today than the one over the role of carbohydrates in our diets. Low-carb diets such as the Atkins diet have captured the public's attention to an extent that few other weight-loss plans have. As a result, more and more people have come to believe that carbohydrates are inherently bad. But that's not entirely the case. Starches and sugars are our major source of energy. Fiber, another form of carbohydrate, also has significant health benefits.

Almost all of the starches and sugars that humans burn for energy come from plants; the only major exception is lactose, the sugar in milk. In effect, each plant is a complex food factory that takes water from the soil, carbon dioxide from the air, and energy from the sun to make glucose, a simple sugar that is later converted into starch. As the plant develops and grows, it also makes various vitamins, minerals, and other phytochemicals, as well as some fat and protein. Consequently, we can get our carbohydrates and most of the other nutrients needed to sustain us from the thousands of different grains, seeds, fruits, and vegetables that can be grown.

Carbohydrates are classified according to their chemical structure and digestibility; they are divided into two groups: simple and complex. Simple carbohydrates, or sugars, can generally form crystals that dissolve in water and are easily digested. Naturally occurring sugars are found in a variety of fruits, some vegetables, and honey. Processed sugars include table sugar, brown sugar, and molasses.

Complex carbohydrates have a range of textures, flavors, colors, and molecular structures. Composed of complex chains of sugars, these carbohydrates are further classified as starches or fiber. Our digestive system can break down and metabolize most starches, which are found in an array of grains, vegetables, and some fruits. Our digestive system, however, lacks the enzymes that are needed to break down most fiber, including cellulose and other woody parts of the plant skeleton, and pectin and other gums that hold plant cells together. But dietary fiber is still important because it promotes smooth colon function and may help prevent some types of cancer, heart attacks, and other diseases.

Energy food

Our body metabolizes simple carbohydrates and starches into glucose, or blood sugar, the body's primary source of fuel. Carbohydrates are high-quality fuels because—compared to proteins or fats—little is required of the body to break them down in order to release their energy.

Glucose, the only form of carbohydrate that the body can use immediately, is essential for the functioning of the brain, nervous system, muscles, and various organs. At any given time, the blood can carry about an hour's supply of glucose. Any glucose that is not needed for immediate energy is converted into glycogen, a large molecule composed of a chain of glucose units, which is stored in the liver and muscles; when necessary, the liver turns the glycogen back into glucose. The body can store enough glycogen to last for several hours of moderate activity.

Glycemic index (GI) researchers are learning that the rate at which carbohydrate-rich foods are digested and absorbed into the bloodstream also affects health. The rate at which a food causes blood sugar to rise can be measured and assigned a numerical value. This measure is referred to as the food's glycemic index (see Glycemic Index). Foods with a low GI such as pumpernickel bread, rye bread, brown rice, bulgur, oatmeal, lentils, yams, apples, pears, and yogurt take longer to digest and cause a slower, more gradual rise in blood sugar. This means that energy is released more slowly, leading to more consistent energy levels. Low-GI foods are better for blood sugar control in diabetics and may help with weight loss. The carbohydrates in high-GI foods such as white bread, white rice, mashed potato, corn flakes, and watermelon are more quickly absorbed and so provide a quicker source of energy. For active people high-GI foods can be a source of quick energy to aid short-duration sports performance and recovery, while lower-GI foods are better for endurance.

When glucose reserves run low, the body turns first to protein and then to fat for conversion into glucose. Burning protein, however, robs the body of lean muscle tissue. In addition, if the body has to burn fat in the absence of carbohydrates, toxic by-products called ketones are released; these can lead to a potentially dangerous biochemical imbalance.

Carbs: not all bad

Many people feel that the lower their carbohydrate intake is, the healthier they will be. A great deal of research shows that this is not the case. Choosing the healthiest carbohydrates, especially the whole grains, is important to your well-being. It is well-known that whole grains are important sources of fiber but newer research shows that health benefits can also be attributed to the vitamins, minerals, antioxidants, and other plant chemicals found in them. A number of important studies have shown that eating whole grains provides protection from diabetes, cancer, and heart disease. In a long-term study of nearly 90,000 women, and in a similar study of about 44,000 men, those who consumed the most cereal fiber had about a 30 percent lower risk of developing type 2 diabetes. The Nurses' Health Study, an ongoing survey monitored by the Harvard School of Public Health, also suggests a lower risk of heart disease and stroke among whole-grain eaters.

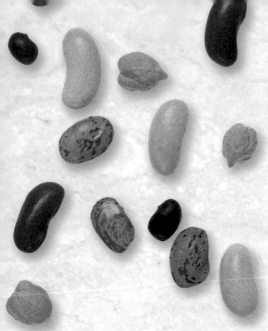

Carbohydrate primer

- Legumes, such as dried beans and peas, provide the best food value per dollar spent.
- Just because you don't see "sugar" listed as an ingredient on a food label doesn't mean it's not there. Look for words ending in "ose" (sucrose, lactose, maltose, fructose, glucose, and dextrose) and anything described as "syrup" (such as corn or malt syrup), as well as honey and molasses.
- Both carbohydrates and proteins provide 4 calories per gram, compared to 9 calories per gram of fat. Sugar and starches become fattening only when they are consumed with fatty additions or are eaten in quantities much larger than the body can readily use, in which case they are converted and stored as body fat.

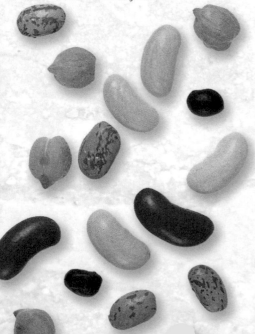

Complex carbohydrates

The human diet worldwide is based on complex carbohydrates. Populations that eat a higher-carbohydrate, low-fat diet generally enjoy good health. Vegetarian, Mediterranean, and Asian diets typically provide a high percentage of calories from complex carbohydrates in foods such as whole grains, lentils, beans, fruits, and vegetables. In North America, too much of the carbohydrate intake is in the form of simple sugars due to the high consumption of refined and processed foods. Another factor has been the proliferation of low-fat foods. Consumers often assume that these are also low-calorie foods. In many cases, fats have been replaced by carbohydrates with no great saving in calories. The many low-fat, high-carbohydrate foods available, including low-fat cookies, cakes, muffins, baked chips, and oversized bagels are all adding to expanding waistlines.

How much do you need?

In 2002, a joint American–Canadian expert report provided a set of reference values for nutrient intakes for healthy Americans and Canadians. It suggests that adults get 45 to 65 percent of their caloric intake from carbohydrates. This translates to roughly 225 to 325 g of carbohydrates each day for a 2,000-calorie diet. Both children and adults should consume at least 130 g of carbohydrates a day. This is based on the minimum amount needed to produce enough glucose for the brain to function. This amount is easily exceeded in the average North American diet. The problem is that the excess usually comes from refined carbohydrates.

Although refined carbohydrates, such as white flour and white rice, are just as good energy sources as whole-wheat flour and brown rice, processing removes many essential nutrients, including the B vitamins, iron, and other minerals, as well as dietary fiber. The best approach is to build a diet around whole or lightly processed grains, legumes, beans, and raw or slightly cooked vegetables and fruits.

Carb loading

Nutrition can have a significant impact on athletic performance and vice versa. Regular exercise increases the body's ability to utilize glucose efficiently and to store glycogen in muscle tissue. Thus, the fitter you are, the greater your ability to store the extra glycogen that is needed for endurance events, such as running a marathon or cross-country skiing. That's why carbohydrates are the preferred fuel for most sports.

Special concerns

Carbohydrates can be worked into almost any diet, but certain diseases may need adjustments. Diabetics must manage the total amount and type of carbs eaten at each meal and snack. Contrary to popular belief, sugar does not cause diabetes, nor do diabetics have to completely avoid sugar.

Those with heart disease need to emphasize high-fiber complex carbohydrates in their diet. Soluble fiber, found in oat bran and fruit pectin, helps lower cholesterol and plays an important role in preventing atherosclerosis, the buildup of fatty deposits in coronary arteries and other blood vessels.

Cancer patients are often advised to increase their carbohydrate intake and decrease fat intake, especially if they have cancers of the breast, colon, uterus, prostate, or skin. Evidence suggests certain fats may encourage tumor growth.

CARDIOVASCULAR DISEASE

EAT PLENTY OF

- Fresh fruits and vegetables, foods rich in vitamin C, beta carotene, and other antioxidant nutrients.
- Fish.
- Soy protein.
- Apples, oat bran, and other soluble fiber foods.
- Whole-grain breads and cereals.
- Nuts.

LIMIT

- Saturated fats in fatty meats, chicken skin, full-fat dairy products, coconut oil, and lard.
- Eggs, whole milk, organ meats, and other high-cholesterol foods.
- Fats, especially those that are saturated.
- Trans fatty acids found in partially hydrogenated margarine and shortenings, processed foods made with partially hydrogenated fats, and baked goods.

AVOID

- Excessive alcohol.
- Tobacco use in any form.
- Salty foods (if you have hypertension).

Heart and blood vessel disease remain leading causes of death in North America despite dramatic reductions in their incidence since the 1960s. Roughly one in five North Americans will suffer a heart attack and a million die every year as a result of a stroke or heart attack. In addition to the risk for premature death, cardiovascular disease represents a heavy financial burden to the health care system.

There have been numerous population studies since the early 1950s that have confirmed beyond any doubt that diet is a major force in both the cause and prevention of heart disease. One of the most extensive research projects is the Framingham Heart Study, which has followed more than 5,000 men and women in this Boston, Massachusetts, suburb for more than 40 years. Another large-scale study, the "Seven Countries Study" compared the incidence of heart disease among men in seven countries and then correlated these statistics with diet, smoking habits, physical activity, and other lifestyle factors.

By carefully analyzing the results, researchers have identified certain risk factors that predispose people to heart disease: heredity, advancing age, and gender (premenopausal women have a lower risk than men and older women) are among those over which people have no control. Tobacco use tops the list of controllable risk factors.

Poor diet is instrumental in most other factors: these include high blood cholesterol, which promotes the buildup of fatty deposits in the coronary arteries and leads to angina and heart attacks; obesity, which increases the risk of heart attack and contributes to other cardiovascular risk factors; high blood pressure, which can lead to a stroke and heart attack; diabetes, a disease that affects the heart, blood vessels, and other vital organs; and excessive alcohol use, which harms the heart and blood vessels.

A HEART-HEALTHY DIET

If the wrong diet can promote heart disease, the right one can reduce the risk. This is true, even in the face of such unalterable risk factors as advancing age and a family history of heart attacks.

There is nothing radical about a heart-healthy diet; in fact, it's the same common-sense balanced regimen that protects against cancer, adult-onset diabetes, and obesity. Complex carbohydrates, especially whole-grain breads and cereals, beans and other legumes, along with ample fresh fruits and vegetables form the foundation. About 10 to 12 percent of daily calories should come from protein foods—lean meat, fish, poultry (without the skin), egg whites, and a combination of grains and legumes (beans and rice, for instance, together make up a complete source of protein). Saturated and trans fats, sugars, and salt should be used sparingly.

Ideally, smart eating should be instilled during childhood, which is when atherosclerosis—the clogging of arteries with fatty deposits—begins. It takes 20 to 30 years—in some cases even longer—for the vessels to become clogged enough to produce symptoms. By that time, however, it may be too late; in a distressing number of cases, the first indication of heart disease is a fatal heart attack.

In addition to encouraging a low-fat diet, it's also a good idea to accustom children to the natural flavor of foods, rather than adding lots of salt. While there are some conflicting reports, numerous studies show that populations with a high intake of salty foods have an

WINE AS MEDICINE?

For years, researchers have tried to determine why the French have fewer heart attacks than their counterparts in other industrialized countries. It would seem that the high-fat diet and pervasive tobacco use for which the French are renowned, would predispose them to more, not less heart disease. Increasingly, researchers have settled on wine as the protective factor, although there is uncertainty over exactly what it is in wine that benefits the heart.

It should be noted, though, that French lifestyle may also play a part. They eat more fresh fruits and vegetables and consume far fewer calories than North Americans. They also eat much less refined sugar and take longer vacations.

increased incidence of hypertension.

A group of researchers in Finland identified excessive iron as another dietary factor that may well damage the heart and blood vessels. Their research found that men with high levels of iron in their blood also had an increased incidence of heart attacks.

While it was already well known that excessive iron damages the heart, liver, and other vital organs, this was the first time that iron levels in the high–normal range were linked to a serious health risk. It reinforces the long-standing

YOU ARE WHAT YOU EAT. Vegetables, beans, whole grains, and lean protein make up a heart-healthy diet.

advice not to take any supplements without first consulting a doctor.

THE CHOLESTEROL FACTOR

Excessive cholesterol circulating in the blood is the major precipitating factor in atherosclerosis. In rare cases, an inherited disorder, familial hypercholesterolemia, causes high blood cholesterol. Without a stringent low-fat diet and cholesterol-lowering drugs, people with this disorder invariably suffer an early heart attack—sometimes during childhood. Far more often, high cholesterol is caused by diet, lack of exercise, and other lifestyle habits.

For most people, moderately elevated cholesterol levels can be lowered by adopting a diet with less than 30 percent (but preferably 20 percent) of its calories coming from fats, mostly the monounsaturated and polyunsaturated types found in plant oils, fish, nuts, and seeds. Doctors have traditionally advised using margarine, especially the kinds made with corn, safflower, and other unsaturated fats, instead of butter. But the trans fatty acids in hardened margarine may raise LDL cholesterol levels even more than butter's mostly saturated fat does. A soft margarine made from nonhydrogenated fats is probably the best choice. Several such brands are now available.

SUPERSTAR FOODS AND NUTRIENTS

Fruits and vegetables. Numerous studies correlate a diet rich in fresh fruits and vegetables with a 25 percent or better reduction in heart attacks and strokes. Researchers believe that it's the ample vitamin C, beta carotene, and other antioxidants in fruits and vegetables that account for the difference. Antioxidants protect cells against damage from the unstable molecules that are released when the body uses oxygen. Oxidation of LDL cholesterol—the type that forms fatty plaque—is thought to be instrumental in initiating atherosclerosis. Fruits and vegetables are also high in bioflavonoids and other plant chemicals that act as antioxidants.

Fish. Salmon, sardines, herring, trout, and other fatty cold-water fish are high in omega-3 fatty acids, which reduce the tendency of blood to clot. This benefit can be had from consuming two or three servings of fish a week. Although fish oil supplements are high in omega-3 fatty acids, they should not be taken without approval by a doctor, because they may increase the risk of a stroke. Omega-3 fats are also found in plant sources including canola, soybean, and flaxseed oil, soft, nonhydrogenated margarines, ground flaxseed, and nuts.

Soluble fiber. Pectin, oat bran, and other types of soluble fiber help lower cholesterol and improve glucose metabolism in people predisposed to develop diabetes. Oats, oat bran, psyllium, flax, lentils, legumes, apples, pears, grapes, and other fruits are high in soluble fiber. A combination of legumes and grains is a prudent low-fat meat alternative.

Whole-grain foods. Several studies have found that diets high in whole-grain foods such as whole-wheat bread and whole-grain cereals reduce the risk of coronary heart disease. They contain a variety of important vitamins and minerals, as well as phytochemicals with antioxidant properties.

Soy. A large body of evidence has shown that adding soy protein to a low-fat diet lowers the risk for heart disease. Soy contains plant compounds called isoflavones that appear to benefit the heart. Together they help to lower cholesterol levels. Soy protein is found in soybeans and products made from these beans, including tofu and soy beverages.

Special margarines. Plant sterols have been shown to help lower cholesterol levels when consumed as part of a heart-healthy diet. They are found in plant-sterol enriched margarines (not available in Canada), vegetable oils, nuts, sesame and sunflower seeds, soy, and legumes.

Olive and canola oil. The omega-6 polyunsaturated fats found in safflower, sunflower, corn, cottonseed, and soybean oils reduce cholesterol levels when they replace saturated fats in the diet.

Monounsaturated fats tend to lower total and LDL cholesterol levels when they replace saturated fats in the diet. They are found in oils such as olive and canola.

Folate. Green leafy vegetables, orange juice, lentils, enriched cereals, and asparagus are good sources of folate, which can lower heart disease risk by helping to regulate homocysteine levels. Homocysteine forms in the body from methionine, a common amino acid, and high levels are considered to be as dangerous a risk factor for heart disease as high levels of cholesterol. Folate works together with vitamins B_6 and B_{12} to keep homocysteine levels from accumulating. B_6 is found in meat, poultry, fish, legumes, nuts, seeds, leafy greens, bananas, and whole grains. B_{12} is found in animal foods such as meat, fish, and poultry.

Nuts. Nuts and seeds, used moderately, are rich sources of fiber, vitamin E, essential fatty acids, and minerals all linked to heart health. Studies have shown that adding nuts to the diet lowers risk of heart disease.

DO SUPPLEMENTS HELP?

Although observational studies suggest that antioxidants from food sources play a protective role against cardiovascular disease, studies using supplements have proved disappointing. One trial found no significant benefits from taking daily supplements of vitamin E, beta carotene and vitamin C in people at high risk. And, the relationship between vitamin E and prevention of heart disease is still not resolved. Some research has even shown that antioxidant supplements may reduce the efficacy of the "statin" type cholesterol lowering drugs.

FOOD AS MEDICINE

A study published in the July 2003 issue of the *Journal of the American Medical Association* suggests that a low-fat vegetarian diet may be just as good as the "statin" drugs at lowering high cholesterol levels. Forty-six adults with high cholesterol levels were put on either a low saturated fat diet, the same diet plus medication, or a strict vegetarian diet that included soy proteins, high-fiber foods, and a margarine containing plant sterols. The researchers found that the subjects on the vegetarian diet lowered their cholesterol levels by almost 29 percent compared with a decrease of 30 percent in those who followed the low-fat diet with medication during that same time. Those following only the low-fat diet had just an 8 percent drop in cholesterol.

Although more research is needed, these positive results underline the great importance of diet as an option for those people who are working to lower their cholesterol levels. There are a number of dietary factors in this vegetarian diet that help lower cholesterol: the soy protein, the plant sterols, and the soluble fiber found in fruits, vegetables, and grains such as oats and barley. ❖

DID YOU KNOW?

HIGH HOMOCYSTEINE LEVELS CAN BE JUST AS DANGEROUS TO YOUR HEART AS SMOKING OR HIGH CHOLESTEROL

Twenty-five percent of North Americans dying from cardiovascular diseases don't have high blood pressure, high LDL cholesterol, don't smoke and aren't excessively overweight. High levels of homocysteines in the blood may be the culprit. Homocysteine is an amino acid known to damage the walls of an artery when it reaches high concentrations in the blood.

CARROTS

BENEFITS

- An excellent source of beta carotene, the precursor of vitamin A.
- A good source of dietary fiber and potassium.
- Help prevent night blindness.
- May help lower blood cholesterol levels and protect against cancer.

DRAWBACKS

- Excessive intake can give skin a yellowish tinge.

Native to Afghanistan, carrots are our most abundant source of beta carotene, a compound that can function as an antioxidant and can also be converted by the body into vitamin A. The more vivid the color of the carrot, the higher the levels of this important carotenoid. One cup of cooked carrots has 70 calories, 4 g of fiber, and about 18 mg of beta carotene. This provides more than 100 percent of the Recommended Dietary Allowance of vitamin A—a nutrient essential for healthy hair, skin, eyes, bones, and mucous membranes. Vitamin A also helps prevent infections.

A U.S. government study found that volunteers who ate about one cup of carrots a day had an average 11 percent reduction in their blood cholesterol levels after only 3 weeks. Lowered cholesterol levels, in turn, decrease the risk of heart disease. The cholesterol-lowering effect is likely due to the high soluble-fiber content of carrots, mostly in the form of pectin.

SEEING IN THE DARK

Carrots will not prevent or correct our most common vision problems, such as nearsightedness or farsightedness. But a deficiency of vitamin A does cause night blindness, an inability of the eyes to adjust to dim lighting or darkness. Vitamin A combines with therotein opsin in the retina's rod cells to form rhodopsin, which is needed for night

TAKE CARROTS TO HEART

Studies show that high doses of beta carotene may help reduce the risk of cardiovascular disease by about 45 percent. Carrots are one of the richest sources of this important carotenoid. Studies also indicate that high doses of beta carotene in pill form will not help prevent heart disease.

vision. Eating one carrot every few days provides enough vitamin A to prevent or overcome night blindness, if this condition is caused by vitamin A deficiency.

COOKED OR RAW?

Naturally sweet, carrots make an ideal high-fiber, low-calorie snack food. Interestingly, cooking actually increases carrots' nutritional value, because it breaks down the tough cellular walls that encase the beta carotene. To properly absorb beta carotene, the body needs a small amount of fat, because carotenoids are fat, not water soluble. Adding a pat of butter or margarine to cooked carrots ensures that the body will fully utilize this nutrient. Cooked and pureed carrots are an ideal beginner food, as they are naturally sweet and high in nutrients.

Carrots also contain other carotenoids, including alpha carotene, as well as bioflavonoids. The beneficial effects of carrots may not be reproduced by taking isolated supplements. Indeed, a number of studies have shown that beta carotene supplements may actually be harmful, particularly to smokers. This is not a problem with an excessive intake of carrots, but it can result in the skin taking on a yellow-orangish tinge. This harmless condition, called carotenemia, disappears in a few weeks of reducing carrot intake. If the yellow skin color persists, or if the white portions of the eyes are also discolored, the problem may be jaundice, a symptom of a liver disorder. ❖

CAULIFLOWER

BENEFITS

- An excellent source of vitamin C.
- A good source of folate and potassium.
- Low in calories and high in fiber.
- An anticancer food.

Cauliflower is rich in vitamin C, folate, and various other phytochemicals linked with good health. A cup of raw cauliflower florets has more than 50 percent of the Recommended Dietary Allowance (RDA) of vitamin C, 15 percent of the RDA for folate, and reasonable amounts of potassium and vitamin B_6. It also has bioflavonoids, indoles, and other chemicals that protect against cancer.

Filling, high in fiber, and low in calories (25 in a cup of florets), this is an ideal snack food for weight watchers. Raw cauliflower has more folate (80 percent is lost in cooking).

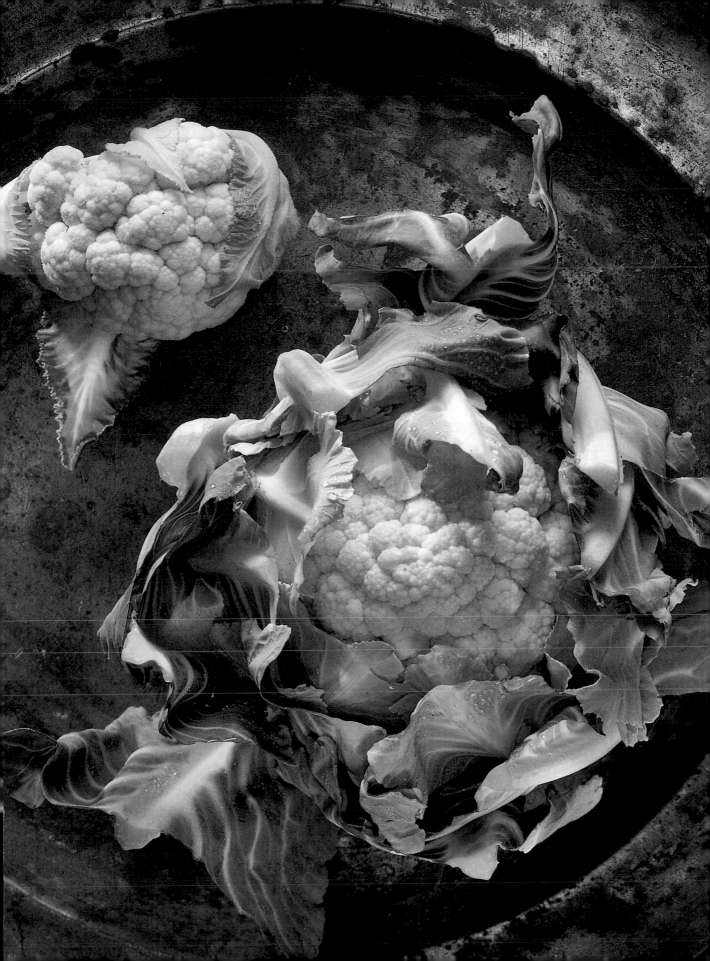

To retain flavor and reduce nutrient loss, cook cauliflower rapidly by boiling in a minimum amount of water or steaming. Too much cooking turns cauliflower mushy and releases sulfurous compounds, resulting in an unpleasant odor and bitter taste. Boiling the vegetable in an open pot helps disperse these compounds. To avoid discoloring the cauliflower, don't cook it in aluminum or iron pots.

When buying cauliflower, look for a head with firm, compact florets. If it is fresh, the leaves will be crisp and green, and the head, or curd, snowy white. Broccoflower is a hybrid of cauliflower and broccoli; it resembles cauliflower but is green and has a milder flavor. Another variety, purple cauliflower, has more beta carotene than the white variety. ❖

CELERIAC

BENEFITS

- Low in calories with small amounts of vitamins C and B$_6$.

DRAWBACKS

- Not readily available in many supermarkets and produce stores.

A winter root vegetable, celeriac is a member of the parsley family and is closely related to celery; in fact, its other names include celery root, knob celery, and German celery. Fresh celeriac resembles a large, round, knobby turnip, but when the tough outer skin is peeled away, the flesh is white, with a flavor and odor similar to celery.

Celeriac has a mild, celerylike flavor and lends itself to a variety of dishes. For example, it is often grated raw into salads, boiled and pureed to add body and flavor to soups and stews, chopped into poultry stuffing, or sliced, dipped in an egg batter, and sautéed to serve as a meat substitute. It is also served as an accompaniment to haddock, salmon, and spicy pork. The French cut celeriac into thin strips, blanch them, and toss them with a mustard-mayonnaise dressing to make an alternative to celery salad.

A half-cup serving of cooked celeriac contains 25 calories, 1.5 g of fiber, 5 mg of vitamin C, and some B$_6$ and phosphorus. It is nutritionally similar to celery, although it contains slightly more folate and iron. ❖

CELERY

BENEFITS

- Low in calories and a source of fiber.
- A good source of potassium.
- In significant amounts may reduce inflammation and protect against cancer.

Dieters tend to eat lots of celery because it is so low in calories, however, it is a misconception that chewing the stalks consumes more calories than the vegetable provides. Two stalks of celery contain less than 10 calories (celery is about 95 percent water by weight), yet their fiber content makes them very filling. Celery is a good source of potassium; it also contributes small amounts of vitamin C and some folate. Although it is not very high in nutrients, it adds a unique flavor to a variety of foods—from soups to salads and poultry stuffing.

Celery leaves are the most nutritious part of the plant, containing more calcium, iron, potassium, beta carotene, and vitamin C than the stalks. The leaves should be salvaged for soups, salads, and other dishes enhanced by the flavor of celery.

MEDICINAL PROPERTIES

Herbalists have advocated fresh celery and celery seed tea to treat gout and other forms of inflammatory arthritis, as well as high blood pressure and edema. Studies indicate that phthalides in celery may reduce the body's levels of certain hormones that constrict blood vessels and raise blood pressure. Polyacetylenes, also found in celery, are said to reduce production of certain prostaglandins, body chemicals that are instrumental in producing inflammation. There is no scientific proof, however, that celery can ease arthritis pain or lower blood pressure and increase urine output.

In theory, celery may help reduce the risk of certain cancers. The polyacetylenes destroy benzopyrene, a carcinogen that occurs in foods cooked at a high temperature. This benefit may be partially offset by celery's high levels of plant nitrates, substances that the body converts into nitrosamines, which are linked with an increased risk of cancer. However, many researchers believe that this is a minor risk because most plants high in nitrates and other potentially cancer-causing substances also contain chemicals that neutralize any harmful effects. Cooking celery by boiling, braising, or steaming lowers nitrate levels. ❖

CELIAC DISEASE

EAT PLENTY OF

- Low-fat milk, eggs, fish, meat, and poultry for protein.
- Vegetables and fruits for vitamins and minerals.
- Legumes, potatoes, and rice for starches, minerals, and protein.

AVOID

- Bread, pasta, cereals, cakes, and other wheat, rye, or barley products.
- Foods using wheat products as a thickening agent or coating, such as breaded foods, meat loaf, frankfurters, sausages, sauces, and soups.
- Beverages containing gluten, such as beer, malted drinks, and chocolate milk.
- Many commercial salad dressings except pure mayonnaise.

Celiac disease, also known as celiac sprue or nontropical sprue, is a disorder that affects about 1 out of every 133 Americans and 1 out of every 200 Canadians. Typically, the disorder becomes apparent when a young child starts eating foods containing wheat, rye, barley, and other cereal grains. The problem is caused by gliadin, one of the proteins collectively known as gluten, found in these grains. Gliadin combines with antibodies in the digestive tract to damage the walls of the small intestine and interfere with the absorption of many nutrients, especially fats and certain starches and sugars.

Children with the disease are usually plagued with such symptoms as stomach upsets, diarrhea, abdominal cramps, bloating, mouth sores, and an increased susceptibility to infection.

Their stool is pale and foul-smelling, and it floats to the top of the toilet bowl, indicating a high fat content. The child's growth may be stunted; some children develop anemia and skin problems, especially dermatitis. Diagnosis is confirmed by an inspection of the small intestine with a special viewing instrument and an intestinal biopsy indicating abnormalities characteristic of celiac disease.

People who develop celiac disease later in life may have had a mild or symptomless form of the disease in childhood. In unusual cases, adults with no prior history of gluten sensitivity develop the condition after surgery on the digestive tract. Women with celiac disease often fail to menstruate (amenorrhea) and may also have problems getting pregnant.

Once the disease has been identified, patients are advised to permanently eliminate any foods that contain gluten from their diet. A registered dietitian can assist in planning nutritionally balanced meals that are gluten-free. Most doctors also prescribe supplements to counter any nutritional deficiencies. If anemia is a problem, iron and/or folate supplements will also be recommended.

AVOIDING GLUTEN

Hundreds of everyday foods contain gluten: breads, cakes, rolls, muffins, baking mixes, pasta, sausages bound with bread crumbs, foods coated with batter, sauces and gravies, soups thickened with wheat flour, and most breakfast cereals, as well as some candies, ice creams, and puddings. Many baby foods are thickened with gluten, although most commercial first-stage foods are gluten-free.

Always read labels on packaged foods. Avoid ingredients such as flour-based binders and fillers and modified starch. Be suspicious of any label that specifies "other flours" because they are likely to include at least some wheat derivatives. Beer is made from barley and should be avoided, along with malted drinks.

Outside the home, order only plain foods, such as broiled fish or meat, steamed vegetables, and a baked potato—all without any sauces or dressings. Even communion wafers contain some gluten. However, gluten-free wafers are now available; check with your pastor.

DO ONE SIMPLE THING

STAY THE COURSE ON A GLUTEN-FREE DIET

When a person with celiac disease first starts a gluten-free diet, the body's healing response time may take several weeks or months. This is because of the time it takes for the lining of the digestive system to regrow. However, the immune system will remember gluten, and any further ingestion of gluten can cause prolonged damage.

Contrary to popular belief, people with celiac disease can eat pasta, bread, and other baked products, but they must look for gluten-free items, such as rice pasta and baked goods made with corn, rice, potato, or soy flours. Gluten-free flour is now available. In general, it is better to prepare most foods at home to assure a healthy diet without risking exposure to gluten.

It was once believed that oats also contained the offending gliadin protein, but some analyses have shown that they do not. Thus, doctors are now allowing patients to experiment with oat products; if they provoke symptoms, however, they should still be avoided. It is important to differentiate between pure oats and oat products that have been contaminated with wheat; care must be taken to avoid the latter. ❖

CEREALS

BENEFITS
- High in complex carbohydrates.
- Many are high in fiber.
- Enriched cereals are high in iron, niacin, thiamine, and riboflavin, along with other B vitamins.
- Iron-fortified infant cereals are ideal introductory solid foods.

DRAWBACKS
- Many commercial varieties are high in salt, sugar, and fat.
- Bran cereals can reduce the absorption of iron, zinc, and other minerals.
- High-bran products may cause bloating and flatulence.

Served hot or cold, cereals can be a healthful, low-calorie breakfast main dish. Many also make popular snacks and can be used as ingredients in meat loaf, muffins, and cookies. Since ancient times oatmeal and other cooked cereal porridges have been valued as much for their economy and ease of preparation as for their nutrition.

The first ready-to-eat cold cereals in North America were developed as health foods by the Western Health Reform Institute in Battle Creek, Michigan, founded by the Seventh-Day Adventists in 1866. The Adventists were seeking a vegetarian alterna-

tive to the traditional cooked breakfast of ham or bacon and eggs. It took another 30 years, however, for cold cereals to gain much of a following. In 1899 Dr. John Harvey Kellogg, the medical director of the Battle Creek Sanitarium (a health institute that specialized in the treatment of digestive diseases), and his brother Will invented a wheat-flake cereal to improve bowel function. A few years later they developed another cereal made of cornflakes. Adding to these developments, one of Dr. Kellogg's patients, C. W. Post, came up with a wheat and barley mixture that he called Grape Nut Flakes. Food companies founded by the Kellogg brothers and Post remain North America's leading producers of cold cereals, with dozens of different brands.

Although prepared cereals are gaining popularity in Europe and other parts of the world, they are generally considered a North American product with one notable exception—the granola-type mixture of oats, wheat flakes, nuts, and dried fruits invented by Dr. Max Bircher-Benner, a Swiss pioneer of the natural health-food movement in Europe. Variations of his muesli, which is served either hot or cold, are now popular in North America, as well as in most European countries.

Wheat, corn, rice, oats, and barley are the most familiar grains used to make cereals. Most flaked cereals are varying combinations of flour, water, sugar, and salt that are mixed into a dough, rolled thin, and then toasted. Some cereal preparations are spun into different shapes, such as tiny doughnuts or cartoon characters; in others, the grains are shredded or exploded.

NUTRITIONAL VALUE

Cereals are one of the most popular members of the complex carbohydrate, or starch, food group. More than 90 percent of all commercial cereals are enriched or fortified with various vitamins and minerals, especially iron, niacin, thiamine, vitamin B_6, and folic acid. Regulations about adding nutrients to cereals differ in the United States and Canada. In Canada enrichment is limited to a few nutrients whereas some American cereals can mimic vitamin pills. Unfortunately though, many of the cereals that hype their vitamin and mineral content are loaded with sugar. Better to eat an unsweetened cereal and take a vitamin pill.

Some cereals have added dried fruits and nuts—but usually not enough to justify their higher cost. An economical and healthful

DID YOU KNOW?

EATING BREAKFAST MIGHT HELP YOU LOSE WEIGHT

People who eat breakfast instead of skipping this meal have more success in losing weight.

approach is to buy plain cereal and add your own fresh fruits, raisins, seeds, nuts, or other ingredients. The granola-type cereals are often high in fat from added oils; many commercial cereals are also high in salt. It's best to make your own. If you use store-bought granola cereal, look for a low-fat brand.

Oat cereals are high in soluble fiber that helps lower blood cholesterol levels, thereby reducing the risk of heart disease. Some cereals, especially those made from whole grains or with added bran, are high in insoluble fiber as well. These help prevent constipation and may also reduce the risk of some cancers, including colon cancer. Whole-grain cereals rich in fiber are a convenient way to add more fiber to your diet. Look for a cereal that contains at least 3 g of fiber per serving. Just don't add too much bran to your diet all at once; it can cause bloating, abdominal discomfort, and intestinal gas and flatulence.

Most cereals are relatively low in calories, but this varies considerably, depending on the ingredients and how they are served. Serving whole milk can more than double the calorie content of many cereals. Using skim or 1-percent-fat milk saves calories and, for older children and adults, it is much healthier than whole milk. When you are comparing the calorie content of cereals, pay at-tention to serving sizes given on the package's nutrition label; some cereals are low in calories only when consumed in very small amounts.

Kids' cereals in particular are often extremely high in sugar. In fact, sugar may top the ingredients on the nutrition table, which means that the product has more sugar than anything else. Check the nutrition tables on other cereals to find a product that offers more fiber and less sugar. ❖

SOMETHING FOR EVERY TASTE. *Cold cereal with low-fat milk provides a flavorful low-calorie breakfast; for a heartier start, try oatmeal or other cooked cereal. Fruits add flavor and extra vitamins and minerals.*

CHEESE

BENEFITS

- High in protein and calcium.
- A good source of vitamin B_{12}.
- Cheddar and other aged cheeses may fight tooth decay.

DRAWBACKS

- Most are high in saturated fat and sodium.
- Some may trigger migraines or allergic reactions in susceptible people.

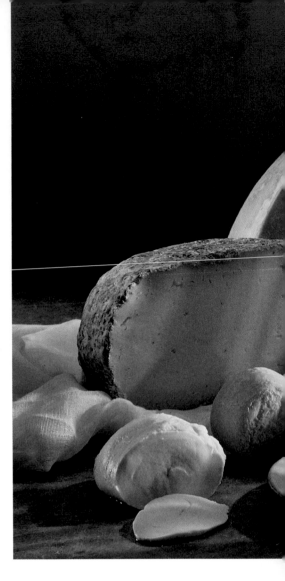

One of our most versatile and popular foods, cheese is used for everything from snacks and appetizers to main courses and desserts. It's an ancient food that can be made from the milk of almost any animal—cows, sheep, goats, yaks, camels, and buffaloes.

Most cheeses are made by adding a mixture of enzymes, known as rennet, to milk to curdle it. The main enzyme in rennet, which traditionally has been isolated from the stomach lining of calves, is chymosin. Today, it can also be produced by inserting the gene that codes for its production into bacteria. This allows for a more ready production of chymosin and can also cater to consumers who do not favor the idea of an animal extract in their cheese. The liquid that remains after the curds have formed is known as whey. When it is drained away, we are left with cottage or farmer's cheese. Or the curds may be mixed with other ingredients, injected with special molds or bacteria, soaked in wine or beer, pressed or molded, or smoked or aged to make any of hundreds of different cheeses.

On average, it takes about 4 qt (3.8 liters) of milk to make 1 lb (450 g) of Cheddar, Muenster, Swiss, or other firm cheese. A typical 1-oz (30-g) serving of cheese contains 115 calories, about 200 mg of calcium, and 9 g of fat. Cottage cheese has the fewest calories—about 90 in a half-cup serving, but it has only half the calcium of milk. Cream cheese, Brie, and other soft cheeses are comparable to hard cheeses in calories and fat, but have less calcium.

DO ONE SIMPLE THING

GO FOR FLAVOR, NOT FAT

Use small amounts of a highly flavorful hard cheese, such as romano, to add taste without adding a lot of fat.

EAT IN MODERATION

Cheese is rich in calcium and protein, making it a staple for vegetarians. But it's also high in fat, cholesterol, and sodium. Most people— especially those with a weight or cholesterol problem—should use it moderately, as an occasional treat or garnish rather than as a staple food. Exceptions include adolescents going through a growth spurt, vegetarians, and thin older women threatened by osteoporosis, a weakening of the bones. Many people who cannot digest milk because of lactose intolerance can eat cheese, especially the hard ones; the bacteria and enzymes used to make cheese also break down some of the lactose (milk sugar).

HEALTH HAZARDS

Doctors often advise patients with heart disease, elevated blood cholesterol, or high blood pressure to reduce the amount of cheese they consume. Because most cheese is high in cholesterol and its fat is highly saturated, it increases the risk of atherosclerosis, the clogging of arteries with fatty deposits. And the sodium it contains can be a hazard for people with high blood pressure.

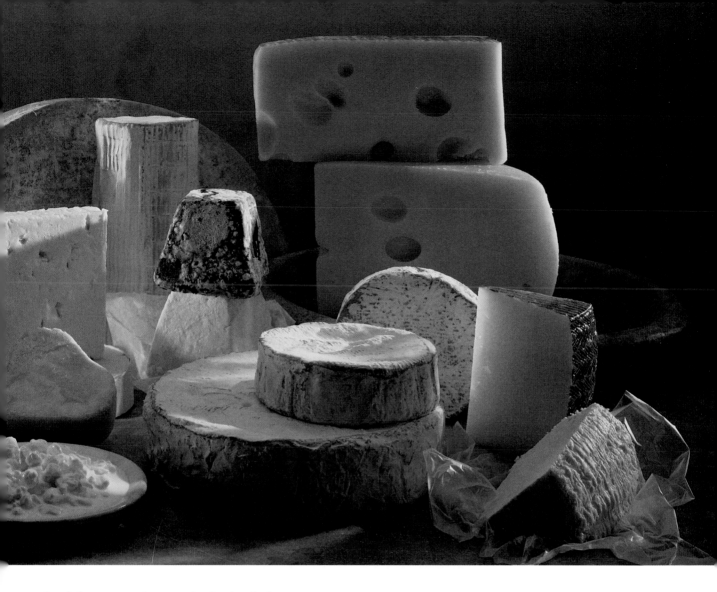

Aged cheese can trigger a migraine headache in some susceptible people. The likely culprit is tyramine, a naturally occurring chemical in Cheddar, blue cheese, Camembert, and certain other ripe cheeses. Tyramine also interacts with monoamine oxidase (MAO) inhibitors, drugs sometimes used to treat depression, and can cause a life-threatening rise in blood pressure. People taking MAO inhibitors should get a list of foods to avoid from their doctor.

People who are allergic to penicillin may react to blue cheese and other soft cheeses that are made with penicillin molds. Also those who are allergic to cow's milk may react to cheese, especially cottage and other fresh cheeses. Cheeses made from goat's or sheep's milk are less likely to be allergenic.

Pasteurized milk must be used to make commercial cheese in both the United States and Canada. Occasionally, however, health-food stores and specialty shops sell imported or homemade unpasteurized cheese. Such cheeses

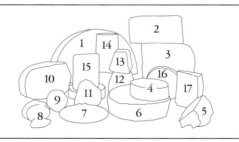

CHEESES FROM AROUND THE WORLD.
Cheddar (1), Emmental (2), Jarlsberg (3), Camembert (4, 6), Ricotta (5), Cottage cheese (7), Mozzarella (8), Crottin de Chavignol (9), Ticklemore (10), Cœur de chèvre (11), Natural pyramide (12), Ash pyramide (13), Chèvre (14), Feta (15), Little Rydings (16), Peccorino (17).

DID YOU KNOW?

CHEESE FIGHTS CAVITIES

Studies have shown that cheese can help you take a bite out of tooth decay. The fat naturally contained in cheese coats your teeth and acts as a natural barrier against bacteria. Also, all cheese contain casein, which provides a natural tooth protectant. And finally, the calcium and phosphorus found in cheese help remineralize tooth enamel.

can harbor dangerous salmonella and other bacteria; a case in point involved several food-poisoning deaths in the United States that were later traced to imported cheese made from raw milk.

LOW-FAT CHEESES

Fat gives cheese its rich texture and delicious taste, but it also adds calories and cholesterol. About 70 to 80 percent of the calories in cheese comes from fat. Even reduced-fat or part-skim milk cheeses can be high in fat; more than 50 percent of the calories in part-skim milk mozzarella come from fat. Historically, low-fat cheeses often lacked flavor, and tended to be high in salt to improve flavor; sodium phosphate may be used to create a smoother texture. Today, there is a broader range of tasty low-fat cheeses on the market. Cholesterol-free imitation cheeses are often made of soy, or tofu; they still can be high in fat and sodium.

Fresh cheeses made from skim milk—for example, nonfat ricotta and cottage cheese—are low in fat and calories. Whipped or blended versions of these cheeses can be substituted for regular cream cheese, which is 90 percent fat. Nonfat yogurt, strained through cheesecloth, is another possible alternative. ❖

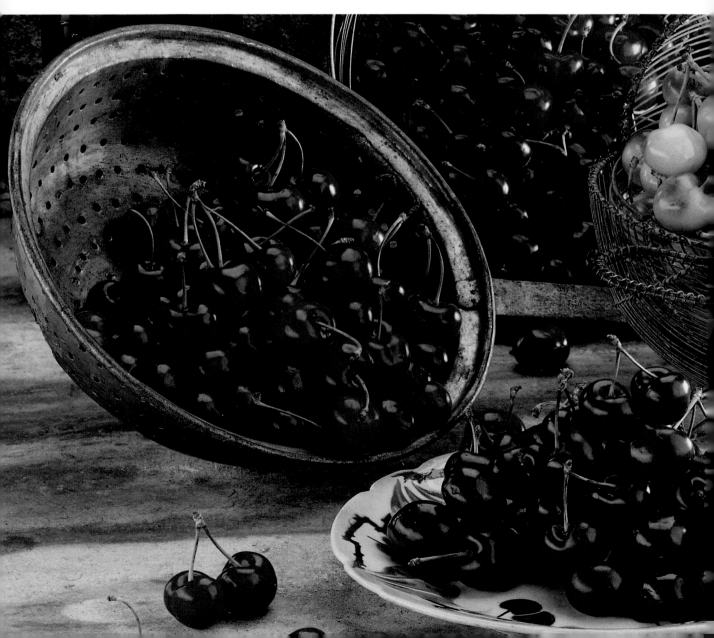

CHERRIES

BENEFITS

- Low-calorie, almost fat-free snack or dessert.
- High in pectin, a soluble fiber that lowers cholesterol.

DRAWBACKS

- Can provoke allergic reactions in susceptible people.
- They spoil quickly and are available for only a few weeks in the summer.

A member of the plant family that includes plums, apricots, peaches, and nectarines, cherries

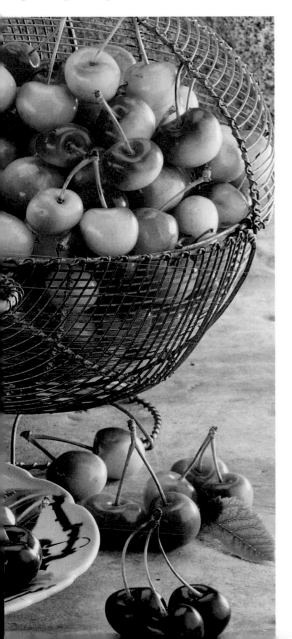

are generally lower in vitamins and minerals than their larger cousins. Still, the flavor and low calorie content of the various sweet varieties make cherries an ideal snack or dessert during the relatively short time they are in season. Sour cherries, which are more nutritious than the sweet types, are used mostly for making jams and other preserves or are baked into pies and other pastries.

NUTRITIONAL VALUE

One cup (250 ml) of sweet or sour cherries contains about 130 calories. Both are a source of beta carotene, vitamin C, and potassium, but sour cherries are much higher in beta carotene. Cherries are a good source of pectin, a soluble fiber that helps control blood cholesterol levels. Cherries are also an abundant source of quercetin, a flavonoid with anticarcinogenic and antioxidant activities.

Traditional folk healers often advocate sour cherries to treat gout, as do some alternative practitioners; these practitioners sometimes suggest the juice of wild chokecherries to prevent or alleviate an attack of gout. There is some evidence to support this claim. Research suggests that a substance in cherries called cyanidin has anti-inflammatory properties, an attribute that might help reduce the swelling and pain of gout. Limited research also shows there is potential of sour cherries in alleviating the symptoms of arthritis.

People who are allergic to apricots and other members of the plum family may also suffer a reaction to cherries with the most likely symptoms being hives and a tingling or itching sensation in or around the mouth.

Some studies also link the flavonoid quercetin with a reduced risk of coronary artery disease, in addition to its other activities.

VARIETIES OF CHERRIES

There are more than 1,000 varieties of cherries worldwide. The most popular sweet cherries in North America are Bing and other dark colored varieties, ranging from deep maroon to almost black, and Lamberts, which are a bright crimson. Queen Annes are yellow with tinges

SWEET AND SOUR TREATS. *The yellowish Queen Anne cherries (right) are very sweet and ideal for a snack, while the scarlet Morello cherries (left) are sour and make delicious pies. Bing cherries (foreground) are best eaten raw, and the versatile Dukes (center, back) can be cooked or eaten raw.*

of red, large, and very sweet. Sour varieties, or pie cherries, are smaller than the sweet types.

When buying fresh cherries, look for plump, firm fruit with green stems. Both sweet and sour cherries spoil quickly and have a relatively short season. Imported cherries are not as flavorful as the local fruit that is picked and marketed at the height of its ripeness. ❖

CHESTNUTS

BENEFITS

- Rich in folate and vitamins C and B$_6$.
- Good source of iron, phosphorus, riboflavin, and thiamine.
- Much lower in fat and calories than almost all other nuts.

DRAWBACKS

- Tend to be expensive and are sometimes difficult to find.

Unlike most other nuts, chestnuts are made up almost completely of carbohydrates and are low in fat and calories. They are also high in a number of important nutrients: A 3- to 4-cup serving of chestnuts provides more than 40 percent of the adult Recommended Dietary Allowance (RDA) of vitamin C, 25 percent of the RDA of folate, and also provides some vitamin B$_6$. The same size serving, which contains 240 calories, 3 g of protein, and 2 g of fat, also contributes more than 10 percent of the RDA for iron, phosphorus, riboflavin, and thiamine.

HIGH IN NATURAL SUGAR

After chestnuts are picked, their starch begins to turn to sugar, giving the nuts their mild, sweet flavor. Chestnuts are almost always cooked, either by roasting or boiling, before they are eaten. When heated, the nuts swell and crack their thin, soft shells, which makes them very easy to peel.

WATER CHESTNUTS

These crunchy vegetables, which are served in many Asian dishes, salads, and soups, are unrelated to chestnuts; in fact, they are not nuts nor do they grow on trees. Instead, they are tubers that grow wild in marshes or the shallow water along lake banks in China and Japan, and other areas in Asia. The Chinese also cultivate water chestnuts as a second crop in their rice paddies.

Most water chestnuts sold in North America are imported from China. They contain moderate amounts of protein and vitamin C, but they are not as nutritious as potatoes and other tuberous vegetables.

Chestnuts are often used in baked desserts. Roasted nuts can be dried and ground into a flour that makes a rich, flavorful crust for tarts or pies. Boiled chestnuts, which have a consistency similar to that of potatoes, can be mashed or pureed to add to cake batter or used as a pastry filling. They are also served as part of a traditional Thanksgiving dinner, either as a side dish or added to turkey stuffing. Marrons glacés, a delicacy available in gourmet shops, are peeled whole chestnuts preserved in a sweet syrup. Chestnuts are also commonly used in soups, salads, and pasta dishes, as well as in some liqueur desserts.

The chestnut develops inside a prickly burr that is gathered after it falls from the tree in early autumn. It should not be confused with the horse chestnut, which is inedible. At one time, the American chestnut tree grew abundantly in the more temperate regions of North America, but a terrible blight in the early 1900s destroyed almost all of these trees. Since then, a hybrid of the American tree and the Oriental chestnut tree has been introduced to North America; however, most of the chestnuts that are now sold in supermarkets are actually imported from Italy and Spain; other major producers are China and South Korea. ❖

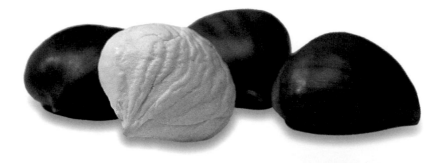

CHILDHOOD NUTRITION

■ FOOD FOR THE GROWING YEARS ■

During the first few years of life, it's vital to meet a child's nutritional needs in order to ensure proper growth and also to establish a lifelong habit of healthy eating.

Eating a meal should be both a healthy and an enjoyable occasion—a fact that many parents may overlook when planning a meal for their growing children. Instead of a fast meal (especially one short in nutritional value) that family members eat at different hours, mealtimes should promote family togetherness whenever possible.

Relaxed dining experiences with good food and conversation (that doesn't involve criticizing table manners or pleading with children to eat) help to foster family relationships, as well as good digestion. You can also involve children in family meals by having them help out with simple mealtime tasks, such as peeling potatoes, preparing salads, or setting the table. If mealtime is a pleasant event, children may practice healthful eating habits later on in life.

The growing years

Between the ages of 2 and 20, the human body changes continuously and dramatically. In general, muscles grow stronger, bones grow longer, height may more than double, and weight can increase as much as fivefold. The most striking changes take place during puberty, which usually occurs between the ages of 10 and 15 in girls and slightly later—between the ages of 12 and 19—in boys. Sexual development and maturity take place at this time, which results in a startling physical transformation.

Children need energy for all the growing years: typically 1,300 calories a day for a 2-year-old, 1,700 for a 5-year-old, 2,200 for a 16-year-old girl, and 2,800 for a 16-year-old boy. (See "Food for Growing Up," page 105.)

The amount of food that a child needs varies according to height, build, gender, and activity level. Left to themselves, most children will usually eat the amount of food that's right for them; however, it is up to the parents to make sure that their children have the right foods available to choose from. Don't fall into the age-old trap of forcing them to eat more food than they want or need. Yesterday's notion of "cleaning your plate" can lead to overeating and weight problems in some cases, or to a lifelong dislike of particular foods. Parents may find it better to serve smaller portions in the first place or to allow children to serve themselves.

Changes in appetite

In most children, appetite slackens as the growth rate slows after the first year; it will then vary throughout childhood, depending on whether the child is going through a period of slow or rapid growth. It is perfectly normal for a young child to eat ravenously one day and then show little interest in food the following day.

Eating patterns change with the onset of the adolescent growth spurt; teenagers usually develop voracious appetites to match their need for additional energy. At the same time, many develop erratic eating habits—for example, skipping breakfast, lunching at school or at a fast-food restaurant, then snacking almost nonstop until bedtime. Although snacking is not the ideal way to eat, a "food on the run" lifestyle won't necessarily cause nutritional problems as long as the basic daily requirements for protein, carbohydrates, fats, and various vitamins and minerals are met. You can generally keep your teenager out of nutritional danger by providing snacks that are high in vitamins, minerals, and protein but low in sugar, fat, and salt. This basically means buying healthful snack foods, such as fresh and dried fruits, juices, raw vegetables, nuts, cheese, whole-grain crackers, unadulterated popcorn, and yogurt—not candy, cake, cookies, potato chips, corn chips, and soft drinks.

Foods for toddlers

After the first year children can eat most of the dishes prepared for the rest of the family. Toddlers, however, have high energy requirements and small stomachs, so they may need five or six small meals or snacks a day. Schedule a toddler's snacks so they don't interfere with food intake during meals. An interval of about an hour and a half is usually enough.

Toddlers often go on food jags—for example, eliminating everything that's white or green. Such food rituals are often short-lived, although they can be annoying or worrisome if they get out of hand. Respect the child's preferences without giving in to every whim; offer a reasonable alternative.

Balance and variety

Children need a wide variety of foods. Carbohydrates—breads, cereals, fruits, and vegetables—should make up the major part of the diet. Protein foods can include meat, fish, milk, soy products (such as bean curd), and combinations of grains and legumes. Milk is an important source of calories, minerals, and vitamins. Children 4 to 9 years old should have 2 to 3 milk-product servings every day (some of the milk may be in the form of cheese or yogurt). Grilled and baked foods are preferable to fried and fatty ones for children of all ages.

The value of dietary fats

Fats are probably the most misunderstood nutrients. Although everyone should avoid excess fat, we all need a certain amount for important body functions. Several vitamins (A, D, E, and K) can be absorbed only in the presence of fat, and fats are necessary for the production of other body chemicals, including the hormones that transform boys and girls into men and women. Despite the benefits of fat intake, excessive fat intake in childhood may lead to obesity and many adult diseases. The current recommendation for fat intake is similar in the United States and Canada. The general recommendation is that children should consume a diet containing no more than 30 percent of energy as fat and no more than

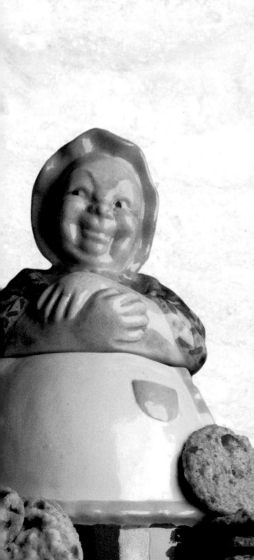

DO ONE SIMPLE THING

PACK YOUR KIDS' LUNCHES

That way you can ensure that they have nutritious choices such as carrot sticks and fruit. While most school cafeterias are providing more healthy offerings for students, such as wraps and salads with low-fat dressings, many still serve fat-laden fries and other fast-food staples. School vending machines are packed with processed foods that also contain unhealthy trans fats. If your kids look forward to a special treat, slip in a homemade cookie, which is healthier than packaged varieties.

FOOD FOR GROWING UP

As children grow, their nutritional needs change; some needs vary between the sexes. The chart below gives an overview of the Recommended Dietary Allowances (RDAs) of certain nutrients for children from ages 1 to 18.

AGES		1–3	4–8	9–13	14–18
VITAMIN A (mcg)	Boys	300	400	600	900
	Girls	300	400	600	700
VITAMIN D (mcg)		5*	5*	5*	5*
VITAMIN E (mg)		6	7	11	15
VITAMIN C (mg)		15	25	45	65–75
NIACIN (mg)	Boys	6	8	12	16
	Girls	6	8	12	14
THIAMINE (mg)	Boys	0.5	0.6	0.9	1.2
	Girls	0.5	0.6	0.9	1.0
RIBOFLAVIN (mg)	Boys	0.5	0.6	0.9	1.3
	Girls	0.5	0.6	0.9	1.0
FOLATE (mcg)		150	200	300	400
VITAMIN B_6 (mg)	Boys	0.5	0.6	1.0	1.3
	Girls	0.5	0.6	1.0	1.2
VITAMIN B_{12} (mcg)		0.9	1.2	1.8	2.4
CALCIUM (mg)		500*	800*	1,300*	1,300*
IRON (mg)	Boys	7	10	8	11
	Girls	7	10	8	15
ZINC (mg)	Boys	3	5	8	11
	Girls	3	5	8	9

Asterisks (*) represent daily Adequate Intake (AI). The term Adequate Intake is used rather than RDA when scientific evidence is insufficient to estimate an average requirement.

Do's and don'ts: encouraging good eating habits

✔ Do set a good example for your child to copy. Share mealtimes and eat the same healthy foods.
✔ Do discourage snacking on sweets and fatty foods. Keep plenty of healthy foods, such as fruits, raw vegetables, low-fat crackers, and yogurt, around for children to eat between meals.
✔ Do allow children to follow their natural appetites when deciding how much to eat.
✔ Do encourage children to enjoy fruits and vegetables by giving them a variety from an early age.
✔ Don't give skim or 1-percent-fat milk to children under the age of 5 unless your doctor prescribes it; at this stage, children need the extra calories in whole milk.
✔ Do ask children to help prepare meals. If parents rely mostly on convenience foods, children may not learn to enjoy cooking.
✔ Don't add unnecessary sugar to drinks and foods.
✔ Don't accustom children to extra salt by adding it to food or placing the shaker on the table.
✔ Don't give whole nuts to children under the age of 5, who may choke on them. Peanut butter and chopped nuts are fine as long as the child is not allergic to them.
✔ Don't force children to eat more than they want.
✔ Don't use food as a bribe.
✔ Don't make children feel guilty about eating any type of food.

10 percent of energy as saturated fat. The transition to this diet should begin after 2 years of age with a gradual reduction in fat intake over time.

Eating their vegetables

Many parents have a battle when it comes to getting children to eat vegetables, but you can win children over by appealing to their taste for bright colors and interesting textures. Choose crisp, raw carrot sticks and other attractive, crunchy veggies. Substitute minced vegetables (zucchini, eggplant, mushrooms) for ground meat in spaghetti sauce, or chop chickpeas with grains and other vegetables to make "veggie burgers."

Iron deficiency

Iron is an essential mineral for normal growth and development for a child. Unfortunately, many children have inadequate stores of iron due to insufficient intake of iron-rich foods. There are two types of iron: heme,

Childhood obesity and TV

Several studies have documented associations between number of hours of TV watched and the rate of obesity. Moreover, heavy TV watching has been associated with higher intakes of calories, fat, sweet and salty snacks, and carbonated beverages in children. This may be due to increased exposure to advertising campaigns for these foods.

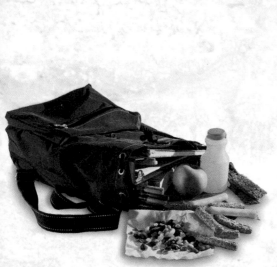

Easy, healthful snacks

Stock up on healthful snacks that children and teenagers can nibble on throughout the day.
- Breads and crackers with spreads such as peanut butter, low-fat cheese, canned tuna or sardines, and lean cold cuts.
- Rice cakes and whole-grain crackers or breadsticks.
- Fresh and dried fruits.
- Yogurt.
- Sticks of carrot, celery, or other raw vegetables, and cherry tomatoes with nutritious dips.
- Plain popcorn.
- Breakfast cereals.
- Water, milk, or fruit juice.

which is easily absorbed by humans, and nonheme iron, which is poorly absorbed. Foods that contain heme iron include meat, eggs, fish, poultry, and seafood while breakfast cereals, legumes, grains, breads, seeds, nuts, dried fruits, and dark green, leafy vegetables contain the nonheme variety. Children should have a variety of iron-containing foods in their diet. In addition, the consumption of vitamin C-rich foods improves the absorption of dietary iron.

A growing epidemic: obesity

In North America, children are becoming obese (defined as being 20 percent or more above desirable weight) or overweight in growing numbers and by earlier ages. The consequence: high blood pressure, high cholesterol, type 2 diabetes, some cancers, sleeping disorders, and orthopedic complications. One study found that the arteries of many American teenagers are so clogged that the kids are at increased risk for a heart attack. Research of this kind led the American Heart Association to establish guidelines urging doctors to intervene in childhood obesity by urging parents to limit foods high in saturated fat for children over 2, encourage kids to consume more fruits, vegetables, and whole grains, and to get at least 60 minutes of physical activity every day.

Overweight children tend to become overweight adults. Parents must foster positive elements, such as healthy eating, positive body image, and active lifestyle early in a child's life. The best approach to controlling weight in obese youngsters is serving smaller portions and encouraging regular, vigorous exercise.

Foods for teenagers

Adolescents need more of everything to keep up with the massive teenage growth spurt: calories and protein for growth and to build muscles; and protein, calcium, phosphorus, and vitamin D for bone formation. For many the demands of school and social life mean that they eat meals away from home; suddenly they are responsible for choosing the major part of their diet. Some may not make the best choices. Others may use food to establish an identity, such as by becoming a vegetarian, without knowing how to maintain proper nutrition. Both obesity and eating disorders can plague adolescents. A sensitive approach is necessary in order to help an adolescent maintain a positive self-image and professional help may be necessary.

Building bone

Calcium is important for forming strong, healthy bones during adolescence and preventing osteoporosis later in life. Youths 10 to 16 years old need 3 to 4 milk-product servings a day—the equivalent of 2 cups of milk and 1 to 2 oz (30–60 g) (2 slices) of cheese or 3 to 4 cups of yogurt—every day. If teens are not drinking milk, they can try a smoothie, fortified soy beverages, cheese on a sandwich, or even chocolate milk.

Snacking and fast food

Teenagers often prefer snacks loaded with fat, sugar, and salt: potato chips, French fries, hamburgers, hot dogs, pizza, and candy bars. These are high in sodium and strike a poor balance between calories and nutrition; a steady diet of them is low in vitamins A and C, calcium, and dietary fiber. Encourage teenagers to choose grilled chicken (not breaded), sandwiches with lean meats, or a slice of vegetarian pizza.

CHILIES

BENEFITS

- An excellent source of beta carotene and vitamin C.
- May help relieve nasal congestion.
- May help prevent blood clots that can lead to a heart attack or stroke.

DRAWBACKS

- Require careful handling during preparation to prevent irritation of the skin and eyes.
- May irritate hemorrhoids in susceptible people.

A popular ingredient in Southwestern cooking, chilies, or hot peppers, add spice and interest to many foods; some of the milder varieties are consumed as low-calorie snacks.

The heat in chilies comes from capsaicinoids, substances that have no odor or flavor themselves but impart their bite by acting directly on the mouth's pain receptors. This results in the teary eyes, runny nose ("salsa sniffles"), and sweating experienced by most people who indulge in the hotter varieties. For those with a cold or allergies, eating chilies can provide temporary relief from nasal and sinus congestion. Capsaicin and other capsaicinoids are concentrated mainly in the white ribs and seeds, which can be removed to produce a milder flavor.

Handle chilies with care. Wear thin gloves and wash all utensils well with soap and water after use. Even a tiny amount of capsaicinoids causes severe irritation if it is transferred to the eyes. Be sure to avoid handling contact lenses after chopping chilies.

PACKED WITH NUTRITIOUS PROPERTIES

Chilies are more nutritious than sweet peppers, and the red varieties generally have a higher nutritional content than the green ones. They are very good sources of antioxidants, especially beta carotene and vitamin C. Just one raw, red hot pepper (1½ oz/45 g) contains about 105 mg of vitamin C, more than 100 percent of the Recommended Dietary Allowance (RDA). Chilies also contain bioflavonoids, plant pigments that some researchers believe may help prevent cancer. In addition, recent research indicates that capsaicin may act as an anticoagulant, perhaps helping to prevent blood clots that can lead to

---

A CONSUMER'S GUIDE TO CHILIES

Chile hotness is rated in Scoville units. The hottest pepper on record is the habanero, which is rated at 100,000 to 350,000 Scoville units. By contrast, the serrano comes in at about 5,000 to 15,000 Scoville units. Scoville units are the measurement of capsaicin level (the oil that makes chiles hot). Pure capsaicin rates 16 million units. Although chiles can vary from pod to pod and plant to plant, listed below is an approximate ranking for several varieties of chiles, with 10 being the hottest:

Rank	Scoville units	Pepper type
10	100,000–350,000	Habanero; Scotch Bonnet
9	50,000–100,000	Santaka; Chiltepin; Thai
8	30,000–50,000	Aji; Cayenne; Tabasco; Piquin
7	15,000–30,000	Chile de Arbol
6	5,000–15,000	Yellow Wax; Serrano
5	2,500–5,000	Jalapeño; Mirasol
4	1,500–2,500	Sandia; Cascabel
3	1,000–1,500	Ancho; Pasilla; Espanola
2	500–1,000	New Mexico; Anaheim; Big Jim
1	100–500	Mexi-bells; Cherry
0	0–100	Mild Bells; Sweet Banana; Pimento

The following is a description of a selection of popular peppers from the mildest to the hottest.

MILD TO MODERATELY HOT:

- **Anaheim.** These long, slender red or green chilies are among the most popular in North America.
- **Ancho.** These dark red, heart-shaped peppers are usually dried.
- **Cherry.** These small, round red chilies are often pickled.
- **Poblano.** Green chilies with a small, tapered shape; they are usually roasted, and may be stuffed or added to a variety of dishes.

HOT:

- **Cascabel.** These round red or green chilies are usually dried.

VERY HOT:

- **Cayenne.** These long red chilies are dried and often ground into a hot pepper spice.s
- **Habanero or Scotch Bonnet.** Shaped like red, yellow, or orange lanterns, these are considered the hottest of cultivated chilies.
- **Jalapeño.** These tapered green or red chilies are sold fresh, canned, or pickled.
- **Serrano.** These small, bullet-shaped green or red chilies are often used in hot salsas.

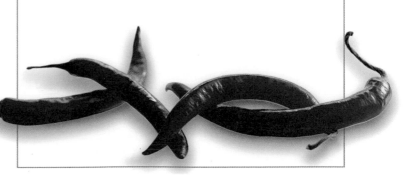

a heart attack or stroke. Incorporated into creams, capsaicinoids alleviate the burning pain of shingles and can help with the pain of arthritis. They may also reduce the mouth pain associated with chemotherapy. Commercially available poultices for relief of lower back pain also contain capsaicin.

Contrary to popular belief, there is no evidence that chilies cause ulcers or digestive problems; however, they may cause rectal irritation. ❖

CHINESE FOOD

See Fast Food

CHOCOLATE

BENEFITS

- Can elevate moods in some people.
- Like other plant foods, it contains various antioxidants.
- It tastes great!

DRAWBACKS

- High in calories and fat.
- May trigger migraine headaches.

The returning crew of Columbus's fourth voyage in 1502 brought the first cocoa beans from the New World to Europe. The Spanish eventually combined them with vanilla, and other flavorings, sugar, and milk to arrive at a concoction that, as one writer noted at the time, people "would die for"; Aztec Emperor Montezuma described it as a "divine drink, which builds up resistance and fights fatigue."

For the first couple of centuries, chocolate was served only as a beverage. A solid form—probably more like marzipan than the chocolate we know—was touted as an instant breakfast in 18th-century France. The stimulant effects of chocolate are due to its caffeine content and were thought to make it a particularly useful food for soldiers standing watch during the night.

The chocolate bar, first marketed in about 1910, captured the public's imagination when it was issued to the U.S. armed forces as a "fighting food" during World War II.

THE SOURCE OF CHOCOLATE

Chocolate is made from the beans found in the pods that grow on the cocoa tree, an evergreen that originated in the river valleys of South America. Native Central and South Americans valued cocoa so highly that they used cocoa beans as currency. Today about three-fourths of the world's chocolate is grown in West Africa and most of the rest in Brazil.

After cocoa beans are harvested, an initial phase of fermentation and drying is followed by low-temperature roasting to bring out the flavor. Various manufacturing processes follow, depending on whether the product is to be solid as chocolate or cocoa powder.

In 1828 the Van Houten family of Amsterdam, seeking to make a better drinking chocolate, invented a screw press to remove most of the cocoa butter from the beans. Not only did it make a better drink, but they also found that by mixing the extracted cocoa butter back into ground cocoa beans, they could make a smoother, fatter solid paste that would absorb sugar; this led to "eating chocolate."

COMPONENTS

Chocolate is not a great source of nutrients, but there is no harm in eating a limited amount of chocolate, especially the dark variety.

An ounce (30 g) of solid chocolate contains about 150 calories and 2 or 3 g of protein. The original bean has significant amounts of vitamin E and B vitamins. These nutrients, however, are so diluted as to be negligible in modern processed chocolate. Sweet or semisweet chocolate contains between 40 and 53 percent fat, or cocoa butter. Both chocolate and cocoa powder supply chromium, iron, magnesium, phosphorus, and potassium, but fat and calories make chocolate an inappropriate source of these minerals except when used in emergency rations.

A chemical composition that prevents it from quickly turning rancid made cocoa butter valuable as a long-lasting food and cosmetic oil.

Chocolate is a solid at room temperature, but since its melting point is just below the human body temperature, it begins to melt and release its flavor components as soon as it is placed in the mouth.

White chocolate, a mixture of cocoa butter, milk solids, and sugar, contains no cocoa solids. Unlike milk chocolate, white chocolate does

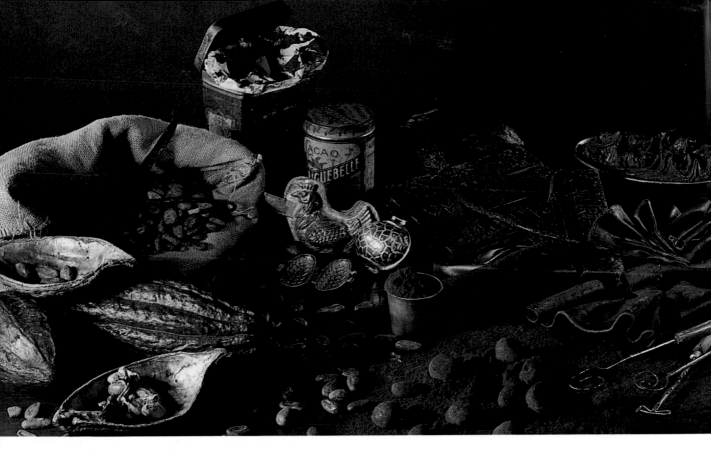

not keep well, because it lacks the compounds that prevent milk solids from becoming rancid over time.

THE FEEL-GOOD FACTOR

Chocolate contains two related alkaloid stimulants, theobromine and caffeine, in a ratio of about 10 to 1. Theobromine, unlike caffeine, does not stimulate the central nervous system; its effects are mainly diuretic. Commercial chocolate products contain no more than about 0.1 percent caffeine and are much less stimulating, volume for volume, than a cup of decaffeinated coffee. Unsweetened baking chocolate for home use is a more concentrated source of caffeine. Chocolate is also rich in phenylethylamine (PEA), a naturally occurring compound that has effects similar to amphetamine. This compound can also trigger migraine headaches in susceptible people.

Some people (often women) have a tendency to binge on chocolate after emotional upsets. No scientific basis for this behavior is known. However, psychiatrists have theorized that "chocoholics" may be people who have a faulty mechanism for regulating their body levels of phenylethylamine; others attribute chocolate cravings to hormonal changes, such as those during puberty or during a woman's premenstrual phase.

After centuries of investigation, chocolate's once-vaunted aphrodisiac qualities can be discounted. But in its myriad modern forms, chocolate is an endless temptation and a culinary source of pleasure.

NEW STUDIES

A report in the February 2003 issue of the *Journal of the American Dietetic Association* sheds some positive light on chocolate. Researchers reviewed a number of studies on the possible health benefits of chocolate, particularly the dark variety, and cocoa. They found the flavonoids in chocolate to have some disease-fighting antioxidant properties—also found in red wine, and some fruits and vegetables—associated with a decreased risk of heart disease.

Chocolate is best tasted on an empty stomach. Never put chocolate in the refrigerator—it will cause the cocoa butter to separate and form a white bloom. When tasting chocolate, let it sit in your mouth for a few seconds to release its primary flavors and aromas. Then chew it a few times to release the secondary aromas. Let it rest against the roof of your mouth so you get the full flavor. ❖

MELTS IN THE MOUTH. *Chocolate comes in a wide variety of shapes, textures, colors, and sweetness—something for everyone.*

DO ONE SIMPLE THING

MAKE DARK CHOCOLATE YOUR CHOICE

Choose dark chocolate over milk chocolate. Dark chocolate contains more antioxidants and less fat. Milk chocolate contains milk fat that is highly saturated.

CHOLESTEROL
■ THE FACTS AND THE MYTHS ■

By now, most people know that high levels of blood cholesterol can lead to blocked arteries. If an artery that supplies blood to your heart becomes blocked, a heart attack may occur. If an artery that supplies blood to your brain becomes blocked, a stroke could occur. Still, confusion abounds over the role of diet in affecting cholesterol.

Although often portrayed as a dietary evil, cholesterol is essential to life. The body needs it to make sex hormones, bile, vitamin D, cell membranes, and nerve sheaths. These and other functions fall to serum cholesterol, a waxy, fatlike compound, termed a "lipid," that circulates in the bloodstream. The liver manufactures about a gram each day, which is all the body requires.

Dietary cholesterol is found only in animal products. The body does not need this cholesterol, but anyone other than a strict vegetarian who excludes all animal products will consume varying amounts of it. Many factors—exercise, genetics, gender, and other components of the diet—influence how the human body processes dietary cholesterol; some people can consume large amounts but have normal blood levels, while others eat very little but have high blood cholesterol. Diet appears to account for about 20 percent of the cholesterol in the body, with the remaining 80 percent produced by the liver.

The Mediterranean diet

Doctors have known since the 1950s that the so-called Mediterranean diet reduces the risk of premature death. The first study showed that heart disease rates can be predicted from cholesterol levels, that an intake of saturated fats increases the risk, and that monounsaturated fats, mainly olive oil, reduces the risk of not only heart disease, but cancer as well.

The same study found the lowest premature mortality rate on the Greek Island of Crete. The Cretans ate very little meat, lots of legumes and fruits, moderate amounts of fish and red wine, and copious amounts of olive oil. Bread, mostly whole grain, was an integral part of their diet. The first clinical evidence suggesting that a Mediterranean diet was advantageous in the West came in 1994 when Dr. Serge Renaud in France undertook to investigate what would happen to patients who had a heart attack and then were counseled to follow a Mediterranean diet.

The patients on the Mediterranean diet were encouraged to eat more fruits, vegetables, and fish, less red meat, and were also asked to replace butter with margarine that was enriched in alpha-linolenic acid. The reason for this was that the traditional Cretan diet features lots of walnuts, olive oil, and a vegetable called purslane, all of which are rich in linolenic acid, a compound that is thought to be protective against heart disease. It didn't take long for results to show up. After just 2 years, the death rate in the intervention group was reduced by 70 percent!

Good versus bad cholesterol

To travel through the bloodstream, cholesterol molecules attach themselves to lipid-carrying proteins, or lipoproteins. Two types of lipoproteins are the major transporters of cholesterol: low-density lipoproteins (LDLs) carry two-thirds of it; most of the remainder is attached to high-density lipoproteins (HDLs). LDLs tend to deposit cholesterol in the artery walls, leading to atherosclerosis and an increased risk of heart disease. In contrast, HDLs collect cholesterol from the artery walls and other tissues and take it to the liver to be metabolized and eliminated from the body. This is why LDLs are often called the "bad" cholesterol and HDLs the "good." A third type, very-low-density lipoproteins (VLDLs), carries a small amount of cholesterol and triglycerides.

A blood cholesterol test measures the amount of cholesterol in the blood. This can be expressed in two ways, in terms of milligrams (mg) of cholesterol per deciliter, or millimoles (mmol) of cholesterol per liter. The multiplication factor 0.026 converts the milligram system to the millimole system. A value below 200 mg/dl (5.2 mmol/l) is considered desirable. If the total is more than 200 mg/dl, LDL and HDL levels should be measured individually. LDL levels should be below 130 mg/dl (3.5 mmol/l); 130 to 159 (3.5–3.9) is classified as borderline high, over 160 (4.0) is considered high risk for coronary artery disease and a heart attack. HDL levels should be at least 45 mg/dl (1.2 mmol/l), and the higher the better. In assessing

EATING TO KEEP CHOLESTEROL IN CHECK

There's no doubt that what you eat influences the levels of cholesterol and other fats in your blood. Numerous studies document that diet high in animal products and other saturated fats tend to elevate cholesterol levels, in contrast to the low levels found in people whose diet consist largely of whole grains, fruits, and vegetables. People with a family history of heart disease should be diligent in following a diet that limits the cholesterol-raising foods and emphasizes the cholesterol-lowering foods indicated below.

FOODS THAT MAY RAISE CHOLESTEROL

- Hard margarine and vegetable shortening, which are high in saturated fats and trans fatty acids.
- Cookies, cakes, pastries, and chocolates, especially those made with saturated tropical oils, or partially hydrogenated oils.
- Full-fat dairy products, such as cheese, cream, and butter; all are high in saturated fats.
- Fatty meats and meat products, such as marbled beef, pork and lamb chops, hamburgers, bacon, frankfurters, salamis, and other cold cuts.

FOODS THAT MAY LOWER CHOLESTEROL

- Whole-wheat, pumpernickel, rye, and multigrain breads and rolls.
- Oatmeal and breakfast cereals that contain oat or rice bran, as well as tofu and other soy products.
- Nonhydrogenated soft margarine, olive oil and canola oil, safflower, sunflower, cottonseed, and soy bean oils.
- Vegetables, such as sweet corn, onions, garlic, lima beans, kidney beans, and other legumes.
- Fruits, such as oranges, apples, pears, bananas, and such dried fruits as apricots, figs, and prunes.
- Nuts such as almonds, walnuts, pecans; seeds such as sesame and sunflower seeds.

cardiovascular risk, doctors calculate the LDL/HDL ratio by dividing the total cholesterol by the HDL figure. A desirable ratio is less than 4.5.

How diet can help

Experts agree that dietary modification is appropriate if the total cholesterol count is greater than 200 mg/dl (5.2 mmol/l) or if the LDL level exceeds 130 mg/dl (3.5 mmol/l). Reducing intake of saturated fats has the greatest effect on lowering blood cholesterol levels. A diet that limits fat intake to 20 percent or less of total calories and restricts saturated fats to 7 percent or less can lower total blood cholesterol an average of 14 percent. Most people can significantly lower intake of saturated fats by cutting down on, or eliminating fatty meats, whole milk, and other full-fat dairy products, as well as tropical oils (coconut, palm, and palm kernel). It is also important to lower intake of trans fatty acids found in partially hydrogenated oils and foods containing them such as cookies, crackers, other commercial baked goods, many snack foods, and some margarines and spreads.

Tobacco should be avoided. Firsthand and secondhand smoke both cause a drop in health-promoting antioxidants such as vitamin C. Tobacco smoke also incourages the immune system to increase LDLs.

DO ONE SIMPLE THING

SPREAD YOUR BREAD WITH MARGARINE CONTAINING PLANT STEROLS

Results from various studies and randomized trials indicate that people age 50 to 59 would reduce their heart disease risk by 25 percent after only 2 years by using these margarines. Plant sterols, although not available in Canada, can also be found in specially produced yogurts, cheese products, and salad dressings.

Stricter diets yield even better results

Try a vegetarian diet. The vegetarian low-fat (less than 10 percent of calories) program developed by Dr. Dean Ornish can lower LDL cholesterol substantially. His program also calls for exercise and meditation.

Be sure to include foods that actually lower cholesterol. It isn't just what you don't eat that matters; consuming foods that have a cholesterol-lowering effect also helps. Flavonoid-rich foods, including citrus fruits and onions, are known to promote healthy cholesterol levels. Soluble fiber is also a weapon against cholesterol. It is commonly found in oats, beans, and flaxseed. The pectin in apples and other fruits lowers cholesterol, as does the soy protein found in tofu, tempeh, and soy milk. It has also been established that regular daily consumption of carrots can lead to a reduction of LDL cholesterol levels.

Eat fish rich in omega-3s. Two or three servings a week of salmon, sardines, and other cold-water fish are linked with a reduced risk of heart attacks and strokes. Initially, it was thought that the omega-3 fatty acids in fish reduced cardiovascular risk by lowering blood cholesterol levels; however, recent studies suggest that their benefit comes from interfering with blood clotting and from possible changes in the way the liver metabolizes other lipids.

Eat lots of soy products. A large body of evidence has shown that adding soy protein to a low-fat diet helps to lower cholesterol levels. Soy protein is found in soybeans and products made from these beans, including tofu and soy beverages.

Look for margarine with plant sterols. Plant sterols have been shown to help lower cholesterol levels when consumed as part of a heart-healthy diet. They are found in plant-sterol enriched margarines, vegetable oils, nuts, sesame and sunflower seeds, soy and other legumes.

At one time, increasing the intake of polyunsaturated fats—corn, cottonseed, safflower, soy, and sunflower oils—was advocated to lower cholesterol, but studies have found that these oils reduce the levels of the protective HDLs at the same time as they lower the harmful LDLs. In contrast, monounsaturated fats found in canola and olive oils, some nuts and avocados have the opposite effect, cutting LDLs without altering HDL levels.

The role of dietary cholesterol is still unclear; recent studies indicate it is not as potent in raising blood cholesterol as saturated fats are. Still, some experts recommend limiting dietary cholesterol intake to 300 mg a day—the amount in one and one-half egg yolks, 4 oz (115 g) of beef liver, or 2 cups of whole milk, a 6-oz (170-g) steak, and 1 cup of ice cream.

Other approaches

Increased exercise, weight loss, and stress reduction can all lower cholesterol or improve the LDL/HDL ratio. Women are protected from developing coronary artery disease during their reproductive years by the estrogen their body produces; but according to the most recent research, estrogen supplements taken after menopause do not offer similar protection.

Moderate alcohol intake lowers the risk of heart attack. This may be due to alcohol's ability to raise HDL, its tendency to reduce the stickiness of platelets, or the presence of antioxidants, such as resveratrol, in red wine. If dietary and other lifestyle changes fail to reduce blood cholesterol, drugs may be prescribed.

DID YOU KNOW?

A VEGETARIAN "APE DIET" CAN LOWER CHOLESTEROL AS WELL AS A STATIN DRUG

A diet modelled on the food groups that apes eat has been shown to lower high cholesterol as effectively as lovastatin, a common anticholesterol drug in the statin group. Or so one study done at the University of Toronto, and published in the *Journal of the American Medical Association*, concluded. The diet, developed for the study, consists of four food groups: nuts (especially almonds), soy proteins, high-fiber foods (like oats and fruits), and a margarine with plant sterols.

CHRONIC FATIGUE SYNDROME

EAT PLENTY OF

- Pasta, rice, and whole-grain cereals and breads for complex carbohydrates.
- Fruits and vegetables for vitamin C.
- Foods rich in essential fatty acids such as fish, flax, nuts and seeds, canola oil, and wheat germ.
- Salty foods (if low blood pressure is part of the diagnosis).

LIMIT

- Caffeine, especially near bedtime.

AVOID

- Alcohol.

Currently one of the most controversial disorders, chronic fatigue syndrome (CFS) often has flulike symptoms, no apparent cause, and no proven cure. It is marked by persistent, debilitating fatigue, as well as other baffling symptoms that include headaches, muscle aches and weakness, tender lymph nodes, sore throat, joint pain, sleep that doesn't lead to feeling refreshed, difficulty concentrating, postexercise exhaustion that lasts for 24 hours, and short-term memory problems. There may also be a chronic or recurring low-grade fever.

There is no laboratory test for CFS, so a doctor must systematically rule out all other medical causes that produce similar symptoms. According to diagnostic criteria set up by the Centers for Disease Control and Prevention (CDC), the chronic fatigue and at least eight other nonspecific symptoms must persist for at least 6 months.

Although some claim that CFS is a new disorder (for example, the "yuppie flu" of the 1980s), doctors since the 1800s have reported similar disorders but given them different names, including hypoglycemia (low blood sugar), chronic Epstein-Barr virus, myalgic encephalomyelitis, and postviral fatigue syndrome. Many theories regarding possible causes have been advanced, but none have been proven. In many cases, CFS develops in the aftermath of a viral illness, such as mononucleosis or the flu, but no single viral cause has been identified. Other possible contributing factors include prolonged stress, hormonal imbalance, low blood pressure (hypotension), allergies,

immune system disorders, and psychological problems. Some experts suggest CFS is a group of ailments that share similar symptoms. In any event, it is estimated that more than one-half million North Americans suffer from the disease. At least two-thirds of the sufferers are white middle-class women. Most CFS patients eventually recover, but it may take a year or more to do so.

MEDICAL TREATMENT

Various medications are prescribed to treat CFS symptoms, but none appear to cure the disorder. Aspirin and other painkillers may alleviate headaches, joint pain, and muscle soreness, and antidepressant drugs help some patients. Some doctors advocate antiviral drugs, such as acyclovir, or injections of gamma globulin, a substance containing antibodies from the blood serum of a number of people, but studies have failed to document their value.

NUTRITIONAL APPROACHES

Although there is no known cure for CFS, certain nutrients in foods may help. Doctors stress the importance of a well-balanced diet.

Start with ample starches. Fruits and vegetables help to provide the carbohydrates the body needs for energy. They also supply the vitamins needed to resist infection.

Avoid alcohol. It lowers immunity, so should be avoided, and caffeinated drinks should be used in moderation to minimize sleep problems.

Eat to strengthen your immune system. Foods rich in zinc, such as seafood (especially oysters), meat, poultry, eggs, milk, beans, nuts, and whole grains, as well as foods rich in vitamin C, such as citrus fruits, berries, melons, kiwis, broccoli, and cauliflower, may help keep the immune system working properly. A robust immune system can help ward off certain viruses, such as flu and colds that may possibly precede the onset of CFS.

Consume more essential fatty acids. Some of the symptoms of CFS include swollen glands and inflammation of the joints, which may be relieved temporarily by foods rich in essential fatty acids. These include fish, nuts, seeds, flaxseed and flaxseed oil, canola oil, wheat germ, and leafy green vegetables.

FIVE-STEP ACTION PLAN

COPING WITH CFS

1. Obtain an accurate diagnosis, preferably from a physician who has experience in treating CFS.
2. Keep a detailed diary of your progress, noting symptoms and how foods and activities affect your physical well-being.
3. Establish a sensible and balanced program of treatment that covers diet and exercise.
4. Don't nap during the daytime; instead get between 7 to 9 hours of sleep each night.
5. Join a support group.

MIGHTY MAGNESIUM

Magnesium is associated with the contraction and relaxation of muscles. Getting more of the mineral may help alleviate muscle tenderness in people with CFS. Good food sources include sunflower seeds, avocados, and amaranth.

One study indicates that low blood pressure may contribute to the fatigue experienced by CFS patients. Usually, blood pressure rises slightly during periods of stress or physical activity. But in some people, blood pressure remains constant or goes down, resulting in fatigue. These people may be salt-resistant and need a higher salt intake to raise blood pressure. Researchers have noted that many CFS patients have low-salt diets, which may explain their hypotension and fatigue. Symptoms became less severe when the patients increased their intake of salty foods.

Some alternative practitioners advocate injections of vitamin B_{12}, along with supplements of vitamins A and C, iron, and zinc, to treat CFS. But a balanced diet is preferable to taking supplements. Another approach that appears hopeful is for patients to take a combination of evening primrose oil and fish oil; in one study, 85 percent reported some improvement after 15 weeks. Caution is needed when taking herbal remedies—many contain potentially harmful stimulants. ❖

CIRCULATORY DISORDERS

EAT PLENTY OF

- Oily fish, such as salmon and sardines, for omega-3 fatty acids.
- Citrus and other fresh fruits and vegetables for vitamin C.
- Seeds, nuts, seafood, and wheat germ for vitamin E.

LIMIT

- Fatty meat and other sources of saturated fats.

AVOID

- Smoking and excessive alcohol use.

The most common circulatory, or vascular, disorders are high blood pressure and atherosclerosis; others include various clotting abnormalities and diseases marked by reduced blood flow. Some of the more common are aneurysms, intermittent claudication, phlebitis, and Raynaud's disease.

ANEURYSMS

These balloonlike bulges form in weakened segments of the arteries, especially the aorta, the

DO ONE SIMPLE THING

EAT MORE ONIONS AND GARLIC

These vegetables are especially helpful in improving blood flow. After chopping garlic, let it rest for 10 minutes prior to cooking it. This will allow the allicin and its potent derivatives to be activated and unleash the full nutritional power of garlic.

body's largest artery, which stems directly from the heart. Many aneurysms are due to a congenital weakness, while others are caused by atherosclerosis and high blood pressure.

A low-fat, low-salt diet is recommended. There is no specific dietary treatment for an aneurysm, but following a low-fat, low-salt diet can help prevent those caused by atherosclerosis and high blood pressure. Consuming ample fresh fruits and vegetables will provide the vitamin C needed to strengthen and maintain blood vessels.

INTERMITTENT CLAUDICATION (LEG PAIN)

Severe leg pain and cramps induced by walking are symptoms of intermittent claudication. A lack of oxygen due to inadequate blood flow causes the pain.

Atherosclerosis is responsible for most intermittent claudication; it is also common in diabetic patients. Adopting a very-low-fat diet and an exercise program (for example, the regimen developed by cardiologist Dean Ornish) has helped many patients. Including onions and garlic in the diet is said to improve blood flow. Patients with severe blockages, however, may require surgery to remove them.

PHLEBITIS

Any inflammation of a vein is referred to as phlebitis; the large, superficial veins in the lower legs are the most commonly afflicted. Although painful, this type of superficial phlebitis is not as dangerous as when veins located deeper in the legs become inflamed, setting the stage for thrombophlebitis. In this condition, clots form at the site of inflammation; pieces may break away and travel to the heart and lungs.

Phlebitis can be treated with aspirin and other anti-inflammatory drugs and by applying warm compresses. Clot-dissolving drugs may be administered for thrombophlebitis; other measures may be required to prevent clots from reaching vital organs.

Eat more fish. A diet that includes several servings a week of fatty fish or other sources of omega-3 fatty acids, as well as foods high in vitamin E, helps reduce inflammation and clot formation. Gamma linolenic acid, a substance in evening primrose and borage oils, has a similar effect; but check with your doctor first, as they may interact with prescribed drugs.

RAYNAUD'S DISEASE

This condition is characterized by periods of numbness, tingling, and pain in the fingers and toes due to constriction or spasms in the small arteries that carry blood to the extremities.

Typically, Raynaud's disease is set off by exposure to the cold; in some people, however, periods of stress may trigger an attack. For unknown reasons, two-thirds of all Raynaud's sufferers are women. Smoking is blamed in many cases. Some victims may also have lupus, rheumatoid arthritis, and other inflammatory autoimmune disorders.

Get your fill of omega-3s. Avoiding exposure of the hands and feet to cold temperatures can usually prevent or minimize attacks. Of course, not smoking and avoiding secondhand smoke is critical. Eating foods that are high in omega-3 fatty acids and vitamin E may help. ❖

CIRRHOSIS

EAT PLENTY OF
- A combination of grains and legumes instead of meat for protein.
- Carbohydrates for energy.
- Cereals, breads, potatoes, and legumes for B-complex vitamins.
- Fruits and vegetables for vitamin C.

LIMIT
- Animal protein, salt, and fats.

AVOID
- Alcohol and salty processed foods.

In cirrhosis, a chronic progressive disease, normal liver cells are replaced by scar tissue. Prolonged, heavy alcohol use is the most common cause, but cirrhosis may also result from hepatitis, inflammation or blockage of the bile ducts, inherited conditions, or a reaction to a drug or environmental toxin.

In its early stages, cirrhosis does not usually produce symptoms, but as the liver is increasingly infiltrated with fibrous tissue, a person may experience fatigue and nausea, and have a poor appetite. In the later stages, jaundice may develop and fine, spidery blood vessels appear on the skin. The liver damage is irreversible, but the progress of cirrhosis can be arrested and the complications treated with diet and other measures.

DIET AND LIVER REPAIR

Stop drinking alcohol. Whether or not alcohol intake is the cause of cirrhosis, it is essential to stop drinking entirely to prevent further liver damage. Although the scar tissue cannot be replaced, the liver does have a remarkable ability to repair itself. To achieve this and regain lost weight, a daily intake of 2,000 to 3,000 calories is necessary. Most people with cirrhosis, however, have little appetite; thus, frequent small meals may be more tempting than three large ones.

Eat plenty of protein. It is important to include sufficient protein in the diet. The recommended daily intake of protein for those with cirrhosis is 0.54 g per pound (1.2 g per kilogram) of body weight. This is more than the amount that is recommended for healthy people. Some evidence supports the use of vegetable protein foods such as those in soy, peas, and legumes, especially for people who develop mental confusion, a condition called hepatic encephalopathy. A good supply of carbohydrates is needed. Moderate amounts of polyunsaturated fats (oily fish, corn oil, safflower oil) also provide needed calories without overburdening the liver. Regular intake of vitamin C in the form of fresh fruits and vegetables will also help, strengthening the immune system.

Replace depleted vitamins and minerals. Nutritional deficiencies are common among cirrhosis patients. Enriched cereals, breads and pasta, and fruits and vegetables will help. Often, a doctor will also prescribe supplements.

FLUIDS AND SALT

The orderly flow of body fluids is an early casualty of cirrhotic damage. In a healthy person, the blood supply circulates through vessels in the liver; but in cirrhosis, rigid scar tissue forms on the liver, hindering the blood from passing freely. As the blood backs up, the pressure in the supplying vessels increases, which forces plasma out of the blood vessels and into the tissues that surround the abdominal cavity. People with cirrhosis often have distinctive abdominal swelling, known as ascites. The volume of blood in the vessels throughout the body is

DANGER SIGNS

If you, or someone you know, has the following symptoms, cirrhosis may be the culprit: weight loss, nausea, vomiting, impotence, jaundice, and swelling of the legs.

therefore decreased, and when the kidneys register the fall in blood flow, they send out a signal for help in the form of the hormone aldosterone. Far from helping, this causes the body to retain sodium (instead of excreting it in the urine in the normal manner), which in turn produces a further damming of fluid and worsens the ascites. The whole body becomes puffy and swollen, and the vicious cycle continues with other complications that arise as the blood seeks a way to bypass the obstruction in the liver. This entails increasing blood flow in vessels in neighboring organs, such as the veins of the esophagus. Some cirrhotic patients suffer from varices (varicose veins) in the esophagus, which can rupture and cause severe bleeding.

People with cirrhosis should eat little salt, especially if ascites is present, and drink about four to six glasses of fluids a day. If varices are present in the esophagus, the food should be soft and thoroughly chewed. ❖

CLAMS

See Shellfish

COCONUTS

BENEFITS
- A useful source of iron and fiber.
- High in easy-to-digest fatty acids.

DRAWBACKS
- High in saturated fats and calories.

The coconut, the seed of a palm tree that grows mostly in tropical coastal areas, yields numerous food and nonfood products. The oil is used in vegetable shortening, nondairy creamers, some spreads, and many commercial baked goods; it is also an ingredient in shampoos, moisturizing skin lotions, soaps, and various cosmetics. The creamy coconut meat that lines the interior of the nut's hard outer shell is eaten raw or used to flavor ice cream, confectionery products, and baked goods. Coconut milk, the sweet white fluid from the heart of the nut, is served as a beverage or used as a marinade. It contains virtually no fat.

Dried coconut meat, or copra, is rich in oil. In fact, more than 90 percent of the fatty acids in coconuts are classified as saturated; remarkably, coconut oil is more highly saturated than

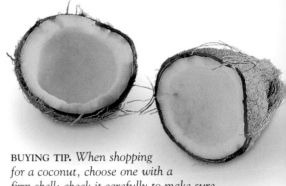

BUYING TIP. *When shopping for a coconut, choose one with a firm shell; check it carefully to make sure there are no dark or soft spots on it.*

the fat in butter or red meat. This high level of saturation results in an oil that resists turning rancid, making coconut oil ideal for commercial baking. However, it is also a major drawback; saturated fats tend to raise blood cholesterol levels. In light of this, people who have elevated cholesterol levels or any other cardiovascular risk factors are typically advised to avoid products made with coconut oil.

On the plus side, the fatty acids are easy to digest, and a half cup of coconut meat has about 1 mg of iron and a fair amount of fiber. ❖

COFFEE

BENEFITS
- Stimulates the central nervous system.
- Can help you stay awake and alert.

DRAWBACKS
- May contribute to difficulty falling asleep and disturbed or reduced sleep.
- Drinking large amounts can cause irritability and jittery nerves.
- Increases excretion of calcium.

Our major source of caffeine, coffee is the substance millions of North Americans use to stay alert. In addition to caffeine, coffee contains nearly 400 other chemicals, including trace amounts of several vitamins and minerals, tannins, and caramelized sugar. Coffee is not entirely calorie-free; while a 6-oz (180-ml) cup of sugar-free black coffee has only 4 calories, some specialty coffee drinks have more fat and calories than a rich dessert. A cup of whole-milk mocha topped with whipped cream is on a par with a hot fudge sundae.

A dedicated coffee drinker might consider reducing caffeine from other sources—for example, giving up caffeinated soft drinks from the diet.

POSSIBLE HAZARDS

Coffee is best consumed in moderation. The following are possible hazards linked to coffee:

- Infertility. A number of studies have found that consuming more than 300 mg caffeine a day is associated with a delay in conception.
- Heart problems. Caffeine prompts a temporary rise in blood pressure; it can also provoke cardiac arrhythmias in susceptible persons.
- Bone loss. Coffee increases calcium excretion in the urine. To compensate for this loss, heavy coffee drinkers should consume extra calcium-rich foods.
- Caffeine withdrawal. Heavy coffee drinkers who stop imbibing coffee abruptly may suffer headaches, irritability, and other withdrawal symptoms for a few days. Cut back gradually.
- Cholesterol problems. Cafestol and kahweol, compounds in coffee, can boost cholesterol synthesis by the liver. These are found in highest concentrations in Scandinavian and Turkish coffees, as well as French-press brews.
- Caffeine is a diuretic, meaning it increases the output of urine. This is a concern for men with prostate problems.

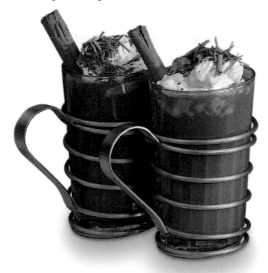

DECAFFEINATED COFFEE

Many people drink decaffeinated coffee to escape the insomnia and jittery nerves caused by caffeine. But even decaffeinated coffee has up to 5 mg of caffeine in a 5-oz (150-ml) cup. People with sleep problems are better off avoiding coffee. ❖

COLD CUTS

See Smoked, Cured, and Pickled Meats

COLDS AND FLU

CONSUME PLENTY OF

- Fruits and vegetables for vitamin C.
- Garlic and hot peppers (chilies), which may act as natural decongestants.
- Fluids to loosen phlegm.

The runny nose, cough, and sore throat of a cold are hard to escape; most people suffer two or three bouts with the enemy a year. That's why it's called "the common cold."

In the winter months, flu (short for influenza) inflicts a similar misery on people; what makes flu worse is the presence of fever, as well as muscle and joint aches. The complications of flu—especially pneumonia—can be serious and thousands of North Americans die from flu or its complications each year.

Colds and flu are highly contagious respiratory infections that are caused by viruses. More than 200 cold viruses (rhinoviruses) have been identified; unfortunately, developing immunity to one does not protect you from the others. There are fewer flu viruses, but they undergo frequent mutations—that is, they change their protein structure just a little—each year as they sweep around the globe. This is why new flu vaccines are produced yearly that protect against the prevailing strains of the virus. Doctors recommend annual flu shots for everyone over the age of 65, people of any age who have a circulatory, respiratory, kidney, metabolic, or immune disorder.

CATCHING THE "BUG"

Colds and flu are spread when virus-laden fluid droplets are released into the air by coughing and sneezing or transferred to surfaces by touch. British researchers have shown that the cold

GRANDMA'S SECRET WEAPON

It seems that the centuries old home remedy of chicken soup for fighting the common cold is not just an old wives' tale. Scientists believe that a 12-oz (355-ml) dose of the soup may reduce inflammation of the lungs. It is thought that chicken soup slows down the activity of white blood cells that can cause the inflammation.

virus is activated at temperatures slightly below 98.6°F (37°C), the normal temperature for humans. So it seems that the old wives' tales about catching cold have a grain of truth: If you sit in a draft, your temperature may drop just enough to activate the cold viruses that have been biding their time in your nasal passages.

When you breathe overly dry air (especially in planes and artificially ventilated office buildings), your nasal passages may form tiny cracks that provide an entryway for viruses. The best defense is plenty of fluids to rehydrate the tender membranes; try using a humidifier or opening the window to improve air quality.

You're more vulnerable to colds and flu when your immune system is depressed. Preventive steps include avoiding alcohol, getting plenty of rest, and reducing stress levels.

THE ROLE OF DIET

While there's no cure for colds or flu, eating properly may help to prevent them, shorten their duration, or make symptoms less severe.

More than two decades of extensive research have failed to substantiate claims that megadoses of vitamin C can prevent or cure colds. While there is no evidence to suggest it will prevent you from getting sick, some studies show it can shorten the length of the cold or lessen the symptoms. Vitamin C is known to have a slight antihistaminic effect, so drinking more citrus juice or taking a supplement may help reduce nasal symptoms.

One of the worst effects of high fever is dehydration. During a cold or flu, drink a minimum of 8 to 10 glasses of fluids a day in order to replenish lost fluids, keep mucous membranes moist, and loosen phlegm. Drink water, tea, and broth. Abstain from alcohol, which dilates small blood vessels and makes the sinuses feel stuffed up. Alcohol may produce adverse effects when taken with many drugs and reduces the body's ability to fight infection.

THROAT SOOTHER. *Add lemon to hot water or weak tea to loosen mucus and ease pain.*

The debate about whether to starve a cold and feed a fever is obsolete; doctors recommend eating when you feel hungry. The following foods may be helpful and comforting.

Chicken soup. Grandma was right! Not only is it soothing and easy to digest, but chicken soup also contains cystine, a compound that helps thin the mucus, relieving congestion.

Spicy foods. Hot peppers, or chilies, contain capsaicin, a substance that can help break up nasal and sinus congestion. Garlic, turmeric, and other hot spices have a similar effect.

The effect of zinc on the common cold remains controversial. Some research shows that sucking on zinc lozenges at the first sign of a cold may help cut the cold's duration and/or severity. Taking zinc supplements over a prolonged period is not a good idea since getting more than 40 mg per day over a long period of time can actually weaken your immune system, making it less able to fight against disease. It is important to ensure that your diet contains zinc-rich foods since zinc is important to a healthy immune system. Food sources of zinc include seafood (especially oysters), red meat and poultry, yogurt and other dairy products, wheat germ, wheat bran, and whole grains.

WHEN TO SEE A DOCTOR

Most colds and bouts of flu go away by themselves, but a doctor should be seen if you have:
- A cough that produces green, yellow, or bloody phlegm.
- A severe headache or pain in the face, jaw, or ear.
- Trouble swallowing or breathing.
- A fever over 100°F (37.8°C) that lasts more than 48 hours. ❖

COLITIS

LIMIT
- Fats, oils, and caffeine.

AVOID
- Foods that provoke symptoms.
- Alcohol in all forms.

Colitis, also called ulcerative colitis or inflammatory bowel disease, is a chronic inflammatory disease that causes bleeding ulcers in the colon and rectum. Symptomatic flare-ups alternate with periods of symptom-free remission. In mild cases of colitis, patients may have normal bowel movements with a mucous discharge;

more commonly, the disease also causes abdominal cramps and bloody diarrhea. When the disease is severe, violent and persistent bloody diarrhea is accompanied by fever, malaise, loss of appetite and weight, and anemia.

Although colitis may strike at any age, it most often develops between the ages of 15 and 30. The cause remains unknown, although infection, the immune system, heredity, and diet have all been implicated.

FOOD AND COLITIS

Modification of the diet is a mainstay of colitis treatment. Because people vary greatly in their response to foods, each person must develop an eating plan based on personal experience.

Start a food diary. Fundamental to the diet plan is a food diary that lets the patient key symptoms to specific foods. It is also important to consult a qualified dietitian to ensure good nutrition. Vitamin and mineral supplements are often needed to compensate for a restricted diet and possible absorption problems.

Avoid foods high in insoluble fiber. Foods that irritate the bowel often include those high in insoluble fiber, which is found in bran, whole grains, nuts, seeds, dried fruits, and the skins of potatoes, fresh fruits, and vegetables. Less irritating are pectin and other types of soluble fiber, which can be obtained from oats, poached peeled fruits, and cooked leafy green vegetables.

Keep fats and oils to a minimum. Fatty foods are hard to digest, so keep fats and oils to a minimum and avoid fried and sautéed foods, as well as such obviously fatty items as bacon, potato chips, and most cheeses.

Avoid caffeine. Depending on how your intestines react, you may want to avoid caffeinated drinks, decaffeinated coffee and colas, alcohol, spicy foods and seasonings (such as horseradish and mustard), and beans, cabbage, and other vegetables that may produce gas.

Stay clear of dairy products. Many people with ulcerative colitis have an intolerance to dairy products during symptom flare-ups; some, however, can use lactose-free products.

Load up on protein and other nutrients. The diet should provide enough calories, protein, and other nutrients to make up for the limitations. Eggs, fish, poultry, and lean meat supply high-grade protein. Red meat, especially liver, is an important source of iron for people who are constantly losing blood from the bowel. Eat as much as you want of pureed, canned, or soft-cooked vegetables and fruits that are strained to remove seeds and skins.

During a severe flare-up, a very-low-residue bland diet (a diet low in fiber designed to avoid producing stool) might include clear broth, weak tea, toasted white bread, soft-cooked eggs, gelatins, and cooked cream of wheat. As healing progresses, soft-cooked fish, poultry, and lean meats can be added, along with baked or boiled skinless potatoes and, eventually, cooked fruits, and steamed vegetables. In severe cases, liquid diets given orally, or intravenously, or by a nasogastric tube, may be necessary to prevent malnutrition. Liquid supplement drinks provide protein, vitamins, and minerals—helpful nutrition during a flare-up.

DRUG THERAPY

The first medication usually tried with ulcerative colitis is 5-aminosalicylic acid (mesalamine), often in combination with a 5-ASA derivative such as sulfasalazine. These drugs reduce inflammation. Anyone taking these medications should consume folate-rich foods, such as liver and leafy greens. Patients who do not respond to this therapy are treated with steroids, usually prednisone or hydrocortisone, which can be given orally, through an enema, or as a suppository. Long-term cortisone therapy can cause weight gain, thinning of the bones, and high blood pressure, so patients have to be carefully monitored. Because steroids promote the retention of fluids, patients taking these medicines should reduce their salt intake; they may also need extra calcium to prevent osteoporosis. ❖

CONSTIPATION

CONSUME PLENTY OF

- Fresh fruits and vegetables, grains, and other high-fiber foods.
- Fluids (at least 8 glasses a day).

LIMIT

- Sugar and refined starchy foods.

AVOID

- Alcohol in all forms.
- Any foods that provoke constipation.

Many people wrongly assume that they are constipated because they don't have a daily bowel movement. In fact, it's perfectly normal for bowels to move as often as three times a day or as infrequently as once in 3 or 4 days. Regularity is different for everyone.

DRINK HOT LIQUIDS

Hot liquids stimulate the bowels. Drink a cup of herbal tea or a glass of hot water with lemon, or a caffeinated coffee in the morning to help ease the effects of constipation.

THE PROBLEM OF HEMORRHOIDS

Chronic constipation, obesity, pregnancy, and an inherited predisposition are common causes of hemorrhoids—varicose veins in the anal area. Most hemorrhoids are symptom-free, but some cause itching, pain, and bleeding, especially during bouts of constipation. Straining to pass a hard stool can rupture one of the distended veins and result in considerable bleeding; more often, the stool contains small amounts of bright red blood. The blood loss itself is usually inconsequential, but any rectal bleeding should prompt medical investigation to rule out colon cancer or polyps.

Avoiding constipation and maintaining a normal weight will often eliminate hemorrhoid symptoms. Some sufferers find that curries, chilies, and other hot, spicy foods increase discomfort during bowel movements; citrus fruits and other acidic foods may also be irritating.

In severe cases, chronic blood loss from hemorrhoids can cause anemia; a doctor may prescribe iron supplements and removal of the hemorrhoids. Eating iron-rich foods can help restore the body's iron reserves.

There are two types of constipation: atonic occurs when the colon muscles are weak and lack tone; spastic (sometimes called irritable bowel syndrome) is characterized by irregular bowel movements. Atonic constipation, the more common of the two, develops when the diet lacks adequate fluids and fiber; a sedentary lifestyle is another common cause. Spastic constipation can be caused by stress, nervous disorders, excessive smoking, irritating foods, and obstructions of the colon.

Drink water. Adults should drink 8 glasses of nonalcoholic fluids every day. When a low-fiber diet coincides with a low-fluid intake, the stool becomes dry and hard, and increasingly difficult to move through the intestinal tract.

Exercise. Regular physical activity helps to stimulate bowel movements, whereas prolonged inactivity can cause constipation. Several medications, especially codeine and other narcotic painkillers, reduce peristalsis, the rhythmic muscle movements that push digested food through the bowel.

Avoid alcohol. Drinking alcohol has a similar effect in some people. Poor toilet habits, such as putting off going to the toilet despite an urge to defecate, can also cause constipation.

Use laxatives sparingly. Excessive laxative use reduces normal colon function. If a laxative is needed, one made of psyllium or another high-fiber stool softener is the best choice.

RECIPE FOR RELIEF

Increase intake of dietary fiber. The insoluble type of fiber that absorbs water but otherwise passes through the bowel intact, is instrumental in preventing constipation. Whenever possible, try to use the whole vegetable; fiber tends to be concentrated in the peelings, stems, and outer leaves—parts that many cooks discard. But any increase in high-fiber food consumption should be gradual and accompanied by more fluids to work with the higher amount of insoluble fiber.

EATING SMART. *A diet rich in whole grains and fiber helps relieve constipation.*

Enjoy a little dried fruit. Avoid adding miller's bran to foods—this can cause uncomfortable gas and bloating; it also reduces the absorption of iron, calcium, and other minerals. Instead, try a few prunes or dried figs. ❖

CONVENIENCE AND PROCESSED FOODS

BENEFITS
- Provide meals for people who don't have time to cook.

DRAWBACKS
- Many are high in fat, salt, and calories.

Technological advances have dramatically enhanced the quality and increased the range of processed foods. Vacuum-packed or frozen pre-cooked meals ready for the microwave oven, instant mashed potatoes and hot cereals, jars of prepared baby foods, and envelopes of soup, dessert, and sauce mixes are just a few of the timesaving foods that many people rely on. In addition, delicatessens and take-out restaurants are everywhere (see Fast Food).

Some critics blame this growing reliance on convenience foods, which are typically high in fat and calories, for the fact that almost one-half of all adult North Americans are overweight. Of these, almost one-quarter are obese.

DO ONE SIMPLE THING

ALWAYS ADD A FRESH SIDE SALAD

When preparing a meal consisting of processed food, like a frozen lasagna, always add a side salad. A fresh green salad provides a wide assortment of valuable nutrients.

The fact is, convenience foods are here to stay; however, anyone who follows the basic rules of variety, moderation, and balance can work them into a healthful, nutritious diet.

CONVENIENCE FOODS

Almost everyone consumes some convenience foods, defined as items that require little or no preparation; from ready-to-eat breakfast cereals, canned or frozen goods, to prepackaged heat-and-serve meals. Nutritionally, some of these products do not measure up to home-cooked meals, but this varies greatly among foods. Instant soups contain a few dehydrated vegetables and many artificial flavorings, emulsifiers, fillers, and preservatives. Homemade or even canned soups are more nutritious and contain fewer additives. Most convenience foods also tend to contain more sugar, salt, and fat than comparable dishes prepared at home.

Processing may strip vitamins and minerals from some foods, but there are exceptions in which convenience foods are actually more nutritious than their fresh counterparts. Vegetables and many fruits harvested and quick-frozen at their peak often have more vitamins than those picked before maturity, shipped long distances, and then allowed to sit on store shelves. Most enriched cereals and breads provide more nutrients than those made with the original grains.

Many food processors have been prompted by consumer demands to enhance the nutritional quality of their products by adding healthful ingredients (for example, calcium to orange juice) or by reducing fat, sugar, and salt. Although some claims of low-fat, no cholesterol, and "lite" may be misleading, an informed shopper who knows how to decipher food labeling can make healthful choices.

THE PRICE OF CONVENIENCE

Most convenience foods carry a higher price tag than the total cost of their ingredients. For many people, however, the extra cost is worth the savings in time and effort. Still, they may worry about the nutritional value of frozen dinners, breakfast bars, and other convenience foods. To answer such concerns, many food manufacturers now produce special products. Some of these are low in calories and sodium, while others are designed to meet the special needs of people with nutrition-related problems like diabetes and food allergies. It's important to check labels and ingredient lists. Also, special health or dietary items tend to be more expensive than the regular lines, even though their components may be similar.

Combining convenience foods with fresh ingredients can save both time and money while increasing interest and nutritional value. For example, you can build a tasty and nutritious meal around a frozen entrée by adding a green salad and seasonal vegetables that take only minutes to prepare.

FOODS FOR CHILDREN

Most parents rely upon at least some convenience items when introducing foods into a baby's diet. Instant cereals and jars of pureed fruits, vegetables, and meats are certainly easier than homemade baby foods. More questionable are the convenience foods that many older children seem to prefer. Favorites like hot dogs and cold cuts are usually loaded with fat, salt, and preservatives; instant puddings may provide milk, but they are also high in sugar, fats, and artificial flavorings and colorings.

When feeding children, emphasize foods made with minimal processing; for example, chicken is a better pick than hot dogs, yogurt is more healthful than puddings, uncoated oat cereals or low-fat granola is a wiser choice than sweetened children's cereals. ❖

CORN

....

BENEFITS

- A good source of folate and thiamine.
- A rich source of lutein.
- Air-popped unbuttered popcorn is low in calories and very high in fiber.

DRAWBACKS

- The niacin in corn is not released in the human digestive tract.
- Corn lacks lysine and tryptophan, two essential amino acids needed to make a complete protein.

Indigenous to the Western Hemisphere, corn is the most abundant grain crop; worldwide, it

DO-IT-YOURSELF
CONVENIENCE FOODS

A growing number of cooks are discovering that they can make their own convenience foods—all it takes is a freezer and planning. Instead of discarding leftovers, for example, make up a frozen prepackaged meal that can be popped in the microwave at a later date. This approach also allows you to control the amount of fat, salt, and other ingredients.

If you're making a soup or stew, double the recipe and then freeze the extra portion. Similarly, buy extra fresh vegetables that are in season and freeze them for later use. Be sure to date the packages, and use the oldest first.

is exceeded only by wheat as a cereal grain. Most of the corn grown in the United States and Canada is field, or dent, corn, which is allowed to mature on its stalk, dried, and used as animal feed or processed into flour to make cereals. Flint corn, another field variety, keeps better than dent corn and is used to make cornmeal. Flour corn has soft, starchy kernels that are easily ground into flour, making it a favorite with Native peoples to make tortillas and other corn dishes.

Sweet corn, which is harvested while still immature, is the type consumed as a vegetable. It can be cooked in several different ways: on the cob or with the soft kernels removed and served fresh, frozen, or canned for future use.

CORN AND NUTRITION

Corn is high in starch and protein, but it lacks two essential amino acids—lysine and tryptophan; as a result, it is not a suitable protein substitute. In undeveloped countries, children are sometimes fed a diet made up mostly of corn, which can lead to two deficiency diseases: kwashiorkor, caused by inadequate protein, and pellagra, resulting from a deficiency of niacin. When corn is consumed along with beans and other legumes, however, it provides a complete protein.

One medium ear of corn contains 83 calories. One cup of kernels provides 13 percent of the Recommended Dietary Allowance (RDA) for folate. It is also a source or potassium, thiamine, and fiber.

Corn is a good source of lutein, a powerful antioxidant that may help lower the risk of age-related macular degeneration, a common cause of blindness in older adults.

Most of the niacin in corn is in the form of niacytin, which is not broken down in the

human digestive tract. Early nutrition researchers were puzzled by the fact that Mexicans and South Americans did not develop pellagra, even though their diets were made up mostly of corn. It was discovered that combining the corn with an alkaline substance releases the niacin in niacytin; thus, mixing cornmeal with lime water to make tortillas prevented pellagra. Similarly, Natives in South America ground corn with alkaline potash to loosen the bran, another practice that released niacin and prevented pellagra.

While corn may not be a complete food, it is by far our most important farm crop; not only is it fed to pigs, cattle, and other meat animals, but it is also used in more than 800 different processed foods. This is why people who are allergic to corn have difficulty finding corn-free processed foods.

POPCORN

A popular snack food, popcorn is a special variety that grows on a cob smaller than those of sweet corn. As the kernels are heated rapidly, the moisture inside them is converted to steam. When the steam pressure builds to a certain point, it bursts the outer shell and the interior turns into a fluffy mass of starch and fiber many times larger than the original kernel. A cup of air-popped plain popcorn has only 30 calories, making it an ideal, high-fiber snack. Popping the corn in oil and adding a tablespoon of butter, however, increases the calorie content more than fivefold, to about 155 per cup. ❖

CRANBERRIES

BENEFITS
- A fair source of vitamin C and fiber.
- Juice helps prevent or alleviate cystitis and urinary tract infections.
- Contain bioflavonoids, thought to protect eyesight and help prevent cancer.

DRAWBACKS
- Must be prepared with large amounts of sugar to make them palatable.

Once served mostly as a condiment at Thanksgiving and Christmas, cranberries are now consumed throughout the year as juice, a dried snack fruit, and an ingredient in muffins and other baked goods. Cranberries belong to the same family as blueberries and huckleberries, but unlike these fruits, they are too tart to

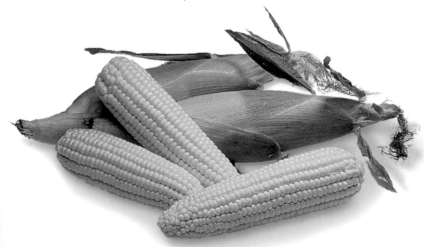

POPULAR YEAR-ROUND. *Cranberries are at their peak when they bounce.*

necessary to cure an established urinary infection. Most commercial cranberry juice is often too diluted to be effective in preventing or treating urinary infections; it also contains large amounts of sugar or other sweeteners. Use a juicer to make your own cranberry juice. To reduce the amount of sugar needed, dilute a cup of concentrated juice with 2 to 3 cups of apple juice and then sweeten to taste.

OTHER BENEFITS

Cranberries provide fiber, along with some vitamin C; they also contain bioflavonoids, plant pigments that help counter the damage of unstable molecules that are formed when oxygen is used by the body. European researchers have found that one of these bioflavonoids, anthocyanin, promotes formation of visual purple, a pigment in the eyes instrumental in color and night vision. Other studies suggest anthocyanin has an anticancer effect. ❖

eat raw. Even when sweetened, cranberries retain a fresh tartness that complements poultry and pork.

Cranberries are a native North American plant. Although they still grow wild in boggy areas, most are cultivated in Massachusetts, Wisconsin, British Columbia, Oregon, Washington, and New Jersey. When buying fresh cranberries, look for firm, bright red fruit. Berries that are at their peak will bounce when dropped; those that don't are likely to be soft and past their prime.

ROLE IN CYSTITIS

Cranberry juice has long been used as a home remedy for cystitis and also to prevent kidney and bladder stones. Originally, this benefit was attributed to quinic acid, a substance that increases urine acidity and prevents the formation of calcium stones. It was also thought that this acidity helped prevent cystitis. Studies show, however, that cranberries also contain a natural antibiotic substance that makes the bladder walls inhospitable to the organisms responsible for urinary tract infections. This prevents the bacteria from forming colonies; instead, they are washed out of the body in the urine. (Interestingly, blueberry juice has a similar protective effect.)

Many urologists and gynecologists now advise patients who suffer recurrent or chronic bladder infections to drink a couple of glasses of cranberry juice daily as a preventive measure. See a doctor, however, if symptoms develop or persist; prescription antibiotics are usually

CRAVINGS

EAT PLENTY OF
- Low-fat starchy foods to satisfy a carbohydrate craving.
- High-fiber foods to avoid feeling hungry.

LIMIT
- Foods you might crave, especially sweets, chocolates, and salty items.

AVOID
- Becoming overly hungry, which can lead to overindulgence.

All of us occasionally have an irresistible urge for a certain food or beverage. But merely having a sudden need for a particular food does not constitute a true craving, nor does indulging in an occasional chocolate, ice cream, or other favorite food. A craving goes much deeper—it's an insistent desire that you can't ignore, even though satisfying it may entail considerable inconvenience or even danger.

Occasional cravings may be in response to stress, hormonal changes, or excessive hunger. More obsessive cravings, however, can stem from a specific illness, addiction, or deep-seated psychological problem.

Recent research suggests that hormonal changes are responsible for many food cravings, especially those that develop during periods of stress, pregnancy, or different phases of a woman's menstrual cycle. Following this theory, fluctuating hormonal levels may influence the brain's production of serotonin and other chemicals—changes that can trigger an intense desire for specific foods. Under these circumstances, a person usually craves chocolate or other sweets; researchers think this is because sugars are a quick source of glucose, which the brain needs for energy. Eating a diet high in whole grain, starchy foods along with moderate amounts of protein may prevent the craving for sweets because these complex carbohydrates and protein are metabolized more slowly than sugars, thus providing a steady supply of glucose.

DID YOU KNOW?

PICA IS THE TERM THAT DESCRIBES BIZARRE FOOD CRAVINGS

For unexplained reasons, some people, especially children, develop intense cravings for nonfood items, such as paint chips, soil, clay, or laundry starch. This phenomenon is known as pica, which comes from the Latin term for magpie—a bird that will eat almost anything.

Pica can have serious consequences, including lead poisoning, intestinal obstruction, worm infestations, and even death if poisonous substances are consumed.

PREGNANCY CRAVINGS

Pregnant women often develop strange food cravings, especially for pickles and other salty foods. In this instance, the craving reflects a physical need. During pregnancy, a woman's volume of blood doubles, and as a result she needs extra sodium to maintain a proper fluid balance. Normally, adding salt to food supplies the necessary sodium. As for other cravings, there's usually no harm in satisfying them in moderation, provided overall nutritional needs are met. But if the cravings are for bizarre indigestible items like laundry starch, soil, clay, and ice, it constitutes pica and may reflect a serious medical or psychological problem, and requires the attention of professionals.

A craving for ice is a common sign of iron deficiency; conversely, the deficiency can be caused by eating starch, clay, and other substances that bind to iron and prevent its absorption. Taking iron supplements to counter the deficiency usually puts an end to the craving.

Cravings are also influenced by cultural traditions, some of which are still practiced in places like the rural American South or among recent immigrants. For example, some folk healers urge pregnant women to eat clay for an easier delivery; others maintain that consumption of soil provides needed iron. Such practices, however, are dangerous for both the mother and her fetus.

TO GIVE IN OR TO DENY?

Some experts believe that food cravings reflect the "wisdom of the body"; we feel an urge to eat particular foods to fulfill a nutritional need. In general, however, we tend to crave foods that are not particularly nutritious, and in such instances, psychological factors are probably more influential than physical needs. For some people, food may fill an emotional void, leading a person to turn to certain foods during periods of stress or sadness. The power of suggestion is another possible trigger, which is why just a brief whiff of a favorite food can result in an intense desire for it.

People often make the mistake of trying to deny a craving. Some may succeed, but more often than not, denial fosters an even stronger desire for the food. Unless the object of the craving poses a serious health risk (for instance, a person with high blood pressure craving salty foods), experts say it is better to satisfy the longing, but to do so in moderation. A healthier approach is to anticipate the craving and to satisfy it in advance. For example, if a woman invariably develops a strong craving for sweets during her premenstrual phase, she can lessen it somewhat by increasing her intake of starchy foods, which raise blood glucose levels. Eating more fruits, which are high in natural sugars, may also satisfy the desire for sweets.

Some medications, particularly steroids and other hormonal preparations, can promote food cravings. These drug-related cravings, however, are usually nonspecific; the person may simply feel ravenously hungry and crave eating in general instead of a particular food.

Avoiding becoming overly hungry can also forestall cravings for sweets or fatty foods. Hunger is the body's way of letting you know it's running short of fuel; it's a powerful instinct that is almost impossible to deny for any length of time. This is one reason why dieters often find it so hard to adhere to an overly restrictive regimen; their resolve may be strong, but it's almost impossible to deny the body's instinct for self-preservation. Eating small, frequent meals is how to avert hunger and the subsequent strong cravings that can lead to overeating. ❖

CROHN'S DISEASE

CONSUME
- Lean meat, fish, and poultry for the protein necessary for healing.
- Under a doctor's supervision, vitamin, mineral, and other nutritional supplements.

LIMIT
- High-fiber foods, especially if the bowel is partially obstructed.

AVOID
- Alcohol in any form.
- Any food that worsens symptoms.

Also known as ileitis, Crohn's disease is a type of inflammatory bowel disease that can affect any part of the intestinal tract, from the mouth to the anus. However, it most commonly attacks the colon and the lower part of the small intestine, or the ileum.

Crohn's disease is a chronic condition that may recur after lengthy periods of remission. Common symptoms are abdominal pain, often in the lower right area, and diarrhea. Typically, diseased portions of the intestine are interspersed with normal segments; fistulas (abnormal passageways between portions of intestines) are common. The diseased portions may become obstructed, an emergency situation. There may also be weight loss, fever, and intestinal bleeding persistent enough to cause anemia. Children with Crohn's disease may suffer stunted growth and delayed sexual development.

There are many theories about the causes of Crohn's disease, but none have been proved. Some scientists believe that the immune system is affected by a virus or a bacterium that triggers an inflammatory reaction in the intestinal wall. Crohn's disease appears to run in families; about 20 percent of those who have the disease have a blood relative with some form of inflammatory bowel disease. Symptoms can flare up in periods of unusual or prolonged stress, but stress doesn't appear to cause the disease.

MEDICAL TREATMENT
Crohn's disease has no cure, but a combination of drugs usually alleviates symptoms. As in the case of colitis, 5-ASA agents are frontline therapy, with sulfasalazine being the most popular choice. When Crohn's flares up, prednisone is commonly used. Drugs that suppress the immune system, such as 6-mercaptopurine or the related azathioprine can also be effective. While these drugs do suppress the immune reaction that contributes to inflammation, they also increase the susceptibility to infection. If all these therapies fail to provide relief, infliximab (Remicade) has been approved as an intravenous treatment. This substance partially neutralizes the activity of a protein called tumor necrosis factor (TNF), which is thought to be responsible for the inflammation associated with Crohn's disease. Crohn's patients sometimes suffer from bacterial overgrowth in the intestine which requires the use of antibiotics.

Surgery is often needed to correct complications, such as an intestinal blockage, perforation, and abscesses. Sometimes it is necessary to remove the diseased section of bowel; unfortunately, this does not prevent recurrences in other portions of the intestinal tract.

NUTRITIONAL APPROACHES
Nutritional deficiencies are common in people with Crohn's disease for several reasons. During a flare-up, symptoms squelch appetite, and a person is unlikely to consume enough food to maintain weight and good nutrition. Nutrition can be a problem even during periods of remission; if the small intestine is damaged by inflammation, vitamins and nutrients are not absorbed properly. Surgical removal of portions of the intestine further impairs the body's ability to absorb nutrients.

Eliminate any foods that provoke symptoms. Although some doctors advise patients to avoid all fried foods, dairy products, spices, and high-fiber foods, there is no specific diet for Crohn's disease. The overall objective is to consume adequate calories, vitamins, and minerals without exacerbating symptoms. Try eliminating any food that seems to create problems for several weeks, and keep a diary of symptoms to determine whether giving it up is helpful. Eliminate only one type of food at a time, such as milk and other dairy products.

Avoid foods high in fiber. High-fiber foods are generally discouraged because they may be irritating to the intestines, and they can also exacerbate diarrhea. High-fiber foods often are improperly digested and pass through to the colon where they can be digested by bacteria.

This may cause bacterial overgrowth, which in turn can exacerbate Crohn's. Alcohol should be avoided as it can worsen intestinal bleeding; it lowers the body's immunity; and it has been known to contribute to malnutrition.

Eat smaller, more frequent meals, and chew carefully. Consuming six or more small meals a day is less likely to provoke symptoms than having three large ones. Eat slowly and chew each mouthful thoroughly. This is good advice for anyone hoping to improve digestion, but it is of particular importance to those suffering from Crohn's disease.

Talk to your doctor about taking nutritional supplements. Even patients who can consume a normal diet may develop nutritional deficiencies because of poor absorption of nutrients; thus, many patients need to take a daily multivitamin and mineral supplement. High-dose vitamins should only be taken under a doctor's supervision. Those who develop vitamin B_{12} deficiency, for example, often need to take it by injection if they lack the intestinal substances to metabolize it.

SPECIAL SUPPLEMENTS

Patients with severe symptoms or who have had extensive surgery may need a special high-calorie liquid formula, either as a nutritional supplement or as a replacement for normal meals. Again, such supplements should be prescribed by a doctor. In unusual cases, an elemental diet—a low-fat, easy-to-digest formula—may be prescribed. Unfortunately, such formulas often have an unpleasant taste, but if the patient is unable to drink it, it can be given through a feeding tube (known as enteral nutrition).

The most severe cases of Crohn's disease may require total parenteral nutrition (TPN), in which all nutrients are given intravenously. TPN is most beneficial for patients who need to rest their intestinal tract so it can heal or who are unable to absorb enough nourishment from their regular diets. This approach is also beneficial in treating a child whose growth is being stunted by inadequate nutrition. Because it can be administered at home, TPN allows for a more normal lifestyle. ❖

CUCUMBERS

BENEFITS

● Low in calories.

Cucumbers belong to the same plant family as melons, pumpkins, and winter squash, but they are not as nutritious. One cup of sliced cucumber provides only about 6 mg of vitamin C and smaller amounts of folate and potassium. The skin contains some beta carotene, but cucumbers are often peeled, especially if they've been sprayed with wax to retard spoilage.

Because cucumbers are approximately 95 percent water, they are very low in calories; a cup of slices contains fewer than 15 calories. Folk healers often recommend cucumbers as a natural diuretic, but any increased urination is probably due to their water content rather than an inherent substance.

In North America cucumbers are used mostly as a salad ingredient or as pickles. Commercially, they are used mainly to make pickles and relishes; cucumber juice contains some alpha hydroxy acids, which improve the effectiveness of facial masks, and other cosmetic products.

In many countries cucumbers are an important staple; worldwide, they rank ninth among vegetable crops with multiple uses. In India and Central Europe, for example, they are diced and mixed with herbs and yogurt to serve as a salad. They are also stuffed and baked or served as a cooked side dish, as well as used in vinaigrettes, tartar sauces, and cold soups. ❖

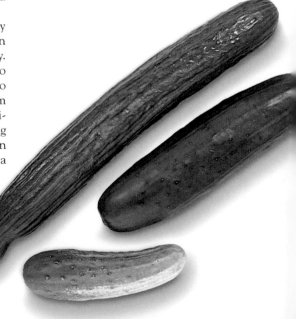

MULTIPURPOSE VEGETABLE. *Cucumbers are eaten whole, pickled, are found in salads, and used to make relishes, as well as a variety of cosmetic products.*

CURRANTS

BENEFITS

- An excellent low-calorie source of vitamin C and potassium.
- High in bioflavonoids.

DRAWBACKS

- Fresh currants are highly perishable and are available for only a few weeks in the summer.

The several varieties of fresh currants are actually berries that are related to gooseberries. The fruit marketed as dried currants is a variety of grape, and thus a type of raisin.

Red and white currants are the most common types available in North America, usually for only a short time during the summer. Black currants (cultivated mostly in Europe) lead both the red and white types in nutritional value. A cup of black currants provides a whopping 220 mg of vitamin C, as well as 360 mg of potassium. This compares with 50 mg of vitamin C and 300 mg of potassium in a cup of red or white currants (also good amounts of these essential nutrients). All types are low in calories, about 70 in a cup of fresh berries. Currants are also a good source of fiber, providing about 2 g per cup.

Because they are quite tart, fresh currants usually are not eaten raw; instead, they are used in baking or to make jams, jellies, and sauces. Diluted and sweetened black currant juice is a refreshing beverage that is very high in vitamin C. The juice can be fermented and made into liqueurs and cordials.

MEDICINAL USES

All varieties of currants are rich in bioflavonoids, pigments that are thought to boost the antioxidant effects of vitamin C; they also help inhibit cancer growth and may possibly prevent other diseases. Europeans have long valued black currants for their antibacterial and anti-inflammatory properties, which are thought to come from anthocyanin, a bioflavonoid in the berry skins. In Scandinavia a powder made from dried black currant skins is used to treat diarrhea, especially that caused by *Escherichia coli*, a common cause of bacterial diarrhea. Europeans also use black currant syrup to ease the inflammation of a sore throat. ❖

CYSTIC FIBROSIS

CONSUME PLENTY OF

- Fish, poultry, eggs, meat, and other high-protein foods for growth.
- Starchy foods and a moderate amount of sweets for energy.
- Fat (as much as can be tolerated) for extra calories.
- Salt to replace that lost in sweat.
- Fluids to prevent constipation.

AVOID

- Low-calorie products.

A genetic disease that afflicts over 33,000 children in North America, cystic fibrosis affects the glands that produce mucus, sweat, enzymes, and other secretions. The most serious consequences of the disease occur in the lungs, pancreas, and intestines, all of which become clogged with thick mucus. As the lungs become congested, they are especially vulnerable to pneumonia and other infections. When the ducts that normally carry pancreatic enzymes to the small intestine become clogged, difficulty in breaking down fats and protein is the result, along with other digestive problems. Abnormal amounts of salt are lost in sweat and saliva, which can lead to serious imbalances in body chemistry.

At the moment there is no cure for cystic fibrosis, although scientists are testing gene therapy as a means of correcting the underlying genetic defect. In the meantime, a combination of an enriched diet, vitamin supplements, replacement enzymes, antibiotics and other medications, and regular postural drainage to clear mucus from the lungs serves as the best treatment, and has greatly improved the outlook for people with cystic fibrosis.

MEAL-PLANNING TIPS

Start with a balanced diet that is suitable for the entire family, then add the extra calories and nutrients that are needed by the person with cystic fibrosis:

- Serve larger portions, especially of high-calorie foods.
- Enrich whole milk by adding a cup of dried milk to each quart or liter.
- Provide frequent snacks, such as dried fruit and nuts, toast with jam or jelly, ice cream, a peanut butter and jelly sandwich, or pizza.
- Offer a high-calorie snack shortly before bedtime.
- Serve juices or nectars instead of water with meals.
- Add extra eggs, which are easy to digest, to puddings, custards, and other high-calorie dishes.

NUTRITIONAL NEEDS

Since diet is critical in managing cystic fibrosis, the treatment team usually includes a clinical dietitian. To grow properly, children with cystic fibrosis typically need to consume many more calories than are normally recommended.

In the past it was almost impossible to meet these markedly increased calorie demands because of the body's inability to digest and absorb fats and protein. The development of improved enzyme preparations to supplement or replace those normally produced by the pancreas has helped solve this problem. These supplemental enzymes, in the form of tablets, capsules, or powder, must be taken with every meal and snack to aid digestion.

Eat larger portions and lots of snacks. There is no special diet for cystic fibrosis; rather, the child is encouraged to take larger portions during meals and have more frequent snacks. Babies with the disease may be given a formula that contains predigested fats.

Eat more protein. For older children, high-protein foods, such as meat, poultry, fish, eggs, and milk, are emphasized—and as much fat as the child can tolerate to help get the extra calories.

EXTRA NUTRITION. *An omelet made with herbs and cheese, and stir-fried shrimp, vegetables, and a generous portion of noodles, provide good amounts of nutrients, protein, and calories.*

Vitamin and mineral supplements are often necessary, but these should be taken only under the supervision of a doctor.

Consume more sodium. Salt is also an essential part of the diet, because cystic fibrosis affects the sweat and salivary glands, causing them to excrete abnormal amounts of sodium and chloride in perspiration and saliva. This situation can be especially critical during hot weather or exercise, when it may be necessary to consume extra salt. Otherwise, adding moderate amounts of salt to flavor foods should be sufficient to maintain adequate sodium levels.

Supplements may be prescribed. If digestive problems develop despite taking enzymes, supplements of predigested fats may be prescribed, and in some cases, calorie-enriched supplements may be necessary. Usually these can be taken by mouth, but in severe cases they are administered at night through a feeding tube. Intravenous feeding is rarely necessary, but if required, it can be given at home.

Some people with cystic fibrosis may also develop diabetes if the pancreas becomes so clogged that it can no longer make adequate insulin, the hormone needed to metabolize carbohydrates. In such cases, insulin injections are added. Constipation and even intestinal obstruction are common in cystic fibrosis. It's important to consume adequate water and other fluids, but high-fiber foods are not recommended. A doctor may prescribe a laxative to prevent constipation.

DIETARY DIFFERENCES

Parents often find it difficult to deal with the dietary recommendations for a child with cystic fibrosis. It's important to understand that the nutritional needs of a person with cystic fibrosis are very different from those of a healthy person. A high-calorie diet with as much protein and fat as can be tolerated is necessary. Prescription enzymes that improve absorption of fats and protein have made a big difference in living with cystic fibrosis. Fats provide more calories per unit than other nutrients, so they are a critical source of energy. The body also needs fat in order to absorb vitamins A, D, E, and K.

In the absence of diabetes, it's not necessary to restrict sugary foods. These simple carbohydrates are more easily absorbed than starches. However, sweet snacks should be accompanied by protein to provide balance and the amino acids needed for growth, immune function, and repair and maintenance of body tissue. ❖

It's important to brush your teeth after eating dates. Both the dried and fresh fruits are very sticky, and because of their high sugar content, they can lead to dental decay if bits are allowed to adhere to the teeth. ❖

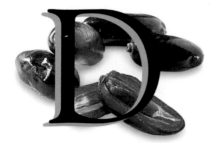

DATES

BENEFITS
- An excellent source of potassium.
- A good source of iron, niacin, and vitamin B_6.
- High in fiber.

DRAWBACKS
- High sugar content and stickiness promote tooth decay.

Prized for their sweet fruits, date palms are among the oldest cultivated trees; they have been grown in North Africa for at least 8,000 years. These desert trees are extraordinarily fruitful, producing up to 200 dates in a cluster.

Fresh dates are classified according to their moisture content, falling into three categories: soft, semisoft, and dry. Most varieties in North America are semisoft, which are marketed fresh, as well as dried after part of their moisture has been evaporated.

With 60 to 70 percent of their weight coming from sugar, dates are one of the sweetest of all fruits. One-half cup (about 12 medium dates) contains about 275 calories—many more than most fruits. They are very high in potassium; 12 dates provide 650 mg, more than a comparable amount of other high-potassium foods, such as bananas and oranges. Twelve dates also provide 15 percent or more of the Recommended Dietary Allowance of iron, niacin, and vitamin B_6, as well as 6 g of fiber. However, dates have almost no vitamin C.

Dates contain tyramine, an organic compound found in aged cheese, certain processed meats, red wine, and other products. Anyone taking monoamine oxidase (MAO) inhibitors to treat depression should avoid dates, because tyramine can interact with these drugs to produce a life-threatening rise in blood pressure. In some people, tyramine can also trigger migraine headaches.

DENTAL HEALTH

CONSUME PLENTY OF
- Calcium-rich foods, such as low-fat milk, yogurt, and cheese.
- Fresh fruits and vegetables for vitamins A and C, and for chewing in order to promote healthy gums.
- Tea, which is a good source of fluoride.

LIMIT
- Dried fruits and other sticky foods that lodge between the teeth.

AVOID
- Sweet drinks and snacks.
- Steady sipping of acidic drinks for prolonged periods.

In addition to brushing and flossing, a healthful diet (with natural or added fluoride) protects teeth from decay and keeps the gums healthy. Tooth decay (cavities and dental caries) and gum disease are caused by colonies of bacteria that constantly coat the teeth with a sticky film called plaque. If plaque is not brushed away, these bacteria break down the sugars and starches in foods to produce acids that wear away the tooth enamel. The plaque also hardens into tartar, which can lead to gum inflammation, or gingivitis.

A well-balanced diet provides the minerals, vitamins, and other nutrients essential for healthy teeth and gums. Fluoride, occurring naturally in foods and water, or added to the water supply, can be a powerful tool in fighting decay. It can reduce the rate of cavities by as much as 60 percent.

DENTAL HEALTH GUIDELINES

Start right by eating right during pregnancy. Make sure that your children's teeth get off to a good start by eating sensibly during pregnancy.

DID YOU KNOW?

FLUORIDE IS STILL CONTROVERSIAL

Over the past 40 years fluoride has been the subject of exhaustive research. Twenty different countries have conducted 140 studies on the safety and effectiveness of fluoridation. The scientific community's overwhelming conclusion: Water fluoridation is absolutely safe and extremely effective when used correctly. One part fluoride for every 1 million parts of water (1.0 ppm) is all that's needed to reduce cavities by up to 40 percent. Despite this, fluoridation still has many skeptics.

DO ONE SIMPLE THING

CHEW GUM SWEETENED WITH XYLITOL

Chew it for at least 5 minutes within 5 minutes after finishing a meal. Gum sweetened with xylitol helps to counter harmful bacteria in your mouth, which promote cavities. A study showed that people who chewed gum with xylitol after meals had far fewer cavity-causing bacteria in their mouth 5 minutes afterward than people who chewed other gums or no gum at all.

Particularly important is calcium, which helps to form strong teeth and bones, and vitamin D, which the body needs to absorb calcium.

You need lots of calcium for healthy teeth and gums. Low-fat dairy products, fortified soy and rice beverages, canned salmon or sardines (with bones), almonds, and dark green leafy vegetables are excellent sources of calcium.

You need vitamin D to help absorb the calcium. Vitamin D is obtained from fluid milk, fortified soy and rice beverages, margarine, fatty fish such as salmon, and moderate exposure to the sun.

Fluoride is key. To a large extent, cavities can be prevented by giving children fluoride in the first few years of life. Fluoride is supplied through fluoridated water (not all municipalities fluoridate their water supply, however), beverages made with fluoridated water, tea, and some fish, as well as many brands of toothpaste and some mouthwash. Fluoride supplements are available for children who don't have access to fluoridated drinking water. It is wise to check to see if the water supply in your area is fluoridated. Excess consumption of fluoride can cause mottling of the teeth.

Also needed are phosphorus, magnesium, vitamin A, and beta carotene. In addition to calcium and fluoride, minerals needed for the formation of tooth enamel include phosphorus (richly supplied in meat, fish, and eggs) and magnesium (found in whole grains, spinach, and bananas). Vitamin A also helps build strong bones and teeth. Good sources of beta carotene, which the body turns into vitamin A, include orange-colored fruits and vegetables and the dark green leafy vegetables.

Children are particularly vulnerable to tooth decay; parents should:
- Provide a good diet throughout childhood;
- Brush children's teeth until they're mature enough to do a thorough job by themselves (usually by 6 or 7 years old);
- Supervise twice-daily brushing and flossing thereafter;
- Never put babies or toddlers to bed accompanied by a bottle of milk (which contains the natural sugar lactose), juice, or other sweet drink;
- Never dip pacifiers in honey or syrup.

THE SUGAR FACTOR

Sucrose, most familiar to us as granulated sugar, is the leading cause of tooth decay, but it is far from the only culprit. Although sugary foods, including cookies, candies, and sodas, are major offenders, starchy foods (such as breads and cereals) also play an important part in tooth decay. When starches mix with amylase, an enzyme in saliva, the result is an acid bath that erodes the enamel and makes teeth more susceptible to decay. If starchy foods linger in the mouth, the acid bath is prolonged, and the potential for damage is all the greater.

Be careful when eating dried fruits. Dried fruits can have an adverse effect on teeth, because they are high in sugar and cling to the teeth. Even unsweetened fruit juices can contribute to tooth decay—they are acidic and contain relatively high levels of simple sugars.

Fresh fruits, especially apples, are better choices. Fresh fruit, although both sweet and acidic, is much less likely to cause a problem, because chewing stimulates the saliva flow. Saliva decreases mouth acidity and washes away food particles. Apples, for example, have been called nature's toothbrush because they stimulate the gums, increase saliva flow and reduce the build-up of cavity-causing bacteria. A chronically dry mouth also contributes to decay. Saliva flow slows during sleep; going to bed without brushing the teeth is especially harmful. Certain drugs, including those used for high blood pressure, also cut down saliva flow.

HELPFUL FOODS

You can protect your teeth by concluding meals with foods that do not promote cavities and may even prevent them. For instance, aged cheeses help prevent cavities if consumed at the end of a meal. Chewing sugarless gum stimulates the flow of saliva, which decreases acid and flushes out food particles. Rinsing your mouth and brushing your teeth after eating are important strategies to prevent cavities.

GUM DISEASE

More teeth are lost through gum disease than through tooth decay. Gum disease is likely to strike anyone who neglects oral hygiene or eats a poor diet. Particularly at risk are people with alcoholism, malnutrition, or AIDS/HIV infection or who are being treated with steroid drugs or certain cancer chemotherapies. Regular brushing and flossing help to prevent puffy, sore, and inflamed gums.

Gingivitis, a very common condition that causes the gums to redden, swell, and bleed, is typically caused by the gradual buildup of plaque. Treatment requires good dental hygiene and removal of plaque by a dentist or dental hygienist. Left untreated, gingivitis can lead to periodontitis—an advanced infection of the gums that causes teeth to loosen and fall out. There may even be more serious consequences of gum disease. Studies have shown a link between poor oral health and heart disease. Bleeding gums apparently provide an entry port for bacteria or viruses that can cause heart problems. Women with tooth or gum problems are also more likely to give birth to premature babies.

Bleeding gums may also be a sign that your intake of vitamin C is deficient. Be sure that your diet includes plenty of fresh fruits and vegetables every day; munching on hard, fibrous foods, such as a celery stick or carrot, stimulates the gums. ❖

DEPRESSION

CONSUME
- A balanced diet including lots of complex carbohydrates, fish, and food sources of vitamins B_6 and B_{12} and folate.

LIMIT
- Alcohol, which can be a depressant.
- Caffeine, which can interfere with sleep and mood.

AVOID
- Foods and drinks that contain tyramine (if you are taking MAO inhibitors).

Throughout a long and productive life, Winston Churchill lived in dread of visitations by the "black dog," as he called his periodic bouts of paralyzing depression. Other writers, seeking to describe the anguish of clinical depression, have told of trying to find the way through a thick yellow fog or being kept from the sunlight by a trailing black cloud. Clinical depression is quite different from the normal "down" reaction to disappointment. Depression is a serious disorder, probably caused by a disturbance in brain chemistry. It can strike out of the blue and—for a few of the more fortunate sufferers—can disappear just as mysteriously. Many sufferers can benefit from medications to lift their mood.

One of the classic signs of depression is a dramatic change in eating patterns. Some people lose all desire to eat; others develop voracious appetites, especially for carbohydrates. People with depression typically have little energy. Other common signs of depression include an unshakable feeling of sadness, inability to experience pleasure, early awakening or multiple awakenings throughout the night, insomnia, excessive sleepiness, other sleep disorders, inability to concentrate, and indecisiveness. Feelings of worthlessness or guilt may be accompanied by recurrent thoughts of death. Anyone who has some or all of these symptoms nearly every day for more than 2 weeks may be suffering from major depression.

Unfortunately, people over the age of 65 are four times more likely to suffer from depression than younger people; however, elderly sufferers do not always exhibit the classic signs. Instead, they may show signs of dementia, complain of aches and pains, and appear agitated, anxious, or irritable. Researchers estimate that almost one-third of widows and widowers meet the criteria for depression in the first 4 weeks after the death of a spouse. Half of these people are still clinically depressed after a year. If you notice symptoms of depression in someone, try to persuade the person to see a doctor.

People with Parkinson's disease, stroke, arthritis, thyroid disorders, and cancer often suffer from depression. But the person may feel depressed because he has a serious illness or because the underlying disease has triggered a chemical change in the brain. Depression also can be a side effect of many medications taken for other existing conditions; these include beta-blockers for hypertension, digoxin and other drugs for heart disease, indomethacin and other painkillers, corticosteroids (including

FISH OILS: A CURE FOR DEPRESSION?

Could eating more fatty fish be a simple way to help alleviate depression? Research points to "yes." Researchers have known for some time that rates of depression are lower in countries where lots of fish is consumed and higher in countries where little fish is eaten. Recently experts have noted that some people who suffer from depression have markedly low levels of omega-3 fatty acids, which are normally found in high concentrations in the brain.

These fatty acids are abundant in fatty fish, especially cold-water fish such as salmon, trout, and mackerel. Low fish consumption and low levels of a potent form of an omega-3 fatty acid called DHA have both been linked with higher rates of postpartum depression.

Recently, a flurry of research studies has supported the notion that consuming more omega-3 fatty acids can help stabilize the mood. When researchers fed omega-3 fatty acids to piglets, the fatty acids had the same effect as the antidepressant Prozac—that is they significantly increased levels of the neurotransmitter serotonin. New studies in people have shown that omega-3 fatty acids can help symptoms of depression as well as bipolar disorder.

More research is needed, but meanwhile, there's no harm in adding more fish to your diet. For people who don't like fish, fish-oil supplements are available in health-food stores. Talk to your doctor before taking them, though, since they can thin the blood. Flaxseeds and flaxseed oil are other sources of omega-3 fatty acids.

prednisone), antiparkinsonism drugs, antihistamines, and oral contraceptives and other hormonal agents.

DIETARY FACTORS

People with depression often fail to take care of themselves, neglecting their appearance and eating irregularly. Nutritious food is needed to cope with any disease, but unfortunately, depressed people are especially likely to be careless about their nutrition. The resulting poor nourishment may impede recovery.

On the other hand, eating the right foods can actually help stabilize mood.

Eat a diet that emphasizes carbohydrates. Meals that are especially rich in carbohydrates have been associated with a calming, relaxed effect. These foods allow the amino acid tryptophan to enter the brain where it is then used to make serotonin. Feel-good food choices include pasta, breads, grains, cereals, fruits, and juices.

Limit sugar consumption. When some sugar-sensitive people eat large quantities of sweets, they may experience an energetic "high" followed by a "low" with weakness and "jitters" when the sugar is metabolized.

Get a lot more of these B vitamins. Vitamins B_6, B_{12}, and folate, all may help certain forms of depression. Vitamin B_6 has been shown to provide some relief to women suffering from PMS-related depression. Part of this may be due to the role of B_6 in helping convert tryptophan to serotonin in the brain. B_6 sources are meat, fish, poultry, whole grains, bananas, and potatoes. Other research has found that many depressed people are deficient in folate and B_{12}. Folate is found in green leafy vegetables, orange juice, lentils, corn, asparagus, peas, nuts, and seeds. B_{12} is found in all animal foods and fortified soy and rice beverages.

Turn to tryptophan. Found in turkey and other animal products, this amino acid is needed to make the mood-critical neurotransmitter serotonin. Research indicates that tryptophan can help induce sleep and may play a role in treating certain types of depression. Tryptophan supplements were touted in the late 1980s as a remedy for depression and insomnia. Tragically, this led to several thousand cases—nearly two dozen of them fatal—of a rare muscle disorder. The problem was caused by a manufacturing error that led to the introduction of a contaminant into the supplements. Consequently, both the American and Canadian governments have banned the sale of tryptophan supplements. Fortunately, you can obtain tryptophan from food. Besides turkey, good amounts of the amino acid are found in almonds, pumpkin seeds, and watercress.

DRUG-FOOD INTERACTIONS

Antidepressant drugs in the class called monoamine oxidase (MAO) inhibitors can have serious side effects when taken with certain foods, especially those containing tyramine and other amines. Alcohol should be avoided altogether. These drugs include phenelzine (Nardil) and tranylcypromine (Parnate). If you are taking one of these drugs, your blood pressure could rise dangerously when you eat foods rich in tyramines.

As a general rule, all protein-rich foods that have been aged, dried, fermented, pickled, or bacterially treated should be eliminated from the diet. Foods that are rich in tyramine include all aged cheeses, dry fermented sausages such as summer sausage, pepperoni, salami, pastrami, smoked or pickled fish, nonfresh meat or poultry, tofu and soy products including soy sauce, beer and ale, any overripe or fermented fruit or vegetable, broad beans, sauerkraut, bananas, soups containing meat extracts or cheese, gravies and sauces containing meat extracts, yeast extracts and meat extracts, protein dietary supplements, and certain wines (including Chianti and champagne).

Coffee, tea, colas, chocolate, weight-loss dietary supplements containing cocoa, yeast, yeast extracts, fava beans, and ginseng contain small amounts of tyramine but are generally safe enough if taken only occasionally and in small amounts.

ANTIDEPRESSANTS AND WEIGHT

Another class of antidepressant drugs, called selective serotonin reuptake inhibitors, can reduce the appetite, leading to a slight but progressive weight loss. These drugs include fluoxetine (Prozac), sertraline (Zoloft), and paroxetine (Paxil). If you are taking one of these drugs, you may need to make a special effort to maintain your optimum weight during treatment.

Tricyclic antidepressants, which can cause weight gain, include imipramine (Tofranil), amitriptyline (Elavil), and nortriptyline (Pamelor). If you are overweight to begin with, or gain weight while taking any of these drugs, ask your doctor to suggest an alternative. ❖

DID YOU KNOW?

CHOCOLATE IS A MOOD ENHANCER

The naturally occurring substance in chocolate called phenylethylamine (PEA) has been found to elevate endorphin levels and act as a natural antidepressant.

DIABETES

EAT PLENTY OF

- Regular meals and snacks to avoid fluctuations in blood sugar levels.
- A balance of carbohydrate, protein, and fat at each meal.
- Low-fat, high-fiber foods to achieve and maintain a normal weight.

LIMIT

- "Empty calorie" foods such as sweets and snack foods, which can contribute to obesity.
- Saturated fats and foods made with hydrogenated fats.

More than 19 million North Americans have diabetes mellitus, a serious metabolic disease that affects the body's ability to derive energy from blood sugar, or glucose. It results when the body cannot produce or properly use insulin, a hormone needed for glucose metabolism. Because all human body tissues need a steady supply of glucose, diabetes can affect every organ. In particular, it can lead to heart disease, kidney failure, blindness, and nerve problems.

TWO TYPES OF DIABETES

About 10 percent of diagnosed diabetes cases are type 1, also called insulin-dependent diabetes mellitus (IDDM), or juvenile-onset diabetes since the disease often develops in children. In this autoimmune disease, the body's mechanisms for protecting itself from foreign organisms are turned against its own tissue. Because diabetes often develops after an infection, such as chicken pox, researchers theorize that after destroying the invaders, the immune system keeps attacking; but having no worthy targets turns on body tissue. The result is destruction of the cells that produce insulin in the pancreas.

THE WEIGHT CONNECTION

The prevalence of type 2 diabetes is increasing as more baby boomers move into the high-risk age groups and become increasingly overweight. Not every overweight person will get diabetes, but 85 percent of type 2 diabetics weigh more than they should. Extra fat, especially abdominal fat in the "apple-shape" body, is associated with insulin resistance. Newly diagnosed, overweight type 2 diabetics may banish the disease by adopting a healthier lifestyle to reach and maintain their ideal weight. Even if they don't reach their ideal weight, any loss makes the disease easier to control with diet and exercise alone.

KEEPING CONTROL. *Diabetes does not demand special meals, just a healthy diet. Clockwise, from top, are pasta with vegetables, a baked potato topped with a vegetable medley, a poached salmon on whole-grain bread.*

MEDICAL PROOF THAT WEIGHT LOSS IS POWERFUL PREVENTIVE MEDICINE

A major clinical trial studied a large group of overweight people at high risk for diabetes. Researchers found that those who lost modest amounts of weight cut their diabetes risk by 58 percent. People over the age of 60 cut their risk even more. Losing just 5 percent of body weight is enough to make a difference.

DRINKING MORE
JAVA MAY REDUCE
THE RISK OF
TYPE 2 DIABETES

According to a recent study in the *Annals of Internal Medicine,* men who drank more than six 8-oz (240-ml) cups of caffeinated coffee a day lowered their risk of type 2 diabetes by about half, and women reduced their risk by nearly 30 percent.

Researchers note that coffee contains potassium, magnesium, and antioxidants that might improve the body's response to insulin. They stress, however, that more research is needed to establish whether it is coffee—or something else about coffee drinkers—that protects them.

PREGNANCY-RELATED DIABETES

Gestational diabetes can complicate pregnancy for both mother and baby. The effects of hormonal changes and weight gain during pregnancy increase demands on the pancreas and can lead to insulin resistance. Gestational diabetes can strike any expectant mother but is most likely in those who are over 30 years of age and overweight, as well as those who have had a previous baby weighing more than 9 lb (4 kg) or a family history of gestational or type 2 diabetes.

All women should have a blood test for diabetes between the 24th and 28th weeks of pregnancy. If gestational diabetes is diagnosed, the mother will need to modify her diet and monitor weight gain carefully; she may require daily insulin injections for the rest of the pregnancy. Although this type of diabetes usually disappears almost immediately after childbirth, women who have had it are at high risk for type 2 diabetes in later years.

MYTH BUSTER

Myth: Diabetics have to give up sweet desserts.

Reality: Contrary to popular belief, there is no need for people with diabetes to cut out sugar entirely. An occasional sweet treat is fine.

People with type 1 diabetes must take insulin daily. They must also strictly control their diet and physical activity to maintain near-normal blood glucose levels.

The most common types of diabetes, affecting over 90 percent of diabetics, is type 2, or non-insulin-dependent diabetes mellitus (NIDDM). Also termed adult-onset diabetes, this form typically occurs in older adults, who are usually overweight. Although these people often have adequate or even high levels of insulin, they cannot use the hormone properly. Unfortunately, because of the growing obesity problem in children, type 2 diabetes is beginning to show up in this population.

The early symptoms of type 2 diabetes may not be noticeable, so it can go undiagnosed until there is a serious complication, such as a heart attack or stroke. It is estimated that almost 6 million North Americans have type 2 diabetes but don't know it. Although they may not experience any symptoms, the disease may be damaging the heart, blood vessels, nerves, kidneys, eyes, and other organs. While much of this damage is permanent, it can be prevented with early treatment. Adults over the age of 50 should have their blood sugar levels tested every 2 years, or more often if they are overweight, or have a family history.

For most people with type 2 diabetes, diet and exercise alone can provide effective treatment; however, some may need oral medications to improve the effect of their own insulin, and a few may need insulin injections.

DIET STRATEGY

Diet is the cornerstone of diabetes management. An appropriate diet can help maintain optimal blood glucose levels and prevent or delay the long-term complications of diabetes. Diabetics should consult a registered dietitian to work out a diet. In addition to managing blood glucose, meal planning should take into consideration age and related health concerns like cholesterol levels or high blood pressure.

Your carbohydrates, fats, protein mix is key. To maintain healthy blood glucose levels, meals and snacks should be balanced to provide a mixture of carbohydrates, fats, and proteins. Adults may need to reduce fat and cholesterol intake to protect against heart and kidney disease. An overweight person needs to focus on weight loss by decreasing caloric intake and increasing daily activity levels.

CARBOHYDRATES

Carbohydrates are the basic currency of glucose. For most diabetics, carbohydrate-rich foods such as vegetables, breads, cereals, and pasta should account for 45 percent to 60 percent of their daily calories. Because the fiber content of these carbohydrates slows down the release of glucose, high-fiber starches, such as barley, oat cereals, beans, peas, and lentils, help suppress any sharp increases in blood sugar levels after meals.

Dietary guidelines allow for simple carbohydrates, like syrups, sugars, and sweeteners, to be included in the diet in moderation. As opposed to recommendations in the past, the emphasis is now on monitoring total carbohydrate consumption at each meal/snack rather than the source of carbohydrate. But all carbohydrates are not equal when it comes to nutrition. Complex carbohydrates such as grains and cereals provide vitamins, minerals, and fiber, whereas sugars and sweeteners provide mostly calories; therefore, complex carbohydrates should make up the bulk of the diabetic diet, and sugars only a small amount.

Soluble fiber—the kind found in oatmeal—may actually help lower blood-sugar levels (it also helps lower cholesterol). And insoluble fiber, found in whole grains and many vegetables, helps you feel full on fewer calories.

PROTEIN

Choose nutritious protein sources. There is no research to support either an increased or decreased protein intake for uncomplicated diabetes, so the recommended amounts for non-diabetics is also appropriate for adults with diabetes. High-quality protein foods (lean meats, meat substitutes, and lower-fat dairy foods) should supply 10 to 20 percent of daily calories.

FAT

People with diabetes should follow a lower-fat diet. High-fat diets contribute to obesity and high cholesterol levels. Saturated fats from animal foods and hydrogenated fats in packaged foods should also be limited. On the other hand, monounsaturated and polyunsaturated fats—such as those found in vegetable oils, nuts, fish, and avocados—are good for the heart and also slow the digestion process, helping to stabilize blood-sugar levels. They may also reduce insulin resistance. ❖

DIARRHEA

CONSUME PLENTY OF

- Water, mineral water, herbal teas, ginger ale, apple juice, broth, or low-sugar sports beverages to replace lost fluids, salts, and minerals.
- Binding foods in the BRAT diet—bananas, rice, applesauce, and toast.
- Skinless baked potatoes, boiled or poached eggs, and other bland foods as the bowels return to normal.

AVOID

- Citrus juices.
- Most other foods, especially salads, fruits, and whole grains, until bowel function normalizes.
- Alcohol, which dehydrates, and caffeine, which stimulates the bowel, for 48 hours after the symptoms disappear.

Acute infectious diarrhea is one of the world's most common ailments. An estimated 5 billion cases occur every year, and in North America, diarrhea is runner-up only to the common cold as a cause for absences from work. Although diarrhea causes fatalities—due to dehydration—it is seldom a threat in affluent, well-nourished societies, except to such vulnerable groups as babies, the elderly, and invalids. In the developing countries, many deaths have been prevented with the use of a homemade rehydration fluid that has been promoted through the World Health Organization (WHO) efforts.

CAUTION

While eating apples or applesauce can help ease diarrhea, drinking apple juice can have the opposite effect. In fact, drinking too much fruit juice of any kind is often the cause of diarrhea in toddlers.

THE DEFINITION

Diarrhea—the frequent passage of loose, watery stool—is not a disease but a symptom of an underlying problem. It is most commonly brought on by food poisoning, especially among travelers. Transient looseness can be caused by overconsumption of laxative foods (such as prunes), heavy use of sugarless chewing gum sweetened with sugar alcohol (such as sorbitol), and over-the-counter indigestion remedies containing magnesium. Emotional stress that causes irritable bowel syndrome may disrupt the normal bowel pattern with alternating diarrhea and constipation; similar symptoms occur in colitis and Crohn's disease, both inflammatory bowel disorders. In many instances, however, diarrhea develops without any identifiable cause. Unless the problem persists or recurs often, this is not a cause for concern.

DIETARY MANAGEMENT

Most cases of diarrhea are minor and short-lived and can be managed at home with simple dietary measures.

Stop solid food and rehydrate. Start by eliminating all solid foods and sipping warm or tepid drinks to prevent any further dehydration. Drinking half a cup of fluid every 15 minutes or so is usually enough. Suitable drinks include water, mineral water, herbal teas, and ginger ale. Clear broths also help replace the salts and other minerals lost in a bout of diarrhea. You can make your own rehydration fluid by mixing ¼ teaspoon (1 ml) of baking soda, with a pinch of salt, and ¼ teaspoon (1 ml) of corn syrup or honey in an 8-oz (250-ml) glass of water or juice. If you choose a commercial sports drink, one with more than 10 percent sugar can aggravate diarrhea.

Slowly introduce low-fiber foods. When you feel like eating (but preferably not within the first 24 hours), start with low-fiber foods such as crackers, toast, rice, bananas, cooked carrots, boiled potatoes, and chicken. Often doctors will recommend bananas, rice, applesauce, and toast (called the BRAT diet), especially for children. Apples and other fruits high in pectin (a soluble fiber) help counteract diarrhea; that's why unsweetened applesauce is a traditional home remedy. Cooked carrots are

> ## WHEN TO CALL A DOCTOR
> Mild diarrhea can usually be self-managed. But call your doctor promptly for any of the following:
> - Diarrhea that lasts more than 2 days (1 day for a child under 2, a frail elderly person, or someone with diabetes) or if it worsens during that time.
> - The appearance of blood, mucus, or worms in the feces.
> - Severe abdominal pain.
> - Diarrhea that is accompanied by vomiting or fever.

also high in pectin. Try them pureed. Although cooked and pureed fruits and vegetables can usually be tolerated, do not eat raw fruits, high-fiber vegetables, or fatty foods until the bowel movements are back to normal. Other suitable foods include salted crackers and chicken-rice soup, which help to replenish depleted sodium and potassium.

Avoid milk products until the symptoms disappear. Some of the organisms that cause diarrhea can temporarily impair the ability to digest milk.

RECURRENT DIARRHEA

Some people have recurrent or chronic diarrhea due to malabsorption of a particular nutrient. For example, in lactose intolerance, the sugar in milk passes intact into the colon, where it is fermented by bacteria, producing hydrogen gas, along with water retention, bloating, and diarrhea. In all cases of recurrent or chronic diarrhea, you should see your doctor as soon as possible.

OTC REMEDIES

Over-the-counter (OTC) antidiarrheal drugs may give some relief when diarrhea has no obvious cause or is due to a minor illness, such as a flu, but many physicians believe that you will heal faster by letting nature take its course. Never use a nonprescription antidiarrhea product for more than 2 days without consulting your doctor. ❖

THE BRAT DIET.
The diet's name is an acronym for its components— bananas, rice, applesauce and toast. These binding foods are often suggested as the first to try after an episode of diarrhea.

DIETING
■ KEEPING THE WEIGHT OFF ■

There's no easy way to lose weight. Whether you decide on a high-protein diet, a low-fat diet, or some other approach, experts agree that the only way to shed excess weight is to cut the total numbers of calories you consume and/or burn more calories through exercise. Simple enough to understand—but often much more difficult to do.

Even as we've become more and more obsessed with diets and dieting, we've become fatter and fatter. In fact, obesity in the industrialized world is reaching epidemic proportions. Sixty-four percent of American adults are overweight, including 23 percent who are obese (defined as having a Body Mass Index [BMI] of 30 or more). In Canada, close to half the population is overweight and one in six people is obese. It seems that even as diet books and low-fat cookies fly off the shelf, the essential messages about how to lose weight safely and permanently aren't sinking in.

Real weight loss

The "secret" to losing weight is this: Burn more calories than you eat. When the body uses more energy than it takes in (remember, food equals energy), it depletes its fat stores. In other words, eat less and your body will burn fat for energy. Of course, what you eat is important, too. A diet based solely on cabbage soup won't provide the nutrition your body needs—and you'll get tired of it soon enough and return to your old eating habits with a vengeance.

Any weight-loss plan needs to center on foods you can keep eating for a lifetime—and of course it helps if those foods will also help protect you from cancer and other diseases. After all, it's not all about losing weight. A diet that is high in meat and low in fruits (Atkins, for example) may lead to short-term weight loss, but is not in keeping with current nutritional knowledge. Excessive meat consumption has been linked with a variety of diseases and a high-fruit diet protects against cancer. Fruits, vegetables, whole-grain foods, low-fat dairy products, and lean protein are the cornerstone of healthy eating, whether or not you're trying to trim your waistline. The foods that your body can easily do without—which happen to be the ones packed with calories—are the ones to cut back on. That means cakes, cookies, fatty meats, whole milk, cream sauces, and the like.

When people want to lose weight, they usually want instant results. Most people who go on crash diets to shed heft fast usually end up putting it back on just as quickly—and often put back more than they lost. Experts suggest a goal of losing about 1 lb (0.45 kg) a week. There are 3,500 calories in 1 lb (0.45 kg) of stored fat, so you'll have to reduce your food intake by 500 calories a day to get there. Or you can eat 250 fewer calories and burn 250 more through exercise.

CAUTION

North Americans spend more than $25 billion each year on commercial weight-loss programs. Beware of any diet regime driven by an obvious profit motive. Fad diets don't work in the long term. Be wary of so-called "fat blockers" and "starch blockers" that claim to absorb fat and block starch digestion. These claims have not been proven. Also be wary of herbal weight-loss products—many of these are loaded with stimulants such as ephedrine that can provoke cardiac arrhythmias and other serious side effects.

Research shows that people who exercise in addition to eating less keep off the most weight for the longest time. Work up to getting at least 30 minutes of moderate exercise (such as fast-paced walking) a day. By exercising you'll raise your metabolism so that you burn more calories, even as you sleep. Exercise also helps you feel better mentally and physically, and may help you stick to your weight-loss plans.

Tips for taking it off

Countless people try the latest fad diets, only to go off the diet when it stops working and eventually try another one, and so on. Don't be one of those people. Instead, follow these basic tips for losing weight safely, naturally, and permanently.

■ **Eat breakfast, and don't skip meals.** Eat more often to avoid a completely empty stomach, which can make you overeat at your next meal. Researchers have discovered a hormone called ghrelin, secreted by the stomach. When your stomach is empty, your ghrelin levels surge, which makes you run for the nearest food. Instead of skipping meals, plan to eat four to six small meals or snacks, spaced 3 to 5 hours apart.

■ **Choose your carbs carefully.** Despite what the popular media might have you believing, you don't need to avoid all carbohydrates in order to lose weight. But you should shy away from simple carbohydrates, such as sugar, white bread, white pasta, and white rice. These foods are quickly turned into glucose by the body, and the influx of glucose causes a rapid rise in the hormone insulin, whose job it is to escort glucose out of the bloodstream and into cells. A surge of insulin is followed by a glucose "crash," which leaves you hungry in no time.

Instead of simple carbohydrates, focus your attention on complex carbohydrates, found in whole-grain foods as well as in vegetables and fruits. To avoid insulin spikes, forgo meals made up mostly of simple carbohydrates or starches without fiber (think mashed potatoes). That means no big plates of white pasta, and no bagel-with-jelly breakfasts. If you're having pasta, have plenty of vegetables or some lean meat along with it, or add white beans to the dish. Instead of white toast with jam for breakfast, have whole-wheat toast with an egg-white omelet.

■ **Eat lower on the glycemic index.** The glycemic index (GI) indicates the rate at which carbohydrate-rich foods are digested. Foods that are digested faster are quickly converted into glucose, leaving you hungry again. Foods with a low GI score include brown rice, lentils, yams, and apples. Those with a high GI number—in other words, foods to avoid if you're trying to lose weight—include cornflakes, white rice, and mashed potatoes. (See Glycemic Index for more details.)

■ **Choose bulky foods.** Foods that don't leave you hungry are higher in bulk and lower in calories. Any food that contains plenty of fiber, water, or air is a "bulky" or "high-volume" food. These include high-fiber fruits and vegetables as well as beans. Instead of eating a handful of raisins, choose water-dense

DO ONE SIMPLE THING

EAT MORE CALCIUM-RICH FOODS

Evidence suggests that calcium may stimulate fat loss by suppressing hormones that cause fat to be stored rather than burned. Adding calcium-rich foods such as milk, yogurt, or other dairy products to a low-calorie diet therefore may make it easier for your body to mobilize fat stores and burn fat.

grapes. Instead of a glass of orange juice, have an orange, which is far less calorie-dense and contains fiber that juice lacks. If you're making chili, add more beans to bulk it up without adding a lot of calories. Instead of French fries, try whipping up some winter squash with skim milk (Whipped foods contain air, which gives bulk without adding calories.) Other low-cal, high-volume foods to favor are broth-based soups. Studies show that people who start a meal with soup eat less at that meal and later in the day. Just be sure to avoid cream soups, which are high in calories.

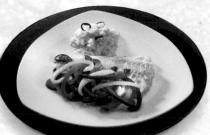

■ **Watch out for low-fat foods.** Some low-fat foods, such as low-fat dairy products, are a real boon to dieters. But food manufacturers often remove fat from cookies and other treats only to replace that fat with sugar. So check the label before you indulge with abandon; a serving probably contains just as many calories as the higher-fat original version.

In other cases, cutting fat from your diet makes sense, since fat is the most concentrated source of calories. Replace some of the meat you eat with fish or poultry. Remove the skin from poultry before you cook it, and banish the frying pan in favor of steaming, grilling, baking, or microwaving. Choose lean cuts of meat and trim off visible fat. And stay away from sausages, bacon, and cold cuts.

A word to the wise: Don't attempt to cut all the fat out of your diet. Research has shown that people are able to stay on a diet longer and are better able to maintain their weight loss when their diets allow at least some foods that contain fat—for example, nuts and olive oil.

■ **Downsize your portions.** We've become used to bigger and bigger portions both at home and when we eat out. If your fast-food restaurant offers super-size or value meals, think twice about where those extra calories will end up! At restaurants, reduce the temptation to clean your plate by setting aside one-third of your meal before you touch it. When eating at home, check the portion size of foods you enjoy. If your pasta portion has grown to two cups, cut it back to one and a half, and your waistline will start to show the difference. To fool your eye into thinking you're getting more food, use a bread plate instead of a dinner plate for your entrée and a small cereal bowl instead of a giant pasta bowl for your pasta.

■ **Drink plenty of fluids—especially water.** Drink water and lots of it. Seltzer, mineral water, and diet sodas are all good choices. Fluids quench your thirst and reduce your appetite as well. Fruit juice is healthy, but adds calories without fiber. Coffee or tea is fine. If you take it with sugar or milk, select skim milk or a nondairy (low-calorie) creamer, and an artificial sweetener. Allow yourself to have an occasional glass of wine or beer if you wish, but be aware that they add more than 100 calories per glass.

■ **Don't deprive yourself.** Let yourself have small portions of your favorite high-calorie foods once in a while so that you don't get frustrated and end up binging.

■ **Keep your eye on the mirror.** Most people on a diet want to see a lower weight reflected on the bathroom scale. But remember, while you're losing fat, if you're exercising, you may be adding muscle, so your weight might remain the same for a while. Instead of relying totally on the scale, check your reflection in the mirror, your clothing size, your energy level, and the notches on your belt.

■ **Never fast.** Fasting, even when plenty of water is consumed, can be very dangerous; it may lead to lowered blood pressure and heart failure. Also, weight loss gained by fasting is rarely sustained once eating is resumed.

DID YOU KNOW?

EATING SOME FAT CAN HELP YOU STAY ON A DIET

Researchers at Harvard Medical School and Brigham and Women's Hospital in Boston studied people on two weight-loss diets. Both diets contained the same number of calories but one was low in fat and the other higher in monounsaturated fats, such as olive oil, canola oil, peanuts, and other nuts. The researchers found that those on the higher-fat regime (45 to 60 g added fat per day) were able to stay on their diet longer and better able to maintain their weight loss.

DIGESTIVE DISORDERS

CONSUME PLENTY OF

- Fresh fruits, vegetables, whole-grain products, and other high-fiber foods to help digestion.
- Fluids (at least six to eight glasses of water, juices, or other nonalcoholic fluids daily).

LIMIT

- Coffee, tea, colas, and other sources of caffeine.
- Refined carbohydrates.
- Fried foods and other high-fat foods.

AVOID

- Any foods or beverages that provoke a flare-up of symptoms.

Digestion refers to the overall process by which food is broken down mechanically and chemically and is converted to forms that can be absorbed into the bloodstream and delivered to cells. Only water, salt, simple sugars such as glucose, and some other small molecules can be absorbed unchanged. Starches, fats, and proteins must be broken down into smaller molecules before they can be used. Specific proteins called enzymes play a significant role in the breakdown of food.

The digestive process actually begins in the mouth. As food is broken into small pieces by chewing, it is mixed with saliva, which moistens it and supplies enzymes that start breaking down carbohydrates. Once the food has been sufficiently chewed, it is carried through the esophagus, which has a ring of muscles at its base that relaxes to open the passage to the stomach. The ring should normally close to prevent food and stomach acid from returning to the esophagus. In some cases the ring fails to close properly and food is regurgitated, a process that is referred to as reflux; this can occur in people with a hiatal hernia. Reflux can cause indigestion and heartburn, the most common digestive disorders.

When food reaches the stomach, it is churned by the stomach's muscular walls and broken down into smaller pieces. In addition, the stomach walls secrete gastric acid and an enzyme called pepsin that breaks down protein. Special mucus-producing cells within the stomach ordinarily prevent it from digesting its own tissues with these strong digestive juices. However, if these mechanisms fail for any reason, an ulcer can arise.

By the time the food leaves the stomach, it already has been converted into a semifluid called chyme. Digestion continues in the duodenum, the start of the small intestine, where bile from the liver and enzymes from the pancreas break down fats and proteins. The intestines are muscular tubes that move food with rhythmic contractions known as peristalsis. The 20-foot-long (6-meter-long) small intestine is lined with millions of hairlike projections called villi. These have surface membranes that allow the digested nutrients to pass through them and into the tiny blood vessels they harbor. Amino acids from proteins and glucose from sugars are absorbed directly into the bloodstream for delivery to cells throughout the body. While smaller fat molecules also go directly into the blood, larger ones enter into the lymph system.

Fiber and other undigested waste products move into the large intestine, or colon, where much of the water they contain is reabsorbed. That's why it is important to drink at least six to eight glasses of water, juices, and other nonalcoholic fluids a day; otherwise, the fecal mass moving through the colon will become dehydrated, resulting in constipation. Fiber absorbs large amounts of water, and it, along with some of the starches from vegetables and fruits, provides the bulk that helps to stimulate the muscles of the colon.

Depending on the contents of a meal and a person's individual metabolic rate, it may take from 2 to 6 hours for a meal to be fully digested and its nutrients absorbed. Simple sugars are broken down rapidly and may enter the bloodstream just minutes after eating. Starches require about an hour or longer to be digested; proteins need 2 to 3 hours. Fat takes from 4 to 6 hours to be digested and absorbed. For this reason, protein and fat will satisfy hunger for longer periods of time than sugars and carbohydrates will. It takes another 8 to 24 hours for the undigested waste to move through the colon.

The intestine has a remarkable ability to heal itself. It replaces its lining every 72 hours and reacts swiftly to expel harmful substances. However, a diet high in refined and nutritionally deficient foods, typically found in Western countries, can lead to digestive problems ranging from unpleasant but minor episodes of indigestion and flatulence to more serious disorders such as diverticulitis.

DIGESTIVE DISORDERS

The digestive system has a relatively small repertoire of symptoms, principally nausea, vomiting, pain (such as heartburn), bloating, cramping, diarrhea, constipation, and flatulence. The onset of such symptoms may simply reflect a normal response to an unusual meal or be associated with some lifestyle factor, such as eating an improper diet or dealing with the stresses of daily life. Excitement, disappointment, fear, anxiety, and other strong emotions can cause some upset in the digestive system. This should not cause alarm if it is transient.

The digestive system has a limited set of symptoms for expressing distress, so the same symptoms may also reflect any one of a number of very serious disorders, including gastritis, or inflammation of the stomach lining; problems in the intestines, such as ulcerative colitis or Crohn's disease (both are inflammatory disorders); diverticulitis, an inflammation and infection of small sacs protruding from the intestinal wall; irritable bowel syndrome, a functional disorder that affects movement within the intestines; or cancer anywhere in the digestive tract. Similarly, nausea and vomiting may be triggered by an adverse reaction to a medication, emotional upset, mild viral infection, ear disorder, migraine headache, and motion sickness, as well as other serious disorders, including a heart attack and intestinal obstruction.

MALABSORPTION DISORDERS

A similar group of symptoms, especially diarrhea and bloating, also indicate a malabsorption problem, which occurs when the digestive tract is unable to properly utilize one or more components of the diet. Depending on the severity of the problem, the person may experience weight loss, muscle wasting, and show evidence of vitamin and mineral deficiencies. While some malabsorption problems are congenital, others may occur because of illness or its treatment. Problems may arise from the digestive tract itself, or from disorders of the heart and blood vessels, the endocrine glands, or the lymph system.

Some malabsorption conditions involve a single nutrient, as in celiac disease, when the body is unable to absorb gluten (a protein found in wheat, rye, and barley), or lactose intolerance, when the body is unable to digest lactose, the sugar in milk. Others involve an array of nutrients. For example, in cystic fibrosis, enzymes needed to digest protein, carbohydrate, and fat are either missing completely or are present only in reduced amounts.

People with malabsorption problems may be in danger of malnutrition. They may avoid certain foods in order to prevent symptoms, failing to get adequate nutrients. Or the side effects of the disorder may lead to malnutrition. For example, when fat is not properly absorbed, it is discharged from the body as waste and takes with it the fat-soluble vitamins A, D, E, and K.

A registered dietitian can help individuals with malabsorption problems plan meals and a doctor may prescribe vitamin and mineral supplements or other treatments. ❖

DO ONE SIMPLE THING

COOK WITH HEALING HERBS

Some herbs are known to help troubled digestion. Ginger, for example, is reputed to ease nausea. Many of the herbs and spices traditionally used in cooking aid digestion, so use plenty of mint, dill, caraway, horseradish, bay, chervil, fennel, tarragon, marjoram, cumin, cinnamon, ginger, and cardamom. Chamomile tea or angostura bitters, a tincture of the bitter gentian root, also may help. A small amount of bitters can promote digestion and alleviate flatulence.

HERBS AND SPICES. *Cinnamon, mint, dill, and ginger are some of the herbs and spices that can help digestion.*

DIVERTICULITIS

CONSUME PLENTY OF

- Fresh fruits and vegetables.
- Whole-grain cereals and bread.
- Fluids (water, juice, milk, soup, and tea).

LIMIT

- White bread, polished rice, cookies, cakes, and other foods high in sugar and refined starches.

Diverticula are small pouches that form in the wall of the large intestine, creating a condition called diverticulosis. The specific cause remains unknown, but the disease occurs most often in people who are over age 60 and overweight. Weakening of the intestinal wall as a person ages is believed to contribute to the formation of the pouches. As pressure builds up in the large intestine—for example, during a bout of constipation—the weakened areas balloon outward, forming pouches.

The pouches or sacs are not a problem in themselves, producing no symptoms until they become infected or inflamed. Infection or inflammation can occur when waste flowing through the intestines is diverted into one of the sacs and becomes impacted. The resulting condition is called diverticulitis, or inflammation of the diverticula. It can be painful and serious, and may lead to complications, such as abscesses, intestinal obstruction, or perforation of the intestinal wall. In addition to abdominal cramps and pain, other symptoms of diverticulitis include gas, flatulence, fever, and rectal bleeding. Constipation may sometimes alternate with diarrhea.

Diverticulitis occurs primarily in the industrialized Western world, where diets that are high in fat and low in fiber are common. Inadequate consumption of dietary fiber can cause stools to become hard and compact, resulting in constipation. This may provoke unnatural contractions of the large intestine, which in turn leads to the formation of diverticula.

THE ROLE OF DIETARY FIBER

A diet rich in vegetables and whole-grain cereals may help to prevent diverticulitis. The ailment is known to be less common among vegetarians than those who include meat in their diet. Vegetarian diets are typically higher in fiber-rich foods, such as vegetables, fruits, cereals, and

FOODS TO AVOID. *Any foods that have hulls, seeds, strings, or other fibrous parts can become trapped in the diverticula, leading to inflammation and other intestinal symptoms.*

grains. However, excessive fiber, particularly too much bran, can create other digestive problems; for example, studies have suggested that it can irritate the colon. It is important to increase fiber intake gradually, giving the body a chance to get used to it. If you have diverticular disease, do not start taking fiber supplements without first discussing this with your doctor.

To date, there is no scientific evidence to support the association between nuts and seeds and inflammation of the diverticula. Individuals with diverticular disease consuming a diet low in fiber demonstrate more disease symptoms than those consuming a liberal diet (including nuts and seeds). However, many practitioners still recommend that foods with indigestible particles such as corn, nuts, and seeds be avoided. In addition, people may find that certain foods cause inflammation and pain and so should avoid them.

Drink plenty of water. Along with a high-fiber diet, increased fluid intake (at least eight glasses every day) produces bulky, soft stools that move easily through the intestinal tract.

If you have diverticular disease, it is important to avoid constipation, which can increase your risk of a diverticulitis flare-up. ❖

EATING TO BOOST ENERGY
■ A NEW MINDSET ■

In our fast-paced, high-stress society, fatigue and even exhaustion have become the norm. More sleep, of course, is the best answer. But the right diet can also help fuel your body for the long haul and keep your energy levels from flagging throughout the day.

Where does energy come from?

The major components of all foods—carbohydrates, proteins, and fats—are the nutrients that provide calories and so give you energy. The human body converts carbohydrates to glucose, its most important source of energy. This is the "blood sugar" that rises after eating carbohydrates. A rise in blood sugar triggers your pancreas to release insulin, a hormone that helps glucose enter the body's cells. Once inside the cell, glucose supplies the energy to fuel your body. A certain amount of unused glucose is stored in muscles and liver as glycogen. Your body draws on these stores whenever your blood sugar drops. Once glycogen stores are full, excess glucose is converted to fat.

Protein can also be converted to energy but is a less efficient source than carbohydrates. While fats are the most concentrated source of calories, they are actually a less efficient source of energy than carbohydrates because they take longer to digest and metabolize.

Despite some extravagant claims, vitamins don't provide energy. They are needed, however, to power many of the metabolic processes that lead to energy production. A diet that includes an ample supply of vegetables, legumes, fruits, and whole-grain products will provide adequate vitamins and minerals. Some fruits also provide sugars that are quickly converted to energy.

Seven strategies for high-energy eating

Eating for optimal energy breaks many of the "rules" people commonly believe—for instance, that carbohydrates are bad, that snacking is a no-no, and that sugar is a good pick-me-up. These seven simple steps will put you on the right path.

1. Eat breakfast. This is the meal that sets you up for the day. It replenishes your body's energy supply after a night's fast and provides the energy needed to stay physically and mentally alert. Breakfast enhances learning and physical performance. It is a critical meal for adults and children alike. Without breakfast, your body is running on empty. Studies have shown that kids who eat breakfast concentrate better, are more creative, and behave better; this applies to adults as well.

2. Get enough iron-rich foods. Iron-deficiency anemia is one of the most common nutritional deficiencies in North America. Iron is essential for producing hemoglobin, the main component of red blood cells. Hemoglobin carries oxygen to your body's cells where it is used to produce energy and perform essential metabolic functions. If your iron stores are low, your red blood cells can't supply as much oxygen to the cells. The consequences

CAUTION

Increasing your iron intake comes with an important caution. Do not take iron supplements unless you know you are iron deficient and cannot correct the deficiency with an appropriate diet. Too much iron can cause indigestion and constipation, and excessive doses can be toxic. If you think that you are tired because of an iron deficiency, check first with your physician.

The glycemic index

Some carbohydrate-rich foods are digested and absorbed into your bloodstream quickly while others are broken down more slowly. The glycemic index (GI) is a tool developed to measure how different carbohydrates affect your blood sugar after they are eaten and digested.

Foods with a low GI such as pumpernickel bread, rye bread, brown rice, bulgur, oatmeal, lentils, yams, apples, pears, and yogurt cause a slower, more gradual rise in blood sugar, take longer to digest, and so release energy more slowly, leading to more consistent energy levels. Low-GI foods are better for blood-sugar control in diabetes and may help with weight loss.

High-GI foods such as white bread, white rice, mashed potato, cornflakes, and watermelon are more quickly absorbed and so provide a quicker source of energy. For athletes or other active people, high-GI foods can be a source of quick energy to aid short-duration sports performance and recovery, while lower-GI foods are better for endurance events. (For more on this, see Glycemic Index.)

of iron deficiency are fatigue, low energy, and difficulty in concentrating. The best food sources are red meats, organ meats, iron-fortified cereal products and whole-grain or enriched breads, dried fruits, green leafy vegetables, beans, nuts and seeds, and blackstrap molasses.

There are two kinds of iron in our food: heme and nonheme. Heme iron, found in red meat, liver, and eggs, is better absorbed than the nonheme iron found in enriched cereals, some dark green vegetables, beans, nuts and seeds, and certain dried fruits, such as raisins.

You can enhance your body's ability to absorb nonheme iron by eating the food along with one that contains vitamin C. For example, if you want to increase the absorption of iron from a bowl of iron-enriched cereal (such as cornflakes), eat it with some strawberries, or accompany it with a glass of orange juice.

3. Focus on complex carbohydrates. Carbohydrates found in breads, grains, cereals, fruits, vegetables, and sweets are digested and end up as the simple sugar glucose. It is this glucose that provides fuel for your brain, muscles, and other body tissues. Complex carbohydrates in whole-grain breads and cereals, lentils, legumes, and other starchy vegetables are the fuel of choice since they are digested gradually and serve as a steady fuel supply for body and brain. In addition, they provide many important vitamins, minerals, and plant chemicals to keep your body well nourished.

4. Go easy on the simple sugars. Candy and sweets, for example, might give you a quick rise in energy but this is generally followed by a "crash" that leaves you even more tired than you were before.

5. Eat small amounts of food throughout the day. Eating small meals and/or snacks throughout the day keeps your blood sugar steady. A low blood sugar is one of the common causes of afternoon fatigue. Smaller meals can also help stave off feelings of hunger. Eating a midday lunch will refuel you for the afternoon. Snacks can be the same as small meals, so a sandwich, soup, cheese and crackers, mini pizzas, yogurt with fruit, or a bean dip and vegetables all make the nutritional grade. Just be sure to eat less at mealtime if you're snacking between meals.

6. Stay hydrated. Everyone needs at least six to eight glasses of fluid per day to be properly hydrated. If you exercise, you need more. Water regulates your body temperature, transports nutrients to your body, and carries waste away. Fatigue is one symptom of mild dehydration. Unfortunately, you cannot depend on thirst as an indicator of your fluid needs and you could be mildly dehydrated without knowing. You should get in the habit of consuming fluids regularly, even if you are not active. Fluids can come from water, juice, sports drinks, lemonade, milk, soups, or watery foods such as lettuce, cucumbers, and fruit.

7. Go easy on caffeine. The proper amount of sleep is vital for feeling energetic. Caffeine is a stimulant that competes with adenosine, a chemical that helps induce slumber. The more caffeine you drink, the less adenosine is available for making you drowsy—and your sleep may suffer.

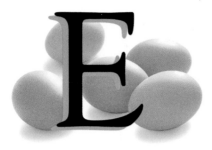

ECZEMA

AVOID

- Foods that trigger or worsen eczema.
- External causes, such as wearing wool clothing next to the skin.

Eczema is an itchy, scaly rash often caused by sensitivity to foods, certain chemicals, or environmental conditions such as dryness. The rash is not always a true allergic reaction, but an immune system reaction to a normally harmless substance. Symptoms vary and can appear anywhere from a few minutes to several hours after exposure to the offending food or substance. Eczema runs in families, often along with a tendency to develop asthma, hay fever, or hives.

THE ROLE OF DIET

Certain foods trigger eczema. Common culprits include eggs, dairy products, seafood, walnuts, and pecans. It is important to be tested for food allergies by a trained physician to avoid dietary limitations that may be unnecessary.

Cow's milk can cause eczema in babies and small children; they may be able to tolerate goat's milk or soy-based products. Many children outgrow their sensitivities by the age of 6, but others have lifelong recurrences.

Consume more antioxidants. Dryness may cause eczema by triggering the formation of free radicals and therefore may be countered by antioxidants such as beta carotene. Preliminary studies indicate that foods rich in this substance can improve eczema. Brightly colored fruits and vegetables including apricots, squash, mangoes, carrots, pumpkin, and sweet potatoes are good choices.

Eat foods rich in essential fatty acids. Foods like vegetable oils, fatty fish, and flaxseed may decrease swelling by helping to generate hormonelike substances called prostaglandins, which reduce inflammation.

Another excellent source of essential fatty acids is evening primrose oil. In an experimental study, patients found that their symptoms improved when they took supplements of evening primrose oil, rich in an essential fatty acid called gamma linolenic acid.

Get lots of vitamin B_6. Some researchers believe a diet rich in vitamin B_6 protects against sensitivity rashes. Good sources include vegetable oil, eggs, oily fish, legumes, brown rice, wheat germ, and leafy green vegetables.

ENVIRONMENTAL TRIGGERS

Chemicals in the environment probably trigger eczema more often than foods do. Common offenders include nickel, which is often used for making costume jewelry, and latex, which is used in household and industrial rubber gloves.

People in certain jobs are at high risk for developing eczema. Acrylic adhesives are a hazard for manicurists and their customers, for dental technicians, and for people who build models as a hobby. Athletes sometimes suffer from skin rashes on the feet caused by the adhesives used in bonding sneakers. Buying another brand of sneakers sometimes solves the problem.

Woolen clothing worn next to the skin can cause a rash. People sensitive to wool should also try to avoid skin-care products based on lanolin, the natural oil that is found in wool.

It makes sense to avoid known triggers. If your rash is worse in either hot or very cold weather, avoid extremes of temperature. Buy only soaps, detergents, and toilet papers that are free of dyes and perfumes. ❖

DO ONE SIMPLE THING

DRINK THREE CUPS OF OOLONG TEA TO RELIEVE ECZEMA

A study suggests that consuming 3 cups of oolong tea a day relieves the symptoms of eczema. It is believed that the polyphenols found in the tea act as antioxidants and suppress allergic responses.

EGGPLANTS

BENEFITS

- Low in calories (unless cooked in fat).
- Meaty flavor and texture lends itself to vegetarian dishes.

DRAWBACKS

- Soak up fat during cooking.
- Provide minimal nutrients.

Eggplants provide very little nutrition, but are among our most versatile vegetables and a component of many popular ethnic dishes, including Indian curries, Greek moussakas, Middle

Eastern baba ghanoush, and French ratatouille. Eggplants are filling, yet low in calories—a cup has 40 calories. Eggplants' spongy texture, however, soaks up fat. Deep-fried eggplants soak up four times as much fat as French fried potatoes.

The tastiest eggplants are firm, with thin skins and a mild flavor. Larger ones are more likely to be seedy, tough, and bitter. Their skins range in color from deep purple to light violet and white.

Eggplants are members of the nightshade family, which also includes tomatoes, potatoes, and peppers. Some have a bitter flavor, which easily can be eliminated with salt before cooking. Slice or cube the eggplant, then sprinkle it with salt. Let it stand for half an hour, then drain it and blot it dry. The salt draws out the excess moisture and reduces bitterness. Eggplants can be stuffed and baked or broiled, roasted, or stewed. If sautéing, use a nonstick pan and minimal oil. ❖

EGGS

BENEFITS
- An excellent source of protein, B vitamins, vitamins A and D, zinc, and iron.
- A source of the antioxidants lutein and zeaxanthin.

DRAWBACKS
- Yolks are high in cholesterol.
- A common cause of food allergy.
- A risk of salmonella if not fully cooked.

The egg is one of nature's best designs, providing everything that a developing chick requires. Its protective shell is not only strong enough to support the mother hen's weight as heat is transferred from her body to the chick, but also

EGG FACTS
- Eggs age more in one day at room temperature than in one week in the refrigerator.
- Egg yolks are one of the few foods that contain vitamin D.
- In North America, each year, 264 million hens produce more than 72.5 billion eggs.

supplies all of the chick's dietary requirements of protein, vitamins, and minerals.

Despite concerns about their high cholesterol content and possible contamination with salmonella, eggs remain a popular and inexpensive source of nourishment. Any fear of salmonella poisoning can be put aside by thorough cooking. Fortunately, an egg's overall nutrient content is not affected by heat.

Eggs are a nutrient powerhouse. Like other animal proteins, those supplied by eggs contain all the essential amino acids. In one 70-calorie egg, you get protein, B vitamins, vitamins A and D, zinc, and iron. Eggs are also an excellent source of vitamin B_{12}, which is essential for proper nerve function. Because vitamin B_{12} is found only in animal products, people who do not eat meat can rely on eggs as an important source of this vitamin.

Eggs are a good source of the antioxidants lutein and zeaxanthin, linked to a reduced risk of age-related macular degeneration, a leading cause of blindness in older adults.

Lecithin—a natural emulsifier found in eggs—is rich in choline, which is involved in moving cholesterol through the bloodstream, as well as in aiding fat metabolism. Choline is also an essential component of cell membranes and nerve tissue. Although the body can make enough choline for its normal needs, some researchers have suggested that dietary sources may be helpful in reducing the accumulation of fat in the liver, as well as repairing some types of neurological damage. Research suggests that choline may be important for early brain development and may improve memory later in life.

THE CHOLESTEROL ISSUE

A large egg contains about 70 calories, 6 g of protein, 5 g of fat (of which less than 2 g is saturated fat), and about 190 mg of cholesterol. Studies show that for most healthy people, it is the total fat, especially saturated fat (found in fatty meat, chicken skin, full-fat dairy products, and coconut and palm oil) and trans fats (found in processed and snack foods), that have the greatest effect on blood cholesterol levels. In general, dietary cholesterol is not as important a factor in raising blood cholesterol as these fats are, but there are some people who are especially sensitive to the cholesterol in foods and do see a rise in their blood cholesterol after eating cholesterol-rich meals. For these people, and for people whose blood cholesterol is already elevated, it is generally suggested to limit egg yolk consumption to 3 to 4 per week.

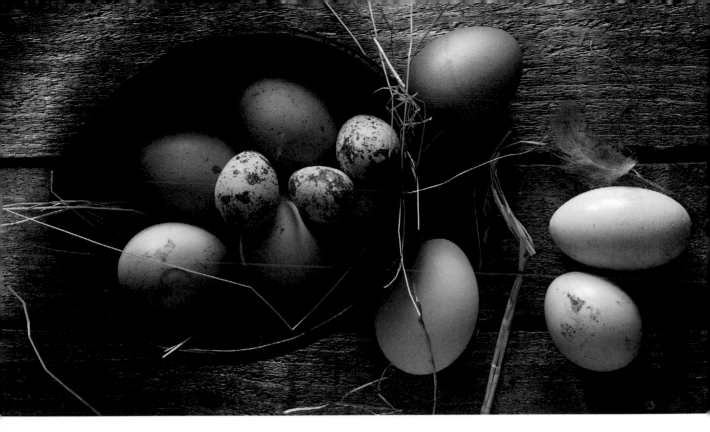

Only the yolks of eggs contain cholesterol; therefore, egg whites need not be restricted. In fact, the whites can be used to replace whole eggs or just the yolks in many recipes without detriment to their taste or texture. For example, you can replace one whole egg with two whites, or you can substitute beaten whites instead of a whole egg to coat foods for frying. You can also buy pourable liquid egg-white products that can be used for baking and omelettes.

CONFUSING EGG LABELS

Labels such as "farm-laid" or "country-fresh" can conjure up misleading images; the hens that laid the eggs may well have been confined to cages. Although the term "free range" may suggest that the chickens are pecking freely in a farmyard, it can be legally applied to the eggs of caged hens if they have daytime access to open runs. In reality, there is very little nutritional difference between free-range eggs and eggs from caged hens.

Whatever the labeling, always open the carton to inspect the eggs before you buy them. Reject any eggs that have cracked or blemished shells. Gently rub your fingers across the top of the eggs to ensure none are stuck to the bottom of the box. It is a myth that brown eggs are more nutritious than white ones, even though many supermarkets charge a higher price for brown eggs. Both are equally nutritious; they just come from different breeds of chicken.

STORING EGGS

Keep eggs in the main part of the refrigerator, which is cooler than the shelves on the inside of the door. Store the pointed end of the egg down, so that the yolk remains centered in the shell away from the air pocket at the larger end. Leave eggs in their original dated carton to keep track of when you bought them. Refrigerated eggs can be kept safely for up to 3 weeks.

EGGS AND ALLERGIES

Eggs are among the foods most likely to trigger allergic reactions. People who are allergic to eggs should be on the lookout for obvious sources, such as mayonnaise and sauces, pancakes, waffles, and bakery items, as well as sherbets and ice cream. They should always check food labels for telltale terms. These include albumin, globulin, ovomucin, and vitellin, which are all ingredients derived from eggs. Those allergic to eggs should also avoid flu shots and other vaccines incubated in eggs.

OMEGA-3 EGGS

Omega-3 fat enhanced eggs are new to the egg world. They are laid by hens fed a diet high in flaxseed. Their yolk is rich in omega-3 fats, the polyunsaturated fats associated with

EGGS OF THE WORLD. *Chicken eggs are most often used in North American homes, but in other parts of the world, quail, duck, and goose eggs are eaten as well.*

DID YOU KNOW?

EGGS ARE A "COMPLETE PROTEIN" FOOD

Protein is composed of 20 different amino acids. Nine of these amino acids cannot be made by the body. These nine are considered essential amino acids and must come from food. Foods that contain all nine essential amino acids are called "complete protein" foods.

THE SALMONELLA SCARE

Occasionally, an egg may be found to harbor salmonella bacteria, which can be passed on by the hen or can enter through cracked shells. Although the risk of food poisoning is relatively low, it is best to avoid eating raw or partly cooked eggs in any form. People at special risk include the frail elderly, young children, pregnant women, and anyone with lowered immunity due to illness.

Caesar salads, fresh mayonnaise, egg-based sauces and dressings, and mousses can all contain raw or partly cooked eggs. To be certain that eggs have been cooked long enough, boil them for at least 7 minutes, poach them for 5 minutes, or fry them for 3 minutes on each side. Both the yolk and the white should be firm. Omelettes and scrambled eggs should be cooked until firm and not runny.

lower risk of heart disease and stroke. These eggs are low in saturated fat and are a better source of vitamin E than regular eggs. Liquid egg products, enriched with the same high-quality omega-3 fatty acids normally found in fish have also become available. These contain 80 percent less cholesterol, 50 percent less fat and calories than regular eggs, and are an excellent source of protein. They can be used anywhere you would use a regular whole beaten egg such as in baking, scrambled eggs, or omelettes. ❖

ENERGY BARS

BENEFITS
- Convenient and portable.
- Some are good sources of protein, carbohydrates, fiber, vitamins, and minerals.

DRAWBACKS
- Many are high in calories, sugar, and/or fats.

Energy bars—the words conjures up visions of high-performance athletes going the distance on the strength of a single bar. These bars have come into the mainstream and are sold in grocery and drugstores, gyms, and health-food stores. People eat them as a performance enhancer, a snack, a high-energy, nutritional pick-me-up, a meal replacement, and a weight-loss tool.

The word energy means the capacity for work or vigorous activity. In the nutrition world, the word energy is synonymous with calories. The truth is that all foods give you energy. Just because a food is called an energy bar, does not mean that eating it will make you more energetic.

Energy bars are not magic foods, but if you're a serious athlete, working out for a long time, or engaging in an endurance sport such as a triathlon or marathon, they can help. If you're trying to increase your caloric intake to support your endurance event and have maximized the amount of regular food you can eat, energy bars can provide the extra calories along with other important nutrients. They're portable, nonperishable, and may be handier, at times, than bagels, yogurt, fruits, or other high-energy snacks. Many athletes find nibbling on them helpful during a long run, and they have proven to be popular with rowers, cross-country skiers, cyclists, and sailors. Energy bars also come in handy for all-day sports events when other foods are not readily available.

While endurance competitors may reap benefits, energy bars aren't much help for recreational athletes. They won't provide extra energy, build muscle, or increase stamina. That has to come from training. If the extra calories provided by these energy bars are not "burned," they can quickly lead to weight gain.

Most people use these products for convenience. For busy people on the go, they can be a great midday snack or a pre- or post-workout snack if you don't have access to fruits or yogurt.

WHAT'S IN A BAR?
All bars are not created equal, and it is important to examine what you are eating and determine if it is right for you. There are high-carbohydrate bars, high-protein bars, 40-30-30 bars, breakfast bars, brain-boosting bars, meal-replacement bars, diet bars, and more. Some are nutritious and some are not.

Look for bars that are low in fat, particularly of the saturated or trans variety. A giveaway for the presence of trans fats is the term "hydrogenated fat" on the label. Some bars are a good source of fiber (aim for 3 to 5 g), as well as important vitamins and minerals.

High-protein bars can be helpful for vegetarian athletes, long-distance runners, and people who require high-protein diets. Go for bars with protein sources such as whey, soy, or casein.

The meal-replacement bars are helpful for people trying to lose weight but should not be used on a regular basis. If you are using the bar as an occasional meal replacement, look for the bars with at least 10 to 15 g of protein.

If you are an athlete, try different bars during your regular workouts before you use them in a competition. Everyone's system is different, so it's important to find what works best for you before you are in the heat of a race.

While energy bars may appear to have the same vitamins and minerals found in fruits, vegetables, and grains, they don't contain the phytochemicals, bioflavonoids, and natural fiber found in foods. ❖

EPILEPSY

AVOID

- Alcohol.
- Any food that appears to trigger attacks or may interact with anticonvulsants.

More than 1.5 million North Americans have some form of epilepsy, recurrent seizures triggered by abnormal electrical impulses in the brain. Some seizures are so mild and fleeting that they are barely noticeable; others last for several minutes, during which the person falls down and is seized by convulsive movements. The frequency of seizures also varies from person to person; some epileptics suffer many seizures each day, while others may go for months between episodes.

Neurologists generally discount any link between diet and epilepsy, with some exceptions. Epileptics who have migraine headaches that are triggered by certain foods often cease to have seizures when the offending foods are eliminated. Some diabetics suffer seizures when their blood sugar levels drop suddenly. Large amounts of alcohol consumed in a short time can cause seizures. Although evidence is sketchy, there have been rare reports of aspartame triggering seizures in epileptics.

THE HIGH-FAT DIET

A rigid diet that appears to halt seizures in children whose attacks cannot be controlled by drugs has been hailed as a recent breakthrough. In reality, however, the diet dates to the early 1900s, when doctors devised a dietary treatment for epilepsy based on the ancient observation that seizures ceased during periods of prolonged fasting. Fasting is hardly a practical long-term treatment for chronic seizures, but researchers found that a high-fat diet mimicked fasting metabolism without starvation.

The ketogenic diet. With the development of effective anticonvulsant drugs, the dietary treatment was dropped. But now neurologists at Johns Hopkins Hospital have refined a dietary treatment for severe epilepsy. After about 24 hours of fasting, the body depletes its reserves of glucose and starts to burn stored fat for energy. However, burning fat in the absence of glucose gives off waste products called ketone bodies, which build up in the blood and are excreted in the urine. Very high blood levels of ketones can upset body chemistry, and even lead to a coma and death. But at lower levels they can eliminate seizures. Carefully structuring the diet by allowing only a sprinkling of carbohydrates can result in a therapeutic level of ketones in the bloodstream.

This regimen, called the ketogenic diet, appears to work best in young children, especially that 20 percent whose seizures are not adequately controlled by drugs. The diet provides about 75 percent of the calories generally recommended for healthy children, and most of these come from fats. A small amount of protein is added to allow for at least some growth, but carbohydrates are kept to a minimum. Fluid intake is restricted. The diet must be carefully tailored and then followed exactly; a small deviation can bring on seizures. To begin, the child is hospitalized for 2 or 3 days of fasting, after which the ketogenic diet is gradually introduced. The diet can be difficult to follow, but after 2 to 3 years, most patients can resume a normal diet and still be seizure-free. ❖

EYE DISORDERS

CONSUME PLENTY OF

- Carrots and sweet potatoes for beta carotene.
- Citrus fruits and broccoli for vitamin C.
- Fatty fish and dairy products for vitamin A.
- Vegetable oils and almonds for vitamin E.
- Seafood, meat, poultry, and beans for zinc.
- Leafy greens, peas, corn, peppers for lutein and zeaxanthin.

LIMIT

- Saturated fats.

The role of antioxidant nutrients and bioflavonoids in vision loss and other degenerative problems associated with aging is becoming increasingly clear. With advancing age, the production of free radicals, those unstable molecules that form when the body uses oxygen, increases. Free radicals can cause eye damage similar to that resulting from exposure to radiation, and can also contribute to such disorders as cataracts and macular degeneration.

AGE-RELATED DISORDERS

Cataracts develop when the lens, the transparent membrane that allows light to enter the eye, yellows, hindering the passage of light rays through it. Vision becomes hazy, cloudy, or blurry; if untreated, the lens may become completely opaque, resulting in blindness.

Although aging is the most common cause of cataracts, they can occur at any time of life, even in infancy. Smoking and diabetes can hasten their development. But a diet that provides ample antioxidants—in particular, vitamins C and E and the carotenoid lutein—appears to slow their progression. At least one study has shown that the prevalence of cataracts in people who took vitamin C supplements for at least 10 years was significantly lower. Vitamins C and E work with antioxidants to ward off free-radical damage.

Macular degeneration, another eye disease that comes with aging, is one of the most common causes of legal blindness among older North Americans. It entails a gradual, painless deterioration of the macula, the tissue in the central portion of the retina. The first symptom is usually blurring of central vision but eventually side vision can also become limited. The cause of macular degeneration is unknown, but recent research suggests that a diet high in antioxidant nutrients may help prevent or slow the disorder. Lutein and zeaxanthin are two antioxidants that may help. These two carotenoids are the dominant pigments found in the macula of the eye and are thought to help filter out some of the harmful light that can damage the retina. Lutein is found in green leafy vegetables such as broccoli, kale, Swiss chard, and watercress, as well as in corn, peas, and egg yolks. Zeaxanthin is also found in greens, red peppers, and corn.

One clinical trial involved more than 3,500 people aged 55 to 80 who already had at least one symptom of age-related macular degeneration. Some were treated with zinc alone, some took the antioxidant vitamins E, C, and beta carotene, some took that mixture plus zinc. Those who took the antioxidants plus zinc had the lowest risk of developing advanced stages of macular degeneration.

DID YOU KNOW?

BILBERRIES CAN HELP

Bilberries are extremely rich in antioxidants, which can help protect vision. Studies suggest that bilberry—available as an extract and in preserves—can help prevent cataracts and even slow or stop their progression.

Research also shows that a diet high in saturated fats increases the risk of age-related macular degeneration. Scientists theorize that saturated fats may clog the arteries in the retina in the same way that they contribute to atherosclerosis in larger blood vessels, such as the coronary arteries. Eating fish more than once a week significantly reduces the risk.

DIABETIC RETINOPATHY

Certain similarities between macular degeneration and diabetic retinopathy—the infiltration of the retina with tiny ruptured blood vessels—suggest that antioxidant nutrients may also be beneficial in this common complication of diabetes. Diet is critical in maintaining tight control of blood glucose levels, which also reduces the risk of diabetic retinopathy.

NIGHT BLINDNESS

The eyes need vitamin A or its precursor, beta carotene, as well as bioflavonoids, to make the pigments that absorb light within the eye. A deficiency in vitamin A, or a failure to utilize it properly, impairs the eye's ability to adapt to darkness and leads to night blindness. This does not entail a total loss of night vision, but rather difficulty seeing well in dim lighting.

Vitamin A deficiency is rare in the Western world, but it remains a major problem in many underdeveloped countries. Organ meats, fortified margarine, butter, and other dairy products are good sources of vitamin A. Dark yellow or orange foods, such as carrots, sweet potatoes, and apricots, as well as dark green leafy vegetables, are the richest sources of beta carotene, which the body converts to vitamin A.

Failing night vision should not be self-treated with vitamin A or beta carotene supplements; the problem may stem from a digestive or malabsorption disorder that prevents the body from using the vitamin. Treatment of the underlying cause usually cures the night blindness. An exception is night blindness caused by retinitis pigmentosa, a genetic disease. However, recent research suggests that vitamin A may, in fact, slow the progressive vision loss of this incurable disease.

CONJUNCTIVITIS

Commonly called pink eye, conjunctivitis is an irritation or infection of the membrane that lines the front of the eyeball and eyelid.

Viruses are responsible for most conjunctivitis, but in recurring cases an allergic reaction may be the cause. ❖

FAST FOOD
■ EATING ON THE RUN ■

Fast-food and take-out restaurants are everywhere in North America, even in hospitals and schools. According to food industry statistics, fast-food restaurants serve more than 60 million North Americans each day.

Some critics blame this growing reliance on fast food, which is typically high in fat and calories, and the supersizing of portions for the fact that more than 50 percent of adult North Americans are overweight. Though defenders note that most fast-food establishments offer some lower-calorie, more-healthful fare, the overwhelming majority of the foods we eat at fast-food chains—the burgers, fries, hot dogs, fried chicken, and pizza—are loaded with fat, salt, and calories, and have very little fiber.

Most fast food is high in saturated fat. Fried foods—especially French fries—also tend to contain significant levels of trans fats, the man-made fats that are created when hydrogen is added to vegetable oil to make it more solid and stable. Trans fats are now believed to be as bad for your health—or even worse—as saturated fats.

Fast-food chains like McDonald's and snack-food manufacturers like Frito-Lay have made commitments to reduce trans fatty acids and saturated fats in their products and to introduce more-nutritious menus or food items. Many fast-food establishments have added a variety of healthier choices to their menus, including salads, grilled foods, baked potatoes, soups, whole-grain buns, fruit cups, low-fat frozen yogurts, and juices. Some

Supersizing

Everyone loves a super value deal. But is it really a bargain when you end up buying unwanted fat, calories, and sodium along with the bigger portion? A decade ago, an original burger, fries, and coke at McDonald's contained 660 calories. Now a super-size value meal contains an incredible 1,450 calories, or more than half of what most people need in a day.

chains also provide a nutrition analysis on their websites or make copies available in their restaurants to help nutrition-conscious diners eat healthfully. And if you log on to www.fatcalories.com, you'll find nutritional information on foods from a number of different fast-food chains.

The safety factor

Occasionally, an outbreak of food poisoning is traced to a fast-food outlet. Any meal that is mass-produced and then allowed to stand for any length of time is vulnerable to contamination. Especially deadly, particularly to young children, is a type of *E. coli* infection contracted by eating undercooked contaminated beef.

It is not wise to take out fast food and then wait several hours before eating it. Any food that is not consumed right away should be refrigerated, and then thoroughly reheated before it is eaten. If you're eating in a restaurant, decline any precooked item that looks like it has been sitting around for a while.

DID YOU KNOW?
NORTH AMERICANS LOVE FAST FOOD

They consume more than 7 billion hot dogs each year, and the average North American consumes more than 100 orders of fries and approximately 150 slices of pizza annually.

SALAD—THE HEALTHIER CHOICE?

You probably think a salad would be the healthier choice at a fast-food restaurant. But think again. You might be surprised to hear that a salad, complete with dressing and toppings, often contains more calories and fat than many of the more traditional fast-food choices. Compare the following.

RESTAURANT	MEAL	CALORIES	FAT (grams)
McDonald's	Chicken Caesar salad with light creamy dressing	379	19.0
	Warm chicken oriental salad with light sesame Thai dressing	335	6.6
	Hamburger	246	7.9
Taco Bell	Taco salad	532	37.0
	Taco supreme	219	14.0
Subway	Roasted chicken salad without dressing	141	3.6
	Roasted chicken salad with packet of ranch dressing	294	18.6
	6-in. (15-cm) roasted chicken sub sandwich	317	5.8
Wendy's	Mandarin chicken salad, plain	155	1.5
	Mandarin chicken salad with roasted almonds, crispy rice noodles, and oriental sesame dressing	596	33.6
	Classic single burger	413	19.0
	Grilled chicken sandwich	302	7.2

When your hectic lifestyle needs a little help from fast food

Many of us lead such busy lives that we can't get by without eating on the run, often in the car. It is possible, however, to make your fast-food choices a little lighter just by being careful which toppings you choose on your menu item. When making your selection, keep the following in mind:

Hamburgers: Basic hamburgers are in the 250- to 350-calorie range, with about 10 to 20 g of fat, while deluxe, all-dressed cheeseburgers weigh in at about 500 calories, with 26 g of fat. Choose a basic hamburger, no cheese, no mayonnaise, no bacon. Order it dressed with mustard, pickle, fresh onion, tomato, and lettuce.

French fries: Of course we all want fries with that, but we must be prepared to pay the nutritional price. Just one medium-size serving of French fries delivers between 360 to 450 calories and a hefty 17 to 22 g of fat. A large order of fries from several chains provides almost 600 calories with 27 g of fat, part of which is trans fat. Try to skip the fries, or eat them only occasionally.

If you must have fries, get the smallest order, and avoid those cooked in anything but vegetable oil (always ask the counter person to verify this). And if possible, order wide, large-cut fries. They are usually slightly lower in fat and salt than the skinny ones because in an entire order of fries, there is less surface area for the oil to cling to. Do not add extra salt, add a little ketchup instead. Ketchup has no fat and only 15 calories per teaspoon.

Hot dogs: The traditional North American hot dog contains about 240 calories, and 16 g of fat. Typically, 60 percent of the calories come from fat, with only a small percentage from protein. Eat hot dogs only occasionally, and watch the toppings: Skip the cheese and chili, stick with mustard, relish, and onions.

Tacos: A regular beef taco with the traditional toppings of lettuce and cheese in a hard taco shell has approximately 180 calories, with 10 g of fat. Stick to one taco, with only the regular toppings.

Pizza: There's no question that pizza is one of our all-time favorite fast foods. Unfortunately, it is also a major source of fat. One 14-in. (35-cm) commercial pizza has anywhere from 22 to 36 g of fat. When eating pizza, try the following:

Stick to one slice. One or two slices of pizza with a side salad or vegetable sticks will boost the nutrition of your fast-food meal while decreasing the fat and calories.

Load up on vegetable toppings. They have the least calories and fat and the most nutrients. Lean meats like chicken and ham are better choices than fatty sausages and pepperoni.

Cut down on cheese. Ask for more sauce and less cheese. If your toppings are grilled vegetables, chicken or seafood, and herbs, try having no cheese at all.

FAST-FOOD HUNTING?

This chart will help you make healthy choices when you're eating fast-food versions of these cuisines and foods.

BEST PICKS	GO EASY ON
Japanese Teriyaki beef, chicken, or shrimp; yakitori chicken; miso soup; stir-fries; sushi; sashimi; noodle soup dishes	Tempura dishes
Italian Pasta with tomato or marinara sauce; salads with low-fat dressings; pizza with lots of vegetables and light on cheese; minestrone soup	Fried veal; chicken parmigiana; double cheese pizza with fatty-meat toppings, cream sauces
Mexican Chicken fajitas, enchiladas, soft-shell beef taco, vegetarian burrito (hold the sour cream and cheese); salsa	Nachos and cheese, guacamole, refried beans, fried taco shells
Greek Lean souvlaki or chicken kebab with salad, dressing on the side	Tzatziki or other high-fat dips, stuffed pastry
Burgers Plain or veggie burger with lettuce, tomato, pickle, and onions; grilled chicken on a bun	Fries, onion rings, mayonnaise, bacon, and cheese toppings
Chinese Soups; mixed vegetables; steamed rice, steamed dim sum; stir-fries	Egg rolls, chicken wings, any deep-fried dishes
Deli Turkey, chicken breast, lean corned beef, pastrami or roast beef sandwiches; dill pickles; green salad	Cheese, sausage, or salami sandwich, potato salad with mayonnaise dressing
Sub Shops 6-in. (15-cm) sub on whole wheat with turkey, beef, chicken, or seafood, lots of veggies, low-fat mayonnaise	Club, meatball, or deep-fried chicken, high-fat sauces
Chicken Roast chicken sandwich or wrap, chicken club, grilled chicken salads, barbequed chicken (remove skin)	Deep-fried, or nuggets, or fingers

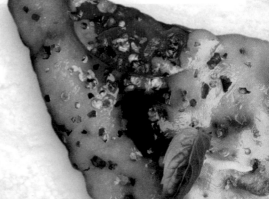

FATS
■ FACTS AND FALLACIES ■

Fat is a dietary evil—or so you probably think. The food industry has exploited this belief in order to sell low-fat and fat-free versions of just about every food product under the sun. But the truth is that fat, in small amounts, is essential to health. Some fats, like those found in fish and olive oil, actually lower our risk of heart disease and even help us stick to a weight-loss plan. The trouble is, these aren't the fats we tend to crave—the saturated fats that give meat, ice cream, and cheese their delicious richness.

What is a fat?

"Lipid" is a general term used to describe substances that usually cannot be dissolved in water but will dissolve in an organic solvent. Fats, oils, waxes, certain sterols and esters all fall into this category. The term "triglyceride" is more specific and applies to fats and oils. These differ in their melting points: at room temperature, fats are solid, whereas oils are liquid. In other respects, they can be considered as a single class of compounds, and for simplicity can be referred to as fats.

Natural fats, whether they are derived from animal or plant sources, are composed of three fatty acid molecules (that's the "tri" in triglyceride) bound to one glycerol (a type of alcohol) molecule. The nature of a fat depends on which fatty acids, drawn from a basic pool of about 25, are attached to the glycerol backbone.

All fats contain the same number of calories by weight; that is, about 250 calories per ounce, or 9 calories per gram. Volume for volume, however, the calorie count can differ substantially. For example, a cup of oil weighs more—and therefore has more calories—than a cup of whipped margarine. The air added to increase the margarine's volume has no calories. In addition, if the whipped margarine is one of the low-calorie versions, a considerable percentage of its weight will come from added water.

A diet rich in high-fat foods results in more weight gain than a diet made up mainly of carbohydrates with some protein. Not only are fats a more concentrated source of calories than the other food groups, but studies indicate that the body is also more efficient in storing fats than carbohydrates and protein.

How we use fats

It is important to distinguish the fat consumed in foods—dietary fat—from fats circulating in the blood or stored as adipose tissue, which is made up of cells specially adapted for that purpose. Even if the diet contains no fat whatsoever, the body will convert any excess protein and carbohydrate to fat and store them as such. When our weight remains steady, it is because we are storing and using fat at equal rates. If our food intake exceeds our need for energy, then no matter what the composition of the diet, we synthesize more fat than we use and gain weight.

The average woman's body is about 20 to 25 percent fat by weight; the average man's is 15 percent. The greater proportion of fat in women is an evolutionary adaptation to meet the demand for extra calories needed to bear and nourish children.

DID YOU KNOW?

ESSENTIAL FATTY ACIDS, LIKE ALPHA-LINOLENIC ACID, HELP KEEP HEART DISEASE AT BAY

Alpha-linolenic acid, an essential fatty acid found in flaxseed, canola, and soybean oil, has been shown to provide numerous health benefits, including helping your heart keep a strong and regular beat. One study showed that in men, the heart-protective effect achieved by consuming this fat was even more significant than reducing saturated fats. Another study showed that women who consumed the most alpha-linolenic acid had a significantly lower risk of dying from heart disease.

Most body cells have a limited capacity for fat storage. The fat cells (adipocytes) are exceptions; they expand as more fat accumulates. An obese person's fat cells may be 50 to 100 times larger than those of a thin person. In addition, overweight infants and children accumulate more fat cells than their thin counterparts. Once in place, fat cells will never go away, although they will shrink if fat is drawn off to be used for energy production. One theory has it that shrunken fat cells emit a chemical plea for replenishment, which could explain why many people spend their lives on a roller coaster of weight loss and gain.

Why we need fats

Fats add flavor and a smooth, pleasing texture to foods. Because they take longer to digest, fats continue to let us feel full even after the proteins and carbohydrates have been emptied from the stomach. Fats also stimulate the intestine to release cholecystokinin, a hormone that suppresses the appetite and signals us to stop eating.

These are likely reasons that people who include a moderate amount of "healthy" fats in their diets are more likely to stay on the diet and lose weight.

Fats also supply the fatty acids that are essential for numerous chemical processes, including growth and development in children, the production of sex hormones and prostaglandins (hormonelike chemicals that are responsible for regulating many body processes), the formation and function of cell membranes, and the transport of other molecules into and out of the cells.

Interestingly enough, fat does not supply energy for the brain and nervous system, both of which rely on glucose for fuel. Like certain vitamins and amino acids, some fatty acids must be obtained from the diet, because the body cannot synthesize them. Our need for essential fatty acids is met by linoleic acid (found in vegetable oils, especially corn, safflower, and soybean oils), which is then converted in the body into arachidonic acid, another essential fatty acid. Finally, fats are needed for the transport and absorption of the fat-soluble vitamins A, D, E, and K. A tablespoon of vegetable oil provides enough linoleic acid and fat to transport all the fat-soluble vitamins we need in a day; any more than this is unnecessary.

Dietary intake

In developing countries fats make up 10 percent of daily calories. In North America daily fat intake has increased from about 30 percent of the daily diet 100 years ago, to 35 to 40 percent today. This is the equivalent of approximately 90 g of pure fat a day and is more than six to eight times what we need. Most experts now recommend that adults restrict their total fat intake to no more than 30 percent of each day's calories. Some authorities believe this number should be lowered to 20 percent, but others feel this is an unrealistic goal for most people.

Saturation

The types of fats we eat may be more important than the total amount of fat we eat. For years nutritionists have recommended unsaturated over saturated fats. In general, saturated fats (but not palm, palm kernel, and coconut oils) are solid at room temperature; most animal fats (beef, butter, and cheeses) are saturated. Monounsaturated fats are liquid at room temperature and solid or semisolid under refrigeration (olive, canola, and peanut oils, and some margarines). Polyunsaturated fats are liquid (corn and sunflower oils) unless hydrogen is added in the process called hydrogenation, as it is in the manufacture of some margarines.

Highly saturated fats raise blood cholesterol levels because they interfere with the removal of cholesterol from the blood. Monounsaturated and polyunsaturated fats, by contrast, either lower blood cholesterol or have no effect on it. When polyunsaturated fats are hydrogenated to make them firm, they become more like saturated fats in their effects on blood cholesterol.

Action plan to reduce your fat intake

✔ Limit meat to 3 or 4 oz (85–115 g) per serving. Buy lean cuts and trim all visible fat before cooking. Buy extra-lean ground beef, or better still, select a lean cut and ask the butcher to grind it for you.
✔ Remove the skin from poultry before eating it. In some instances, this can be done before cooking.
✔ Don't buy prebasted turkey; it's often injected with coconut oil, butter, or other fats.
✔ Broil, bake, grill, or roast meat, fish, and poultry. Use a roasting rack to drain off the fat as the meat cooks.
✔ Cook stews and soups in advance; chill and skim off the congealed fat, and reheat.
✔ Avoid fried foods. Use a nonstick pan and vegetable oil spray for sautéing. Sauté in broth, wine, tomato or fruit juice instead of oil.
✔ Buy low-fat (1 percent) or skim milk, low-fat cheese, cottage cheese, and yogurt.
✔ Toss salad with fat-free dressings or make your own with lemon juice or vinegar, mustard, herbs, and spices. If oil is called for, use olive oil.
✔ Buy a low-fat or even a fat-free substitute for mayonnaise.
✔ Cook rice in a fat-free broth; flavor it with chopped fresh herbs and scallions instead of butter.
✔ Mash potatoes with low-fat yogurt or buttermilk; add chives and parsley for extra zip.
✔ Choose broth-based soups instead of cream soups.
✔ Spread sandwiches with spicy mustard, horseradish, or cranberry sauce instead of mayonnaise or butter/margarine.
✔ Eliminate the use of nondairy creamers and toppings; these products are usually high in saturated fats because they are made with palm oil or coconut oil.
✔ Choose English muffins, bagels, or pita instead of croissants, muffins, doughnuts, or danishes.
✔ Serve sherbet, sorbet, gelato, or frozen yogurt instead of premium ice cream or consider other low-fat dessert alternatives, such as fresh fruits, gelatins, meringues, and angel food cake.
✔ Measure oil, don't eyeball it. The ¼ cup of oil you drizzle over salad or put in your frying pan contains 46 g of fat and about 400 calories. If you measure it, you will use less.
✔ Use buttermilk instead of mayonnaise or sour cream. Buttermilk may sound high in fat but it is as low as 1 percent milk. Use it in baking or as a base for salad dressings. Evaporated 2 percent milk can taste as creamy as regular cream. It can be used for rich-tasting desserts.
✔ Reduce the fat in baking quick breads and muffins by substituting applesauce, banana, or other pureed fruit for part of the fat.
✔ Order your cappuccino or latte "skinny," made with low-fat or skim milk.

A primer on fats

Fats and oils contain many different fatty acids that affect the body in various ways. They fall into two main categories: saturated and unsaturated fats. Food fats almost always contain both saturated and unsaturated fatty acids and are classified as saturated, monounsaturated, or polyunsaturated depending on which fatty acids are present in the greatest concentration. Studies show that the type of fat you eat may be as important as how much you eat.

■ Saturated fats generally come from animal sources—meat, poultry, eggs, and dairy. The plant sources of saturated fats are coconut oil, palm oil, and palm kernel oil. A diet high in saturated fats can raise blood cholesterol levels.
■ Unsaturated fats can help lower LDL-cholesterol levels when they replace saturated fats in your diet. There are two types of unsaturated fats: monounsaturated and polyunsaturated.
■ Monounsaturated fats, which are liquid at room temperature, have been found to lower LDL-cholesterol levels. They are found predominantly in olive, canola, and peanut oils, as well as avocado, some nuts, and seeds.
■ There are two kinds of polyunsaturated fats: omega-3 and omega-6 fats.
■ Omega-3 fats are found in fatty fish such as salmon, mackerel, herring, and sardines, as well as flaxseed, walnut, and canola oils and some newer products such as omega-3 eggs. These fats help prevent blood clotting, which can

OIL IN THE FAMILY

All fats are a mixture of saturated, monounsaturated, and polyunsaturated fatty acids (though we usually call them by the name of the fatty acid they have the most of). Look for the least saturated (red), and a good mixture of everything else. Polys (yellow and green) lower cholesterol, while monos (blue) only lower cholesterol if you eat them in place of saturated fats. Alpha-linolenic acid (green) is an omega-3 polyunsaturated fat that may protect the heart. Canola, soy, and flaxseed oil are good sources. Many researchers recommend a mix of alpha-linolenic acid and linoleic acid (yellow). (Linoleic is a polyunsaturated omega-6 fat.) If you don't want the details, just stick with canola for cooking. It is among the lowest in saturated fat and it has a good mix of alpha-linolenic and linoleic acids.

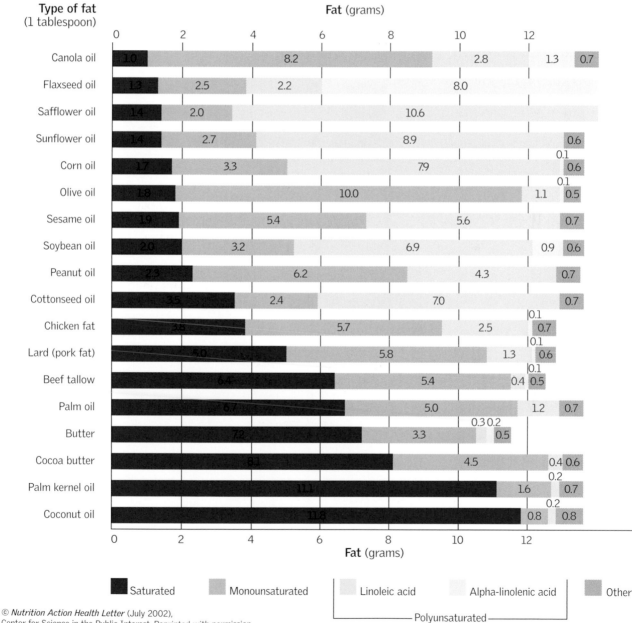

Type of fat (1 tablespoon)	Saturated	Monounsaturated	Linoleic acid	Alpha-linolenic acid	Other
Canola oil	1.0	8.2	2.8	1.3	0.7
Flaxseed oil	1.3	2.5	2.2	8.0	
Safflower oil	1.4	2.0	10.6		
Sunflower oil	1.4	2.7	8.9		0.6
Corn oil	1.7	3.3	7.9	0.1	0.6
Olive oil	1.8	10.0	1.1	0.1	0.5
Sesame oil	1.9	5.4	5.6		0.7
Soybean oil	2.0	3.2	6.9	0.9	0.6
Peanut oil	2.3	6.2	4.3		0.7
Cottonseed oil	3.5	2.4	7.0		0.7
Chicken fat	3.8	5.7	2.5	0.1	0.7
Lard (pork fat)	5.0	5.8	1.3	0.1	0.6
Beef tallow	6.4	5.4	0.4	0.1	0.5
Palm oil	6.7	5.0	1.2		0.7
Butter	7.2	3.3	0.3	0.2	0.5
Cocoa butter	8.1	4.5	0.4		0.6
Palm kernel oil	11.1	1.6	0.2		0.7
Coconut oil	11.8	0.8	0.2		0.8

Polyunsaturated: Linoleic acid — Alpha-linolenic acid

© *Nutrition Action Health Letter* (July 2002), Center for Science in the Public Interest. Reprinted with permission.

trigger a heart attack or stroke. They also help lower triglycerides, which can decrease your risk for heart disease.

■ Omega-6 fats are found in foods that come from plant sources and are liquid at room temperature. Food sources include safflower, sunflower, corn oil, some nuts and seeds such as almonds, pecans, brazil nuts, sunflower seeds, and sesame seeds. These fats should be eaten in moderation since they still will contribute to your total calorie intake.

■ The omega-3 and omega-6 fats in your diet provide the two essential fatty acids that your body cannot produce on its own. Omega-3 fats provide alpha-linolenic acid and omega-6 fats provide linoleic acid. These two fatty acids are essential to health and must be provided by foods you eat.

■ Experts now believe that the ratio of omega-6 fats to omega-3 fats in our diets is too high. While omega-6 fatty acids do not increase levels of LDL ("bad") cholesterol, they may decrease levels of HDL ("good") cholesterol. They appear to contribute to the production of some cell-damaging free radicals. You can shift your ratio by getting more omega-3 fatty acids from fish and other sources.

■ Trans fats are a particular kind of fat created when a vegetable oil undergoes a process called hydrogenation. This process is used to make liquids more solid and is commonly used by industry to prolong shelf life. Trans fats act similarly to saturated fats by raising LDL cholesterol levels. These trans fats are found in partially hydrogenated vegetable oils and some margarines. They are also found in a wide variety of packaged foods such as crackers, cookies, and commercially baked products and in many commercially fried foods. (See "What Are Trans Fatty Acids?" page 76.)

■ Researchers are examining the properties of "conjugated linoleic acid," or CLA. This is a type of polyunsaturated fat that may be very beneficial to health. It is found in small amounts in dairy foods and meat and is also available as a supplement. Preliminary studies have shown that CLA may help reduce body fat, increase muscle mass, and even inhibit the growth of certain cancers. More research is needed before an increased intake can be recommended.

7 sources of good-for-you fats

- Olive oil
- Canola oil
- Nuts, especially almonds and walnuts
- Seeds
- Fatty fish
- Avocados
- Flaxseed oil

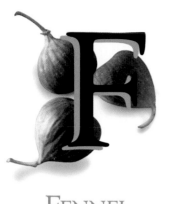

Fennel

BENEFITS

- Leaves are a good source of beta carotene and vitamin C.
- A good source of potassium and fiber.
- Low in calories.

DRAWBACKS

- The oil in fennel seeds can irritate skin.

Filling, yet low in calories, fennel is an ideal food for people trying to lose weight. Although it has a distinctly different flavor, its stalks can be mistaken for celery. Both vegetables are members of the parsley plant family, and like celery, fennel contains fiber and is low in calories—a 1-cup serving has only 25 calories. Fennel is much more nutritious than celery, however; a 1-cup serving is a good source of potassium and fiber and contains some vitamin C, iron, calcium, and folate; the leaves contain beta carotene and vitamin C.

The sweet, licoricelike flavor of fennel is similar to that of anise. The licorice flavor goes especially well with fish; try baking fish on a bed of fennel stalks. All parts of the plant are edible, and it can be prepared in many ways: raw in salads or braised or sautéed as a side dish. Stuffed bulbs are a flavorful vegetarian entrée; the chopped leaves make a colorful and nutritious garnish for other vegetable dishes.

Physicians through the ages have prescribed fennel for a variety of ailments: to stimulate milk production in nursing mothers; aid digestion and prevent bad breath; treat kidney stones, gout, liver and lung disorders. Ancient healers prescribed the seeds to prevent obesity; modern herbalists advocate fennel tea as a diet aid. Aromatic fennel seeds are indeed one of our oldest spices; they also are used to make a refreshing tea that is said to alleviate bloating, flatulence, and other intestinal problems. ❖

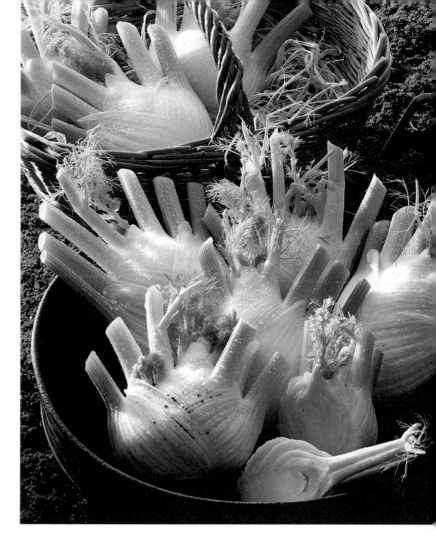

Fever

TAKE PLENTY OF

- Fluids.
- Frequent small, light, bland meals.

Although normal body temperature is generally spoken of as 98.6°F (37°C), human temperature tends to vary over the course of the day, from about 97.6°F (36.4°C) in the morning to about 99.5°F (37.5°C) in the late afternoon—and what's normal for one person can vary above or below the average temperature by as much as one degree. Although minimal increases may simply be caused by hot weather or being bundled up in too much clothing, most people can feel a difference in their body temperature that they will call a fever once it reaches 100.5°F (38°C) or 101°F (38.5°C).

Fever is not a disease in itself, but rather a symptom of some underlying problem, most commonly an infection. Depending on the cause, a fever is often accompanied by other

A COUSIN OF CELERY. *Fennel may look like celery with a fat bulb, but it has its own distinctive flavor that is an asset to a variety of dishes.*

symptoms, such as sweating, shivering, thirst, flushed skin, nausea, vomiting, and diarrhea.

A fever alone does not necessarily require treatment—it is one of the body's natural ways of fighting disease and, generally, should not be suppressed unless it is very high or accompanied by other symptoms. When fever-lowering medication is indicated, either acetaminophen or aspirin may be effective. But aspirin should never be given to anyone under the age of 18 without a doctor's approval; aspirin given during a viral infection increases the risk of developing Reye's syndrome, a potentially life-threatening disease affecting the brain and liver. Keep in mind that children's fevers can rise rapidly, so even a high temperature over 102°F (39°C) does not necessarily reflect the severity of an illness.

NUTRITIONAL NEEDS

Drink lots of fluids. Sweating, the body's response to high temperature, results in the loss of fluid, which is worsened if there is diarrhea or vomiting. So it is important to drink at least eight glasses of fluid daily to prevent dehydration. If a feverish person does not feel thirsty, it may be easier to sip a bit of fruit juice diluted with an equal volume of water every few minutes rather than to drink a whole glass at once. Or the person, especially if a child, can be given a frozen fruit juice bar to suck on.

Warning: Feverish infants can get dehydrated very quickly, because they have a large body surface in proportion to their fluid volume. When babies have high temperatures, parents should give frequent bottles of plain water or a commercial infant rehydration product. You can easily make your own rehydrating solution by dissolving ½ cup of dry, precooked baby rice cereal in 2 cups of water with ¼ tablespoon of salt. The mixture should be thick, but still pourable and drinkable.

Don't starve a fever. There is no medical basis for the saying "feed a cold and starve a fever." If anything, you need more calories than normal if you have a raised temperature because your metabolic rate rises as the fever rises. So if you feel like eating, eat.

If diarrhea is also a problem, try the BRAT diet (bananas, rice, applesauce, toast). When diarrhea is a problem, solid foods should be avoided until the bowels stabilize. Then, small servings of bland foods, such as ripe bananas, applesauce, white toast dipped in chicken or beef broth, chicken-rice soup, rice cereals, boiled or poached eggs can be eaten. ❖

CONSULT A DOCTOR IF:

• An infant under the age of 3 months has a fever that is higher than 100°F (38°C).

• A child or adult under 60 has a fever above 103°F (39.5°C).

• An adult over 60 has a fever over 102°F (39°C).

• A fever of 101°F (38.5°C) persists for more than 3 days.

• A child or adult has a fever of 101°F (38.5°C) that is accompanied by severe headache, nausea and vomiting, a stiff neck, change in alertness, or hypersensitivity to light.

FIBER

BENEFITS
- Helps prevent constipation.
- Relieves the symptoms of diverticulosis and hemorrhoids.
- May help reduce risk of colon cancer.
- Soluble fiber plays a role in lowering elevated blood cholesterol levels.
- Useful as a means of controlling weight.

DRAWBACKS
- Too much fiber can cause bloating and other digestive problems.
- Some high-fiber foods can cause gas.
- Excessive fiber may interfere with the absorption of iron, zinc, and other minerals.

Dietary fiber (also called roughage) is the indigestible component of plant foods. The effects of fiber appear to have been known since biblical times, but only in recent years have scientists begun to understand its importance in the daily diet as a means of preventing disease and maintaining health. Although fiber is not a magic bullet that can prevent or cure everything from cancer to indigestion, research does suggest that the typically low-fiber diets consumed in Western industrialized countries may contribute to such widespread illnesses as coronary artery disease, diabetes, and diseases of the large intestine, including cancer.

The typical North American diet is estimated to provide about 15 g of fiber a day. There is no recommended allowance for fiber but many experts suggest you aim for between 25 to 35 g each day.

DIETARY SOURCES

Most dietary fiber comes from fruits, vegetables, dried beans, peas and other legumes, flax, cereals, grains, nuts, and seeds. The outer layer of a grain, which contains the most fiber, is removed in the refining process. This explains why whole-grain products, such as brown rice and whole-wheat bread, are good sources of fiber.

Fiber falls into two broad categories: soluble and insoluble. Most plants contain both kinds of fiber although certain foods are richer in one than the other. The soluble fibers dissolve in water and become sticky. These are found in lentils, legumes, oat bran, oatmeal, flax, psyllium, barley, and pectin-rich fruits such as apples, strawberries, and citrus fruits. Insoluble fiber does not dissolve, passing through the digestive tract chewed but otherwise largely unchanged. It is found in wheat bran, whole-wheat products, brown rice, the skins of fruits, vegetables such as carrots, broccoli, and peas.

INCREASING FIBER INTAKE

- Eat 5 to 10 servings of fruit and vegetables daily. Leave the skins on when possible.
- Eat breakfast. Breakfast is one of the best fiber opportunities of the day. Aim to get 5 to 10 g by eating fiber-rich cereal, whole-grain toast, and fresh or dried fruit.
- Snack on high-fiber fruit. Pears, berries, or apples, and dried fruit such as prunes or apricots are excellent high-fiber snacks.
- Serve vegetables raw or steamed. Eat the higher-fiber vegetables such as corn, peas, potatoes (with skin on), sweet potatoes, broccoli, brussels sprouts, and turnip.
- Use whole-grain cereals and breads, whole-wheat pasta, and brown rice.
- Try bulgur or barley and other higher-fiber grains.
- Add extra bran. Add bran to muffins, pancake batter, casseroles, meat loaf or as a crispy coating for chicken or fish.
- Eat legumes more often. Try lentil soups, stews, or casseroles.
- Have beans for lunch. One-half cup baked beans contains 8 g of fiber. Eat it with a slice of whole-wheat bread for another 2 g of fiber and you are almost halfway to your suggested daily amount.
- Eat more salads. Add nuts, seeds, or chickpeas or kidney beans to salads.
- Enjoy baked goods made with whole grains. Choose baked goods that are made with whole-wheat flour, bran, oatmeal, raisins, or sesame seeds.

ROLE IN GOOD HEALTH

As it passes through the digestive tract, fiber acts as a sponge, absorbing many times its own weight in liquid. The result is that stools are softer and bulkier and can pass through the intestines more rapidly and be expelled more easily, thus decreasing the likelihood of constipation. This quick passage also helps prevent related bowel disorders, such as diverticulosis and hemorrhoids, which can occur from the increased pressure created by hard stools. It has also been theorized that fiber protects against cancer of the colon by causing the stools to pass more quickly, thus reducing contact with cancer-causing agents. In addition, some researchers speculate that the increased water content of high-fiber stools is also protective because it dilutes these carcinogens. This remains unproved, however, and there may be other substances in high-fiber foods that protect against cancer. Two important studies published in 2003 show that high intake of dietary fiber is associated with a lower risk of colorectal cancer (see Bran).

Some of the soluble fibers—pectin, oat bran, and others—can lower blood cholesterol levels; in turn, this decreases the risk of coronary artery disease and heart attacks due to atherosclerosis, the buildup of fatty plaque in arteries.

Although insoluble fibers have little or no effect, some soluble fibers also help to control blood-sugar levels in people with diabetes. Increasing fiber will not cure diabetes, but a diet that is high in complex carbohydrates and fiber can allow some diabetics to better manage their blood sugar.

Because it is filling and low in calories, eating fiber is helpful when you're trying to lose or control your weight. It provides a welcome feeling of fullness, although this tends to wear off rather quickly as it passes through the digestive system. The best way to use fiber for weight loss is to consume a balanced diet that also includes modest amounts of protein and fat in each meal. Because the body metabolizes these more slowly than fiber, you will not become hungry again as quickly.

HOW MUCH IS TOO MUCH?

Increasing the amount of fiber in the diet should be done gradually. Suddenly increasing fiber in the diet from 10 to 30 g a day, for example, can provoke such unpleasant symptoms as bloating and gassiness. Consuming a large amount of fiber at once can lead to abdominal

A LITTLE FIBER MAKES A BIG DIFFERENCE

One analysis of 67 different studies concluded that for every gram of soluble fiber you add to your diet, you can expect a decrease in LDL ("bad") cholesterol of 2.2 mg/dl (0.05 mmol/l).

cramps or even a bowel obstruction, particularly among older or sedentary persons who already have sluggish bowel function.

Fiber pills are not a good alternative to consuming fiber through what you eat. Pills and other types of supplements lack the nutrients and substances found in high-fiber foods, and it is possible that these, too, are instrumental in disease prevention, not just the fiber itself.

Too much bran and other insoluble fibers can prevent the digestive system from absorbing certain minerals properly, particularly calcium, iron, and zinc. This is rarely a problem and is unlikely to occur unless more than 35 g of fiber per day are consumed.

Fiber may be directly anticarcinogenic. Wheat bran, for example, binds nitrite, making it unavailable to form cancer-causing nitrosamines. Fiber also may prevent carcinogens from entering cells. ❖

FIGS

BENEFITS

- A rich source of potassium, calcium, and iron.
- High in fiber.

DRAWBACKS

- Fresh figs spoil quickly.
- Dried figs are high in calories; their high sugar content and stickiness contribute to tooth decay.
- Can cause diarrhea.
- May be contaminated by molds and their toxins.

Figs have provided sugar in the Mediterranean diet for at least 6,000 years. Introduced to North America in about 1600, figs were planted throughout California by Spanish missionaries in the 1700s but were not cultivated commercially until the 20th century.

Not fruit but flower receptacles, figs bud like other fruit blossoms on the bare branches. The true fruits are the seedlike achenes that develop, along with the inconspicuous flowers, inside the fleshy bulb.

Neither bees nor wind contribute to the pollination of figs. Instead, a unique species of wasp, only about ⅛ in. (3 mm) long, pollinates the flowers as it enters and exits through the small pore on the rounded end of the fig. Commercial fig growers depend on this symbiotic relationship and foster it by tying wild figs containing wasp eggs to the branches of their cultivated trees. This method of ensuring fertilization has been used at least since it was recorded in ancient times by a pupil of Aristotle.

Traditionally, figs were ripened by rubbing their skins with oil, which stimulated production of the maturing agent, ethylene. North American fig growers no longer follow this practice, as it detracts from the taste of the fruit.

Because fresh figs typically bruise easily and spoil rapidly, most are dried or canned. Although high in calories—180 in five pieces—dried figs are a highly nutritious snack food, contributing about 15 percent or more of the Recommended Dietary Allowance (RDA) for calcium and iron, as well as 6 g of fiber, more than 590 mg of potassium, and reasonable amounts of vitamin B_6. Consuming figs with a citrus fruit or another source of vitamin C will increase the absorption of their iron.

Fresh California figs are available only for a short time after they are harvested in late summer or early fall. Examine the figs carefully before buying them; the fruit should be soft but not mushy, with no bruises or signs of mold.

Both fresh and dried figs are high in pectin, a soluble fiber that helps lower blood cholesterol. Figs may also have a laxative effect, so they are especially beneficial to people who suffer from chronic constipation; in others, however, overindulging can provoke diarrhea.

Fig bars are more nutritious and lower in fat and sugar than most cookies; two bars contain less than 100 calories. Because their fruity centers tend to stick to teeth—like plain dried figs—it's important to brush after eating. ❖

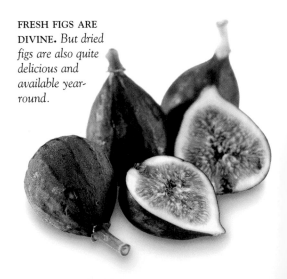

FRESH FIGS ARE DIVINE. *But dried figs are also quite delicious and available year-round.*

FISH

BENEFITS

- An excellent source of complete protein, iron, and other minerals.
- Some are high in vitamin A.
- Contains omega-3 fatty acids.

DRAWBACKS

- Some may harbor PCBs, mercury, and other pollutants.
- Often expensive.

Although a forkful of fish is a gold mine of concentrated nutrients, North Americans consume an average of only 15 lb (6.8 kg) a year, compared to the annual per capita intake of beef and chicken of close to 100 lb (45 kg). While these statistics seem to indicate a clear culinary preference for beef and chicken, there are important health benefits to be gained from eating more fish and less meat.

The average Western diet provides about twice as much protein as necessary; in itself, this might not be a problem except that our typical protein choices of red meat and dairy products come packed with large quantities of saturated fats. In contrast, fish and shellfish are rich in protein with fewer calories, and less fat per serving than most meats. The fats in fish are particularly high in polyunsaturates, which remain liquid even when chilled. (If fish had a lot of saturated fat, it would congeal into a solid mass and prevent them from moving in their cold-water habitat.) And although some shellfish do contain cholesterol, they are low in saturated fats and are no more likely to increase blood cholesterol than skinless poultry.

HEALTH BENEFITS

Eating fish three times a week has been associated with a significant decrease in the rate of heart disease. This became apparent when scientists noted that coronary artery disease—a leading cause of death in North America—was almost nonexistent among the indigenous people of Greenland, Japanese fishermen, and First Nations of the Pacific Northwest. The one factor that these three groups had in common was a diet that relied heavily on fish for protein. When researchers looked at the effects of diets in other populations, they found that men who ate fish regularly two or three times a week were much less likely to suffer heart attacks than men who shunned fish.

In the recent Physicians Health Study, the male participants who ate fish at least once a week were 52 percent less likely to die of a heart attack than men who ate fish once a month or less. It's not yet known whether the effect is due to one factor or many, but evidence so far points to the beneficial action of fish oils. Fish oils are rich in a type of unsaturated fatty acid known as omega-3. These fatty acids decrease the stickiness of blood platelets, making it less likely that they will clump together to form clots. They also increase the flexibility of red blood cells, enabling them to pass more readily through tiny vessels, reduce inflammation of the artery walls, and lower levels of triglycerides in your blood.

A study of more than 43,000 men, published in 2003, showed that men who ate about 3 to 5 oz (85–140 g) of fish one to three times a month were 43 percent less likely to have an ischemic stroke, the most common type of stroke, which is caused by blood clots.

The human body uses omega-3 fatty acids to manufacture prostaglandins, chemicals that play a role in many processes, including inflammation and other functions of the immune system. Several studies have found that a diet that includes fish oil equivalent to the amount in an 8-oz (230-g) daily serving of fish could relieve the painful symptoms of rheumatoid arthritis. Researchers believe that the beneficial effect was due to omega-3 fats, especially eicosapentaenoic acid (EPA). This fatty acid seems to promote the production of forms of prostaglandins and other substances that are less active in inflammation than those derived from saturated and polyunsaturated fats. The anti-inflammatory effects of omega-3 fats are being studied as a possible treatment for Crohn's disease and ulcerative colitis.

Some studies also suggest that people who eat fish regularly (especially varieties rich in omega-3s) are less likely to suffer from a decline in age-related thinking skills such as memory. Other studies link low levels of omega-3s to higher rates of depression.

A study from Australia involving more than 3,500 older adults found that eating fish just one to three times per month appeared to protect participants against age-related macular degeneration, the leading cause of blindness in older adults.

> ### WHERE ARE THE OMEGA-3s?
>
> The best source of omega-3 fats are salmon, mackerel, herring, sardines, anchovies, and trout. You'll also find them in halibut, bluefish, ocean perch, bass, red snapper, and smelts.

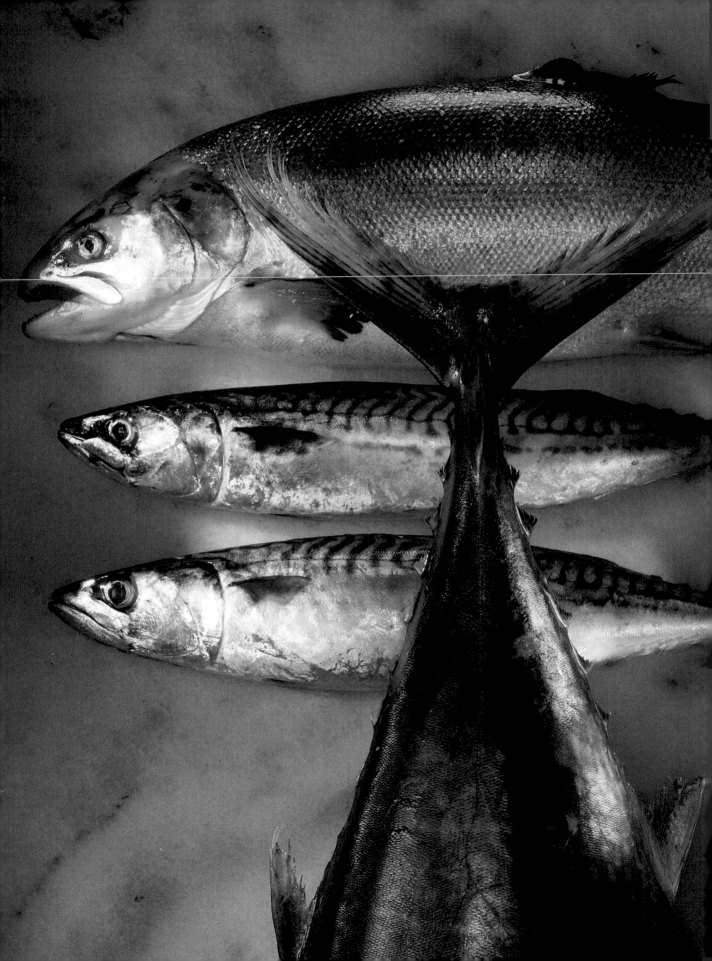

A HEALTHY CATCH. Oily fish, such as tuna (tail up), salmon (top), and mackerel (lower pair), are high in health-giving omega-3 fatty acids.

NUTRITIONAL VALUE

All fish are rich in nutrients, especially protein, niacin, vitamin B_{12}, zinc, magnesium, and more. Oily fish are particularly rich in vitamins A and D. In addition, the bones in canned salmon and sardines are an excellent source of calcium.

Fish are high in protein because they carry a massive bulk of muscle on a much more spindly skeleton than land animals do. Contrary to popular belief, it's not necessarily true that the darker the flesh, the oilier the fish; the dark color is, in fact, due to the presence of myoglobin, a pigment that stores oxygen in the muscles. The flesh of salmon and trout gets its appealing pink color from astaxanthin, a carotenoid pigment derived from the crustaceans and insects the fish feed on. The diet of farmed fish is often fortified with carotenoids to enhance the pink color of the flesh.

There is no difference in nutrient content between fish that are farmed and those caught in the wild. However, some farmed fish, such as salmon and trout, have a texture that is mealier than that of their wild counterparts. There is some concern that farmed fish may contain PCBs since these substances are more likely to be found as contaminants in coastal waters.

HOW MUCH IS ENOUGH?

The mounting evidence about fish-linked cardiovascular benefits led the American Heart Association to include eating two servings of fish a week in its updated dietary recommendations. Some experts suggest up to three servings of fish a week are needed to provide the benefits attributed to omega-3 fatty acids.

Fish oil supplements may be advisable for some people, but check with your doctor first since they can "thin" the blood. Look for a product with a combination of DHA and EPA (two omega-3 fatty acids). Avoid fish liver oil capsules, which are a concentrated source of vitamins A and D. These vitamins can be toxic when taken in large amounts for long periods.

HEALTH RISKS

Some raw fish preparations, particularly sushi (see Sushi), can harbor parasites. Dutch "green" herring and Scandinavian gravlax (pickled salmon) are also raw, but the pickling process used in herring and properly made gravlax eliminates worms and eggs.

Oily fish, like fresh herring and mackerel, must be cooked or processed soon after they are netted. If kept too long before cooking they are susceptible to bacterial growth, which can cause scombroid poisoning, characterized by a rash and stomach upset.

Shellfish from waters polluted by human waste bring a threat of viral hepatitis as well as bacterial infections that can cause severe gastrointestinal upset. Shellfish farms are required to meet strict health standards to ensure that their products are safe, but bacterial contamination still occurs. The old rule of eating raw oysters only in the "R" months does have some validity since bacteria are more likely to survive in warmer waters. Thorough cooking destroys the bacteria that can contaminate oysters.

Coastal waters are, at times, tinged red by a species of algae (*Karenia brevis*) in a phenomenon known as "red tide." Shellfish from red tide areas should not be eaten because they concentrate a toxin produced by the algae. Eating contaminated shellfish brings on symptoms of poisoning within 30 minutes: facial numbness, breathing difficulty, muscle weakness, and sometimes partial paralysis. Ciguatera poisoning is similar, and is caused by a toxin produced by a species of plankton. The plankton are consumed by fish, which then pass the poison on to the humans. In some cases, the effects of this toxin have lasted more than 20 years.

Large, long-lived fish, such as tuna, shark, king mackerel, and swordfish, may accumulate heavy-metal contaminants—especially mercury—which are toxic to the human nervous system and can be dangerous for unborn babies. Because of this potential hazard, women should either avoid these fish completely during pregnancy or eat them no more than once a month. In terms of canned tuna, albacore tends to be higher in mercury than light tuna. Some consumer groups recommend that pregnant women eat no more than 6 oz (170 g) of light tuna every 4 days—10 days for albacore.

Some species of fish caught in certain areas may show high levels of PCBs and other industrial pollutants; they are best avoided. Pregnant women are advised not to eat striped bass, especially from the northeastern regions, which may accumulate oil residues. Check with your local

DID YOU KNOW?

FARMED SALMON CONTAINS HIGH LEVELS OF POLLUTANTS

One major study suggests that eating farm-raised salmon more than once per month, depending upon its country of origin, could slightly increase your risk of cancer. Farm-raised salmon contain significantly more dioxins, PCBs, and other pollutants than do salmon caught in the wild. Researchers blamed the feed used on fish farms for concentrating ocean pollutants. Wild salmon were given a clean bill of health—they have much lower levels of pollutants.

FISH FACTS AND FOOD VALUES

NUTRIENTS PER 3 OZ (85 G)	DID YOU KNOW?

WHITE FISH, SUCH AS COD, HADDOCK, SOLE, AND FLOUNDER

Calories: 100–160 Protein: 17–23 g Fat: 0.8–1.3 g Iron: 0.3–1.1 mg	These fish are rich in vitamin B_{12}, and they contain a low to fair level of omega-3 fatty acids.

OILY FISH, SUCH AS HERRING, MACKEREL, SALMON, AND TROUT

Calories: 180–215 Protein: 18–21 g Fat: 5.6 g (salmon) to 14.3 g (herring) Iron: 0.8–1.0 mg	Oily fish are an excellent source of omega-3 fatty acids and vitamin B_{12}. Some of these fish also contain small amounts of calcium.

CANNED FISH, SUCH AS ANCHOVIES, SARDINES, AND TUNA

Calories: 100–210, depending on whether the fish is canned in oil or water.
Protein: 17.7–23 g
Fat: 2.1 g (tuna in water) to
    8.4 g (sardines in oil)
Iron: 0.5 mg (tuna in water)
    to 3.6 mg (anchovies)
	Canned tuna contains only small amounts of omega-3 fatty acids. Canned salmon and sardines, eaten with the bones, are good sources of calcium. Anchovies are high in sodium and purines; they should be avoided by those with gout or high blood pressure. Similarly, sardines contain purines and should not be consumed by people with gout.

SMOKED FISH, SUCH AS SALMON, MACKEREL, AND KIPPERS (HERRING)

Calories: 100–180 Protein: 18.6 g Fat: 7.8–15.1 g Iron: 1.2 mg	Smoked fish, while tasty, tend to be packed with sodium; thus, they should either be consumed occasionally in very small amounts or avoided entirely by people with high blood pressure.

FROZEN FISH STICKS

Calories: 150–215 Protein: 8.6–13.3 g Fat: 7.6–12.8 g Iron: 0.3 mg	Fish sticks are an extremely popular frozen food product, especially with children, who might not otherwise be willing to try fish. However, as they are dipped in batter, or fried, and then served with tartar sauce, they tend to be high in fat. To lower the fat content, try baking them in an oven rather than frying in oil, and flavoring them with lemon instead of a high-fat sauce.

CAVIAR, BLACK AND RED, GRANULAR

Calories: 215–225 Protein: 21–23 g Fat: 12.8–15.6 g	Beluga caviar is the highest quality caviar, and also the most expensive; the sturgeon that produce these eggs can weigh as much as 3,500 lb (1,588 kg) and can be up to 100 years old. Caviar is highly perishable and should be bought fresh, stored in a refrigerator, and served in a tub of ice. It is very high in sodium and calories; a mere teaspoonful contains 40 calories. This delicacy should be avoided by those trying to watch their weight or anyone with high blood pressure.

FUGU: DINING WITH DEATH

The Japanese specialty fugu—puffer fish, or blowfish—can turn a dinner into a fatal game of Russian roulette. The ovaries, roe, and liver of the puffer fish contain a deadly toxin. A slip of the knife during preparation can allow this poison to contaminate the flesh. This toxin, tetrodotoxin, is so powerful that consuming just a drop quickly brings on paralysis, followed by death. Fugu is never served in Japanese homes, and restaurant chefs must endure long apprenticeships before they are entrusted with preparation of the dish. Despite these precautions, fugu is the major cause of fatal food poisoning in Japan, causing dozens of deaths every year, according to official statistics.

---

health department before eating fish caught in local streams and lakes. They may contain pollutants that are harmful.

Caution: Flake fish before serving to children to prevent bones from getting stuck in the throat.

BUYING FISH

Both the United States and Canada have developed state-of-the-art regulations to ensure that the processing of fish is safe and sanitary and that companies can easily detect potential problems and move quickly to react, prior to the food's coming to market. But when it comes to choosing your fish, the following guidelines should be observed:

• When buying fresh fish, look for bright, glossy skin; clear, bulging eyes; tight scales; and firm flesh. There should be only a clean, briny aroma—no whiff of iodine, ammonia, or strong "fishiness" should be present. Buy fish only at markets that keep them covered (both top and bottom) with ice.

• Buy canned tuna that is packed in water; oil-packed tuna is higher in calories.

COST AND PREPARATION

Although fresh fish can be expensive, it is economical to use. If you buy a whole fish, use the head and bones to make stock for low-fat soup. Combine fish with carbohydrates to stretch a small amount: a single poached salmon steak can be flaked into spinach noodles, or fillets of cod can be mixed with herbed mashed potatoes for a family meal of fish cakes. Fish needs little preparation, and cooks quickly. Steaming, poaching, baking, and grilling all preserve flavor without adding calories. Avoid dishes that demand lavish amounts of buttery sauces that spoil the low-fat value of the fish. ❖

FLATULENCE

CONSUME PLENTY OF
- Yogurt made with live cultures.
- Peppermint and fennel teas.

LIMIT
- Fatty foods.
- Dried beans and other legumes, onions, broccoli and other members of the cabbage family, and any other foods that exacerbate the problem.
- Fruits and fruit-based sweeteners, such as sorbitol and fructose.

AVOID
- Milk if you are lactose intolerant.
- Carbonated drinks, chewing gum, and drinking straws, which all encourage swallowing air.
- Bran and high-fiber laxatives.

Excessive gas, or flatulence, causes uncomfortable abdominal bloating, which can be relieved only by bringing the gas up from the stomach (burping) or expelling it through the anus. Although it is embarrassing, this experience is the completely natural result of intestinal bacteria acting on undigested carbohydrates and proteins. The average person has more than 13 episodes a day, most of which pass unnoticed. It's only when certain malodorous gases are released that the problem becomes unpleasant.

Flatulence seems to worsen with age, and some individuals are simply more susceptible to gas than others. Eating smaller portions, chewing food thoroughly, and not gulping liquids should minimize episodes. Some experts also believe that reducing the amount of air in the digestive tract may help to prevent flatulence, so they advise against drinking carbonated beverages, chewing gum, or drinking through a straw, which promotes swallowing air.

Some foods are especially notorious gas producers; topping the list are those that produce methane gas when fermented by intestinal bacteria. Soybeans, kidney beans, lentils, and dried peas can result in unpleasant-smelling flatus.

Soak dried beans first. Except for lentils and split peas, which do not need to be presoaked, soaking dried beans for at least 4 hours (preferably 8 or more hours) before cooking them in plenty of water helps to reduce the indigestible sugars, raffinose and stachyose, that cause gas.

Avoid vegetables from the cabbage family. Many people also experience flatulence after eating onions and brussels sprouts, broccoli, cauliflower, and other members of the cabbage plant family; you may be able to reduce gas production by adding such spices as anise, ginger, rosemary, bay leaf, and fennel seeds during cooking. Some cooks add kombu seaweed, available in Asian markets and natural food stores, to cooking water for the same purpose.

Increase fiber intake very gradually. Passing gas can be an uncomfortable side effect of a well-intentioned move toward a healthier, high-fiber diet. Nutritionists suggest increasing fiber intake gradually, and they recommend avoiding bran and high-fiber laxatives. In addition, sorbitol, fructose, and other sweeteners can cause flatulence in some people, as can high doses of vitamin C.

Other approaches. Beano, a product made from natural enzymes, is available in pharmacies as drops or tablets. It helps reduce flatus when a few drops are sprinkled on gas-producing food or a tablet is taken before a meal. A cup of peppermint or fennel tea after a meal sometimes helps improve digestion and reduce flatulence. Some people find that eating yogurt made with live cultures cuts down on gas production. Yoga, particularly the knee-to-chest pose, is also said to alleviate the condition.

Sometimes flatulence is due to a medical disorder; if the problem is severe and persists, it could be a symptom of food allergies, Crohn's disease, intolerance to milk, or irritable bowel syndrome (IBS). ❖

FLAX

BENEFITS
- A good source of fiber and alpha-linolenic acid.
- Contains lignans.

DRAWBACKS
- Pregnant and breast-feeding women should not eat large quantities of flax.
- People who are on tamoxifen should speak to their physician and/or exercise caution before adding flax to their diet.

Flaxseed, traditionally known as linseed, is a tiny seed packed with a variety of components that can play an important role in your diet.

Flax is a great source of soluble fiber. It can help lower cholesterol levels and consequently

CAUTION

Flax may not be for everyone.

• **If you are taking tamoxifen or a similar drug:** Lignans, contained in flax, have anti-estrogen properties similar to these drugs. Since there is no published research regarding their interaction with flax, people who are on this therapy should speak to their physician and/or exercise caution before adding flax to their diet.

• **If you are pregnant or breast-feeding:** You should not eat large quantities of flax, since the effects on a fetus or nursing infants are unknown.

lower heart disease risk. Studies at the University of Toronto showed that 25 to 50 g of flax per day helped lower blood cholesterol significantly. The insoluble fiber in flax is also helpful in preventing constipation.

Flax is a rich source of alpha linolenic acid (ALA). ALA is an essential fatty acid, also considered a "heart healthy" fat. Because your body cannot manufacture this fatty acid, you must consume it as foods. Omega-3 fatty acids help reduce the thickness of blood so the heart doesn't have to work as hard to push the blood through the blood vessels. They also lessen the stickiness of blood platelets, reducing their tendency to clump together to form clots.

Flax may protect against some cancers. Flax contains lignans, which convert in the body to compounds that are similar to the body's own estrogen but have much weaker activity. They can occupy estrogen receptors in cells and block the effects of more powerful estrogens. That is why numerous studies are currently looking at the role flax may play in lowering the risk of hormone-linked cancers such as of the breast or colon. Animal studies have already shown that flax can reduce tumor size and can even influence the incidence of tumor development. Human studies are limited, but one study showed that the tumor growth in breast-cancer patients was reduced when they were given daily muffins containing 25 g of ground flax. Patients on tamoxifen should not consume large amounts of flax.

Flax contains no gluten, is very inexpensive, and has a pleasant nutty flavor. There is no recommended daily amount, but many studies use one to two tablespoons of ground flaxseed daily.

You can eat whole flaxseeds but they tend to come out the way they went in. Ground seeds are preferable for nutrient absorption. You can grind your own in a blender or food processor, or you can buy it already ground. Once ground, store what you don't use in an airtight, opaque container in the fridge or freezer.

Flaxseed oil provides omega-3 fatty acids but not the fiber and the lignans of the seeds. Flax oil should be kept in the fridge and has limited shelf life; check best-before date. It breaks down with heat so is not a good choice for cooking.

To use flaxseed:

• Add it to cereal, muffin batters, breads, pancake mixes, and cookie mixes;
• Stir ground flaxseed into yogurt or smoothies, juice or applesauce;
• Sprinkle on salads for a nutty flavor;
• Add to casseroles, meatballs, or meat loaf;
• Make a pesto sauce with fresh basil, garlic, ground flaxseeds, flaxseed oil, and grated Parmesan cheese;
• Use flaxseed oil in salad dressings or drizzle over steamed vegetables just before serving. ❖

FLOUR

BENEFITS
• A concentrated source of starch.
• Enriched flours are a good source of iron and B vitamins.

DRAWBACKS
• Substantial vitamins, minerals, and fiber are lost during milling.

People have been grinding various seeds, as well as dried fish and other foods, to make flour for thousands of years. Initially, the seeds were roasted and ground between two stones to make them easier to eat; eventually, water was added to the flour, and the paste baked into a type of crude bread. As agricultural societies developed, they devised increasingly sophisticated methods of grinding and sifting grains and seeds. Today, huge, fully automated mills are responsible for producing tons of flour, which are then transformed into breads, pasta, pastries and other baked goods, and thickening agents and other food additives.

NUTRITIONAL VALUE
In general, flour is a more concentrated source of calories than its source material because the moisture has been removed. For example, 1 lb (450 g) of potato flour contains 1,600 calories, compared with 350 in a pound of raw potatoes; one cup of cornmeal has about 400 calories,

while a cup of cooked corn only has 100. This increased density of calories is the reason food relief organizations often prefer to provide flour made from grains, legumes, tubers, or dried fish rather than the raw products.

On the other hand, many nutrients are lost in flour milling and processing. Wheat flour, our most common variety, is milled by using steel rollers to crack the grain. The bran and germ are then sifted out and the remaining part of the seed (the endosperm) is passed through a series of rollers and sifters to make a fine, powdery product. Removing the bran and germ from wheat reduces the fiber and the amounts of the 22 vitamins and minerals found in the whole grain. Because of this depletion, wheat flour is usually enriched with iron, riboflavin, thiamine, niacin, and folic acid (important nutrients that might not be provided otherwise). Manufacturers may also add vitamin B_6, calcium, and magnesium; the label specifies whether or not the flour is enriched and what nutrients have been restored or added.

Whole-grain flour, which is made by restoring the germ and bran at the end of the process, provides more fiber, protein, vitamin E, and trace minerals than enriched white varieties do. Depending upon the type of flour, other ingredients are added; these include salt and baking soda or baking powder to make self-rising flour, extra gluten for special baked products, or bleaching agents such as benzoyl peroxide for whiteness.

TYPES OF FLOURS

Almost any type of grain or seed can be ground into flour, although those with a high fat or moisture content must first be defatted and roasted or dehydrated. Because most grains lack gluten, the protein that makes flour ideal for baking, they are usually mixed with varying amounts of wheat flour, which is high in gluten. Some of the more common flours include the following:

Amaranth is higher in protein, including the amino acid lysine, than most other flours.

Arrowroot, made from maranta roots, is one of the most digestible flours.

Barley, a soft, bland flour, is used for unleavened baked goods.

Buckwheat, made from the same seeds as kasha, is high in lysine.

Cornmeal is not as nutritious as many other types of flour, but it provides a complete protein when combined with beans and other legumes.

Cottonseed flour is made from hulled seeds

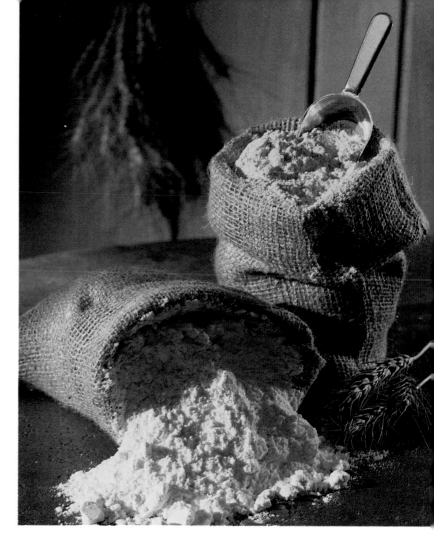

after oil is extracted and contains very high levels of protein.

Fish flour is produced from whole dried defatted fish; it contains very high levels of calcium and protein.

Oat, which is high in soluble fiber, is used mostly in cereals and breads.

Potato, made from steamed and dried potatoes, is used in baking and is also a common thickening agent.

Rice is manufactured mostly from broken polished grains; typically, this flour is used to make noodles, cookies, and unleavened baked goods.

Rye is high in fiber as long as the bran and germ have been retained. It is usually combined with wheat flour to form a mixture used in bread-baking.

Soy, made from soybeans, is often combined with wheat flour to increase the protein content of baked goods.

Triticale is a hybrid of wheat and rye and is also very high in protein; triticale is often mixed with wheat flour to increase its nutritional content. ❖

FLAVORFUL FLOURS. *By combining whole-grain and refined flours, bakers can produce a tastier, more nutritious product that still has a fine texture.*

FOOD AND FITNESS
■ TO BOOST ENDURANCE ■

Regular physical activity does wonders for your health, your shape, and your mood. No matter what your age, health, and level of fitness, there's a form of exercise to suit you.

Exercise burns calories; it also keeps bones healthy, improves cardiovascular performance, enhances digestion, tones the muscles and the skin, and increases your chance of getting a restful night's sleep. In addition to its physical benefits, exercise activates the brain to release endorphins, morphinelike natural painkillers that soothe pain and create a sense of emotional well-being. Endorphins are responsible for the "runner's high" that many athletes experience. They help to explain why exercise has a positive impact on your state of mind and ability to manage stress.

Exercise is energizing

The paradox of exercise is that by expending energy you can increase energy. By improving the heart's performance and ability to pump blood, aerobic exercise makes your body more energy-efficient, and you consume less oxygen when going about normal daily activities. In effect, it is like tuning up a car's engine and getting better gas mileage. If you are unused to regular exercise, however, you may feel a bit stiff or sore and fatigued at first. Start slowly, perhaps adding only 10 minutes of activity three times a week, and gradually build up the intensity and duration of your workout. After a few weeks of following a regular exercise regimen, most people report a surge of energy.

Exercise burns fat

In this sedentary society you need to schedule regular exercise to keep your body trim and improve your health. If you eat more food than your body uses up in energy, the surplus calories are stored as fat. The only way to lose weight and keep it off is to combine a healthy low-calorie diet with regular aerobic exercise, such as brisk walking, jogging, cycling, swimming, or aerobic dancing. By speeding up breathing and raising your heart rate, aerobic exercise helps to burn body fat. Undertaking an exercise program, however, doesn't give you a license to eat all the French fries, fudge, and brownies you can lay your hands on. On the contrary, a balanced diet is essential to provide the energy you need to sustain a regular exercise program.

Move it to lose it

When you exercise aerobically, your body first burns the glucose circulating; it then turns to the glycogen stored in the muscles and the liver, as well as some fatty acids. Thus, an exercise session longer than about 20 minutes burns more fat and helps to shed weight and keep it off. Endurance training increases the amount of fatty acids being burned. Therefore, the best way to promote fat burning is steady,

WHAT DOES A HIGH-CARBOHYDRATE DIET LOOK LIKE?

A 132-lb (60-kg) athlete training 2 to 4 hours daily would need
about 360 to 600 g of carbohydrate per day. Use these
numbers to total your carbohydrates for the day:

FOOD	GRAMS OF CARBOHYDRATE	FOOD	GRAMS OF CARBOHYDRATE
3 pancakes	50	1 cup apple juice	30
1 large potato	50	1 banana	27
1 cup cooked rice	45	3 tbsp. raisins	25
1 medium bagel	42	1 apple	21
1 cup yogurt (low fat)	42	1 cup cereal	20
1 cup cooked pasta	40	2 rice cakes	16
1 pita bread	33	1 tbsp. jam	14
2 slices of bread	30	1 cup milk	12

sustained effort, in which you exercise for long periods—at least 25 to 30 minutes at a time—at 30 to 40 percent of your maximum capability.

Fuel for sport

The food you eat fuels your performance, at the gym, on the playing fields, or even at home and work. The right combination of food and exercise will give you the added edge. Here are some fit tips:

1. **Carbohydrates are the body's preferred source of fuel for physical activity and are an integral part of an athlete's training program.** Breads, grains, cereals, pasta, fruits, and vegetables provide high-octane fuel for muscles and speed up restocking of muscle fuel after exercise. If you aren't eating enough carbohydrates, you will tire more quickly. The exact amount of carbohydrate required depends on an individual's training and personal requirements. Daily carbohydrate requirements for athletes training heavily can range from 2.7 to 4.5 g per pound (6–10 g per kilogram) of body weight. For example, a 132-lb (60-kg) athlete training 2 to 4 hours daily would need about 360 to 600 g of carbohydrate per day.

2. **Fluids are critical to high performance.** During high activity, fluid losses increase the risk of cramps, heat exhaustion, or heat stroke. Drink before, during, and after an event as part of your exercise routine. Get into the habit of drinking lots of fluids even on days when you aren't working out. Water, sports drinks, fruit and vegetable juices, or mineral water are good choices. Cold water or sports drinks are recommended for workouts, training sessions, and competitions. Alcohol and caffeine are dehydrating and don't count as part of your hydrating fluid intake. Drink 14 to 20 oz (400–600 ml) 2 hours before a workout and 5 to 12 oz (150–350 ml) every 15 to 20 minutes during exercise.

3. **Time your meals.** If you're running a race or competing in an event, have a low-fat, high-carbohydrate meal 2 to 3 hours beforehand. Eat foods you are familiar with and that you digest easily. Fruit, yogurt, bagels, a smoothie or a bowl of cereal are good choices. If you have food in your stomach when you are working out, blood is diverted

Sports drinks

Sports drinks hydrate and nourish your body during exercise and replenish lost fluids after exercise. Besides water they contain carbohydrate and electrolytes like sodium and potassium. The added carbohydrate fuels your muscles, and the sodium and potassium replace losses from sweat. The sodium also helps your body absorb and retain water and triggers your thirst mechanism to make you drink more. During exercise that is intense or lasts longer than 45 to 50 minutes, these drinks containing 6 to 8 percent carbohydrate are easily absorbed into your body and can provide energy to your working muscles that plain water cannot. Sports drinks are usually more helpful for longer periods of exercise but many people prefer them to water because they have more flavor. Some research has shown that sports drinks help you recover your fluid losses after exercise more quickly than water.

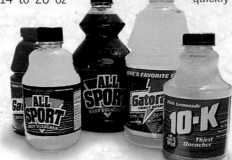

away from your digestive tract to your working muscle leading to cramps and a heavy feeling. If you exercise first thing in the morning, you have enough reserved energy from the day before to sustain 60 to 90 minutes of exercise. If you find it difficult to eat breakfast before an early morning workout, have a carbohydrate-rich snack before bed the night before. If you exercise later in the day and it has been longer than 4 hours since your last meal, have a snack 45 to 60 minutes before you begin. Your food choices and preferences may vary depending on the time of day you are exercising, the sport you are doing, and the level of intensity of your workout. You'll quickly learn which food combinations work best for you.

4. Try carbo loading before endurance events. Carbohydrate loading is appropriate for athletes entering marathons, triathlons, or long-distance bike races. For events that last less than 90 minutes nonstop, a regular high-carbohydrate diet is sufficient. Loading involves reducing training somewhat 3 to 4 days before a race and increasing carbohydrates to 70 to 80 percent of total calories during this time.

5. Replenish carbohydrate after exercise. After exercise, it is important to replenish the glycogen in muscles. Eat a carbohydrate-rich meal/snack within 30 minutes after a workout. This is when your muscles are most receptive to incoming carbohydrates. Eating carbohydrate-rich foods within the first 1 to 4 hours after a hard workout is especially important if you are doing two or more events in a day. Foods like bagels, fruit, and cereal are also easy to eat. Juices and sports drinks are good sources of carbohydrate immediately after exercise if you don't have an appetite for solid foods. They will also help you to rehydrate.

6. Replace the sodium and potassium lost during exercise with food. Eat potassium-rich fruits and vegetables including bananas, oranges, cantaloupe, and tomatoes. Replace the sodium lost through sweat by lightly salting your food after exercise.

7. Physical activity may increase your need for some vitamins and minerals. However, if you are eating sufficient calories to meet the demands of your activity and the calories are coming from nutritional foods, you probably don't need any supplements. Supplements won't give you added energy unless you are deficient to begin with.

8. No need for more protein. Protein is important to help build and repair body tissues and muscle. Many athletes believe that because muscles are made of protein, eating large servings of protein foods will help build larger muscles. This is not true. Training, not protein supplements, is the best stimulus for muscle growth. Athletes do have an increased protein requirement, but this can be met by a well-planned and well-balanced diet. The best way to build muscle is to eat enough food to replace the energy used during the day. The daily protein recommendation for endurance athletes is 0.54 to 0.64 g per pound (1.2 to 1.4 g per kilogram) of body weight, whereas for resistance and strength trained athletes it can be as high as 0.73 to 0.77 g per pound (1.6 to 1.7 g per kilogram) of body weight per day.

Meeting Your Protein Needs

An endurance athlete needs 0.54 to 0.64 g of protein per pound (1.2–1.4 g per kilogram) of body weight per day. So, a 154-lb (70-kg) athlete would need 84 to 98 g of protein per day. Here are the approximate protein values of some foods. You can see how easily you could meet your needs through a varied diet.

FOOD	GRAMS OF PROTEIN
3 oz (85 g) canned tuna	22
3 oz (85 g) cooked meat, fish, or chicken	21
1 veggie burger, about 3 oz (85 g)	17
1 cup cooked lentils	16
3 oz (85 g) firm tofu	13
2 oz (60 g) almonds	12
1 cup milk	8
1 cup yogurt	8
1 oz (30 g) cheddar cheese	7
1 egg	6
¾ cup oatmeal	4
1 slice bread	3
½ cup vegetables	2

When eating to train, consume plenty of:

■ Starchy foods, such as pasta, legumes, brown rice, potatoes, and whole-grain breads, for complex carbohydrates to provide a steady source of energy.
■ Fluids, before, during, and after exercise.
■ Fruits and vegetables for vitamins and minerals, especially potassium.
■ Vegetables and legumes for vitamins and minerals.
■ Lean meat, fish and poultry, low-fat milk and dairy products, and other high-protein foods to maintain muscles.

Creating a sport program

✔ Don't try to cram exercise into a crowded schedule. Instead, substitute it for a less important activity, such as watching television. Increase exercise by walking at least part of the way to and from work, or try working out at lunchtime.

✔ Pick an exercise you enjoy. Try cross-training to ward off boredom. Take a brisk walk one day, go to the gym and lift weights the next. Enroll in a yoga class for stretching and flexibility, or go swimming, and so on.

✔ Whatever your exercise plan, begin slowly and build gradually. Anyone over 40, over-weight, or with high blood pressure, heart, bone or joint disease, diabetes, or who is a smoker, should see a doctor first.

✔ If you prefer to exercise alone, go to a gym and try various equipment. Then consider buying an exercise machine to use at home.

FOOD POISONING

CONSUME PLENTY OF

- Diluted sweetened drinks to replace lost body fluids and provide energy.
- Bananas, rice, cooked apples, and dry toast (the BRAT diet) for 24 to 48 hours after symptoms have subsided.

AVOID

- Overhandling any food.
- Having raw and cooked foods touch, such as on food preparation surfaces.
- Raw or undercooked eggs, such as in mayonnaise, sauces, mousses, cold desserts, or unbaked cake batters.
- Old leftovers or foods that are past their expiration date.

Next to the common cold, food poisoning is our most prevalent infection, afflicting perhaps as many as 90 million North Americans.

In all, more than 250 diseases can be spread through contaminated food. The term "food poisoning" is now generally applied to illness (most often gastroenteritis, but occasionally nervous system complications) resulting from bacterial or viral contamination of food. Bacteria, including those that can cause foodborne illness are found naturally all around you. They are invisible, so you cannot rely on sight or taste to detect them. Bacteria can cause disease either through their rapid multiplication inside the body (bacterial infection) or through toxins that they may produce (bacterial intoxication). While heat destroys bacteria in food, some toxins, such as those produced by staphylococcal organisms, are heat stable. Infestation with parasites from raw or undercooked meat and fish can also cause food poisoning. Thanks to strict regulations controlling food processing, and the use of additives, illness due to deliberate adulteration of foods is a thing of the past.

There are many opportunities for contamination to occur along the trail of harvesting, processing, packing, transporting, and displaying food for sale. Most cases of food poisoning are caused by bacterial contamination, usually traceable to faulty handling and preparation in the home, or in restaurants, or food-service outlets. The microorganisms that are most often responsible are *Clostridium botulinum, Clostridium perfringens, Escherichia coli, Listeria monocytogenes, Salmonella* strains, and *Staphylococcus aureus.*

TYPICAL SYMPTOMS

Food poisoning usually causes nausea and vomiting, diarrhea and cramps, headache, and sometimes fever and prostration. The infection can be serious in vulnerable people, especially in infants and young children, people with chronic illness (including AIDS and other immune system disorders), and the frail elderly. Call the doctor if someone you know in these groups has symptoms of food poisoning. Otherwise, most cases clear up without medical help.

Botulism is a rare but grave form of food poisoning caused by a nerve toxin from *C. botulinum.* Symptoms of nerve and muscle impairment are double vision and difficulty in speaking, chewing, swallowing, and breathing; any of these call for immediate medical attention.

The body rids itself of the organisms that cause food poisoning through vomiting and diarrhea. Unpleasant though they may be, it's best to let nature run its course. Don't tax your digestive system with food until it's able to handle it. Prevent fluid depletion by sipping a mixture of apple juice and water or weak tea.

When you're confident that your system has settled down, reintroduce foods on the BRAT diet (see Diarrhea). Then try other bland foods, such as soft-cooked chicken and mashed potatoes. Avoid fresh fruits for a few days.

SIMPLE PRECAUTIONS

Foods of animal origin are the most susceptible to contamination. The muscles of healthy animals are free of bacteria, but they provide a rich culture medium for the growth of bacteria picked up in handling and processing. The skin prevents bacteria from penetrating the flesh of a living animal, but microorganisms can be transferred from the skin to the muscle when the carcass is cut up. Meats that are dressed with skin, such as poultry, are the most prone to spoilage, because bacteria remain on the skin despite thorough washing after slaughter.

Be careful when handling meat, fish, shellfish, and especially poultry. Wash hands thoroughly with hot water and soap before starting any food preparation, and repeat as necessary throughout the process. Also, remove rings, and make sure fingernails are clean both before and after food preparation.

Use hot, soapy water to thoroughly wash food preparation surfaces, such as chopping boards and countertops. Never allow cooked food to touch an unwashed surface where traces of raw food remain. Wash plates and utensils used for raw meat or poultry before using them for cooked meat or other food. Wash and sanitize your meat thermometer after each use.

Always keep raw foods away from other foods, and separate starchy foods and dairy products to prevent cross-contamination. Ensure raw foods don't contaminate cooked foods, either directly by contact or indirectly (for example, by letting meat juices touch other foods). Place raw foods in sealed containers.

Wash your dishcloth or sponge with hot water and soap after every use. This will avoid the possibility of cross-contamination and the spread of bacteria.

Keep food refrigerated. If you don't intend to eat food immediately after preparing it, refrigerate or freeze it. Never leave food for longer than 2 hours at temperatures between 45°F (7°C) and 140°F (60°C), which are ideal for bacterial growth. Always cook hamburger to an internal temperature of 160°F (70°C).

Discard food that smells bad or is discolored. Don't use food from damaged cans or containers. Never taste foods that look "off"; don't even sniff them. Most important, never buy or use a can if the ends are bulging. This is most likely caused by the pressure of gases produced by bacterial metabolism.

You cannot see or smell most bacteria that might make you sick. Tasting is risky and will not tell you if a food is unsafe. For some bacteria, such as certain varieties of *E. coli*, even a tiny taste may make you sick. That is why the best advice is: When in doubt, throw it out!

GOOD VERSUS BAD GERMS

It may seem puzzling that the bacteria and yeasts used in fermentation produce healthful foods, while some of their relatives cause various forms of sickness. The reason is that the beneficial bacteria (for example, *Lactobacillus acidophilus* and *L. bifidus* in some yogurts) inhibit the growth of unwanted organisms, crowding out potentially harmful members of the Clostridium, Bacillus, and Streptococcus families. Clearly, not all bacteria are alike; some are dangerous, while some are helpful. ❖

WHAT'S YOUR POISON?

If you have symptoms of food poisoning, try to figure out when you ate a suspect meal, as this can help determine which bacteria is responsible. If a fever develops or the symptoms persist for more than a couple of days, consult your doctor.

MICROORGANISMS	SYMPTOMS
CAMPYLOBACTER JEJUNI	
Infection usually stems from contact with infected animals or contaminated food (in many cases, from raw or undercooked poultry).	Fever, nausea, abdominal pain, and diarrhea, which may be bloody. Symptoms typically come and go; there may also be an enlarged liver and spleen.
CLOSTRIDIUM BOTULINUM (BOTULISM)	
Home-canned foods, improperly packed and sterilized canned products, and contaminated vegetables, fruits, fish, and condiments. More rarely it is found in beef, pork, poultry, milk products, unpasteurized honey, and garlic bottled in oil.	Within 18 to 36 hours, double vision and difficulty with muscular coordination, including chewing, swallowing, breathing, and speech. Progressive muscle weakness and paralysis can lead to respiratory failure and death.
CLOSTRIDIUM PERFRINGENS	
Outbreaks have often been associated with contaminated meat.	Severe diarrhea, abdominal pain, bloating, and flatulence appear in 8 to 24 hours.
ESCHERICHIA COLI (E. COLI)	
Undercooked beef or unpasteurized milk. Most cases have been traced to contaminated ground beef, but a few cases have been linked to rare roast beef.	Bloody diarrhea and vomiting. In severe cases, seizure, paralysis, and even death. Symptoms appear within 24 to 48 hours. patients may require hospitalization.
LISTERIA MONOCYTOGENES	
Organism found in the soil and intestinal tracts of humans, animals, birds, and insects. Infection usually follows eating contaminated dairy products and raw vegetables.	Adults may develop meningitis, with headache, stiff neck, nausea, and vomiting. Eye inflammation and swollen lymph nodes sometimes develop; in unusual cases, the heart is involved. Symptoms usually appear in 8 to 24 hours.
SALMONELLA	
Infected meat-producing animals, undercooked poultry, and raw milk, eggs, and egg products.	Within 12 to 48 hours, nausea, abdominal pain, diarrhea, vomiting, and fever; symptoms typically last 1 to 4 days.
STAPHYLOCOCCUS AUREUS	
Commonly spread by food handlers with skin infections who transmit the organism to such foods as custards, cream-filled pastries, milk, processed meat, and fish; poison is caused by a toxin rather than the bacterium.	Within 2 to 8 hours, severe nausea and vomiting. There may be also diarrhea, abdominal cramps, headache, and fever. Shock, prostration, and electrolyte imbalance may occur in extreme cases.
TRICHINELLA	
Raw or undercooked pork that has been fed contaminated meat; bear meat.	Within 24 to 48 hours, fever and diarrhea, with pain and respiratory problems.

FOOD SAFETY
■ STORAGE AND PREPARATION ■

The techniques used to clean, store, and prepare food not only affect its taste, texture, and nutritional value, but are also instrumental in preventing spoilage and food-borne illness.

By using the proper methods to prepare and store foods, you can keep them wholesome and nutritious; preserve their appetizing appearance, taste, and texture; and use them economically. Exposure to heat, light, moisture, and air can cause some foods to spoil or deteriorate, and many lose flavor, texture, and nutritional value if kept too long. Improper handling and storage also raise the possibility of food poisoning.

Use the two-hour rule in your home and while shopping. Refrigerate or freeze all perishables within two hours of purchase or preparation. If the weather is hot, reduce that time to one hour and use a cooler for perishables. The highest risk foods are meat, fish, shellfish, poultry, eggs, dairy products, mayonnaise mixtures and moist foods such as poultry stuffing. It is especially important that these foods be handled carefully and most importantly, kept at the right temperatures—hot foods hot, cold foods cold.

Food storage

Heat and humidity greatly increase the risk of food spoilage, so you should never store foods in warm places, such as near the stove or refrigerator. To minimize the risk of contamination and accidental poisoning, always keep food and cleaning products in separate areas.

Because even canned foods deteriorate with time, you should stack cans in the order of their date of purchase so that the oldest can is used first. Practice "first in, first out" for all food products. Store them away from moisture in a 50°F to 70°F (10°C to 21°C) temperature range. Dry goods should be kept in a cool, dry pantry and used before the expiration date.

Always read labels carefully. They often contain important storage information and recommended "use by" dates. When in doubt about shelf life, call the company (many have toll-free numbers). Remember, when in doubt about any food, toss it out!

Grains and nuts

Grains, flours, and other foods packed in materials easily penetrated by insects—for example, cardboard boxes, paper bags, and cellophane packages—should be transferred to plastic, metal, or glass containers with

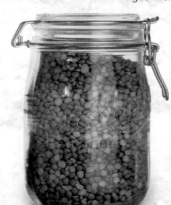

tight-fitting lids. (Even then, insect eggs in the flour or grains may hatch. To kill the eggs before storage, put the product in a microwave oven set on High for 2 to 3 minutes.) Under normal storage conditions, the shelf life of white flour is about one year from the time it is milled. Flour can be frozen for long-term storage if carefully wrapped in moisture- and vapor-proof material.

Whole-grain flours spoil within a few weeks because their fats turn rancid. Storing them in a freezer extends their life.

Cake mixes last about one year at room temperature, after which time the quality starts to decline.

Bread, cereals, and crackers are normally best kept in closed containers at room temperature. Cereals, like other foods made

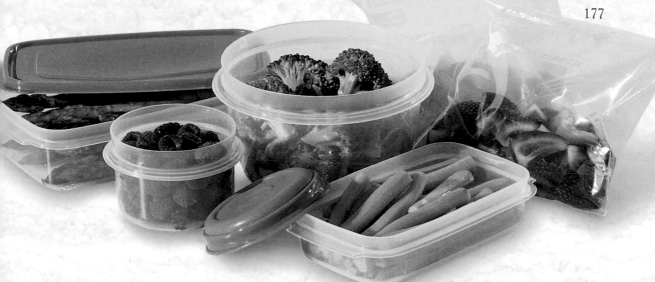

from grains, should be stored in a dark place because they will lose riboflavin if left exposed to light.

Yeast breads will keep for a few days if wrapped in plastic or foil and stored in a cool, dark place, such as a bread box. In hot weather, refrigeration may be required to prevent mold.

Unshelled nuts can be kept at room temperature for 3 to 6 months; shelled nuts may become rancid unless refrigerated or frozen. Discard any that smell musty or are moldy.

Baking powder generally lasts 12 to 18 months or expiration date on container. To test for freshness, mix 1 teaspoon baking powder with ⅓ cup hot water. If it foams vigorously, it still has rising power. Store tightly covered in a dry place. Make sure measuring utensils are dry before dipping into the container.

Baking soda should be stored tightly covered in a dry place. If using as an odor catcher, change it four times a year.

Produce

Raw fruits and vegetables often slowly lose their vitamins when kept at room temperature, but tropical fruits deteriorate rapidly if stored in the cold. Most produce is best stored at about 50°F (10°C); if refrigerated, put it in the crisper section; the restricted space slows down moisture loss. Avoid storing fruits and vegetables for long periods in sealed plastic bags; they cut off the air supply, causing the produce to rot. Paper and cellophane are better storage materials, because they are permeable. Keep juice in a small container so that vitamins are not lost through exposure to oxygen.

In regions where winter temperatures average 30°F (–1°C) or less, fruits and vegetables bought in bulk can be stored in a cool basement or root cellar. Carrots, cabbage, and lettuce keep well at about 32°F (0°C). To prevent rot caused by dampness during storage, wash produce just before using.

Leave the stems on berries until you're ready to use them, and refrigerate peas and beans in their pods. Cut the green tops off root vegetables, such as carrots, beets, parsnips, and turnips, or they will continue to draw nourishment from the roots.

When stored below 40°F (4°C), potatoes develop a sweetish taste from the conversion of starch to sugar; the sweetness disappears when the

Food storage and preparation tips

■ To store fresh herbs, wash them and stand them upright in a glass containing an inch or two (2.5–5 cm) of cold water. Cover with a plastic bag and refrigerate.

■ To freeze berries, place them in a single layer on a cookie sheet, freeze, then pack in airtight containers.

■ Fruits, vegetables, and grains left to soak in water can lose vitamins and minerals. Wash vegetables and fruits under running water to remove soil, insects, and water-soluble pesticides just before using them.

■ The skins of fruits and vegetables are especially concentrated in nutrients, but also are more likely to be tainted with bacteria or pesticide residues. While some nutrients are lost by peeling, this is not significant. Discard the coarse outer leaves of many green vegetables for the same reason.

■ Store cottage cheese upside down in its original container. It will keep longer.

■ Eggs are porous and will absorb refrigerator odors. Store them in their carton, not in the refrigerator door compartment.

■ Before returning an opened ice cream carton to the freezer, press plastic wrap on the surface of the ice cream to prevent ice crystals from forming.

Handling meat and fish safely

✔ Wash poultry under running water and pat it dry with paper towels before preparation. Some experts recommend washing with diluted vinegar to reduce the risk of bacterial contamination.

✔ Rinse fish and pat dry.

✔ Use a meat thermometer to ensure that the food reaches a safe temperature in the middle. This is the only way to tell if your food has reached a high enough internal temperature to destroy harmful bacteria.

✔ A thermometer in a rare-cooked roast or broiled steak should register 140°F (60°C). Bacteria exist only on the surface of raw meat. Therefore, roasts and steaks can be eaten rare, providing the surface of the meat is well cooked.

✔ Ground meats or ground poultry should always be well cooked and reach a temperature of 160°F (70°C). Poultry is cooked when the leg joints move easily and the juices run clear. Fish should flake easily with a fork. Pork should have no pink color.

✔ Never refreeze ground meat or poultry.

✔ When basting or applying a sauce during grilling or broiling, brush the sauce on the cooked surface only. Be careful not to recontaminate fully cooked meat or poultry by adding sauce with a brush previously used on raw or undercooked foods.

Thermometer know-how

1. Take temperature of thin foods like burgers within one minute of removal from heat, larger cuts like roast, after 5 to 10 minutes.

2. Insert thermometer stem/indicator into the thickest part of the food, away from bone, fat, or gristle.

3. Leave thermometer in food for at least 30 seconds before reading temperature.

4. When food has an irregular shape, like some beef roasts, check the temperature in several places.

5. Always wash thermometer stem thoroughly in hot, soapy water after each use.

tubers are returned to room temperature. Potatoes are often packaged in burlap bags or covered with mesh that protects them from light while still allowing air to circulate. Store potatoes in the dark, because exposure to light causes poisonous alkaloids, such as solanine and chaconine, to form.

Freezing raw fruits and vegetables causes the water they contain to form ice crystals that break down cell membranes and walls, resulting in a mushy texture and a loss of nutrients. Deterioration of fruits and vegetables can also be caused by enzymatic activity; blanching prevents this problem. Immerse vegetables for a few seconds in rapidly boiling water to deactivate their enzymes, then plunge them into cold water to stop the cooking process. Most fruits are not suitable for blanching, but you can prevent browning and deterioration by packing them in a solution of sugar, either with or without ascorbic acid.

All produce should be wrapped air-tight to prevent freezer burn, which causes dry patches that have a rough texture and "off" taste. Frozen vegetables should be cooked straight from the freezer; thawing encourages the destructive activity of residual enzymes and microorganisms. Do not refreeze foods that have been thawed.

The home-canning process preserves foods by rapid heating of hermetically sealed containers. The heat destroys microorganisms and stops enzyme action, and the vacuum seal prevents contamination. An improperly canned food may cause serious food poisoning. Cans and jars that have bubbles, incomplete seals, or gas escaping on opening must be discarded.

Surprisingly, some commercially processed foods may be more nutritious than fresh. Produce for freezing or canning is often harvested in peak condition and processed quickly to preserve its appearance and nutritional value. Many fresh fruits and vegetables, on the other hand, are picked before ripening and matured under refrigeration; they never reach peak flavor. Look for vine- and tree-ripened varieties, and buy produce in season.

Meat, poultry, and fish

■ Store meats and fish in the coldest part of the refrigerator. Wrap meat for freezing in freezer paper. Avoid using gas-permeable plastic wrap; it allows moisture to evaporate and causes freezer burn.

■ Shellfish cannot be kept more than a few hours at refrigerator temperature, but they last 2 or 3 days on ice or at a temperature below 32°F (0°C).

■ Hot dogs and cold cuts stay fresh until their expiration dates if they are refrigerated unopened in their original vacuum-sealed bags. Once opened, they should be rewrapped in an airtight bag and used within a few days.

■ Cured and smoked meats are best stored in their original wrappings; make sure that cold cuts bought from the deli counter are wrapped well and used within a day or two. Meat with discoloration, an off smell, or any sign of mold must be discarded.

■ Never defrost meat, poultry, or fish at room temperature. Defrost on the bottom shelf of the refrigerator. If using the microwave to defrost, cook immediately.

Dairy products

■ Fresh milk and cream should be tightly sealed to prevent tainting by odors from other foods. Milk retains its nutritional value better in cartons, because exposure to light destroys some of the vitamin A and riboflavin.

■ Store nonfat powdered milk in a tightly closed container at room temperature in a place where it's not exposed to light.

■ Keep soft cheese and butter tightly covered and refrigerated. Because of concerns about chemical contamination, some people keep plastic materials away from fatty foods, including cheese and butter (see Pollutants). Foil is a good wrapper. Butter freezes well in its original wrapping.

■ Hard cheeses. It's not necessary to refrigerate hard cheese and other ripened cheeses, which keep well covered in a cool, dark cupboard.

Oils

Storage times vary according to the oil and method of processing; some companies claim up to one year opened and two years unopened, depending on the oil, and recommend refrigerating after opening. Oils that have a shorter storage life include walnut, sesame, hazelnut, and almond oils. These are better stored in the refrigerator. Check the label for storage information. Fats turn rancid on exposure to air and pick up odors from other foods. Store tightly sealed oils in a dark cupboard or the refrigerator. Exposure to light and warm temperatures rob oils of vitamins A and E. The cloudiness that forms in some refrigerated oils clears at room temperature.

Margarine, like butter, should be well covered and refrigerated; stores for future use may be frozen. You can refrigerate commercial mayonnaise after opening it. Use homemade mayonnaise as soon as it's made; however, discard leftovers to reduce the risk of food poisoning by *Salmonella* bacteria.

Sugars

Corn syrup and molasses keep well at room temperature, because they are too sugary for bacteria to thrive. However, natural maple syrup and artificially flavored syrups are susceptible to molds; refrigerate them after opening. Refrigerate opened jams and spreads.

White sugar, left unopened in its original package, can be kept for many years in a cool, dry place. Store sugar in an airtight container or freezer bag.

Brown sugar should be stored in an airtight container to retain its moisture and prevent it from hardening. Tightly close the bag or transfer to an airtight container. If your sugar hardens, place a slice of apple or orange in the container to help bring back its original consistency. Or heat the hardened sugar for 20 to 30 seconds in the microwave just before using.

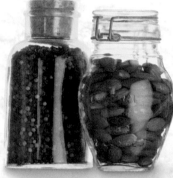

Spices and herbs

The average shelf life of spices and herbs, properly stored, can be 1 to 2 years for leafy herbs, 2 to 3 years for ground spices and 4 years for whole spices. Air, light, moisture, and heat speed flavor and color loss of herbs and spices. Store in a tightly covered container in a dark place away from sunlight, such as inside a cupboard or drawer. For open spice rack storage, choose a site away from light, heat, and moisture. Avoid storing above or near the stove, dishwasher, microwave, refrigerator, sink, or a heating vent. Check freshness of spices and herbs by look, smell, and taste. A visual check for color fading is a good indicator of flavor loss.

COLD STORAGE TIMES

PRODUCT	REFRIGERATOR (40°F/4°C)	FREEZER (0°F/−18°C)
Bacon	7 days	1 month
Butter	1–3 months	6–9 months
Chicken or turkey, whole	1–2 days	1 year
Commercial mayonnaise	2 months	Don't freeze
Eggs, fresh, in shell	3–5 weeks	Don't freeze
Ground beef, turkey, veal, pork, lamb	1–2 days	3–4 months
Hot dogs, unopened package	2 weeks	1–2 months
Luncheon meat, unopened package	2 weeks	1–2 months
Margarine	4–5 months	1 year
Milk	7 days	3 months

FRENCH FRIES

See Fast Food

FRUITS

BENEFITS

- Excellent sources of vitamin C, beta carotene, and potassium; lesser amounts of other vitamins and minerals.
- Contain various polyphenols, which may protect against cancer and other diseases.
- High in fiber and low in calories.
- A source of natural sugars that provide quick energy.

DRAWBACKS

- Some provoke allergic reactions and asthma attacks in susceptible people.

For much of human history, fruits have been a favorite food, and with good reason: they're tasty, easy to digest, a good source of quick energy, and packed with vitamins and minerals.

Anthropologists theorize that apes and early humans alike favored the sweet-tasting fruits, because both species observed that such foods were less likely to be poisonous than those that were bitter. Early hunter-gatherers foraged for wild fruits and berries, but as agrarian societies developed, humans learned to cultivate fruit-bearing bushes and trees. They also developed methods to dry many fruits so that they could be enjoyed during the off-season.

NUTRITIONAL VALUE

Today fruits are lauded for their nutritional value as well as for their pleasing flavor.

Fruits are rich in antioxidants. Numerous studies demonstrate that people who eat ample amounts of fruits (health experts recommend 5 to 10 servings a day) enjoy a reduced incidence of cancer, heart attacks, and strokes. A large study found that men and women who ate five to six servings of fruits and vegetables every day had a lower risk of ischemic stroke, the most common type of stroke. Another large Harvard study found that those who ate eight or more servings a day of fruits and vegetables had a lower risk of heart disease compared to those who ate fewer than three servings. Researchers believe that the high amounts of antioxidants, especially vitamins C and A (in the form of its precursor, beta carotene), in most fruits protect against these and possibly other diseases.

DID YOU KNOW?

EATING PEARS AND APPLES MAY HELP SHED WEIGHT

One study suggests that adding pears and apples to your daily diet may help you lose weight faster. Researchers studied the impact of fruit intake on overweight women who ate just 10 oz (300 g) per day of apples or pears, while following a low-calorie diet. They found that the women who ate fruits lost more weight than the women who didn't.

Antioxidants work by preventing the cell damage caused by free radicals, unstable molecules that are released when the body uses oxygen. Fruits are also high in polyphenols, phytochemicals with antioxidant properties that may prevent or retard tumor growth.

Citrus fruits are among the richest sources of vitamin C. Nutritionists recommend at least one daily serving of an orange, grapefruit, tangerine, or other citrus fruit. A serving is one medium-size fruit or an 8-oz (240-ml) glass of pure juice. Other fruits that are high in vitamin C include cantaloupes and other melons, kiwifruits, strawberries, raspberries, mangoes, and papayas. Cranberry juice is another excellent source.

Brightly colored fruits are high in beta carotene. Fruits with orange or deep yellow flesh—including apricots, cantaloupes, and mangoes—get their color from the yellow-orange pigment beta carotene, which the body converts to vitamin A. Other carotene pigments, such as lycopene in red fruits, or bioflavonoids such as quercetin in grapes, are thought to protect against heart disease. In fact, recent studies indicate that quercetin or resveratrol may be the ingredients in wine responsible for the noted reduction in heart disease and stroke among moderate wine drinkers.

Many fruits are high in potassium, an electrolyte that is essential to maintaining a proper balance of body fluids. Adequate potassium also appears to reduce the risk of developing high blood pressure. People taking diuretic drugs, which increase the excretion of potassium in the urine, are advised to eat extra servings of bananas, melons, apricots, and dried fruits to maintain adequate levels of this mineral.

Most fruits are low in calories and high in fiber, a fact that enhances their appeal to people who are weight conscious. Apples, pears, and many other fruits contain pectin, a soluble fiber that helps regulate blood cholesterol levels. Berries, citrus, and dried fruits are especially high in both soluble and insoluble fibers.

THE PESTICIDE ISSUE

Because fruit trees are particularly vulnerable to a variety of worms, flies, and other destructive insects, most growers use pesticide sprays to keep them in check. Many people worry that residues of these pesticides pose a substantial health risk. Experts stress, however, that the pesticides used on fruit trees in North America meet specific safety standards and that the health benefits of eating fruits outweigh any risk. Even so, fruits should be washed well before eating, and some should be peeled. These include apples that have been sprayed with a wax to extend their shelf life and to make them more attractive. The wax itself is harmless, but it seals the skin and prevents pesticide residue from being washed away.

Citrus fruits are often coated with fungicides and other pesticides to prevent mold growth and fruit fly infestation. Ordinarily, this practice would not pose a problem because the peels are discarded. But if you are using the zest of fresh citrus peels, wash the fruit thoroughly. This is also a good precaution to follow before squeezing the juice from citrus fruit. Don't use soap when washing produce. You may consume the soap residues.

Imported fruits may be more hazardous than those grown locally, because pesticides that may be banned in North America may be used abroad. There are safety standards for imported foods, which are also subject to inspection, but not every batch of imported food can be tested for pesticide residues. Consequently, consumer groups warn against eating imported fresh produce. It's probably unnecessary to go this far, but it is a good idea to be extra diligent about washing imported fruits and other produce before eating them.

Anyone who is uncomfortable eating foods that have been treated with pesticides can shop for organic produce that has been grown without the use of these substances. Be prepared to pay more for organic produce, however, and don't expect it to look as perfect as foods that have been grown using pesticides. Also make sure you inspect the foods carefully for moldy or blighted spots; these may harbor natural cancer-causing agents. ❖

TEN WAYS TO EAT MORE FRUIT

1. At breakfast top your cereal with sliced bananas, kiwifruits, fresh berries, or dried fruit such as raisins or apricots and drink a small glass of juice. Try something new like dried cranberries or sliced mango.

2. Fill a cantaloupe or other melon with low-fat cottage cheese.

3. Carry single-serving cans of unsweetened fruit for snacks at work.

4. Pack your briefcase, backpack, or glove compartment with easy-to-carry fruit such as apples, pears, bananas, clementines, or dried fruit.

5. Make a smoothie with yogurt, milk, or soy beverage mixed with a variety of fresh or frozen berries.

6. Mix a bowl of low-fat yogurt with fruit.

7. Add 1 cup (250 ml) fresh or frozen berries to pancake batter. Top pancakes with applesauce or rhubarb compote instead of syrup.

8. In restaurants, order fruit as a starter or dessert.

9. Don't throw out overripe bananas. Peel and freeze them and use them later for banana bread or muffins.

10. Add fruit such as apples, pears, and mandarin orange sections to green salads.

FUNCTIONAL FOODS
■ ENHANCED FOR HEALTH ■

The link between diet and health continues to grow, and researchers have begun looking at benefits that certain foods may provide beyond their basic nutritional value. Recent years have seen a growing interest in functional foods—foods that have specific components, naturally occurring or added, that may reduce the risk of certain diseases. Whole as well as fortified, enriched, or enhanced foods can fall into this category.

Unmodified whole foods such as fruits and vegetables are the simplest example of a functional food. For example, broccoli, carrots, or tomatoes may be considered functional foods because they are particularly rich in compounds that have been linked with reduced risk of various diseases. Modified foods, including those fortified with nutrients or enhanced with specific phytochemicals or botanical extracts, are also functional foods. There is hope that these can play a role in prevention and treatment of conditions like cancer, diabetes, high blood pressure, heart disease, arthritis, and others.

The functional-food market is one of the fastest-growing segments of the U.S. food industry, and is also growing rapidly in Japan and England. In other countries, such as Canada, growth is slower because of current regulatory constraints.

Some types of fortified functional foods have been around for a long time. For example, we fortify milk and margarine with vitamin D to prevent vitamin D deficiency diseases such as rickets. We add iodine to salt to prevent goiter. But the recent explosion of research into the role of food and nutrients and disease has resulted in huge interest by food companies to develop and market foods as medicine. For example, in the United States, products like cereal with added psyllium to lower cholesterol, tea with St. John's wort for mood improvement, and chips with kava-kava to promote relaxation are now found on store shelves. Since these products are not regulated, a consumer has no way of knowing how much of the supposed "active ingredient" they contain. Herbal medicine experts decry the

Definitions

Functional foods: Foods or food components that have shown benefits in reducing the risk of chronic disease beyond basic nutritional functions. Other terms that have been used interchangeably with functional foods are designer foods, medicinal foods, and pharma foods.

Fortified foods: A type of functional food that has been enhanced, or fortified, with nutrients or other food components, to help prevent or treat disease. Calcium-fortified orange juice is an example of a fortified food. Fortified foods can also be called enriched or enhanced foods.

Nutraceuticals: Products isolated from food and sold in medicinal forms to help prevent or treat disease, such as omega-3 fatty acids, or phytoestrogens.

addition of herbs to products such as soft drinks and snacks as an attempt to exploit people's growing interest in alternative medicine. These products are not available in Canada, where ingredients such as kava are banned.

There are many areas of controversy surrounding functional foods. Some believe that they will distract people from eating healthy diets. Some blast manufacturers for making health claims for which, in many cases, there is little or no scientific support. Others believe that there is plenty of evidence to show that certain functional foods could be the answer to reducing the prevalence of chronic disease and the cost of treatment. Regardless of the controversy, strong consumer interest in functional foods will most likely drive continued development of this market. Here is a list of some food components that are the focus of current research.

■ **Omega-3 fatty acids.** These have been linked to the treatment and prevention of a large variety of diseases, including heart disease and stroke, lupus, diabetes, inflammatory bowel disease, arthritis, and breast, colon, and prostate cancer. Foods containing omega-3 fatty acids include fatty fish, fish oils, and flaxseed. Some eggs now contain omega-3 fatty acids.

■ **Soy protein.** Research supports soy protein's role in the reduction of blood cholesterol levels. It remains unknown whether the effect comes from the isoflavones (hormonelike plant compounds) in soy or some other components—perhaps sterols. Isoflavones are now being studied for their potential anti-cancer properties. They may also guard against osteoporosis. Soy protein can be found in a variety of soy foods, including soybeans, soy nuts, tofu, and soy beverage.

■ **Probiotics and prebiotics.** Probiotics are active bacterial cultures that can help restore gut function and improve immune response. They are found in yogurt and other fermented foods. Prebiotics are substances that stimulate the growth of specific beneficial bacteria in the colon. Fructooligosaccharide (FOS) and inulin, both of which are found in chicory root, are good examples. They can be extracted from the root and added to processed foods.

■ **Lutein.** This carotenoid (a type of antioxidant) has been linked to age-related macular degeneration, the main cause of vision loss in older people. It is in foods such as eggs, corn, spinach, kiwifruits, oranges, broccoli, and chard.

■ **Psyllium.** In the United States, psyllium is being added to cereals and other foods for its cholesterol-lowering soluble fiber.

■ **Oats.** Oats have been widely studied for their ability to lower cholesterol levels. They contain a cholesterol-reducing soluble fiber known as beta-glucan.

■ **Stanols and sterols.** In the United States, these cholesterol-lowering compounds, which are derived from wood oils, are being added to margarines such as Benecol.

THE LINK BETWEEN DIET AND DISEASE

Proportion of disease onset linked to diet

Arteriosclerosis	50%
Hypertension	50%
Stroke	50%
Diabetes	50%
Coronary heart disease	40%
Cancer	35%–50%

When in doubt, stick with nature's functional foods

As researchers and food companies continue to look at new ways to link food products with disease prevention and treatment, remember that nature has provided us with an abundance of functional foods. Fruits and vegetables, as well as whole grains, legumes, nuts, and seeds are examples of foods naturally packed with phytonutrients that we know can lower the risk of cancer, heart disease, hypertension, and many other chronic diseases. No matter what the future of functional foods brings, you can't go wrong sticking with the basics.

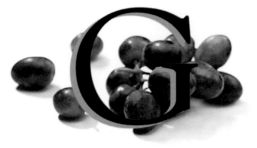

GALLSTONES

EAT PLENTY OF
- Small meals at regular intervals.
- Breakfast daily.

AVOID
- Weight gain.
- Excessive alcohol.

The gallbladder seems to serve no purpose other than to store and concentrate bile, a substance produced by the liver to digest fats in the small intestine. Removal of the organ appears to have no effect on digestion. Bile fluid contains high levels of cholesterol and the pigment bilirubin, both of which precipitate as crystals to form stones; these may be as fine as beach sand or as coarse as river gravel. Most gallstones are hardened cholesterol; the rest are made up of bilirubin plus calcium.

Gallstones can develop in both sexes, but they are most common in overweight middle-aged women. They also tend to run in families. Women, especially those who have borne children, are thought to be particularly vulnerable because of the high levels of blood cholesterol and bile that develop late in pregnancy and in the weeks following childbirth. It is believed, too, that the female hormones progesterone and estrogen, whether occurring naturally or taken in oral contraceptives, may play a role in gallstone formation. Crash weight-loss diets are believed to be another precipitating factor; many people appear to develop gallstones after a period of yo-yo dieting, with repeated cycles of weight loss and gain, or after a single dramatic weight loss.

Many people never know they have gallstones because they have no symptoms. For some, however, the presence of gallstones can cause pain in the upper right abdomen when the gallbladder contracts to release bile after a meal, and inflammation of the gallbladder (cholecystitis) that brings on sudden, severe pain extending to the back and under the right shoulder blade, with fever, chills, and vomiting. If stones obstruct the flow of bile, the skin and the whites of the eyes become jaundiced. Left untreated, stones can lodge in the bile duct and cause inflammation of the liver or pancreas.

For frequent painful attacks, the usual treatment is the surgical removal of the gallbladder, called cholecystectomy; the procedure can be performed by conventional surgery or by laparoscopy, which involves only a tiny incision and a brief hospital stay. Medications have been used with mixed success to dissolve gallstones, but the stones often recur if the person stops taking the drug. Another option is a procedure called lithotripsy, which uses shock waves to break up the gallstones.

GALLSTONES AND NUTRITION

Eat small, frequent meals—especially breakfast. For years, people with gallstones have been warned to eliminate fats and cholesterol from their diets. This advice was based on the observation that most stones are formed of cholesterol. In fact, there's little evidence that a low-cholesterol diet will lower the risk of gallstones. Some clinicians even claim that the occasional fatty meal causes the gallbladder to empty itself, which may be beneficial.

Although a diet high in fiber and low in fats is recommended for general health, there are no scientific grounds for believing that high fiber intake can favorably influence cholesterol metabolism, at least as far as gallstones are concerned. It is known, however, that the bile is more likely to form stones after the long period of fasting that occurs overnight, while we sleep. Because of this, some doctors recommend that people with gallbladder problems should eat a substantial breakfast, which will cause the bladder to empty itself and flush out any small stones and stagnant bile. Other doctors go even further, and advise patients to eat frequent small meals to maintain this filling and emptying cycle.

Consume plenty of starchy foods with lots of fruits and vegetables. People with gallstones should avoid foods that cause them discomfort. Their diet should emphasize starchy foods, with lots of fruits and vegetables, moderate servings of protein, and small amounts of fat. Alcohol should be used in moderation, if at all, especially if the gallbladder disease also affects the liver and pancreas. ❖

GARLIC

BENEFITS

- May help lower high blood pressure and elevated blood cholesterol.
- May prevent or fight certain cancers.
- Antiviral and antibacterial properties help prevent or fight infection.
- May alleviate nasal congestion.

DRAWBACKS

- Causes bad breath.
- Can cause indigestion, especially if eaten raw.
- Direct contact irritates the skin and mucous membranes.

Herbalists and folk healers have used garlic to treat myriad diseases for thousands of years. Ancient Egyptian healers prescribed it to build physical strength, the Greeks used it as a laxative, and the Chinese traditionally used it to lower blood pressure. In the Middle Ages, eating liberal quantities of garlic was credited with providing immunity to the plague. Of course, just because garlic has been used for a long time does not mean that it has been used effectively for a long time. Current research on garlic has curbed the optimism fostered by earlier studies.

Louis Pasteur, the great 19th-century French chemist, was the first to demonstrate garlic's antiseptic properties, information that was put to use during World Wars I and II by the British, German, and Russian armies. Since then, numerous studies have confirmed that garlic can be effective against bacteria, fungi, viruses, and parasites. Today, many proponents of herbal medicine prescribe garlic to help prevent colds, flu, and other infectious diseases.

THE STUDY OF GARLIC

Garlic has been intensively studied in recent years, with more than 500 papers having been published in medical journals since the mid-1980s. The subject of most of these studies has been the sulfur compounds that form when allicin undergoes a variety of chemical reactions. Allicin is not found in fresh garlic but forms when cells are disturbed by cooking, cutting, or chewing. Ajoene, allyl sulfides, S-allyl cystein (SAC), and other products of this allicin cascade have been associated with anticancer, anticlotting, antifungal, antihypertensive, antioxidant, and cholesterol-lowering effects.

Some garlic supplements tout their allicin "content." This is not accurate because allicin is an unstable substance. Claims about "allicin yield" or "allicin potential" are somewhat more appropriate, but not by much. Manufacturers usually determine "yield" by mixing crushed tablets with water and measuring the amount of allicin released. This is not an appropriate model for what happens in the body.

Garlic supplements must be protected from contact with stomach acid since it would immediately destroy alliinase and make the release of allicin impossible. This is usually done by encapsulating in gelatin or coating the pill with cellulose or polyacrylic acid derivatives that dissolve only in the less acidic conditions of the intestine. A fitting test for allicin release is one sanctioned by the U.S. Pharmacopoeia (method 724A), which simulates the conditions encountered by a pill as it travels through the digestive tract. When this test is applied to garlic supplements, the results are astounding. More than 80 percent of products tested release less than 15 percent of their claimed allicin potential. Clearly they do not deliver a therapeutic allicin dosage.

Whether garlic is therapeutic at all can only be determined by human trials. It may be impressive to learn that some garlic extract retards cholesterol oxidation in cells; but that does not mean this happens in the body. Numerous studies of garlic's effects on health have been carried out. Early studies suggested a cholesterol-lowering effect and received much publicity. Unfortunately more sophisticated studies curtailed the initial optimism.

When researchers analyzed the results of the garlic studies, they found, much to their disappointment, that garlic's ability to reduce cholesterol was minimal, and the effect on blood pressure was insignificant. Still, some companies keep promoting supplements based on the early studies.

EFFECT ON HEART DISEASE

While garlic may not reduce cholesterol, it may still have an effect on heart disease. "Ajoene," one of the breakdown products of allicin, may reduce the risk of heart attacks by preventing the formation of blood clots.

PROMISING STUDIES ON GARLIC AND CANCER

The situation is more encouraging with respect to cancer, perhaps because most studies investigated the effect of raw or cooked garlic instead

AN EDIBLE ANTIBIOTIC

Garlic contains compounds that act as powerful natural antibacterial, antiviral, and antifungal agents. It has been shown to inhibit the fungi that cause athlete's foot, vaginal yeast infections, and many cases of ear infection. It may be as effective against certain fungi as antifungal medications. Laboratory studies have shown that garlic extract can neutralize *Helicobacter pylori,* the bacterium that causes most ulcers. (It's unclear, however, whether garlic has this effect in the body.)

of supplements. A meta analysis showed that consuming an average of six or more cloves a week lowered the risk of colorectal cancer by 30 percent and stomach cancer by 50 percent when compared with the consumption of less than one clove a week. Even the risk of prostate cancer may be reduced. A National Cancer Institute study of men in Shanghai showed that eating a clove a day reduced risk by more than 50 percent. There is a caveat to these types of studies though. Consumption of specific foods is determined by means of questionnaires and peoples' memories may not be all that reliable. Furthermore, heavy garlic consumption may just be the hallmark of a mostly vegetarian diet.

There is no consensus on how much garlic should be consumed to make use of its anticancer effect and neither is there agreement on whether cooked or dried garlic confers the same benefits imparted by eating garlic raw. It does seem clear though, that to activate garlic's full nutritional power, it should be chopped or crushed and then left to stand for 10 minutes before cooking. This allows allicin and its potent derivatives to be activated.

TREATING GARLIC BREATH

While there is no guarantee that garlic will have an effect on health, it most assuredly will have an effect on the breath. Eating parsley might help to reduce this unpleasant odor, possibly because of its chlorophyll content. Garlic may cause indigestion, especially if eaten raw. Handling raw garlic can irritate the skin and mucous membranes. Garlic (both fresh and supplements) may enhance the effects of blood-thinning medications. ❖

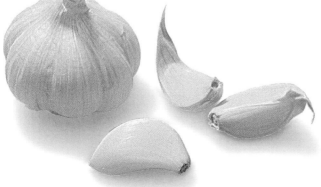

GASTRITIS

CONSUME
- Regular meals with a balance of starchy foods, fruits, vegetables, and low-fat protein.

AVOID
- Fatty foods, tomato-based products, chocolate, alcohol, caffeine, and peppermint, which can cause acid reflux.
- Spicy foods if they irritate you.
- Frequent use of aspirin or other arthritis pain relievers.

An inflammation of the stomach lining, gastritis is usually signaled by indigestion, either with or without bleeding in the digestive tract. Acute gastritis often develops when people are subjected to sudden stress, such as from extensive burns or other severe injury or illness; it may also develop after surgery, leading to stress ulcers and severe intestinal bleeding.

Chronic inflammation can occur with long-term use of certain medications (such as aspirin and arthritis drugs), gastrointestinal disorders (for example, Crohn's disease), alcoholism, or viral infections. It has recently been discovered that many cases of gastritis are caused by a bacterium, *Helicobacter pylori*. This organism has also been linked to peptic ulcers and is the only germ currently known to be able to survive in the acidic environment of the human stomach.

Gastritis is more common with age and most sufferers complain of indigestion, heartburn, nausea, and belching. Other people have no noticeable symptoms, which can be dangerous if gastritis is caused by erosion of the stomach lining with bleeding—normally a result of aspirin or other medication.

Usually, people with acute gastritis caused by illness or injury have already been hospitalized for treatment of their underlying condition; therefore, symptoms of gastritis are managed in the course of their intensive care.

Avoid spicy or acidic foods. Although foods are not the cause of gastritis, people with symptoms should avoid spicy or highly acidic foods, which can irritate the stomach lining. They should also avoid fatty foods, tomato-based products, chocolate, beverages containing caffeine, decaffeinated tea and coffee, peppermint, and alcohol. These foods relax the valve between the stomach and esophagus and make it easier for the stomach contents to back up into the esophagus, causing further irritation.

If you need a pain reliever, ask your doctor to prescribe a nonirritating alternative to aspirin or other nonsteroidal anti-inflammatory drug (NSAID). For gastritis caused by *H. pylori*, the doctor may prescribe antibiotics. Antacids can sometimes soothe the irritation until the inflammation subsides. ❖

GASTROENTERITIS

CONSUME

- Fluids, such as chicken broth or soup, for rehydration.
- Bananas, rice, applesauce, toast (the BRAT diet) to maintain nutrition.
- Solid foods gradually, as symptoms subside.

AVOID

- Alcohol and caffeine, which stimulate the lower bowel.
- High-fiber foods, which may irritate an inflamed bowel.
- Frequent use of aspirin or other arthritis pain relievers.
- If traveling abroad: unpeeled fruits and vegetables, uncooked foods, unboiled tap water, and ice cubes in drinks.

An inflammation of the lower digestive tract, gastroenteritis has many causes: infection with a virus, bacterium, or parasite; ingestion of toxic substances; allergy or intolerance to food; and medications, often antibiotics that alter the normal bacterial population of the lower tract. Also, people with eating disorders, such as anorexia and bulimia, may develop gastroenteritis as a result of laxative abuse.

Thanks to clean water supplies, gastroenteritis due to cholera and typhoid fever is now rare in the industrialized nations. By contrast, gastroenteritis caused by parasites, such as giardia and amoebas, can strike in any country. Parasites can be transmitted in a variety of ways, such as through unsanitary food handling, contamination of drinking water, and close physical contact with an infected person.

Gastroenteritis caused by common bacteria or viruses is often referred to as "stomach flu." Provided the infecting organism is a bacterium or virus and not a parasite, symptoms—like those of diarrhea and food poisoning—usually clear up within a few days, without any special treatment. Nausea and vomiting are not much more than a temporary inconvenience to other-wise healthy adults and older children. On the other hand, in vulnerable groups—babies, the elderly, and people with a suppressed immune system—gastroenteritis can be severely debilitating and requires medical attention.

When vomiting and diarrhea persist longer than 48 hours, your doctor may prescribe a medication to quell nausea, as well as an antibiotic if it seems advisable. Tests may be warranted to identify and isolate the cause of gastroenteritis, such as food sensitivity or exposure to toxic substances. If diarrhea is bloody, your doctor may investigate the possibility of a parasitic infection or bacillary dysentery.

If you have stomach flu, give your digestive system a rest from solid food, but drink plenty of liquids. Sipping ginger ale can help to calm any surges of nausea. Chicken broth with rice is a palatable rehydration remedy; the broth replaces fluid, as well as sodium and potassium to restore the balance of electrolytes, and the rice has a binding effect on the bowel. Don't drink alcohol or beverages containing caffeine; they stimulate the digestive tract and can actually worsen diarrhea.

Reintroduce solid foods gradually. As your bowel settles down, try with small portions of the BRAT diet—bananas, rice, applesauce, and toast. (See Diarrhea.) The bananas provide potassium and carbohydrates; rice is easily digested and provides energy; unsweetened applesauce contains pectin, a soluble fiber that helps add bulk to the stool; and dry toast provides energy in the form of carbohydrates but doesn't overtax the digestive system with fiber that could be irritating to an inflamed bowel.

Your ability to digest lactose may be temporarily affected. After about 48 hours you should be able to tolerate other simple solid foods, such as steamed or boiled potatoes, cooked vegetables, and a boiled or poached egg. Leave dairy foods until last; the fat in cheese is difficult to digest and stays in the stomach longer than other foods, and some infections can temporarily interfere with your ability to digest lactose, the sugar found in milk and dairy products. Many people find they can tolerate low-fat yogurt even when other dairy foods provoke digestive problems. Keep up your fluid intake with water and juices, and resume a normal diet as soon as you feel up to it.

Because some drugs can cause severe gastroenteritis, contact your doctor if any digestive upset occurs while you are taking an antibiotic or other medication. The doctor may decide to switch you to another medication or therapy. ❖

A VIRUS BY ANY OTHER NAME

In recent years outbreaks of an illness called the Norwalk Virus have made the news. In fact, Norwalk is viral gastroenteritis and has the same symptoms. It is most often caused by contaminated food or water. Cruise ships, swimming pools, recreational lakes, wells, and even municipal water supplies may become contaminated and cause outbreaks. Shellfish and salad ingredients are the foods most likely to be a problem. Fortunately, the virus doesn't multiply in food and is destroyed through cooking. Stick to well-cooked food and bottled drinks without ice, especially when traveling, to avoid this illness.

GENETICALLY MODIFIED ORGANISMS
▪ GMOs ▪

The availability of genetically altered foods continues to be a hotly debated issue with powerful lobbies on both sides. Corn that resists attacks by insects, canola that is tolerant of herbicides, and cheese that can be made without using animal rennet have been some of the advances introduced by genetic modification, but some people worry that possible long-term effects may not have been adequately assessed.

For centuries, food growers have tampered with plant and animal genetics by crossbreeding in order to bring out desirable traits while suppressing less desirable ones. The refinement of such techniques has enabled farmers to produce increasingly abundant crops.

In recent years, food biotechnology has added a new dimension, thanks to genetic modification. Genetically modified (GM) foods or genetically modified organisms (GMOs) are terms that refer to a change in the code or organization of the genetic material of an organism. One method to achieve this change is "genetic engineering"—the practice of moving one gene or group of genes from one organism to another.

The production of GMOs is regulated in the United States and Canada. To date, each country has approved at least 40 plant varieties derived by genetic modification. Soybeans, corn, and canola are the most widely produced GM crops and furnish a number of ingredients that are used in highly processed foods. In fact, about 70 percent of processed foods contain at least some GM ingredients.

Improving on nature

Genetic engineering enables research botanists to add desirable hereditary traits to almost any plant. Possibilities include producing more nutritious foods; for example, corn with increased high-quality protein, or a type of rapeseed that synthesizes more of the unsaturated fatty acids of canola oil.

Agricultural scientists are also trying to alter plants to make them more productive or more able to withstand adverse growing conditions, such as drought. This type of genetic engineering has tremendous potential in overcoming world food shortages; conceivably, arid desert areas may one day produce drought-resistant grains.

Another approach involves engineering plants to be resistant to disease, herbicides, and pests. One modification alters a plant's taste to make it less attractive to insects, allowing farmers to reduce pesticide use. Another is aimed at developing a plant resistant to new kinds of herbicides that do not harm the crops and beneficial insects.

Cheese producers have also benefited from genetic modification. The classic way to make cheese involves using rennet extracted from calf stomachs to curdle milk. But chymosin, the major enzyme in rennet can also be produced through genetic engineering. The bit of DNA, the gene, that gives the instructions for the formation of chymosin has been isolated from calf cells and copied, or "cloned." Inserting this gene into the genetic machinery of certain bacteria (*Escherichia coli*), yeasts (*Kluyveromyces lactis*), or fungi (*Aspergillus niger*) causes them to dutifully churn out pure chymosin. Approved in 1990 by the Food and Drug Administration in the United States, chymosin became the first product of genetic engineering in our food supply. It is 100 percent identical to that found in calf stomach, but because it does not come from animals, it is acceptable to consumers who do not want meat products in their cheese.

Extraordinary precautions were taken before chymosin, made by recombinant DNA technology, was marketed. Regulators ensured that no toxins of any kind had been introduced and that no live recombinant organisms were present. Cheese made with it is completely indistinguishable from that produced with animal rennet. In any case, chymosin itself is degraded during cheese making and none is left in the finished product. Today, in North America, more than 80 percent of cheese is made using chymosin.

The downside

Despite the benefits of genetic modification, some people are concerned that this type of manipulation may create adverse consequences.

Gene transfer to nontarget species. For instance, scientists will often incorporate an antibiotic-resistant gene (or tracer) into the genetic material that is being introduced into a plant. If the modified cell is able to survive antibiotic treatment, it means that it has become resistant to that antibiotic and has probably taken on other characteristics carried in the newly added genetic material. So far, evidence that antibiotic-resistant tracers can be transferred to a nontarget species such as a disease-causing microorganism is sketchy, but theoretically, it could happen.

Reduced effectiveness of pesticides and herbicides. There is some concern that insects will become resistant to the pesticides produced by crops that have been genetically modified to produce their own pesticides, or that the herbicide resistance of a GM crop will be transferred to a weed. Another concern is that these crops may harm beneficial insects along with the intended crop-damaging pests.

Unintended harm to the organism or other organisms. Comparatively, animals subjected to genetic engineering do not fare as well as plants. For example, sheep injected with genetically engineered hormones to increase wool growth become more vulnerable to the heat. Pigs and chickens treated with special growth hormones develop painful bone and joint problems. Also, there are ethical issues involved in tampering with animal genes.

Allergic reactions. Concern has been raised that allergens may be transferred through genetic modification. This is unlikely to occur because the structures of proteins introduced by genetic modification are compared with extensive data bases of the structures of known allergens.

It's a question of benefits versus risks

The potential benefits of genetic modification are numerous. Sweet potato is an important crop in Africa but is very susceptible to feathery mottle virus. Inserting a set of genes from chrysanthemums that code for naturally insecticidal compounds called pyrethrins has the potential of increasing yields dramatically. The use of pesticides on cotton has already been

DID YOU KNOW?

YOUR SUPERMARKET IS FILLED WITH GENETICALLY ALTERED FOODS

An estimated 60 to 70 percent of foods available in North American supermarkets contain at least a small measure of a crop that has been genetically engineered. Corn, soybeans, and oil from canola or cotton are the most prevalent genetically modified crops.

dramatically reduced by incorporating a gene that protects it from insects. While there are environmental concerns about pollen drift and crossbreeding with non-GM plants, there has not been a single adverse health effect.

The labeling issue

The labeling of genetically modified foods has become a thorny issue. In response to consumer concerns, some producers would like the opportunity to label their products as containing no GMOs. But some people might interpret it as suggesting that there is a reason to avoid GMOs.

Genetically modified foods on the market have been approved by both the United States' and Canada's stringent regulatory agencies. They have been assessed for their effect on human health as well as environmental safety. Not a single case of human disease has ever been attributed to a GM food. If consumers demand labels, then the information they contain has to be verifiable. This presents a problem because there may be nothing to verify since there is no chemical difference between, for example, soy oil made from genetically modified soybeans and the oil made from non-GM beans. We may also see producers labeling everything in sight as GMO-free, including products where genetic modification is not even an issue.

If we go in the other direction and focus on labeling foods that are sourced from genetically modified plants, we run into other problems. A bag of soybeans, canola, or corn grown with the aid of this technology can be labeled like this. But what about a frozen dinner that has corn starch as an ingredient? The starch may have come from corn with a gene inserted to produce the insecticidal Bt toxin. Yet this starch cannot be distinguished from starch that comes from non-GM corn. Should it be labeled? What about meat from animals raised on genetically modified feed? Or eggs from chickens similarly raised? If regulations are introduced requiring foods that contain GM components to be labeled, what will be the maximum amount allowed to be present before labeling is required?

Do we have a right to know what we're eating?

There is much in our food supply that we are not informed about. There are no food label declarations about the number of insect parts or rat droppings allowed per serving (although there are regulations about these), or the specific pesticides or fertilizers used, or toxins introduced by traditional crossbreeding, or whether the food was grown hydroponically. What about labeling lima beans as a source of natural cyanide?

The labeling of food contents is a contentious issue. Perhaps one way out of this GMO conundrum is to label foods not according to the process by which they were produced, but according to the contents of the final product. If a genetically modified food is nutritionally or compositionally different from its traditional counterpart, it should be labeled. Obviously the labeling issue is not a simple one and the debate will no doubt continue.

GINGER

BENEFITS

- May prevent motion sickness.
- Can help to quell nausea.
- Ginger wine may help to relieve menstrual cramps.

DRAWBACKS

- Raw or candied ginger may irritate oral tissue and other mucous membranes.

The use of ginger for flavoring foods dates back to the earliest civilizations. The Chinese were using ginger as long ago as the 6th century B.C., and Arab traders introduced the spice to the Mediterranean before the 1st century A.D. Transported from the Middle East to Europe by the Crusaders, ginger was an ingredient in almost every recipe found in a 1390 cookbook that was compiled at the English royal court. Spanish settlers brought ginger to the New World in the 1500s.

The Zingiberaceae family includes ginger and two other popular spices—cardamom and turmeric—as well as the banana, an unlikely distant cousin. Cardamom is widely used in tropical cuisines; in addition, it lends fragrance to Scandinavian breads and pastries. Turmeric, a major ingredient in commercial curry powders, is also used in Asia to dye fabrics yellow and in Western countries to improve the color of some margarines and dairy products.

FLAVORFUL FOLK REMEDY

Ginger has a long and honored tradition in folk medicine, and for good reason, according to modern research that is exploring the scientific basis for ginger's effects.

Cancer. Recent studies have shown that beta ionone, a terpenoid found in ginger, has decided anticancer properties. Tumors induced in laboratory animals grow much more slowly if the animals are pretreated with beta ionone.

Nausea and motion sickness. Various forms of ginger—nonalcoholic ginger ale or beer, pills, and candied ginger root—have been used to counter the nausea and vomiting of motion sickness. This practice is particularly well established in Germany, where it is a government-approved treatment for motion sickness and heartburn. A recent study found that ginger was as effective as prescription medication in preventing motion sickness, without causing the drowsiness the drug sometimes does.

Sipping flat ginger ale or sucking candied ginger, which has a more concentrated flavor, may help to quell spells of nausea due to morning sickness, food poisoning, gastroenteritis, or cancer chemotherapy. Ginger is available in capsule form for those who find that the candy is too strong or irritates the mouth.

Pain. Because ginger blocks the pro-inflammatory prostaglandins (hormonelike chemicals), it may also be useful in helping people who suffer from the pain of:

- Migraines. These headaches are thought to be caused by inflammation in blood vessels in the brain. At least one study suggests that taking ginger at the first sign of a migraine can help to reduce the symptoms.
- Arthritis. Prostaglandins contribute to joint swelling in people with arthritis. Studies have shown that people with either osteoarthritis or rheumatoid arthritis experienced less pain and swelling when they took powdered ginger daily. ❖

DO ONE SIMPLE THING

RELIEVE A COLD WITH GINGER TEA

A comforting way to relieve the chills and congestion of a cold: Make ginger tea by simmering one or two slices of fresh ginger root in water for 10 minutes; add a pinch of cinnamon for extra flavor.

ROOT REMEDY. *Adding a slice or two of peeled raw ginger to bean dishes is said to reduce the flatulence these foods often cause.*

GLYCEMIC INDEX
■ AN EVOLVING STORY ■

Despite its growing popularity as a tool to help people improve their health, there are still many controversies and misconceptions surrounding this food classification system.

The glycemic index (GI) is a classification of carbohydrate foods according to the effect they have on the level of blood sugars. Regulating blood sugars is a key strategy in preventing and controlling certain diseases, particularly diabetes.

Over 20 years ago, researchers at the University of Toronto studied more than 50 carbohydrate-rich foods and their effect on blood glucose. The glycemic index was developed by measuring how much a person's blood glucose increased 2 to 3 hours after eating a carbohydrate-rich food compared to a reference food, which was either pure glucose or white bread.

A food that is digested and absorbed quickly has a high GI value, causing a rapid increase in blood sugar. A food that is digested and absorbed slowly has a low GI value. Foods can have a low GI (less than 55), an intermediate GI (55–70), or a high GI (higher than 70). There are currently more than 750 published GI values of various foods.

Glycemic index and health

We used to believe that foods high in sugar, such as cakes and cookies, chocolate, and fruit, were harmful for diabetics because they were quickly digested, leading to a rapid rise in blood sugar. Complex carbohydrates like potatoes, rice, and pasta were thought to break down more slowly, resulting in a more gradual rise in blood sugar. But some sugars actually have a lower glycemic index than many more-starchy foods. Therefore high-sugar foods in moderate servings have no greater effect on blood glucose than many starchy foods and can be included as part of a diabetic meal plan. Researchers are also finding that a low-GI diet may help lower the risk of developing diabetes and heart disease in healthy people.

FACTORS THAT AFFECT THE GLYCEMIC INDEX

Some processing methods and nutrients can affect the GI value of a food.

FACTOR	MECHANISM	EXAMPLES
Cooking or processing starch	Changes the structure of starch and the granules become swollen (gelatinized). Less-gelatinized starch has a lower GI.	Al dente pasta has a lower GI than overcooked pasta.
Sugar	Prevents gelatinization of starch.	Frosted flakes have a lower GI than corn flakes.
Fiber	Slows down interaction between starch and enzymes.	Rolled oats, beans, lentils, apples have lower GIs.
Protein and fat	Slows down rate of carbohydrate digestion.	Fat and protein-containing foods like milk and legumes have low GIs.
Acid in foods	Slows rate of digestion and absorption.	Vinegar, lemon juice, and acidic fruits lower the GI.

In sports medicine, high-GI foods have been used as a source of quick energy to help short-duration sports performance and recovery, while low-GI foods have been used in endurance sports. An interesting theory in another area of research is that low-GI foods can aid in weight loss because they help to control insulin levels. The hormone insulin promotes the storage of fat and also inhibits the breakdown of stored fat for energy.

Current controversies

Although many large health organizations, including the World Health Organization, support the use of the GI for people with diabetes, many others have questioned its value. The controversy stems from the difficulty in applying the GI system in a practical and understandable way to help people improve their health.

One of the biggest issues is that many foods that are considered healthy choices have a higher GI than foods that are considered to be nutritionally less desirable. For example, mashed potatoes have a higher GI than table sugar, and it is definitely confusing to find that unrefined whole-wheat bread has almost the same GI as white bread.

This is where the concept of glycemic load (GL) comes in. It assesses the effect of carbohydrate foods on blood sugar by taking into account the GI but giving a fuller picture than the GI alone. The GI tells you how rapidly a particular carbohydrate turns into sugar. It doesn't tell you how much of that carbohydrate is in that food. Both have an important effect on blood sugar. For example, the carbohydrate in watermelon has a high GI. But there isn't a lot of it, so the GL is relatively low. Despite examples like watermelon, most foods that have a low GL have a low GI. Foods with an intermediate or high GL can have a low to high GI. A GL of 20 or more is considered high, 11 to 19 is medium, and 10 or less is low. (See "Glycemic Index (GI) and Glycemic Load (GL) of Some Common Foods," next page.)

Other issues

GI values vary from one study to another, for a number of reasons. Their values are determined by measuring blood sugar responses after particular foods are eaten. But one person's glycemic response can differ considerably from another's. It may vary even in the same person from day to day. Even the state of food can change its GI. For example, small differences in a banana's ripeness can double its GI. And the GI of boiled potatoes can be increased by 25 percent just by mashing them.

In addition, when you combine foods (adding butter or sour cream to a baked potato, for instance, or having the potato with a serving of meat) the GI of the combined foods becomes much different from the GI of the potato by itself. The reasson is that fat and protein slow gastric emptying, making the GI of the whole dish different than the GI of just a single food.

The bottom line

Remember that the GI is only one measurement of a food and its contribution to health. A low-GI diet will include many foods recommended in a healthy diet—fruits and vegetables, whole grains, and legumes. These foods are lower in fat, high in fiber, and are a rich source of vitamins, minerals, and antioxidants. And some high-GI foods, like potatoes, contain many essential nutrients and are good sources of energy.

With further research, the glycemic index, an interesting and valuable concept, may become an easier tool to apply. In the meantime, the general principles of a healthy diet—variety, balance, and moderation—still apply.

GLYCEMIC INDEX (GI) AND GLYCEMIC LOAD (GL) OF SOME COMMON FOODS

FOOD	GI	SERVING SIZE	GL
Grains and Cereals			
Bagel, white	72	2½ oz (70 g)	25
Barley, pearled	25	5 oz (150 g)	11
Bread, rye, whole meal	58	1 oz (30 g)	8
Bread, white	71	1 oz (30 g)	10
Bread, whole grain, pumpernickel	46	1 oz (30 g)	5
Bread, whole wheat	67	1 oz (30 g)	8
Cereal, All-Bran	50	1 oz (30 g)	9
Cereal, corn flakes	80	1 oz (30 g)	21
Cereal, muesli	66	1 oz (30 g)	16
Rice, long grain, white	60	5 oz (150 g)	24
Rice, long grain, white, instant	68	5 oz (150 g)	25
Spaghetti, white	42	6½ oz (180 g)	20
Sweet corn	60	5 oz (150 g)	20
Dairy			
Milk, skim	32	8½ oz (250 ml)	4
Yogurt	36	7 oz (200 ml)	3
Legumes			
Chickpeas	33	5 oz (150 g)	10
Kidney beans	42	5 oz (150 g)	10
Lentils	22	5 oz (150 g)	4
Fruits			
Apple	39	4 oz (120 g)	6
Apple juice, unsweetened	41	8½ oz (250 ml)	12
Banana	46	4 oz (120 g)	12
Grapes	43	4 oz (120 g)	7
Vegetables			
Baked potato	60	5 oz (150 g)	18
Baked potato, mashed	74	5 oz (150 g)	15
Sweet potato	48	5 oz (150 g)	16
Carrots	92	3 oz (80 g)	5
Miscellaneous			
Coca Cola	53	8½ oz (250 ml)	14
Gatorade	78	8½ oz (250 ml)	12
Sponge cake	46	2 oz (63 g)	17

CAUTION

Don't rely on half the story. If you looked only at the GI figures, you might never eat carrots again. They have almost the same GI as sugar—very high. But that's only half the story. A carrot has just 4 g of carbohydrates and when the formula for determining the GL is used, carrots come up as winners!

GOOSEBERRIES

BENEFITS

- A good source of vitamin C, potassium, and bioflavonoids.
- Fair amounts of iron and vitamin A.
- High in fiber, low in calories.

DRAWBACKS

- Their tartness is usually offset with large amounts of added sugar.
- Gooseberry bushes harbor a fungus that kills some types of pine trees.

Still not very popular in North America, gooseberries are prized for their acidic tartness in Europe, where they are made into pies, jams, jellies, and sauces for poultry. New, sweeter-tasting varieties have been developed, which are more palatable for eating raw.

Gooseberries have many nutritional benefits. They are high in fiber (about 4 g in a cup of raw berries), vitamin C (50 mg per fresh cup), and potassium (250 mg per cup). They are also rich in bioflavonoids—plant pigments that help prevent cancer and other diseases. Some of these nutrients are lost in processing; a cup of canned gooseberries loses more than half of its vitamin C, as well as some potassium. The canned berries are also high in calories, yielding 180 calories per cup, compared to 65 for the fresh fruit.

Folk healers in the past recommended gooseberry juice to treat liver and intestinal disorders. They also believed that a tea brewed from

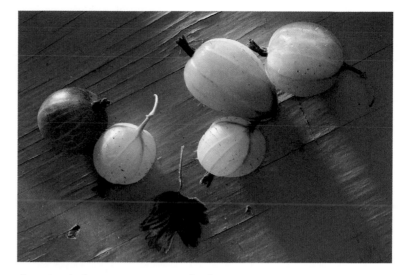

the plant's leaves was a remedy for urinary tract and menstrual disorders. Old herbal medicine books refer to the fruit as feverberries and recommend it for inflammatory disorders. However, there is no scientific evidence that gooseberries or their leaves have any special medicinal qualities.

Gooseberries carry fungi that are transmitted to pine trees and other types of fruit bushes. As a result, efforts are now under way to develop more disease-resistant strains of gooseberries. ❖

A BERRY OF MANY HUES. *Although green gooseberries are the most familiar, some of the more than 700 varieties are red and different shades of blue.*

A GOOSEBERRY PRIMER

- The origin of the name "gooseberries" has nothing to do with geese, even though their acidic flavor goes well with roast goose. Instead, the term comes from the Old English words for the berries—groser, grosier, and grozer. Gooseberries have been cultivated in Europe, and especially in England, since the 15th century.
- There are some 50 different species and more than 700 varieties of gooseberries. Although the gooseberry originated in Europe and western Asia, the United States and Canada now have the most species.
- Gooseberry bushes can attract a fungus that is devastating to white pine forests. For this reason, gooseberries are not cultivated near these forests, also, the berries are regularly inspected to prevent the spread of the fungus.

GOUT

CONSUME PLENTY OF

- Fluids to dilute the urine and prevent the formation of kidney stones.
- Fresh fruits and vegetables (except those high in purines) for vitamins, minerals, and dietary fiber.

LIMIT

- Vegetables high in purines, such as cauliflower, asparagus, green peas, spinach, and mushrooms.

AVOID

- Organ meats, game, anchovies, sardines, herring, meat extracts, and other high-purine foods.
- Alcohol, especially red wine and beer.
- Diuretics and aspirin-based drugs.
- Skipping meals, crash diets.

Marked by swelling, inflammation, and excruciating tenderness in the joints, gout most commonly affects the joints at the base of the big

THE TRUTH ABOUT CHERRIES

Cherry juice—especially black cherry juice—is an old folk remedy for gout that's still popular today. But does it work? Nothing definitive has been proven. However, a study published in the *Journal of Nutrition* in June 2003 reported that eating cherries did indeed lower uric acid levels in the urine of the women in the study, which could explain any anti-gout effect.

When cherries aren't in season, you might consider purchasing cherry fruit extract, available at health-food stores, or drinking half a cup of cherry or blueberry juice a day. Blueberries and strawberries may have effects similar to those of cherries.

Eating pineapple or taking bromelain, an anti-inflammatory enzyme found in pineapple, is also said to work against gout, but it hasn't been shown that bromelain can be absorbed intact into the bloodstream.

toe, other foot joints, knees, ankles, wrists, and fingers. The slightest touch—even that of a bedsheet—may prove to be unbearably painful during an attack of gout.

In North America, gout afflicts about 21 out of every 1,000 people, about half of whom are overweight. It is uncommon in women, especially before menopause.

Mistakenly, gout has had a persistent reputation for being the penalty to be paid for high living and overindulgence. In fact, gout is actually a type of arthritis that is caused by an inherited defect in the kidney's ability to excrete uric acid. This waste product of protein metabolism comes both from the digestive process and from the normal turnover of cells.

When deposits of uric acid crystals build up in the synovial fluid that surrounds the joints, the human body's immune system attempts to eliminate these crystals through the process of inflammation; unfortunately, this causes attacks of intense pain that can continue for days or even weeks if the condition is left untreated. Over time, uric acid crystals accumulate in the form of lumpy deposits under the skin of the ears, the elbows, and near the affected joints.

Gout attacks usually occur suddenly and unpredictably. The good news is that there are now several drugs available that will stop the pain and prevent any future attacks. Colchicine, a drug derived from the autumn crocus flower, is one of the fastest acting and most effective of these. Unfortunately, it can also cause severe nausea and diarrhea, which necessitate stopping the drug immediately. Before these side effects develop, however, the gout attack has usually abated, and the gout sufferer no longer needs to continue taking the medication.

Other, less toxic drugs are given on a long-term basis to prevent the onset of attacks; a flare-up is likely if these drugs are stopped, however. To reinforce the beneficial effect of drug treatment, people with gout should make dietary changes to help reduce their production of uric acid.

MANAGING GOUT WITH DIET

Lose weight gradually. Many people who have gout are obese; losing weight—especially fat around the abdomen—often prevents future attacks. Weight loss should be gradual, however, because a rapid reduction can raise blood levels of uric acid and provoke gout. Fasting increases the blood levels of uric acid, therefore, people with gout should avoid skipping meals. High-protein, low-carbohydrate diets should be avoided since these diets encourage the formation of ketones, metabolic by-products that hamper the body's ability to excrete uric acid.

You may have to modify your drug therapy. Sometimes gout is brought on by using aspirin or diuretics for high blood pressure. These medicines may interfere with normal kidney function and the elimination of uric acid. Your doctor may change treatment if you experience severe joint pain while on a drug therapy.

Avoid foods that are high in purines. Foods with a high content of naturally occurring chemicals called purines promote overproduction of uric acid in people with a tendency for gout. High-purine foods include anchovies, sardines, liver, kidney, brains, meat extracts, herring, mackerel, scallops, game, beer, and red wine; these should be avoided completely. Moderately high purine content is found in whole-grain cereals, wheat germ and wheat bran, oatmeal, dried beans and peas, nuts, asparagus, cauliflower, peas, and mushrooms; eat these in moderation.

Consume plenty of liquids. Try to drink at least 2 qt (2 liters) a day to dilute urine and prevent kidney stone formation. Although beer and wine, as products of fermentation, are the only alcoholic drinks known to be high in purines, any alcohol can interfere with the elimination of uric acid. Gout sufferers should drink only distilled alcohols in small amounts. Caffeinated beverages can also increase the production of uric acid and impair its removal from the body.

Eat fish rich in omega-3s. The omega-3 fatty acids in fish have been found to reduce pain and inflammation in people with rheumatoid arthritis and may have a similar benefit in gout, but this may be countered by the purine content of the fish.

Gout sufferers also may have hypertension, heart disease, diabetes, and high blood cholesterol. Counseling by a registered dietitian may help in designing appetizing, healthful meals that strike a balance between these health concerns and the enjoyment of food. ❖

GRAINS

BENEFITS

- An excellent source of starchy carbohydrate and dietary fiber.
- A good source of niacin, riboflavin, other B vitamins and iron.
- More economical than meat, fish, and other diet staples.

DRAWBACKS

- An incomplete source of protein.
- Gluten in some grain products provokes malabsorption symptoms in people who have celiac disease.

In this era of the low-carb diet, the health benefits of grains—whole grains, that is—are sometimes overlooked. Since prehistoric times, grain products have been one of the basic foodstuffs of agrarian societies. Almost every culture has a staple grain around which its cuisine is centered. Today, thanks to modern agricultural techniques and efficient transportation, we can sample a huge variety of grain products. Despite this proliferation of grains from around the world, we still tend to make the greatest use of our native wheat, which is ground into flour and made into bread and other baked goods. To a lesser extent, we also consume corn, rice, oats, barley, and millet, and many exotic grains.

Whole grains are rich in complex carbohydrates, fiber, and many vitamins and minerals.

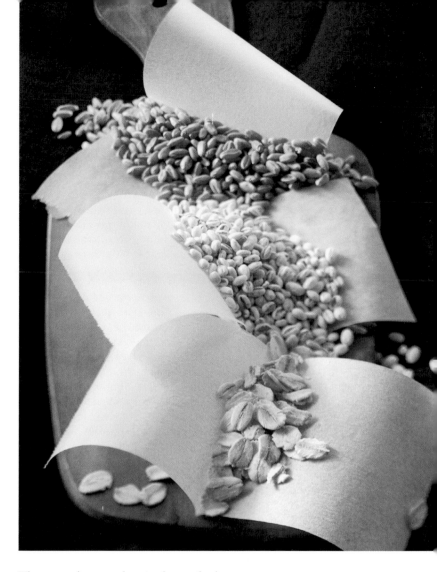

WHOLE GRAINS. *Grains such as wheat, barley, and oats can be added to soups and meat loaf to give the dishes a nutritional boost.*

THE WHOLE TRUTH
Whole Versus Refined Grains

Many of the valuable nutrients in grains are contained in the germ and outer covering that are removed during refining. In contrast, products made from whole grains retain most of their nutritive value; their high fiber content also adds texture and is filling. Refined grain products, including flours, breads, and breakfast cereals, are fortified with iron, thiamine, riboflavin, folate and niacin. Despite the additions, refined products still have less vitamins, minerals, and dietary fiber than whole-grain products. Whole grains contain B vitamins, vitamin E, and an assortment of phytochemicals including lignans, saponins, and plant sterols.

When shopping for whole grain breads and cereals, read labels carefully. Look for the words "whole-wheat flour" as the first ingredient. A product simply labeled "wheat flour" is actually white flour.

They are also very low in fat, and when eaten in combination with beans and other legumes, grains are a good source of complete protein.

Nutritionists urge us to eat more grain products as a healthy substitute for high-fat foods, and recommend we include plenty of grain-based starches, such as breads, cereals, pasta, and rice in our diets, along with dried beans, peas, and other legumes.

DIABETES, HEART DISEASE, AND CANCER PROTECTION

There is a growing awareness of the importance of the quality, as much as the quantity, of grains in the diet. An increased consumption of whole grains reduces the risk of developing type 2 diabetes and cardiovascular disease.

Data from the Physicians Health Study, in which more than 86,000 male physicians participated, showed a significant reduction in the risk of death from cardiovascular disease and death from all causes in the men eating the greatest quantity of whole-grain cereals compared with those of the men eating the fewest servings of whole-grain cereals.

The Iowa Women's Health Study followed almost 35,000 women aged 55 to 69 and found that the more whole grains eaten, the lower the risk of dying from heart disease. Another study found that adults with the highest intake of whole grains were 35 percent less likely to develop type 2 diabetes than those with the lowest intake. There is also growing evidence that eating whole grains instead of refined varieties can reduce your risk of developing cancer.

COMMON GRAIN PRODUCTS

Barley, a staple food in the Middle East, is known to North Americans mainly as a soup ingredient. It has a somewhat sweet taste that makes it an interesting addition to casseroles, pilafs, and salads. Barley is a source of soluble fiber as well as B vitamins and minerals such as zinc, iron, magnesium, and phosphorus.

Bulgur is cracked and roasted whole-wheat kernels; it has a nutty flavor and can be used to make pilaf or stuffing. Couscous is made from durum wheat, the hardest type, which contains the most gluten. It cooks fast and is light, making it a good choice for quick meals. Wheat berries are the whole kernels of wheat and can be used as a cereal or in baked goods.

Corn, or maize, and millet, an ancient grain of Asia and North Africa, are gluten-free; people with celiac disease can eat products made from them. Millet is made into tasty flat breads and can also be used in pilaf or as a stuffing for vegetables. Toasting millet in a dry skillet before cooking adds a nutty flavor.

Kamut is related to the wheat family, has more fiber and protein than many grains. Its buttery flavor makes it great in salads.

Oats are used in breakfast cereals and baked goods. Oat bran is high in soluble fiber, which can help lower blood cholesterol levels. It also helps the body utilize insulin more efficiently, an important asset in controlling diabetes.

Quinoa, an ancient grain, is lower in carbohydrate and higher in protein than most grains. This fluffy grain is sold as whole grain or as pasta and is great in salads. It is tolerated by people on gluten-free diets.

Rice is the staple food for about half the world's population. Brown rice is preferable, because it is unrefined and high in B vitamins and fiber. It also has some calcium and phosphorus. Long-grain brown rice is closer in taste to the refined white rice that most North Americans customarily eat. Short-grain brown

---

HOW GRAINS ARE PROCESSED

The methods in which grains are processed vary according to the specific grain and geographic area. The following techniques are used in industrialized countries.

Cracking. The grains are put through machines that crack or break them into smaller pieces, which cook more quickly than whole seeds.

Extracting oils. The oil-bearing germ of the grain is pressed or heated to extract the oil.

Extracting starches. The grain is first soaked in a solution containing sulfur dioxide or sodium hydroxide, ground to remove the bran, and then spun in a centrifuge machine to separate out the starch.

Flaking. The grains are cooked, dried, and rolled through machines to produce flakes of the desired shape and size. Sugar and flavorings may be added to make cereals.

Milling. The grains are sent into grinders or rollers to remove the hulls, bran, and seed germ; at this time, they may also be cracked or crushed into meal or flour.

Parboiling. The grains (usually rice but sometimes wheat) are boiled in water before milling.

Polishing and pearling. After the hulls are removed, an abrasive is used to shape the kernels.

Puffing. The grains are placed in hot rotating cylinders, or puffing guns. Alternatively, the grains are milled and made into a dough that is puffed in an oven.

Rolling. The grains are compressed between large rollers to flatten them, as in rolled oats, or to convert them into flakes.

Shredding. The grains (usually wheat) are cooked, dried, and then squeezed through a grooved cylinder to form long strands.

---

rice has a heartier texture and a nuttier flavor. White rice is stripped of its outer layers and is mostly starch with a little protein; some types are fortified with thiamine.

Rye contains some gluten, which is the reason rye bread and pumpernickel breads tend to be heavy and moist.

Wheat is one of the most widely consumed grains in the world. If, during milling, the bran (outer husk) and germ (located at the base of the grain) are removed, the end product is less nutritious than if left whole. Whole-grain wheat or whole wheat is a better choice, containing the bran as well as the germ of the wheat. The germ of the wheat kernel is a concentrated source of many nutrients including B vitamins, iron, zinc, phosphorus, potassium, and fiber. ❖

GRAPEFRUITS

BENEFITS

- High in vitamin C and potassium.
- Pink and red varieties contain beta carotene and lycopene, both powerful antioxidants.
- Low in calories.
- Contain bioflavonoids and other plant chemicals that protect against cancer and heart disease.

DRAWBACKS

- Can provoke an allergic reaction in people sensitive to citrus fruits.
- Grapefruit juice can reduce the effectiveness of certain medications.

Flavorful and nutritious—it's easy to understand why grapefruits are no longer just a breakfast option. Half a grapefruit provides more than 45 percent of the adult Recommendedmended Daily Allowance (RDA) of vitamin C; it also has 175 mg of potassium and 1 mg of iron. The pink and red varieties are high in beta carotene, which the body then converts to vitamin A.

A cup of unsweetened grapefruit juice has 95 mg of vitamin C, more than 100 percent of the RDA, and most of the other nutrients found in the fresh fruit. In the past, many people shunned the unsweetened grapefruit juice because of its tartness, but a naturally sweet juice can be made by using the red or pink grapefruits.

Over the years a number of fad diets have promoted the grapefruit as possessing a unique ability to burn away fat. There is no truth to these claims; no food can do this. People following grapefruit diets lose weight because they eat little else—a practice that can lead to nutritional deficiencies. Even so, grapefruits are a good food to include in a sensible weight-loss diet; a serving contains less than 100 calories, and its high-fiber content satisfies hunger.

Grapefruits are especially high in pectin, a soluble fiber that helps lower blood cholesterol. In addition, recent studies indicate that grapefruits contain other substances that prevent disease. Pink and red grapefruits, for example, are high in lycopene, an antioxidant that appears to lower the risk of prostate cancer. Researchers have not yet identified lycopene's mechanism of action, but a 6-year Harvard study involving 48,000 doctors and other health professionals has linked 10 servings of lycopene-rich foods a week with a 50 percent reduction in prostate cancer.

Other protective plant chemicals found in grapefruits include phenolic acid, which inhibits the formation of cancer-causing nitrosamines; limonoids, terpenes, and monoterpenes, which induce the production of enzymes that help prevent cancer; and bioflavonoids, which inhibit the action of hormones that promote tumor growth. Some people with rheumatoid arthritis, lupus, and other inflammatory disorders find that eating grapefruit daily seems to alleviate their symptoms. This may occur because plant chemicals block the prostaglandins that cause inflammation.

Those people who are allergic to other citrus fruits are likely to react to grapefruits, too. The sensitivity may be to the fruit itself or to an oil in the peel. ❖

INSTEAD OF WHITE, BUY PINK OR RED GRAPEFRUITS. *Pink or red pomelo grapefruits are high in lycopene, an antioxidant associated with reduced risk of prostate cancer.*

CAUTION

Grapefruit juice should not be used to take certain medications. Compounds in the juice enhance the effects of the drug, possibly resulting in adverse effects. Drugs to watch out for include the blood-pressure lowering medication felodipine, as well as drugs for anxiety, depression, high blood pressure, elevated lipids, and more. As a precaution, it is best to avoid taking any drug with grapefruit juice until you have asked your doctor or pharmacist if it is safe to do so.

GRAPES

BENEFITS

- High in pectin and bioflavonoids.
- Contain phytochemicals that may reduce risk for heart disease, cancer, and strokes.
- A fair source of iron and potassium.
- A low-calorie sweet snack and dessert.

DRAWBACKS

- Since they are often treated with sulfur dioxide to retard spoiling, grapes may present a problem for sulfite-sensitive people.
- Natural salicylates may provoke an allergic response.

One of the oldest and most abundant of the world's fruit crops, grapes are cultivated on six of the seven continents. Most of the 60 million metric tons grown worldwide annually are fermented to produce wine. Grapes are also made into jams and spreads, used in cooking, and eaten raw as a snack food.

Grapes are divided into two general categories: European, which encompasses most of the varieties used for table food and wine, and American, which have skins that slip off easily and are used mostly to make jams, jellies, and juice. The European type is the more nutritious of the two, but neither ranks high on the nutritional scale when compared to other fruits. A cup of European table grapes provides about 20 percent of the Recommended Daily Allowance (RDA) for vitamin C, about four times that found in the American varieties. Most types provide fair amounts of potassium and iron.

Low in calories, grapes are favored for their sweet, juicy flavor. Another reason for eating grapes may be found in research on the disease-prevention role of bioflavonoids and other plant chemicals. Anthocyanins found in red and blue grapes have numerous health benefits including lowering heart disease and cancer risk. Grapes contain quercetin, a plant pigment that is thought to regulate the levels of blood cholesterol and also reduce the action of platelets, blood cells that are instrumental in forming clots. Some researchers theorize that it is quercetin that lowers the risk of heart attack among moderate wine drinkers. The skin of grapes contains resveratrol, a phytochemical that is linked to a reduction of heart disease as well as a lowered risk of cancer or stroke. Grapes also contain ellagic acid thought to protect the lungs against environmental toxins. To reap the full benefit of grapes, it is best to select red or purple varieties, which seem to contain the highest concentration of healthful compounds. Commercially grown grapes are usually sprayed with pesticides and are treated with sulfur dioxide to preserve their color and extend shelf life; they should always be washed before being eaten. People with asthma should either avoid grapes or look for those that have not been treated with sulfur. Grapes naturally contain salicylates, compounds similar to the major ingredient in aspirin. Salicylates have an anticlotting effect and may account for the benefits of wine with respect to heart disease. People who are allergic to aspirin may react to grapes and grape products. ❖

BENEFICIAL GRAPES. *You don't need to drink wine to derive protection from heart disease. Red grapes offer similar benefits.*

DID YOU KNOW?

RAISINS ARE VERY HIGH IN CALORIES

Raisins are a highly concentrated source of nutrients and calories; a cup contains a whopping 440 calories while providing 3 g of iron, 1,090 mg of potassium, and 6 g of fiber. It takes about 4½ pounds (2 kg) of fresh grapes to produce 1 lb (500 g) of raisins.

GRILLED FOODS
■ EXAMINING THE RISKS ■

Grilling has been a popular method of cooking for thousands of years. Grilled foods retain a lot of flavor and cooking them doesn't require added fats. Vegetables cook quickly on the grill with little loss of moisture or vitamins. In short, grilling is a truly healthful cooking method—with one potentially major caveat.

Caveman cooking

Involving direct exposure of food to the source of heat, grilling or broiling is the modern and controlled version of man's oldest culinary technique—namely, roasting over an open fire. The intense flavor of grilled food results from the numerous chemical reactions that take place when a food surface is subjected to very high temperatures. Grilling—whether by gas flame, electric element, or charcoal—demands temperatures four to six times higher than can be reached in an oven; an electric broiler heats to about 2,000°F (1,090°C) and a gas flame to about 3,000°F (1,650°C), compared with a maximum of 500°F (260°C) for domestic ovens. Unfortunately, the high heat that causes the appealing caramelization of browning has a less desirable aspect: the outside of the food may become unpalatably charred before the inside is cooked through. Grilling is best reserved, therefore, for quick-cooking foods, such as fish and the thinner cuts of meat and poultry. It is an excellent method of preparing such vegetables as eggplant, zucchini, peppers, and mushrooms; apples, peaches, and other fruits are also delicious when grilled. Pre-grill preparation requires little more than a light brushing with oil to prevent food from sticking to the grill or drying out, followed by a dusting of herbs.

The downside of grilling

At grilling temperatures, the surface fat on meat quickly burns away, releasing acrid fumes and creating a risk of fire. There's a further hazard to grilling. Cancer-causing substances called polycyclic aromatic hydrocarbons form when the fat from meat drips onto hot coals and are deposited onto

CAUTION

Even if there are lots of hungry guests waiting for burgers from the barbeque, don't take them off the grill until they're thoroughly cooked. Ground beef could have come in contact with *E. coli* 0157 bacteria, which is present in the intestines of cattle, and may infect the meat during processing. Potentially harmful bacteria are killed when the meat is adequately cooked, but can survive in meat that is rare. Always cook hamburgers until the juice runs clear and be sure not to place cooked hamburgers back on the same platter that held raw meat.

the food through smoke. You can minimize exposure to the fumes by partly baking or parboiling the food, then finishing it off with a few minutes on the grill to achieve a crusty exterior and succulent interior. Choose lean cuts, and trim all visible fat from meat. Whether you're using an oven broiler or an outdoor grill, place a broiling pan to catch melted fat under a spatterproof metal shield.

Heating meat, poultry, and fish to a high temperature also creates substances called heterocyclic amines (HCAs), which have been linked to cancer in animals. HCAs can also form in foods—especially red meat—that are fried or broiled. This may be one reason that frequent consumption of red meat has been linked, at least in some studies, with an increased risk for certain cancers, such as colon cancer.

Other potentially toxic compounds are generated by chemical reactions that take place when foods are cooked at high temperatures. Carcinogenic nitrosamines, for example, form when foods that contain nitrite as a preservative are heated.

There's no direct evidence that substances causing cancer in animals necessarily cause the disease in humans, but there is enough epidemiological evidence to suggest that foods cooked at a high temperature should be consumed in moderation.

Combine protective foods and nutrients as a precaution

The risks of eating grilled foods can be modulated by combining them with certain protective nutrients. Vitamins C and E, for example, block the chemical reaction that generates nitrosamines. As antioxidants, these vitamins, as well as beta carotene, can neutralize some carcinogens. Wheat bran binds with nitrite and makes it unavailable for nitrosamine formation. So, you can balance your grilled breakfast bacon with a glass of vitamin C-rich citrus juice and fortified whole-grain cereal or a bran muffin for vitamin E.

Substances found in vegetables and fruits bind directly to carcinogens, such as the polycyclic hydrocarbons, and prevent them from reacting with DNA. Bioflavonoids, the pigments in many fruits and vegetables, appear to block many carcinogens. Fiber may bind with or dilute carcinogens and speed their elimination from the digestive tract. When you barbecue, serve lots of leafy greens and whole grains along with the meat or fish to ensure a healthy mixture of fiber and vitamins. Make a vegetarian barbecue; add low-fat cheese to satisfy a desire for protein. Grilled fruits end a meal with a colorful cocktail of vitamins, fiber, and flavor.

A warning about marinades

Marinades can add exotic flavors. A small amount of honey or other sugar in the marinade will hasten the caramelization process because simple sugars brown at lower temperatures than proteins and starchy foods do. But don't make the mistake of assuming that a marinated meat is cooked just because the outside is browned. And despite the instructions in many recipes to marinate for hours, there's nothing to be gained from prolonged marination. The marinade cannot penetrate past the surface of the meat, no matter how long the meat is soaked. In addition, the acid of the marinade will eventually tenderize the surface of the meat by denaturing the surface proteins. When left too long in the marinade, your meat will come off the grill with a flavorful but mushy outer layer that contrasts unpleasantly with the inner texture.

Minimizing your cancer risk

Charcoal-grilling foods, especially fatty meats, can create compounds that are potentially carcinogenic. The factors involved are the charring of the food and the smoke produced when fat drips on the coals, which is then carried back up to the meat. To minimize the risks, take the following steps:

1. Avoid flare-ups, since burning juice or fat can produce harmful smoke. If smoke from dripping fat is too heavy, move the food to another section of the grill, rotate the grill, or reduce the heat.
2. Cook meat until it is done without charring it. Remove any charred pieces—don't eat them.
3. Don't place the heat source directly under the meat. For example, place coals slightly to the side so the fat doesn't drip on them. Keep a water bottle handy for coals that become hot or flare up.
4. Cover the grill with punctured aluminum foil before you cook. The foil protects the food from the smoke and fire.
5. Keep meat portions small so they don't have to spend as long on the grill.
6. Defrost frozen meats before grilling. In trying to get the frozen meat cooked, there is a tendency to burn the surface.

GUAVAS

BENEFITS

- An excellent source of vitamin C.
- High in pectin and other types of soluble dietary fiber.
- Good amounts of potassium and iron.

DRAWBACKS

- Fresh fruit is expensive and not widely available.
- Sulfites in dried guavas may provoke an asthma attack or allergic reaction in susceptible persons.

A small tropical fruit that originated in southern Mexico and Central America, the guava now is native to the Caribbean and South America and is grown in Florida, California, Hawaii, southern Asia, and parts of Africa. The fruit can be round, ovoid, or pear-shaped and ranges in size from 1 to 4 in. (2.5–10 cm) in diameter. The thin skins, which vary in color from pale yellow to yellow-green, have a slightly bitter taste, so the fruit is usually served peeled. Most varieties have meaty deep-pink flesh, although some are yellow, red, or white. Ripe guavas have a fragrant, musky aroma and a sweet flavor, with hints of pineapple or banana.

By weight, guavas have almost twice as much vitamin C as an orange: One medium guava provides 165 mg, compared to only 75 mg in a fresh orange. One guava also contains 256 mg of potassium and 5 g of fiber; much of it is in the form of pectin, a soluble fiber that lowers high blood cholesterol as well as promoting good digestive function. Folate, phosphorus, and carotene are also present.

About half of the guava fruit is filled with small, hard seeds. Actual seed counts have ranged from 112 to 535. Although in good varieties the seeds are fully edible, most people discard them. If the seeds are eaten, they contribute extra fiber and lesser amounts of the same nutrients found in the flesh.

A VERSATILE FRUIT

With only about 60 calories per fresh guava, the fruit makes an easy, interesting, nonfattening dessert. Simply cut the fruit in half, scoop out the seeds, then spoon out the flesh. A dash of lime juice or lemon juice contrasts nicely with the sweet flavor. Alternatively, you can peel, seed, and chop or slice guavas to add to a fruit salad. Pureed guava flesh in combination with orange or other citrus juice makes a refreshing drink or cold summer soup. Unripe guavas, which are a little too tart and astringent to be eaten raw, can be blended and cooked with defatted meat juice to make a low-calorie sauce for roasts and poultry dishes.

Look for fresh guavas during the late fall and early winter. When selecting guavas, choose fruits that are firm but not hard. A guava is ripe when the skin yields slightly when pressed. As with almost any fruit, flavor is best when the guava is allowed to ripen on the tree, but green mature fruit will ripen at room temperature. Placing the fruit in a brown paper bag with a banana or apple will hasten ripening.

Gourmet sections in supermarkets carry increasing numbers of guava products—jams, jellies, dried sheets, nectar, and a type of fruit paste called guava cheese. Canned guava is also available, but it is usually processed with large amounts of sugar. Dried guavas are often treated with sulfites, which may provoke asthma attacks or allergic reactions in susceptible persons. Dehydrated guavas are powdered and added to ice cream, candies, and fruit juices for extra flavor. ❖

GUAVA'S CLAIM TO FAME

The city of Tampa, Florida, has paid homage to the guava by nicknaming itself "Big Guava." The variety of the fruit grown here is yellow and pear-shaped. The historic Ybor City district of Tampa even has guava-cooking contests featuring such delicacies as pickled guavas, jellies, and guava cheese, which is eaten like candy. Ybor City also honors the lowly guava by celebrating Guavaween, fashioned after Mardi Gras, instead of Halloween.

EXOTIC FRUIT. *The acid-sweet taste and pungent aroma of guavas evoke images of a tropical paradise. Although the entire fruit is edible when fully ripe, many people discard the seeds and skins.*

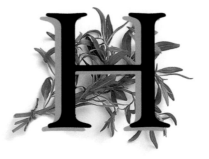

HAIR AND SCALP PROBLEMS

EAT PLENTY OF

- Fruits and vegetables.
- Whole grains.
- Lean meat, fish, and poultry and low-fat dairy products.

Baldness and dandruff are among the most pervasive hair and scalp problems. Hair loss may be either the result of illness or a normal genetic response to testosterone, the male sex hormone. Dandruff—excessive scaling of the scalp—affects more than 50 percent of the population. It may be due to stress or a chronic or recurrent skin disorder, such as seborrheic dermatitis, but the most likely cause is infection by *Pytyrosporum ovale* fungus. This fungus is found naturally on the scalp but some people are more affected by it than others. It feeds on the skin's natural oils and causes irritation and shedding of dead skin.

Hair is composed of the protein keratin. Other nutrients that contribute to hair and scalp health include niacin, biotin, zinc, and vitamins A, B_6, and C. A varied diet based on the basic food groups should provide ample amounts of these nutrients. Because hair is inert material, shampoos and rinses enriched with protein or other nutrients cannot affect hair growth or make hair "healthier."

HAIR LOSS

A healthy human head has from 80,000 to 150,000 hairs, each of which passes through three phases of growth independently of all the others. At any time, 90 percent of the hairs are in the growing stage (anagen), which lasts anywhere from 1 to 5 years. Growth is followed by a resting phase (telogen); this ends after a few months, after which the hair is shed (catagen) to allow new growth. A daily loss of 50 to 200 hairs is a normal part of the cycle.

Although baldness is mediated by hormonal factors, it tends to run in families; your risk may be deduced from the number of bald males among members of both parents' families.

Abnormal hair loss may be precipitated by metabolic disorders (including diabetes, thyroid disease, and crash diets); damage to hair shafts caused by harsh treatments; stress brought on by illness; hormonal changes of pregnancy; medical treatment, including cancer chemotherapy; and very severe scalp disorders.

When diet is involved, the cause may be a grossly excessive intake of vitamin A or a deficiency of iron, biotin, zinc, or protein. Such deficiencies are rare, although an excessive intake of raw egg whites can lead to a depletion of biotin.

Hair loss due to stress or drug treatment is generally temporary. Hair that falls out during a crash diet soon regrows once nutrition returns to normal. Hair lost in patches usually grows back without treatment, but in some instances, corticosteroid injections may be needed. The only medicines for baldness are minoxidil (Rogaine), a topical medicine, and finasteride (Propecia), an oral prescription drug.

DANDRUFF

Many people shed flakes of dandruff, especially in winter, when the scalp may be dry. But some people have a hereditary tendency to develop skin problems that are triggered by a sensitivity to specific foods. Because the offending food varies from one person to the next, the only reasonable advice is to avoid foods that seem to make dandruff worse. Some cases of dandruff may respond to flaxseed oil, which seems to help itchy skin conditions such as psoriasis and eczema. Take 1 to 2 teaspoons a day. You'll need to wait several weeks or months to see an effect.

To control mild dandruff, doctors usually recommend shampooing daily until the dandruff is

MYTH BUSTER

Myth: Hair analysis cannot determine nutritional deficiencies—any such claim is worthless.

Reality: Scientific analysis of hair can confirm the presence of certain toxic elements—even years later. (Hair analysis was used 150 years after Napoleon's death to confirm that he suffered chronic arsenic poisoning.)

DID YOU KNOW?

SOME FOODS PROMOTE DANDRUFF

Some people's dandruff improves when they shun foods that cause the face and scalp to flush; typical offenders are hot liquids, heavily spiced foods, and alcohol.

under control, followed by twice weekly for maintenance. Dandruff shampoos contain zinc pyrithione, tar, or selenium sulfide, all of which work as exfoliants to hasten the shedding of the dead cell layer from the scalp. If these do not work well, shampoos that contain the antifungal medication ketoconazole can be tried. ❖

HAMBURGERS

See Fast Food

HAY FEVER

EAT PLENTY OF

- Fatty fish and other foods high in omega-3 fatty acids for their anti-inflammatory effect.

AVOID

- Honey and bee pollen capsules.
- Any food in the same plant family as sunflowers (the Compositae family).
- Fermented foods or those with molds if fungi spores trigger symptoms.

Hay fever is a seasonal allergy triggered by the inhalation of pollen or, less commonly, molds. Medically known as seasonal or allergic rhinitis, the popular name of hay fever is a misnomer: Although symptoms may occur during the haying season, hay itself is not the culprit, nor is there a fever.

Ragweed is one of the most common offenders, but in susceptible people, tree, grass, and flower pollens can also cause the sneezing, runny nose, tearing eyes, itchiness, and other hay fever symptoms. In general, these symptoms are more irritating than serious. This is not the case for people with asthma, however; for them, hay fever can provoke repeated, sometimes life-threatening attacks.

Stay away from foods in the sunflower plant family. Although foods aren't ordinarily associated with hay fever, people with certain types of seasonal allergies may experience symptoms after eating particular foods. For example, plants in the sunflower, or Compositae, family have antigens that cross-react with members of the Ambrosiaceae family, which includes ragweed. Thus, a person whose hay fever symptoms are triggered by ragweed may react to ingestion of any of a broad variety of herbs and vegetables in the sunflower family.

Watch out for honey. Contaminants or pollens in some foods can also trigger the onset of hay fever symptoms. This is especially true of honey, which may harbor bits of pollen, and bee pollen capsules, a food supplement and natural remedy that is sold in health-food stores.

Eat more omega-3s. There is no special diet that will alleviate hay fever symptoms, although some recent reports suggest that eating fatty fish and other foods that are high in omega-3 fatty acids may reduce the inflammation that is part of an allergic reaction. More research is necessary to confirm this; in the meantime, consumption of fish is still an important part of a varied and balanced diet.

MOLD AS THE CULPRIT

In some people seasonal allergies are triggered by mold spores instead of (or in addition to) pollen. Typically, these people suffer a flare-up of hay fever symptoms when it is cool and damp: usually, beginning in the spring, improving somewhat during the summer, and then worsening again during the damp fall season. Although most mold spores are outdoors, some also grow in dark, moist indoor areas, especially in basements, shower stalls, refrigerator drip trays, air conditioners, and garbage cans. Symptoms generally occur after inhaling the spores, but in some people eating foods and beverages that harbor molds also provokes a flare-up.

Items that should be avoided include:

- Alcoholic beverages, especially beer, wine, and other drinks made by fermentation processes.
- Breads made with lots of yeast or the sourdough varieties.
- Cheeses, especially blue cheese.
- Dried fruits, including raisins and others that are allowed to dry outdoors.
- Mushrooms of all kinds.
- Processed meats and fish, including hot dogs, sausages, and smoked fish.
- Sauerkraut and other fermented or pickled foods, including soy sauce.
- Vinegar and products made with it: salad dressings, mayonnaise, ketchup, and pickles. ❖

IF YOU SUFFER FROM RAGWEED HAY FEVER…

You should avoid the following plant foods:

- Artichokes
- Chamomile (used in herbal teas and medicines)
- Chicory
- Dandelions
- Endives
- Escarole
- Jerusalem artichokes
- Oyster plants (salsify)
- Safflower (used in many vegetable oils and margarines)
- Sunflower seeds and oil
- Tansy (used in some herbal medicines and folk remedies)
- Tarragon

HERBS
■ ENHANCE YOUR DIET ■

Many people think of herbs as medicine used only by alternative practitioners who do not use conventional medical practices. But in fact, herbal medicine is a precursor of modern pharmacology. About one-fourth of all prescription medicines come from herbs and other plants. And many physicians and researchers are taking a new look at traditional herbal remedies.

Unfortunately, there are some misconceptions about the benefits and safety of herbal medicines. Many people assume that because herbal remedies are made from natural ingredients they are safer than synthetic drugs. In reality, some herbal medicines—just like their pharmaceutical counterparts—can have adverse effects. Some are even highly toxic. In addition, herbal remedies are not subject to the same rigorous testing and standards that are required for pharmaceutical products.

A long history

Every society has relied on the healing power of herbs to treat illness, and in some cultures, herbal medicine still prevails. Traditional Chinese healers and Ayurvedic practitioners, for example, continue to use ancient herbal remedies, although these may be combined with modern medical treatments. In Western societies most medicines are synthesized, including many that were originally made from herbs. But there are exceptions: digitalis, the oldest effective heart medication, is still made from foxglove; morphine and codeine are derived from opium poppies; and vincristine, used to treat leukemia, comes from the Madagascar periwinkle.

Medicinal herbs

Interest in medicinal herbs has grown dramatically in recent years. Consumers now have a wide variety of herbal supplements to choose from to help prevent and treat many diseases, including heart disease, cancer, arthritis, low immunity, depression, common colds, and menopausal concerns. But along with greater choice has come a lot of confusion. With store shelves filled with such a vast array of products, how does a consumer choose wisely? Use the checklist at left.

Popular medicinal herb products

The list of medicinal herbs continues to grow. The following are getting a lot of attention:

Aloe vera. The leaves of this succulent plant exude a soothing gel that is effective when used externally to treat minor burns (including sunburn), cuts, insect bites, and stings. Some herbalists recommend taking the juice internally as a tonic or to treat inflammatory digestive disorders, but there is little research on its internal use.

Smart consumer checklist for purchasing herbal products

✔ Start cautiously. Just because herbs are natural doesn't mean they're always safe.
✔ Choose the right form. There are five common ways herbs are sold:
1. Teas are the least expensive and mildest; best choice for those with poor digestion.
2. Tinctures are the strongest with the longest shelf life and are easily absorbed.
3. Capsules are convenient, but have a shorter shelf life. Check expiration dates.
4. Tablets mask the taste of herbs, but binders and fillers may dilute the medicine.
5. Standardized herbs come in many forms, but are often expensive. Potency is assured.
✔ Start with lowest recommended dose.
✔ Teas and tinctures should be taken on an empty stomach for better absorption.
✔ Capsules and tablets should be taken with meals.
✔ Seek advice. If in doubt, ask a doctor.

Bilberry. Bilberry extract is the leading herbal remedy for maintaining healthy vision and treating various eye disorders, including macular degeneration, as well as treating night blindness and poor vision from daytime glare. Bilberry's medicinal properties are derived mainly from one of its major components, anthocyanins, which are powerful antioxidants.

Echinacea. Some preparations made from the purple coneflower can increase immune function and help reduce the severity of viral infections such as the common cold. Studies differ on the effectiveness of echinacea, which isn't surprising. There are many species of the plant, and the chemical composition of a product will differ depending on whether the leaves, stems, or root were used in the preparation, and the solvent used. Since it does increase immune function, people with autoimmune diseases such as arthritis, multiple sclerosis, or lupus may react adversely to echinacea.

Feverfew. This herb reduces the frequency and intensity of migraines by preventing the release of prostaglandins, which dilate blood vessels and cause inflammation. Though it is effective as a preventative, it cannot relieve a migraine once it occurs.

Ginkgo biloba. This herbal remedy is said to improve memory problems related to aging. Recent studies show that it does increase blood flow to the brain, as well as to the arms and legs, by regulating the tone and elasticity of blood vessels. Current research is looking at whether ginkgo's ability to prevent blood clots may help prevent heart attacks and stroke. Because it has an anticoagulant effect, ginkgo should not be taken concurrently with "blood thinners."

Ginseng. The Chinese have long used ginseng to strengthen the immune system, alleviate fever and pain, promote wound healing, overcome depression and fatigue, and treat impotence. There is little scientific evidence to back up the claims.

Hawthorn. This herb, used in the past as both a diuretic and a treatment for kidney and bladder stones, is currently one of the most widely prescribed heart remedies in Europe. It can dilate blood vessels, increase the heart's energy supply, and improve its pumping ability.

Licorice. This well-studied herb stimulates the adrenal glands, reduces inflammation, and can increase the level of interferon, a virus-fighting substance made by the immune system. It is helpful for respiratory problems, coughs and sore throats, and has been used to treat chronic fatigue, fibromyalgia, and other disorders affected by the body's levels of cortisol, the main adrenal hormone. High doses can deplete potassium reserves and raise blood pressure (except for the form of licorice called DGL).

Milk thistle. Well known for treatment of liver-related disorders, this herb protects the liver from toxins including drugs, poisons, and other chemicals. It may be effective in the treatment of cirrhosis and hepatitis, and can reduce liver damage from excessive alcohol. It can promote the regeneration of healthy, new liver cells.

Nettle. One of the benefits of nettle is its ability to control hay fever symptoms such as nasal congestion and watery eyes. It is a good source of quercetin, a flavonoid that has been shown to inhibit the release of histamine. Nettle acts as a diuretic, so it can help rid the body of excess fluid.

St. John's wort. Used to treat cases of mild depression, it is believed to boost levels of serotonin, which affects mood and emotions. The herb may also be helpful for conditions related to depression, such as anxiety, stress, premenstrual syndrome, fibromyalgia, and insomnia. It can cross-react with a number of prescription drugs and reduce their effectiveness.

MYTH BUSTER

Myth: Basil causes cancer.

Reality: When estragole, a naturally occurring compound in basil, is fed to test animals in large doses, it causes cancer and therefore can be accurately labeled as a carcinogen. The dose of estragole ingested from even vast quantities of basil would be way too small to cause concern.

Culinary herbs

Culinary herbs are not as potent as medicinal herbs, but many confer some health benefits. They provide a wide variety of active phytochemicals that promote health and protect against chronic diseases.

Basil. A mainstay in many dishes, basil is also used in larger quantities as a tonic and cold remedy.

Chives. These tiny onion relatives contain sulfur compounds that may lower blood pressure if eaten in large amounts.

Coriander. Pungent fresh leaves or seeds may be chewed to ease indigestion.

Dill. Widely used in pickles, salad dressings, and fish dishes, dill is also eaten to alleviate intestinal gas. Europeans often give babies weak dill tea to relieve colic.

Mint. Chewing the leaves can freshen breath; mint tea is a digestive aid.

Oregano. Brewed as tea, it is said to aid digestion and alleviate the congestion.

Parsley. When consumed in portions of at least 1 oz (30 g), this herb contains useful amounts of vitamin C (fresh parsley only), calcium, iron, and potassium. Parsley is also high in bioflavonoids, monoterpenes, and other anticancer compounds.

Rosemary. Its leaves contain an oil used in liniments to relieve muscle aches. Rosemary tea is said to alleviate headaches.

Sage. Sage tea can be used as a digestive aid; as a mouthwash or gargle to ease painful gums, mouth ulcers, or sore throat. Some research indicates that sage oil can boost acetylcholine levels in the brain, improving memory.

Thyme. Brewed as tea to quiet irritable bowels, as a gargle for a sore throat, or as syrup for a cough or congestion.

HERPES

EAT
- A well-balanced, nutritious diet, with plenty of whole grains, fresh fruits and vegetables, and high-quality protein for a strong immune system.

LIMIT
- Alcohol and caffeine.

AVOID
- Smoking.
- Excessive sun exposure.

A common and highly contagious infectious disease, herpes is caused by strains of the herpes simplex virus and is noted by painful and itchy blisters. Type 1 herpes, or oral herpes, causes cold sores or fever blisters around the mouth. In some cases, this type of herpes infects the eyes and can result in blindness or, even more seriously, can spread to the brain and result in life-threatening herpes encephalitis. Type 2, or genital herpes, is sexually transmitted and causes sores in the genital and anal areas. Engaging in oral sex with an infected person can cause mouth and throat blisters that are difficult to differentiate from type 1 herpes.

Regardless of the type or location, herpes blisters usually rupture into open weeping sores that crust over and eventually heal within a few days or weeks. Some people also experience a mild fever, swollen lymph nodes, and fatigue. Even after healing, the virus remains dormant in the body; some people never have another attack, while others have repeated but milder eruptions sporadically throughout their lives.

Recurrences may be triggered by hormonal changes, physical or emotional stress, fever, exposure to the sun, or other environmental factors. Certain foods and drugs precipitate recurrences in susceptible people. If you have frequent attacks, analyze your lifestyle and try to figure out what specific triggers may have precipitated them.

Although there is no known cure for herpes, some sufferers have reported relief when taking lysine, an amino acid supplement usually sold in health-food stores in the United States (but not in Canada). To help reduce the frequency of herpes attacks, some advocates of natural medicine recommend taking 500 mg to 1,000 mg of L-lysine daily, on an empty stomach. This amino acid is also found in meat, fish, chicken, and dairy products. In more severe herpes cases, doctors prescribe acyclovir, an antiviral medication that can be taken orally or used as a cream. Acyclovir can shorten the duration of an attack and help prevent a recurrence.

Warning: A pregnant woman who has had herpes should inform her obstetrician immediately. An active infection may be transmitted to the baby during delivery and can cause blindness, retardation, even death. A cesarean delivery can prevent transmission.

SELF-CARE

If you have a warning symptom before an outbreak of oral herpes, prompt use of aspirin and ice packs sometimes forestalls the recurrence. Once the lesions appear, compresses of cold water or milk may ease the discomfort. To help protect others from infection, avoid kissing anyone or sharing dishes or utensils during outbreaks.

For genital outbreaks, warm baths or saltwater compresses can help ease inflammation. Keep the infected area clean and dry. Wash your hands after contact with the sores to avoid spreading infection to other parts of your body. Type 2 herpes is very contagious; those infected should never have sexual contact with noninfected persons during an attack. Always tell any prospective sexual partner that you are infected with herpes. Latex condoms may lower, but cannot eliminate, risk of sexual transmission.

Eat a nutritious diet. To help prevent recurrences, strengthen your immune system to resist disease by eating a well-balanced diet with plenty of whole grains, fresh fruits and vegetables, and get enough protein. Don't smoke; avoid excessive alcohol and caffeine. Balance your lifestyle with regular exercise and adequate rest to alleviate stress. Avoid excessive sun exposure, and always wear a sunscreen. It is important that you do not take high doses of vitamin C; studies indicate these can actually provoke a recurrence of herpes. ❖

DO ONE SIMPLE THING

EAT FOODS RICH IN LYSINE

Foods high in the amino acid lysine, found in meat and fish, milk and dairy products, may help to reduce the frequency of herpes attacks.

THE YOGURT APPROACH

Anecdotal evidence suggests that *Lactobacillus acidophilus*, found in certain yogurts containing live or "active" cultures and also sold in capsule form, may help prevent recurrences of cold sores. You may need to take supplements to get a therapeutic dose.

HIATAL HERNIA

EAT

- Small, frequent meals.
- High-fiber foods, such as whole-grain cereals and breads, fresh fruits, salads, and raw or lightly cooked vegetables.

LIMIT

- Coffee and alcohol, including wine, especially before bedtime.

AVOID

- Gaining excess weight.
- Large meals and carbonated beverages.
- Fatty foods, chocolate, and peppermint.
- Alcohol.
- Smoking.
- Any food that produces symptoms.

Under normal circumstances, the hiatus is a small opening in the muscular diaphragm at the juncture where the esophagus meets the stomach. A hiatal hernia develops when the opening widens and allows the upper part of the stomach to protrude upward through the hiatus. Some hiatal hernias are present at birth. Most of them, however, develop during life as the opening of the hiatus becomes stretched, often as a result of pregnancy or excessive weight gain, both of which place upward pressure on the stomach. Severe coughing, vomiting, straining when moving the bowels, or sudden physical exertion may also stretch the hiatus.

Although hiatal hernias are quite common, occurring in almost half of the North American population, most people are unaware of the condition because they don't experience symptoms. A hiatal hernia is usually diagnosed after recurring bouts of indigestion and heartburn, typically as a result of acid reflux into the esophagus. The condition is usually not considered serious. There are, however, exceptions in which frequent exposure to stomach acids causes severe esophageal damage. In such cases, surgical treatment is necessary.

DIETARY APPROACHES

Avoid large meals that overly distend the stomach. Eat four or five small meals spread over the course of a day. In addition, try to avoid drinking carbonated beverages, which may increase discomfort. After eating, do not lie down, stoop, or bend over for at least an hour, because this may promote reflux. Do not try to eat or drink anything for at least 2 hours before going to bed at night, when attacks are most likely to occur.

Avoid substances that relax the diaphragmatic muscle. Alcohol, including wine, is one such muscle relaxant; in particular, abstain from any alcoholic beverage in the evening.

Avoid spicy and acidic foods. Eliminate foods that tend to irritate your stomach or provoke a bout of indigestion. The culprits vary from one person to another, but common offenders include spices, citrus fruits, tomatoes, onions, garlic, pickles, and vinegar. Coffee in any form increases stomach acidity, as does tobacco. Chocolate and peppermint tend to relax the hiatal sphincter; fatty foods stay in the stomach longer than other foods and can also provoke indigestion. Small sips of water or a warm herbal tea may be useful when you feel a bout of regurgitation coming on, but avoid antacids that contain peppermint.

Eat lots of fiber and drink plenty of fluids. Constipation can worsen a hiatal hernia because straining distends the abdomen. Eat plenty of high-fiber foods, such as whole-grain cereals and breads, as well as fresh vegetables and fruits. Daily exercise and an adequate fluid intake are also important.

People who experience frequent nighttime symptoms of a hiatal hernia can try raising the head of their bed 3 to 6 in. (8–15 cm).

If lifestyle modification and conservative medical treatment do not alleviate symptoms, prescription drugs or surgery may be recommended to reposition the stomach below the diaphragm and to narrow the hiatal opening. ❖

HIVES

AVOID

- Foods that have previously caused hives or other allergic reactions.
- Foods and medications colored with Yellow No. 5 (tartrazine) if you are sensitive to this additive.
- Foods that contain salicylate if you are allergic to aspirin.

Medically known as urticaria, hives are the itchy red welts that develop as a result of reactions to foods and other provoking substances. For example, certain medications—aspirin, as well as penicillin and related antibiotics—can

TIPS FOR DEALING WITH HIATAL HERNIAS

- Don't lie down after you eat. Try to wait at least 3 hours before taking a nap or going to bed for the night.
- Don't exercise right after eating. Walking is fine, but wait 2 to 3 hours before strenuous exercise.
- Don't wear tight-fitting clothes. They put extra pressure on your stomach.
- Relax. Stress slows down the digestion, which makes acid reflux worse. Try deep breathing, yoga, or meditation to deal with daily stress.

cause hives in some people. Even those without known allergies can develop hives after being stung by an insect or touching stinging plants, such as nettles, poison oak, or poison ivy. Hives may be accompanied by other symptoms of allergy, including swelling of the eyes and other parts of the body. Many food allergies provoke swelling and itching of the lips and mouth.

Warning: If hives are accompanied by swelling of the throat and difficulty breathing, speaking, or swallowing, seek immediate medical help. These symptoms may signal anaphylaxis, a potentially fatal medical emergency.

WELL-KNOWN CAUSES OF HIVES

The blotchy rash of hives can follow ingestion of almost any food, but among the most common causes are shellfish, nuts, and berries. A person who is allergic to aspirin (acetylsalicylic acid) should also be wary of foods that contain natural salicylates. These include apricots, berries, grapes, raisins and other dried fruits, tea, and foods processed with vinegar. Among the other well-known triggers of hives are emotional stress; exposure to sunshine, heat, or cold (even ice cubes in drinks); and viral infections.

Hives generally develop within hours after exposure to a trigger, but in unusual cases, they may appear several days later. This delayed reaction can make it difficult to identify the offending substance. Delayed reactions are most common with medications; if you develop a rash while taking any drug, report it to your doctor immediately. Medication-related rashes usually start around the head and spread progressively downward. Sometimes a drug allergy develops abruptly after months or even years of taking a medication. Always mention your sensitivity to the pharmacist and any doctor who may prescribe medications for you.

Check food labels to avoid tartrazine. Although food additives are often blamed for causing allergic reactions, only tartrazine (Yellow No. 5), a common coloring agent, has been found to cause hives— and in fewer than 1 out of 10,000 people. All product labels must list food colorants; people who are sensitive to tartrazine should read labels on food products, medications, and vitamin supplements.

NATURE'S BANDAGE

In the days before antibiotics, doctors sometimes treated wounds with honey. Why? Honey has considerable antibacterial properties. It's still considered an excellent wound dressing in some cases, and it dries to form a natural bandage. Several studies of surgical wounds have shown that honey speeds healing. Some manufacturers even sell honey-infused dressings for hard-to-heal wounds. A form of honey called manuka honey, produced in New Zealand from the manuka tree, is said to have antiulcer properties, probably because it kills the bacteria that cause most ulcers.

DEALING WITH HIVES

An outbreak of hives may fade within minutes or persist for days or weeks. If you can link a particular food to hives, avoid it and consult a doctor. When hives persist for more than a few days, a doctor may prescribe an antihistamine medication, as well as a lotion to reduce itching and relieve inflammation. If you get hives repeatedly, the doctor may suggest that you keep a food diary; once you identify the suspect foods, eliminate them from your regular diet, then reintroduce them one at a time to pinpoint the problem.

Eat foods that are high in niacin. Since hives and other allergy symptoms are triggered by the release of histamines, it may be useful to increase consumption of foods that are high in niacin (vitamin B_3), which is believed to inhibit histamine release. Good sources of niacin include poultry, seafood, seeds and nuts, whole grains, and fortified cereals and breads. Choose these carefully, however, because some foods that are good sources of niacin are among those that tend to provoke an allergy.

Avoiding the culprit foods that trigger an allergic reaction is the safest way to prevent an outbreak of hives. If you have had a severe allergic reaction to any substance, ask the doctor whether you need to carry special medication to be used if the reaction occurs again. It's also a good idea to have an identification tag or card that specifies your sensitivity so that emergency medical personnel can be alerted if you become incapacitated. ❖

HONEY

BENEFITS
- A source of quick energy.
- Adds flavor to foods and beverages and improves the shelf life of baked goods.

DRAWBACKS
- Contains more calories volume for volume than sugar.
- Contamination with *Clostridium botulinum* spores may be dangerous for babies under a year old.

Our inborn taste for sweet foods led Stone Age humans to forage for the sweetness of honey. Although bees were first domesticated in artificial hives in Egypt and India about 4,500 years ago, it wasn't until about A.D. 1000 that beekeepers began to understand the interplay

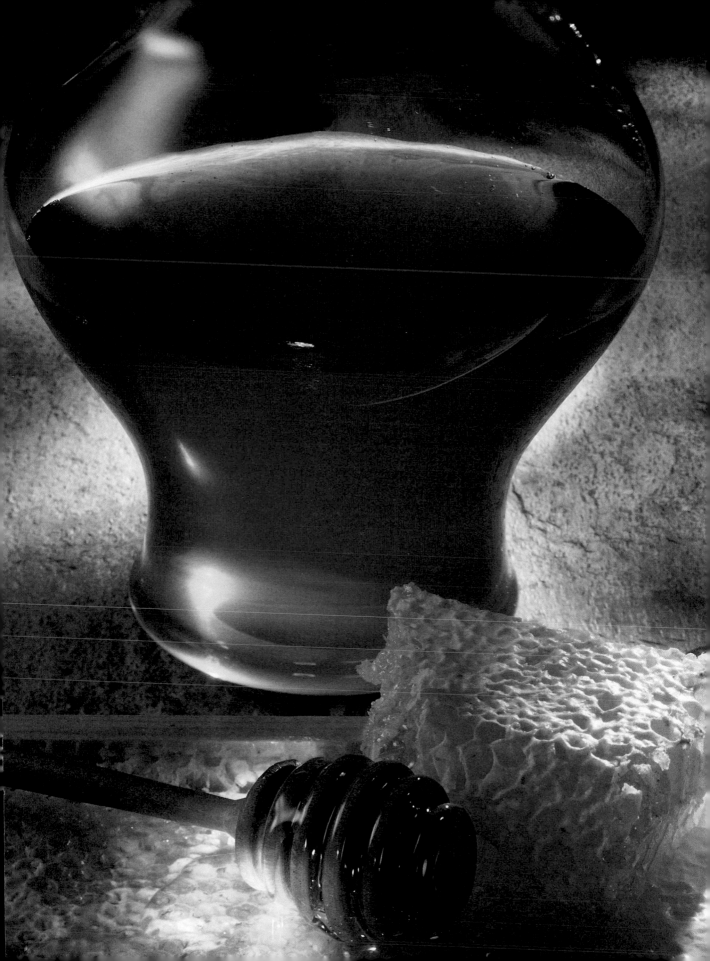

MYTH BUSTER

Myth: Propolis is a potent antioxidant that boosts the immune system and fights viruses and bacteria.

Reality: There is only one true use for propolis, the resinous substance collected by bees from certain plants: To seal holes in a bee's honeycomb and prevent intruders from entering the hive. Propolis consists of dozens of compounds, including fatty acids and flavonoids, which have antifungal and antibacterial effects. But there is little evidence to justify claims that propolis has antibacterial effects superior to antibiotics, or that propolis stimulates the immune system. Some people recommend using propolis to treat ulcers and skin problems caused by fungi. Studies have shown that the mild antimicrobial effects of propolis may be due, in part, to the residue of solvents used to extract the active ingredients. There is no evidence to suggest that propolis is effective in treating any human condition.

between bees and flowers that is required to produce honey.

Honey remained the staple sweetener in Europe until the 1500s, when granulated sugar (more easily stored and transported) became available. But sugar could not entirely replace honey's more complex flavors, and honey remains a popular food.

Bees native to the Americas live only in tropical zones and lack stingers. They scavenge not only in flowers but also in fruits and animal droppings to make honeys that taste strange and are often unsafe. A single Old World species, *Apis mellifera,* was brought to North America by colonists in the 1600s and now produces virtually all of our honey.

FROM FLOWERS TO HIVES

Plants and honeybees have a symbiotic relationship. As the bees gather nectar, they carry pollen with them from one flower to another, thus ensuring cross-fertilization. The bees concentrate the flower nectar into honey, which is stored in their hives. Honeybees also collect and store pollen, which provides developing and young worker bees with protein and vitamins similar to the nutrients in dried beans and peas. While it is food for bees, pollen does nothing for humans that legumes can't do better, and it may trigger life-threatening allergic reactions in susceptible people.

As a bee gathers nectar, it's kept in a sac where enzymes begin a refining and filtering process. When the bee returns to its hive, a chain of workers greets it; each one pumps the nectar in and out of the honey sac until it becomes honey concentrated enough to resist bacteria and molds. It is then stored in a comb to ripen until it is needed for food.

Leguminous plants, especially clover, are commonly cultivated for bee foraging. Other crops favored for the tang of the honey they produce include linden, sage, and thyme.

The liquid honey that is most popular in North America is removed from the comb by centrifugation, it is then pasteurized, strained, filtered, and bottled. Solid honeys are put through controlled crystallization before packaging.

HONEY AS FOOD

Despite all the claims that honey is a wonder food, its nutritional value is very limited; honeys are mostly sugars—fructose and glucose, with some sucrose. Some types provide minute amounts of B complex and C vitamins. Honey does contain some antioxidants, however, mostly polyphenols, but fruits and vegetables are much better sources. Some new studies are looking into the antimicrobial and wound-healing properties of honey.

Volume for volume, honey is higher in calories than sugar; a tablespoon of honey contains 64 calories, compared to 46 in a tablespoon of sugar. This is partly because a tablespoon of honey weighs more than the same volume of sugar. Honey can be substituted for sugar at the ratio of 1 measure of honey for every 1¼ units of sugar; the liquid in the recipe may need to be decreased, however, to compensate for the water that is present in honey. Breads and cakes that are sweetened with honey do stay moister than those that are baked with sugar, thanks to the water-attracting (hygroscopic) properties of honey.

RISK FOR BABIES

Spores of *Clostridium botulinum* have been found in about 10 percent of honeys sampled by the Centers for Disease Control and Prevention (CDC) in the United States. Although not dangerous to adults and older children, infants should not be fed honey because *C. botulinum* can cause serious illness in the first year of life. ❖

HOT DOGS

See Fast Food

HYPERACTIVITY

CONSUME
- A variety of foods to provide a nutritionally complete diet.

LIMIT
- Caffeinated beverages.
- Hot dogs and other foods that contain large amounts of food additives and preservatives.

AVOID
- Self-treatment with high-dose vitamins and minerals.
- Diets that eliminate entire food groups.

About 2 to 4 percent of all children suffer from hyperactivity (or attention deficit disorder), with boys outnumbering girls about fivefold. Parents often describe the hyperactive child as being in perpetual motion—always on the move, disruptive, impulsive, and unable to concentrate. Many researchers theorize that an imbalance in brain chemistry is responsible for the abnormal behavior, but a precise cause has not been identified.

In recent years, diet has been suggested as a possible cause of hyperactivity—a claim discounted by many experts. Although some nutritional deficiencies can certainly affect behavior, these almost never occur in industrialized countries, where malnutrition is seldom a problem. Also, dozens of studies have failed to prove that diet plays any role in hyperactivity. Still, many parents and even some physicians believe that, at least for some children, there is a link. The diet hypothesis was first proposed in 1973 by Benjamin Feingold, a California allergist, who blamed hyperactivity on sensitivity to certain food additives and salicylates, compounds found in fruits, some vegetables, and in aspirin. Dr. Feingold recommended eliminating from the child's diet all foods that contain certain preservatives and artificial flavors and colors, as well as any natural sources of salicylates. Half of his hyperactive patients improved on this diet, and soon many doctors and parent groups were supporting the diet.

Although some reports suggest that an additive-free diet helps a few children, Dr. Feingold's finding of marked improvement in a significant percentage of cases has not been duplicated in scientific studies. Some pediatricians advise parents to try eliminating foods that are especially high in preservatives, dyes, and other additives—for example, hot dogs and other processed meats and some commercial baked goods—to see if there is any improvement. But avoiding all foods that contain natural salicylates is more problematic; there is no evidence that this actually helps, and it can lead to deficiencies of vitamin C, beta carotene, and other nutrients.

Caffeine has been linked to hyperactivity. Experts doubt that it actually causes the problem, but it may add to the restlessness of a hyperactive child. In any event, eliminating caffeine from a child's diet won't hurt.

Orthomolecular therapy—the use of markedly high doses of vitamins and minerals to treat behavioral and other problems—is advocated by some practitioners for hyperactivity. There is no evidence that this helps, but it is known that self-treating with megadose vitamins and minerals can cause serious nutritional imbalances and toxicity.

SUGAR CLEARED AS THE CULPRIT

Hyperactivity has often been blamed on a high intake of sugar. Again, there is no scientific proof of this. In fact, one study conducted by the National Institute of Mental Health in the United States found that children given a sugary drink were less active than a control group that ingested only sugar-free drinks. Some researchers theorize that the calming effect noted in the group given drinks containing sugar may be related to the fact that sugar prompts the brain to increase the production of serotonin, a chemical that reduces the brain's electrical activity. Even so, this is not a good enough reason to give your child loads of sweets—sugar provides calories but is completely devoid of other nutrients; it also promotes tooth decay. ❖

HYPOGLYCEMIA

CONSUME
- Small meals that provide a balance of protein, carbohydrates, and fats.

LIMIT
- Carbohydrate-only (especially sugary) meals and snacks.

AVOID
- Consuming alcohol without food.

Glucose, or blood sugar, is the body's major source of energy; it is also the only form of energy that the brain can use effectively. During digestion and metabolism, the liver converts all of the carbohydrates and about half of the protein in a meal into glucose, which is released into the bloodstream. In response to rising blood glucose levels, the pancreas secretes extra insulin, the hormone that enables cells to use the sugar to produce energy.

Low blood sugar, or hypoglycemia, occurs when the amount of insulin in the blood exceeds that needed to metabolize the available glucose. It is seen often when a person with diabetes takes too much insulin, but it can also occur in other circumstances, such as an overconsumption of alcohol; taking large amounts of aspirin or acetaminophen, beta blockers, and some antipsychotic drugs; or when tumors develop that secrete insulin.

REACTIVE HYPOGLYCEMIA

This condition occurs when blood sugar levels plummet 1 to 2 hours after a meal. Symptoms include dizziness, headache, hunger, trembling, palpitations, and irritability. Many people who experience vague, unexplained symptoms assume that they have reactive hypoglycemia, but the condition is not common. This is because the human body has a very sensitive feedback system that controls insulin secretion. Reactive hypoglycemia can only be diagnosed by monitoring blood glucose levels after ingestion of a known dose of glucose.

Eat small, frequent meals with a mix of carbs, fats, and protein. A diet made up mostly of carbohydrates may produce mild symptoms of hypoglycemia even though the blood sugar levels are usually in the low-normal range. Here's what happens: A person may skip breakfast or have only simple carbohydrates—for example, a glass of orange juice and a sweet roll. The pancreas will secrete a fair amount of insulin to process the glucose in this meal, but since the meal contains no protein or fat, which are metabolized more slowly, the body will burn the glucose in 2 or 3 hours. Sensing a need for more energy, the brain sends out powerful hunger signals. A sweet snack will satisfy this hunger and provide a quick burst of energy, but again, the pancreas will pump out enough insulin to quickly metabolize the glucose. If the scenario is repeated throughout the day, a pattern is established.

The cycle can be broken by consuming regular meals that include small amounts of protein and fats along with starches. These take longer than sugars to be digested and converted into glucose, and they allow for a steady release of energy. Avoid having a breakfast of a bagel with jam, for instance, and have a bagel with cream cheese instead. Include foods that are higher in soluble fiber such as lentils, oats, barley, apples, and citrus fruits since they are absorbed more slowly, and avoid sweets. Choose whole grains (such as whole-wheat bread) over refined grains (such as white bread or pasta) as often as possible. You may also want to consume foods with a low glycemic load (see chart, page 194).

INSULIN OVERDOSE

A much more serious type of hypoglycemia occurs when a diabetic takes more insulin than is needed to metabolize the available glucose. The onset of symptoms of an insulin reaction—hunger, tingling sensations, sweating, faintness, impaired vision, mood changes, palpitations, and a cold, clammy sensation—can be reversed by immediately eating a tablespoonful of sugar or honey, sucking on a hard candy, or drinking a glass of orange juice or a sugary drink. Do not ignore insulin reactions. ❖

DO ONE SIMPLE THING

HAVE ONE OF THESE QUICK-FIX FOODS IMMEDIATELY TO RAISE YOUR BLOOD GLUCOSE:
- ½ cup of any fruit juice
- ½ cup of a regular soft drink (not diet)
- 1 cup milk
- 5 or 6 pieces of hard candy
- 1 or 2 teaspoons of sugar or honey

DID YOU KNOW?

HYPOGLYCEMIA CAUSED BY BINGE DRINKING CAN BE FATAL

Excessive alcohol consumption, especially binge drinking, can cause hypoglycemia because the body's breakdown of alcohol interferes with the liver's efforts to raise blood glucose. This type of hypoglycemia can be very serious or even fatal.

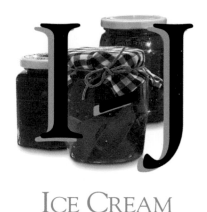

ICE CREAM

BENEFITS
- A good source of calcium.
- Provides protein and digestible, high-calorie nutrition during an illness.

DRAWBACKS
- High in saturated fat and sugar.

Federal standards decree that ice cream must be made with a minimum of 10 percent cream, milk or butter fat. Manufacturers may add various other ingredients, as well as enough air to double its volume. In general, the least expensive ice creams contain the minimum 10 percent fat and the maximum air, while the premium commercial brands have double the fat and half the air.

It is fat that gives ice cream its smooth texture; manufacturers of nonfat and low-fat ices and frozen yogurts compensate for the lack of fat by increasing the sugar—by up to twice the amount—and beating in less air. Therefore, although these products contain less fat, in the end they are not necessarily lower in calories.

Both soft ice cream and ice milk are 3 to 6 percent fat and 30 to 50 percent air. Sherbets are usually made with a small amount of milk fat and milk solids or, sometimes, egg white. Fruit ices, on the other hand, tend to be made with fruit pulp or juice, sugar, and water, with the possible addition of pectin or ascorbic acid. Most of these products contain about 200 calories per cup. Even a half cup of fat-free frozen yogurt with artificial sweetener has about 80 calories.

Ice cream has substantial amounts of calcium and protein, as well as some vitamin A and riboflavin. The price for these useful nutrients, however, is a large helping of saturated fat, with its adverse implications for heart disease, certain cancers, and other conditions. Fruit sorbets—which are high in sugar but fat-free—are a better choice when you want to end a meal with a frozen dessert. Low-fat frozen yogurt is a good substitute for ice cream; a half cup topped with fresh fruit and toasted wheat germ can satisfy cravings for a frosty treat and supply useful amounts of calcium, vitamins, and fiber.

Additives. Storing ice cream presents a problem in the form of "heat shock." When ice cream is removed from the freezer, its surface melts. When the ice cream is refrozen, ice crystals form, resulting in a crunchy texture that terrifies ice cream lovers. The problem can be countered by adding microcrystalline cellulose, a highly purified wood derivative that sops up the water as ice cream melts and prevents it from refreezing into crystals. Cellulose is indigestible and comes out in the wash, as it were. Guar gum, locust bean gum, or carrageenan, all from plant sources, can also be used for the same purpose. Other additives used in ice cream include emulsifiers such as lecithin, mono- and diglycerides, or polysorbates that make for a smooth texture by dispersing the fat globules. ❖

IMMUNE SYSTEM
■ YOUR BODY'S SECRET WEAPON ■

The immune system protects the body from attack by microorganisms, abnormal cells, and chemicals. Its army includes macrophages, T cells, and B cells. Most often, the external threats are infections caused by invading bacteria, viruses, and fungi, while abnormal or cancerous cells pose the major internal threats. In addition, this complex system oversees the repair of tissues that are injured by wounds or disease.

Once in a while the immune system mistakes a harmless foreign substance for an enemy, resulting in an allergic reaction, such as hives, hay fever, or asthma. Less commonly the immune system—mistaking an internal signal—attacks normal body tissue, leading to an autoimmune disease, such as type 1 diabetes, rheumatoid arthritis, or lupus.

The most remarkable characteristic of the immune system is its "memory" for foreign substances and organisms. Confronted with a virus or other invading organism, the system creates an antibody that will recognize it and mount an attack against it at any future encounter. This mechanism, called acquired immunity, is what makes vaccinations work.

System failure or why we get sick

If the immune system is such a wonder, why do we get sick? The simplest explanation is that often there is a lapse between the time an invading organism enters the body and the time the immune system conquers it. In the interim the invader can make its mark, killing cells. How sick you become depends largely on how strong a defense your immune system can launch. Infection, cancer, and other illnesses develop when the immune system is weakened by any number of stressors, including viruses and other invading organisms, malnutrition, and the consequences of aging. Fortunately, antibiotics and sulfa drugs can wipe out most bacterial infections in otherwise healthy people; progress is also being made in the development of antiviral drugs. At times doctors purposely lower immunity to treat an autoimmune disease or to prevent rejection of donor organs.

Dietary influences

The right diet is critical to a strong immune system. The following are the building blocks you need to keep your defenses strong. It's best to get them from food. Supplements are usually not necessary unless you are taking therapeutic doses for a specific condition. However, if you don't eat well in general or have a health problem, you may want to discuss supplements with your doctor.

■ **Proteins are central to the proper functioning of the immune system.** The amino acids they provide are used to make antibodies and other immune compounds that attack foreign invaders and prevent infection. Almost all North Americans have more than enough protein in their diets.

■ **Omega-3 and omega-6 fatty acids help in immune function.** Omega-3 fatty acids, abundant in cold-water fish as well as in flaxseed, are especially beneficial in controlling inflammation and the harmful effects of rheumatoid arthritis and other autoimmune disorders. Research suggests that omega-3 oils help reduce acute inflammation, which occurs as part of the immune response to attack or injury. Omega-3s activate parts of the immune system that rein in attack cells to stop them when their job is done.

■ **Vitamin E is a T cell enhancer.** Vitamin E, found in oils, nuts and seeds, margarine and avocados, may enhance T cell activity and assist in the production of antibodies.

■ **Vitamin C to fortify.** Vitamin C, found in many fruits and vegetables, assists in building and maintaining mucous membranes and collagen, as well as strengthening the blood vessel walls, and is thought to enhance the function of the immune cells. Vitamin C supplements may help reduce the duration of a cold. Red peppers and kiwifruits are excellent sources of vitamin C.

■ **Vitamin A is key.** Found in liver, fish, milk, cheese, and eggs, vitamin A reduces the incidence and severity of infectious illnesses by helping to keep mucous membranes healthy and intact and also hikes antibody response and increases white blood cell proliferation. Beta carotene, once consumed, can be converted to vitamin A in the body.

■ **Zinc is a trace mineral with many important functions, including supporting immunity.** A deficiency of zinc has been associated with slow wound healing. The best food sources are foods of animal origin, including seafood (especially oysters), meat, poultry, and liver, as well as eggs, milk, beans, nuts, and whole grains. But an excess of supplementary zinc can actually depress the immune system.

■ **Selenium is a trace mineral essential for a strong immune system.** The best sources of selenium are Brazil nuts, seafood, some meats and fish, as well as bread, wheat bran, wheat germ, oats, and brown rice.

■ **Iron is an absolute must.** Iron is required for the manufacture of B cells and T cells and ensures that cells get the oxygen they need to function properly and resist disease. Best sources are red meat, eggs, dried fruits, enriched grains, and cereals and legumes.

■ **Antioxidants to protect against free radicals.** Research suggests that the antioxidant properties of carotenoids, such as lycopene (found in tomatoes and tomato products) and beta carotene (found in orange, red, and yellow plant foods, as well as dark green vegetables) may protect immune cells from destructive free radicals, molecules that can harm cells and damage the DNA.

There are no "quick fix" diets for the immune system

Some unscrupulous practitioners exploit the importance of the immune system and the difficulty of understanding its complexity by publicizing methods to boost "immune power." These practitioners recommend a program to "cleanse" the body, followed by megadoses of vitamins, minerals, and amino acids, to restore immune power. There is no evidence that such regimens boost immunity, and high-dose supplements can be dangerous.

More immune boosters

Garlic and onions may stimulate the fighting power of macrophages and T cells because of their powerful sulfur compounds, which may also block enzymes that allow organisms to invade healthy tissue.

Some studies suggest that **moderate exercise** may help improve immune function, especially in people who were previously sedentary.

Some evidence indicates that **shiitake mushrooms** may boost immunity, but the practical significance of this is unknown.

Probiotics, friendly bacteria that can be found in some fermented milk products such as **yogurt and kefir,** may help improve immune responses against viruses.

Blueberries, blackberries, and grapes contain anthocyanins, powerful antioxidants that have potent immune stimulating properties.

Certain **whey proteins,** specially processed to provide a high dose of the amino acid cysteine, enhance immune function. Cysteine is used by the body in the synthesis of glutathione, one of the most important compounds of the immune system.

EGCG, a powerful antioxidant compound found in green tea, may have the ability to inhibit the growth of cancer cells as well as neutralizing harmful free radicals.

IMPOTENCE

CONSUME PLENTY OF
- Foods rich in zinc, such as seafood (especially oysters), meat, poultry, eggs, milk, beans, nuts, and whole grains.

LIMIT
- Alcohol and saturated fats.

AVOID
- Nicotine and all drugs except those prescribed for you.

Although psychological factors certainly affect male sexual function, recent studies show that most cases of impotence are due to an underlying disease or lifestyle factors. Diabetes, atherosclerosis, paralysis, or, less commonly, hormonal imbalances are among the organic causes of impotence. The use of a number of drugs—including alcohol, nicotine, illegal substances, as well as prescription medications—can lead to impotence. Nicotine impedes the blood flow by constricting the small arteries, including those that bring blood to the penis. Medications that commonly cause impotence include antihypertensives, acid-suppressants for ulcers, antidepressants, and sleeping pills. In most cases, an alternative drug can be prescribed.

While diet does not have much of an effect on impotence, medications can help. The most popular drug is sildenafil citrate (Viagra), which boosts the activity of an enzyme, cyclic guanosine monophosphate (cGMP), which is the key to having an erection.

DIETARY FACTORS

Zinc is absolutely key. Zinc is among the minerals thought to be essential to good reproductive health. While zinc intake may not have a direct effect on potency, it may be important for male sexual health, since very high levels are found in the seminal fluid. Good sources of zinc include seafood (especially oysters), meat, poultry, eggs, milk, beans, nuts, and whole grains. Zinc supplements are not recommended; in high doses they can interfere with the absorption of calcium and copper.

Watch your weight. It's important to maintain a normal weight; obesity predisposes a person to diabetes, which is one of the leading causes of impotence. Studies have shown that obesity puts men at greater risk for erectile dysfunction. Also, a diet low in saturated fats helps prevent atherosclerosis, the buildup of fatty plaque that clogs not only the large vessels around the heart but also the penile artery. ❖

INDIGESTION AND HEARTBURN

TAKE
- Small meals at regular intervals.

LIMIT
- Alcohol, caffeine, and coffee in all forms.
- Tomato-based and other acidic foods.

AVOID
- Fatty foods.
- Eating within 2 hours of bedtime.
- Tobacco use of any kind.

Almost half of all adult North Americans have indigestion occasionally, but for some, it is a daily trial. The most common symptom of indigestion is heartburn, a burning chest pain that occurs when stomach acid and other contents flow backward, or reflux, into the esophagus. Unlike the stomach, the lining of the esophagus has no protective lining of mucus-producing tissue, so the acid produces irritation and even ulcerations. Obesity and pregnancy may lead to heartburn because of increased intra-abdominal pressure, which tends to force the stomach fluids up into the esophagus. A hiatal hernia is another possible cause.

Heartburn caused by reflux can usually be controlled with a few lifestyle changes, starting with adopting a low-fat diet that includes a balance of protein, starches, and fiber-rich vegetables and fruits. (Fatty foods take longer to digest and thus slow down the rate of food emptying from the stomach.) Coffee, including decaffeinated brands, promotes high acid production; so does tea, cola drinks, and other sources of caffeine. Citrus fruits and juices can also cause problems. There is no evidence that spicy foods—except possibly, red and black pepper—cause indigestion, but people who find that a spicy meal is followed by discomfort would be better off shunning such seasonings. Reflux is made worse by foods such as chocolate or peppermint that relax the sphincter muscle connecting the esophagus to the stomach.

Avoid large meals, especially late in the day. Try not to eat in the two hours before bedtime. Sit up straight after meals; bending over or lying down increases pressure on the stomach and promotes reflux. Stop smoking; nicotine relaxes the sphincter muscle. Limit alcohol intake to an occasional glass of wine or beer.

The use of nonprescription antacids to treat heartburn by neutralizing stomach acid is questionable; the problem is not too much acid, but acid in the wrong place. If you find that they do help, follow instructions and never take them for longer than recommended. "Proton pump inhibitors" such as omeprazole are very effective drugs for acid reflux. ❖

INFERTILITY

EAT PLENTY OF
- A balanced diet with plenty of fruits and vegetables, lean meat, fish or poultry, whole-grain breads, cereals, and grains, as well as low-fat dairy products.

LIMIT
- Coffee and other sources of caffeine.

AVOID
- Alcohol and smoking.
- Becoming overweight or underweight.

Defined as the inability to achieve a pregnancy after at least a year of trying, infertility affects more than 20 percent of North American couples. Experts cannot explain why the infertility rate has almost doubled in the last 25 years, but at least three factors stand out: the growing trend for couples to delay marriage and parenthood until their most fertile years are past, the rise in sexually transmitted diseases, and a puzzling drop in sperm production.

Many couples assume that infertility rests with the woman; in fact, men are just as likely to be infertile. In 40 percent of cases, the problem lies with the male, and in 40 percent of cases, with the female. The cause can't be identified in the remaining 20 percent, or both partners may be contributing factors. While nutrition is not a leading cause of infertility, consuming a healthful diet enhances the chance of conceiving and delivering a healthy baby.

FEMALE INFERTILITY
The leading cause of female infertility is the failure to ovulate, which may be influenced by the diet, hormonal imbalances, and a variety of other factors. Women who are very thin or markedly overweight often do not ovulate

because the amount of body fat is closely associated with estrogen levels. Women who have very little body fat—professional athletes, dancers, models, and chronic dieters—often stop menstruating and ovulating. Women who are obese may have abnormally elevated levels of estrogen, which can also result in a failure to ovulate.

Conception and weight. Any woman who is considering becoming pregnant should try to achieve her ideal weight before conception. This should be done by eating a balanced diet; a woman who is underweight when she conceives is likely to have such problems as anemia during pregnancy. The baby may be smaller than normal and is more at risk for health problems. Conversely, dieting during pregnancy could be dangerous to the fetus. An overweight woman should diet before trying to conceive; this also lowers her risk of developing high blood pressure or diabetes during pregnancy.

Essential nutrients. Women who take oral contraceptives are likely to experience temporary infertility until their hormonal levels return to normal and they again start to ovulate. Long-term use can result in reduced reserves of folate (a B vitamin that is especially important in fetal development); vitamins B_6, B_{12}, C, and E; and calcium, zinc, and other minerals. Therefore, the woman's diet should emphasize foods that are rich in these nutrients—fruits and vegetables for vitamin C; milk for calcium; and fortified breads and cereals, lean meat, poultry, and seafood for the B vitamins as well as iron, zinc, and other minerals.

Alcohol and smoking are known to reduce fertility in both women and men; a recent study indicated that coffee may have a similar effect.

MALE INFERTILITY
A low sperm count is the major cause of male infertility, and for unknown reasons, men worldwide are producing fewer sperm than a few decades ago. Some scientists believe certain pesticides, which have estrogenlike effects, may be linked to the declining count. Alcohol and tobacco use lower sperm production and should be avoided if there is difficulty conceiving.

Zinc. Inadequate zinc may lower male fertility; a recent study found that men who consumed 1.4 mg daily produced fewer sperm and had lower levels of the male hormone

FOLIC ACID HELPS PREVENT BIRTH DEFECTS

Doctors advise women who are pregnant, or who may become pregnant, to consume lots of folate-rich foods or take folic acid supplements to lessen the risk of having children with neural tube defects such as spina bifida. Good dietary sources of folate include fortified breakfast cereals, leafy greens, legumes, and orange juice.

testosterone than men whose daily zinc intake was 10.4 mg—the zinc Recommended Dietary Allowance (RDA) for adult men is 11 mg.

Vitamin C. Inadequate intake of vitamin C may impair male fertility. One study correlated low levels of vitamin C with an increased tendency of sperm to clump together, a problem that all but disappeared after 3 weeks of taking vitamin C supplements.

Folic acid. Researchers studied a group of healthy men who had low intakes of fruits and vegetables and did not take supplements. Their study suggests that low levels of folic acid in these men were associated with decreased sperm count and decreased sperm density. The vitamin's role is unclear, but researchers believe normalizing folate levels through diet may offset diminished sperm levels. The best food sources of folic acid are dark green vegetables (such as broccoli, spinach, romaine lettuce, peas, and brussels sprouts), orange juice, liver, dry peas, and beans. Other evidence suggests that vitamin B_{12} (found in all animal products) may improve sperm count and motility, even in men who are not B_{12} deficient. ❖

IRON OVERLOAD

LIMIT
- Organ meats and iron-fortified foods.

AVOID
- Iron supplements
- Alcohol, if there is liver damage.
- High doses of vitamin C.

The human body needs a steady supply of iron, but only in tiny amounts—about 10 mg to 15 mg a day for healthy adults. In fact, hemochromatosis, the most common form of iron overload disease, can cause irreversible heart and liver damage.

The body can utilize two types of iron—heme, which comes from animal sources, and nonheme, which comes from plants. The body absorbs 20 to 30 percent of heme iron, compared with 5 to 10 percent of nonheme. When the body's iron reserves are low, the absorption of nonheme iron increases. Consuming iron-rich plant foods with meat or with good sources of vitamin C boosts nonheme iron absorption. By the same token, some substances—for example, tea, bran, and the oxalates found in spinach and kale—decrease the body's absorption.

Genetic factors influence iron absorption. About 10 percent of whites and up to 30 percent of people of African descent carry a gene that predisposes them to store extra iron. The presence of a single gene does not cause problems, but if a person inherits the gene from both parents, he is likely to develop iron overload, or hemochromatosis. Men and postmenopausal women are especially vulnerable.

An iron overload does not produce symptoms until a damaging amount has accumulated in muscle tissue (including the heart), the liver, bone marrow, the spleen, and other organs; this usually occurs during middle age. One of the first indications is a ruddy complexion; the person may also suffer fatigue, joint and intestinal pain, and an irregular heartbeat. As the liver becomes damaged, jaundice may develop.

A blood test can be used to diagnose an iron overload; in some cases, a liver biopsy may also be ordered. Treatment involves periodic removal of a pint (0.5 liter) or so of blood, which reduces iron levels by forcing the body to use some of its stores to make new red blood cells.

Even moderately elevated iron levels may set the stage for heart disease. One study reported that men whose blood iron levels were in the high-normal range were more likely to develop coronary artery disease than those with low-to-normal levels. This supports the theory that excessive iron may injure the artery walls and promote the formation of fatty deposits. This damage may be due to iron's ability to catalyze oxidation processes. Controversy continues over iron and heart disease risk, with some studies showing that only heme iron was linked with heart disease and others finding no link. Some researchers also think that iron may contribute to the joint pain and damage that many women endure following menopause. The message continues to be that you should only take supplements if you are iron deficient.

Foods high in vitamin C, which enhances iron absorption, should not be consumed with iron-rich plant foods by those who are predisposed to store extra iron. Unless prescribed by a doctor, supplements containing iron and large doses of vitamin C should not be taken. Some experts now advise that anyone who is contemplating taking a vitamin C supplement should first have a blood test to measure iron levels. ❖

CAUTION

Cut down on these iron-rich food sources if you are genetically predisposed to storing extra iron:
- Oysters
- Liver
- Lean red meat, especially beef
- Iron-enriched cereals
- Dried beans and whole grains
- Eggs, especially yolks
- Dried fruits
- Dark green leafy vegetables

IRRADIATION
▪ EXTENDING SHELF LIFE ▪

Wouldn't it be wonderful to wave a magic wand over the food supply and make it safe to eat? Since that's not possible, we can do the next best thing: food irradiation. Exposure of foods to X-rays and other forms of ionizing radiation kills the molds, bacteria, and insects that cause spoilage. It delays the ripening of fruits and berries, so extends shelf life. In addition, irradiation inhibits the sprouting of potatoes and other foods, which means that they stay fresh longer. Previously, heat and the use of chemicals (formaldehyde, alcohol, or various pesticides) were the major methods of sterilization, but each had its drawbacks. Heat sterilization entails cooking foods, so they are no longer fresh; chemicals that kill bacteria and other microorganisms often make foods inedible. Irradiation would seem to be an ideal means of sterilization, but the public has been slow to accept it.

Radioactive foods?

Despite assurances that irradiation with X-rays or certain isotopes does not make foods radioactive, some consumer and environmental groups remain unconvinced. They worry that any radiation exposure poses a potential environmental hazard, even if the foods themselves are not made radioactive. They also fear the radiation may foster the development of dangerous mutant organisms or "unique radiolytic products." The latter refer to compounds such as 2-alkylcyclobutanones, which form when animal fat is irradiated. Some studies have shown that such compounds can cause strand breaks in DNA, which raises the prospect of cancer. Most researchers, however, do not attach much importance to this finding. As in cooking, the benefits of irradiation greatly outweigh the risks. There are roughly 50 million cases of food-borne illness in North America every year and a large number of these are caused by *E. coli* and salmonella, which could be controlled by irradiation. Foods such as wheat, flour, potatoes, and spices have been irradiated in many countries for decades without any link to harmful effects.

The government mandates that only certain forms of irradiation can be applied to foods to ensure that they don't absorb the radioactive material. X-rays, which pass through an object without leaving behind radioactive material, and exposure to certain cobalt and cesium isotopes are all acceptable methods. These methods of cold sterilization allow most irradiated foods to retain their fresh appearance and taste. When meat, fish, and seafood are exposed to the high doses of radiation needed to destroy parasites, salmonella bacteria, and other organisms, however, the flesh of some meat may darken, and fish and seafood may become mushy. Irradiation can also oxidize the fats in whole grains, causing them to taste rancid.

Beneficial effects

In general, irradiation preserves more nutrients—particularly niacin, riboflavin, thiamine, and other B-group vitamins—than other sterilization methods do. But very high radiation doses, such as those needed to sterilize meat, will destroy some of the fat-soluble vitamins A, E, and K. The effects of irradiation on vitamin C remain unknown; some studies show no loss of this nutrient, while others indicate major losses.

Irradiated foods must bear this international symbol

Advocates of irradiation emphasize that the technique can increase food supplies in many underdeveloped parts of the world, especially in the tropics, where food spoilage destroys much of the food produced. Irradiation could conceivably solve chronic food shortages in these areas.

DID YOU KNOW?

IRRADIATION HELPS TO PROTECT PEOPLE WITH COMPROMISED IMMUNE SYSTEMS

Food irradiation adds an extra measure of food safety for AIDS patients and others with lowered immunity; these people are cautioned not to eat uncooked fruits and vegetables and to make sure that all meat, fish, eggs, and other foods that may harbor disease-causing bacteria or parasites are cooked until well-done. Even after these precautions are taken, food-borne diseases are a major hazard for people with compromised immunity. High-dose irradiation can eliminate these dangers.

IRRITABLE BOWEL SYNDROME

TAKE PLENTY OF

- Nonalcoholic, caffeine-free fluids.
- Smaller meals.
- High-fiber foods (if constipation is a problem).
- Binding foods (if diarrhea is a problem).

LIMIT

- Alcoholic beverages.

AVOID

- Fried and other fatty foods.
- All sources of caffeine.
- Gas-producing foods, such as beans.

Afflicting up to 20 percent of all adults, irritable bowel syndrome (IBS) is often characterized by abnormal muscle contractions in the intestines, resulting in too little or too much fluid in the bowel.

Symptoms vary markedly from one person to another. Some people experience urgent diarrhea. Others experience the type called spastic colon, with alternating bouts of diarrhea and constipation, as well as abdominal pain, cramps, bloating, gas, and nausea, particularly after eating. Still other symptoms may include mucus in the stool and feelings of incomplete evacuation after moving the bowels. Some people may also complain of fatigue, anxiety, headache, and depression.

There are no tests for IBS, which is diagnosed by ruling out colitis, cancer, and other diseases. Although it may be aggravated by food intolerances or allergies, no specific cause has been established. It may be worsened by stress and emotional conflict, but it is not a psychological disorder. Various dietary factors can play a major role in exacerbating or calming IBS.

A doctor may prescribe medications to quell abnormal muscle contractions and alleviate diarrhea. However, self-care, stress reduction, and dietary modification are the mainstays of therapy. Some recent research suggests that bacterial overgrowth in the bowel may be a cause of IBS. In one study, 78 percent of IBS patients were found to have bacterial overgrowth in the small intestine, and antibiotics eliminated the disease in half of the patients who got rid of the overgrowth.

TRACKING YOUR TRIGGERS

The first step in learning to control IBS symptoms is recognizing the factors that may trigger symptoms. A diary that records IBS symptoms along with all foods and beverages ingested and stressful events can help pinpoint possible culprits. A woman should determine whether symptoms flare up during certain times of her menstrual cycle. When tracking IBS symptoms, jot down the nature and location of any pain, as well as the frequency and consistency of stools and any related problems, such as headaches. Your diary should also note all medications taken, including supplements. A doctor should review this diary to help identify specific contributing factors.

DIETARY MODIFICATION

Because IBS differs from person to person, it's essential to develop an individualized regimen to treat your symptoms. To begin, avoid foods that your diary suggests are causing problems.

Eat several small meals a day instead of large ones. This can reduce the meal-stimulated increase in bowel contractions and diarrhea.

Eat slowly. Eating too quickly may increase swallowed air, which promotes irritating intestinal gas. Also, poorly chewed foods can be more difficult to digest.

Drink lots of water. To maintain adequate fluid, drink at least eight glasses of water or other beverages daily, but avoid such potential bowel irritants as alcohol and caffeine.

Avoid fatty foods. Most doctors advise against eating fried and other fatty foods because fat is the most difficult nutrient to digest. Many people find that it helps to avoid beans and other gas-producing foods.

Watch your fiber intake. Whole-grain products and other high-fiber foods can pose problems for some IBS sufferers who have chronic diarrhea. On the other hand, if constipation is the predominant symptom, a diet that includes ample fresh fruits and vegetables, whole-grain breads and cereals, nuts and seeds, and other high-fiber foods is usually recommended. Insoluble fiber (see Fiber) helps to bulk up stools and ease elimination, relieving IBS-associated constipation. Foods high in soluble fiber absorb water and are helpful for bouts of diarrhea. If constipation is persistent, ask your doctor about taking ground psyllium seeds or another high-fiber laxative. Avoid chronic laxative use, which can lead to problems with vitamin and nutritional deficiencies.

Avoid sugar alcohols. The sugar substitutes sorbitol, lactitol, mannitol, and maltitol are used in a variety of foods and can trigger IBS symptoms in some people. For others, the lactose in dairy products and possibly fructose can exacerbate symptoms. ❖

JAMS AND SPREADS

BENEFITS

- Jams and jellies contain simple sugars for quick energy.
- Peanut butter provides useful amounts of protein, B vitamins, and minerals.

DRAWBACKS

- Jams are less nutritious than fresh fruit.
- Peanut butter is high in sodium and fat.
- Other types of commercial spreads are often low in nutritional value but high in sodium and fat, as well as price.

Jams were developed in ancient times as a means of preserving fruits that would otherwise quickly spoil. When preserved, fruits resist spoilage because they lack the water that microorganisms need in order to grow. Surface molds can be prevented by sealing homemade preserves with an airtight layer of paraffin.

Fruits boiled in sugar will gel via the interaction of fruit acids and pectin, a soluble fiber that is drawn out of the fruit cell walls by cooking. Apples, grapes, and most berries contain enough natural pectin; other fruits, such as apricots and peaches, need to have it added. Low-calorie, reduced-sugar jams are gelled with a special pectin that sets at lower acidity and with less sugar. These products are often sweetened with concentrated fruit juice and thickened with starches.

For nutritional value, there's no comparison between jams and fresh fruits, because most of the vitamin C and other nutrients in fruits are destroyed by intense cooking. While fruit preserves contain substantial amounts of pectin—a soluble fiber that helps control blood cholesterol levels—this benefit is offset by their high sugar content. Simple sugars, however, make jams a source of quick energy.

PEANUT BUTTER

The majority of the peanuts grown in North America are ground into peanut butter. The high fat content of peanuts makes them easy to grind into a paste, but the oil quickly turns rancid when exposed to oxygen and light. Many commercial peanut butters are made with preservatives, stabilizers, and added salt and sugar; you can avoid these ingredients by buying fresh-ground peanut butter made solely from nuts. The oil that rises to the top of the jar can be poured off to reduce the fat content. It's best to store peanut butter in a glass container in the refrigerator, where the darkness prevents the loss of B vitamins and the cold retards oil separation. Peanut butters that don't separate usually contain hydrogenated vegetable oils. This means they are full of trans fatty acids, which are bad for the heart.

Peanut butter can be a valuable nutritional resource for children, who need extra dietary fat for proper growth and development. One tablespoon contains about 95 calories, with 5 g of protein, 8 g of polyunsaturated fat, and significant amounts of B vitamins, calcium, potassium, and magnesium, along with 100 mg of sodium and traces of iron and zinc.

OTHER SPREADS

The supermarket shelves are stocked with many types of spreads, ranging from soft processed cheese products to chocolate-flavored nut butters and whipped marshmallow. Most of the cheese-based products provide small amounts of vitamin A and calcium but are high in sodium, fat, and cholesterol. Chocolate and marshmallow spreads offer little more than calories. ❖

JAUNDICE

LIMIT
- Fatty and sugary foods.

AVOID
- Shellfish that may have been exposed to polluted water.
- Unpeeled fruits and vegetables that may be contaminated by human waste.
- Foods that are sold or prepared in unsanitary conditions.
- All alcoholic beverages.

A yellowing of the skin and the whites of the eyes is the hallmark of jaundice. This condition typically occurs when bilirubin, a pigmented component of bile, builds up in the blood. Bilirubin is a by-product produced by the liver as it breaks down red blood cells to recycle their iron. It is mixed with bile, a digestive juice that is made by the liver, and is eventually excreted from the body in the urine or stool. Jaundice develops if the bilirubin is allowed to accumulate in the body.

There are three general types of jaundice: the most common is due to hepatitis or some other liver disorder; another, known as obstructive jaundice, usually results from gallstones or another gallbladder disease; and the least common involves some sort of abnormality in bilirubin metabolism.

Each year more than 27 million North Americans are afflicted with liver and gallbladder disorders, but not all of these people develop jaundice. Among those who do, hepatitis—an inflammation of the liver—is the likely cause. Five major forms of viral hepatitis have been identified to date; the liver inflammation may also be due to alcohol or drug abuse, adverse reaction to a medication, as well as bacterial, parasitic, or fungal infections of the liver. Some strains of viral hepatitis are highly contagious and can enter the human body through water or food (especially shellfish) that has been contaminated by human waste. Hepatitis can also be spread through blood transfusions from an infected person or by direct contact with infected body fluids or the use of contaminated syringes.

In addition to jaundice, the symptoms of hepatitis include fever, fatigue, nausea, vomiting, diarrhea, and loss of appetite. The urine may be dark in color due to increased bilirubin content, and the stools may be light, clay-colored, or whitish, an indication that bilirubin is not being excreted from the intestinal tract. In a few cases, hepatitis may be serious enough to result in liver failure, coma, and death.

Jaundice may also be due to Gilbert's syndrome (a disorder of bilirubin metabolism), which affects 3 to 5 percent of the population and may be misdiagnosed as hepatitis. In Gilbert's syndrome, chronic jaundice is the only abnormality and does not signify liver disease. Several other rare forms of jaundice are inherited disorders.

INFANT JAUNDICE

It is not uncommon for a baby to develop jaundice during the first few days after birth, especially if the infant is premature. This is known as physiological jaundice, and is usually caused by a liver that is not fully functional. There are usually no other symptoms, and the condition typically clears up within a week, as the liver matures. Exposing the baby to ultraviolet light hastens the process, as the light changes bilirubin to a form that is more readily excreted.

Feeding the infant soon after birth and continuing with frequent feedings helps to reduce the risk of jaundice by stimulating the intestinal tract to produce frequent stools, which increases the excretion of bilirubin. In a few cases the newborn may be reacting to the mother's milk, and breast-feeding must be discontinued for a day or two in favor of a formula. After this resolves the problem, the mother may resume breast-feeding safely.

DIETARY APPROACHES

Any modification of the diet depends on the underlying cause of the jaundice. With a nutritious, well-balanced diet and rest, viral hepatitis resolves itself—although it may take several weeks. Unfortunately, many people find it difficult to eat at the very time that they need extra calories to help the liver recuperate and regenerate its damaged cells. Many individuals report that their appetite decreases and nausea increases as the day progresses, suggesting that breakfast may be the best tolerated meal.

Eat a diet high in protein. When recovering from hepatitis, a person should consume a healthy diet with sufficient protein daily, from both animal and vegetable sources. The best sources are lean meat, poultry, fish, eggs, dairy products, and a combination of legumes and grain products. If the appetite is poor, intersperse several small meals a day with a nutritious snack (such as a milk shake or an enriched liquid drink). Fried and very fatty foods, which are difficult to digest, should be avoided; a small amount of fat is acceptable, however, to provide needed calories and add flavor. In general, the fats in dairy products and eggs are easier to digest than those in fatty meats and fried foods.

Avoid sweets and alcohol. Because they may squelch the appetite for more nutritious foods, it is best to avoid sweets. Alcohol should not be consumed, because it places added stress on an already sick liver. It may be tolerated after recovery, but some liver disorders mandate total abstinence from alcohol for life. There is some evidence that herbal preparations based on milk thistle may help treat liver dysfunction. ❖

JUICES

BENEFITS
- Provides a concentrated form of fruits and vegetables.

DRAWBACKS
- Juicing removes pulp and fiber.
- Juices can be high in calories.

By now just about everyone knows that fruits and vegetables are loaded with vitamins, minerals, and hundreds of other substances that protect against cancer and other diseases. Mainstream physicians and alternative practitioners alike are urging their patients to eat more fruits and vegetables, preferably raw or with minimal processing in order to preserve their nutrients. Most guidelines call for 5 to 10 servings of fruits and vegetables each day—more than what most North Americans now consume.

DRINK YOUR FRUIT AND VEGETABLES

Fruit and vegetable juices are one way to add fruits and vegetables to your diet as well as keep your body hydrated. They provide fluids as well as all the nutrients of the fruits and vegetables they were made from. However, if you are watching your calories, juice may not be your best choice. Despite the nutrition in every glass, the calories from the natural fruit sugar can add up quickly. In addition, the fiber of the fresh fruit and/or vegetable makes the whole foods more filling and satisfying than the juice. For example, one fresh orange has about 60 calories and 3 g of fiber. One cup of fresh orange juice has about 110 calories and less than 1 g of fiber.

When you buy juices, choose the unsweetened varieties that do not have added sugars. Watch for words such as fruit drink or fruit punch. These drinks are not generally nutritionally equivalent to fruit juice. They tend to be higher in sugar (usually corn syrup) and other additives with less actual fruit juice.

Vegetable juices tend to have less sugar than fruit juices. The only caution with canned or bottled vegetable juice is a higher salt content. Check labels carefully, and select a salt-reduced juice. ❖

CAUTION

Fruit juice should not be given to infants under 6 months according to a report from the American Academy of Pediatrics. Juice, while rich in some nutrients, does not have the important nutrients that breast milk or infant formula have. If a baby drinks juice instead of milk, it would be difficult to get the nutrients necessary for growth and development. And drinking a bottle of juice is filling, so the baby won't want to drink milk. In addition, drinking lots of juice can lead to diarrhea, poor weight gain, and tooth decay. As children grow, the same can be true. While the sweet taste of juice is appealing to kids, it should not replace more nutritious foods in their diet. Children should be encouraged to eat whole fruits instead.

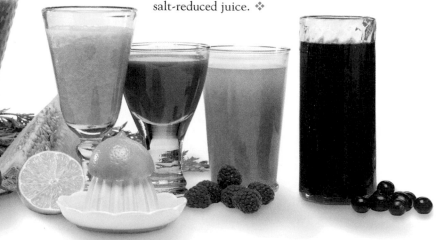

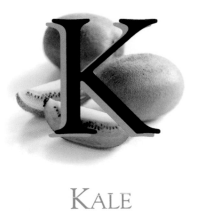

KALE

BENEFITS

- An excellent source of beta carotene and vitamin C.
- A good source of folate, calcium, iron, and potassium.
- Contains bioflavonoids and other substances that protect against cancer.

DRAWBACKS

- May cause gas in some people.

A member of the cabbage family, kale looks like collards but with curly leaves. It is a hardy autumn vegetable that grows best in a cool climate; in fact, exposure to frost actually improves its flavor. Although the types of kale that form leafy red, yellow, and purple heads are used more often for decorative purposes (both in the garden and on the table) than as a food, all varieties are edible and highly nutritious.

Kale—like its relatives in the cabbage family—is an excellent source of vitamin C and beta carotene, which the human body converts to vitamin A; in fact, a 1-cup serving of cooked kale contains almost a day's supply of vitamin A and well over 50 percent of the daily requirement of vitamin C. Other nutrients found in a cup of kale include 20 mcg (micrograms) of folate, 100 mg of calcium, 1 mg of iron, and 310 mg of potassium. It also provides more than 1 g of fiber and has only 50 calories; yet, it is filling, making kale an ideal, highly nutritious food for anyone who is weight-conscious.

In addition, kale contains more iron and calcium than almost any other vegetable; its high vitamin C content enhances the body's ability to absorb these minerals. Serving kale with a lemon dressing or in the same meal as another acidic citrus fruit further boosts absorption of the iron and calcium.

Bioflavonoids, carotenoids, and other cancer-fighting compounds are abundant in kale. It also contains indoles, compounds that can lessen the cancer-causing potential of estrogen and induce production of enzymes that protect against disease.

The typical way of preparing kale is to cook it. To preserve its rich stores of beta carotene and vitamin C, cook kale quickly in minimal water; it can be steamed, chopped, and stir-fried with other vegetables, or simmered until tender in broth to make a tasty soup. Kale shrinks considerably during cooking; it takes about 3 cups of raw greens to make a 1-cup serving. Even cooked, kale produces gas in some people. ❖

KIDNEY DISEASE

CONSUME PLENTY OF

- Liquids to replace lost fluids and maintain fluid balance.

LIMIT

- Foods high in oxalates (citrus fruits, berries, rhubarb, leafy green vegetables, beets, peppers, and chocolate), to prevent kidney stones.
- Salt to reduce fluid retention and prevent high blood pressure.

AVOID

- Over-the-counter painkillers, vitamin pills, and calcium supplements, which have side effects and interactions that cause kidney damage.

Kidney disease may be either a primary condition, such as kidney stones, or a consequence of other disorders, such as hypertension, atherosclerosis, or diabetes—all of which can severely damage the organs' blood vessels. Older men are susceptible to kidney infections stemming from enlargement of the prostate. Pregnant women and diabetics are vulnerable to infections of the urinary tract. Side effects from drugs are common and preventable causes of serious kidney disorders. For example, acetaminophen, aspirin, and other nonsteroidal anti-inflammatory drugs (NSAIDs) and calcium with vitamin D supplements are among the nonprescription drugs that can damage kidneys;

combining aspirin and acetaminophen is especially damaging. Whenever you see your doctor, be sure to mention any over-the-counter medications or vitamin supplements you have been taking, even if occasionally.

Healthy people should not wait for problems to crop up; rather, they should try to follow a diet that will help prevent kidney disorders. Drink plenty of liquids to flush the urinary system and replace lost fluids, and consume a low-fat diet that emphasizes starchy foods, vegetables, and fruits.

Diet is crucial in treating kidney problems. If you have a serious kidney disease, your doctor will probably refer you to a clinical dietitian for advice concerning changes to your diet. The allowable types and portions of foods differ, depending upon the type and severity of the kidney disorder.

KIDNEY STONES

Approximately 1 in 10 North Americans receives treatment for kidney stones each year; men outnumber women about three to one. Some people suffer their first attack after taking up a steady exercise program, such as jogging, and failing to drink enough fluids to replace the amount lost in sweat. At least half of those who suffer one attack will have a recurrence.

Kidney stones form when crystalline minerals—normally flushed away in the urine—stick together to form clumps, ranging in size from a grain of sand to coarse gravel. The cause may be gout or another metabolic problem, or it may be a structural or metabolic abnormality within the kidney. When kidney stones block any part of the urinary system, especially the ureters or bladder, they cause intense pain. Stones may pass through the system; others must be removed surgically or by sound-wave treatment (lithotripsy).

In order to prevent recurrences, it is important to determine the cause of the kidney stones. Most are formed of calcium oxalate or calcium phosphate. Less commonly, stones may form from uric acid crystals, especially in people with gout. A fourth type, cystine stones, occurs in fairly rare metabolic diseases.

FLUIDS FOR HEALTHY KIDNEYS. *Liquids are extremely important when it comes to the proper functioning of the kidneys. Water, lemonade, and juices all help to prevent the formation of stones.*

Fluids, fluids, and more fluids. Regardless of the type of stone, it's essential to drink enough liquids to maintain fluid balance and flush away the minerals that accumulate to form stones. Most people with stones could reduce the risk of recurrence by increasing their fluid intake (plain water is best) so that they excrete about 2 qt (2 liters) of urine a day.

Another beverage to consider is fresh lemonade, sweetened with as little sugar as possible. Lemons are loaded with citric acid, which has been shown to decrease urinary calcium excretion. Although most stones contain calcium, it's not a good idea to cut down on dietary calcium unless your doctor specifically orders it. If the body fails to get enough calcium, it will rob the bones to get the mineral, thus increasing the danger of osteoporosis.

Phosphorus-rich foods contribute to the formation of calcium phosphate stones. The balance of phosphorus and calcium in the diet is very delicate, however, and restricting the intake of one may interfere with the other. A dietitian's or doctor's guidance is necessary when changing your intake of either essential mineral to maintain balanced nutrition.

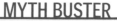

MYTH BUSTER

Myth: People with kidney stones should cut down on calcium-rich foods.

Reality: There is recent evidence that adequate calcium intake actually reduces the risk of calcium oxalate stones because calcium combines with oxalate in the digestive tract and prevents oxalate from being absorbed.

Cut down on foods high in oxalate. Oxalate-rich foods include rhubarb, beets, nuts, tofu, chocolate, tea, berries, red currants, tangerines, wheat bran and wheat germ, most of the dark green leafy vegetables, sweet potatoes, baked beans, lentils, and beer. It doesn't pay to take a drastic approach, however; eliminating all these foods depletes the diet of essential vitamins and minerals. A doctor or dietitian will provide a list of foods that can be eaten in moderation with little risk of causing a recurrence. People with gout should keep to a low-purine diet to reduce the risk of uric acid stones.

Kidney stones are rare in strict vegetarians. While the connection between stones and protein is not fully understood, it is known that protein increases the acidity of urine, which probably plays a role. Many people could reduce the risk of recurrence of stones by decreasing their daily protein intake to between 0.363 and 0.454 g per pound (0.8 and 1.0 g per kilogram) of body weight. It's easier to reduce protein intake if you cut down on animal products. Combining complex carbohydrates such as rice and beans can supply the essential amino acids.

NEPHRITIS

Inflammation of the kidney—known medically as nephritis—may result from a bacterial infection or a number of other causes, including side effects of drugs. Infections sometimes arise elsewhere in the body and reach the kidneys through the bloodstream, or enter the body through the urinary tract and travel up through the bladder to the kidneys. Kidney infections, like stones, require a doctor's intervention and must be treated with antibiotics. No special dietary measures should be necessary; however, people with kidney infections should drink plenty of fluids. A daily glass of cranberry juice helps prevent recurrence of urinary tract infections in susceptible persons.

KIDNEY FAILURE

Kidney failure may be either a temporary response to acute shock or injury or a severe long-term state necessitating drastic treatment. Acute kidney failure may be caused by severe infection, burns, diarrhea or vomiting, poisoning (including drug effects or interactions), surgery, or kidney injury. When the problem is resolved, function usually returns to normal. Chronic kidney failure may be caused by untreated hypertension, poorly controlled diabetes, or an inborn condition. Severe chronic, or end-stage, kidney failure requires regular dialysis—in which a machine removes waste products from the blood—or where possible, kidney transplantation.

Diet is extremely important in the management of kidney failure. General recommendations include restricting phosphorus, potassium, protein, and salt. Fluids must be monitored. With too little, the electrolytes are out of balance; with too much, fluid retention causes edema and electrolyte problems, and contributes to high blood pressure and perhaps congestive heart failure. Protein needs must be adjusted as kidney function, dialysis, or stress levels change.

Studies show that if protein is limited to about 0.5 g per pound (1 g per kilogram) of body weight per day, the patient on dialysis will receive the essential amino acids but reduce the risk of further kidney damage. Proteins from fish, egg whites, and legume and grain combinations are preferable to those in meat because they contain less saturated fat.

Kidney failure requires highly specialized medical care. No changes in diet should be made without a doctor's approval. Consult regularly with a specialist dietitian who will monitor the diet and make any necessary adjustments in the amounts of nutrients, including vitamin and mineral supplements. ❖

KIWIFRUITS

BENEFITS
- An excellent source of vitamin C.
- A good source of potassium and fiber.
- Can be used as a meat tenderizer.

On the outside a kiwifruit looks like a fuzzy brown egg; on the inside its bright green flesh is sprinkled with a ring of small, black seeds. It has a distinctive, somewhat tart flavor with overtones of fruits and berries.

The kiwi originated in China and was known as the Chinese gooseberry until New Zealand fruit growers renamed it for their national bird and began exporting it. Kiwis were once considered an exotic fruit, but they are now grown in California and have become increasingly plentiful. Kiwis are harvested while green and can be kept in cold storage for 6 to 10 months, making them available for most of the year. Ripe kiwis are eaten raw; even the skin can be consumed if it is defuzzed.

A large kiwi provides about 80 mg of vitamin C and the fruits are richly endowed with phytochemicals. A large 4-oz (115-g) fruit contains more than 100 mg. It also provides a good amount of potassium and pectin, a soluble fiber that helps control blood cholesterol levels. Kiwis contain both lutein and zeaxanthin, antioxidants associated with eye health. A 4-oz (115-g) serving has only 70 calories.

An enzyme (actinidin) that is a natural meat tenderizer is found in kiwi. The fruit can be used as a marinade to tenderize tough meats. Rubbing the meat with a cut kiwi and waiting 30 to 60 minutes before cooking will tenderize the meat without imparting any flavor from the fruit. This enzyme also will keep gelatin from setting and will curdle milk and cream; these

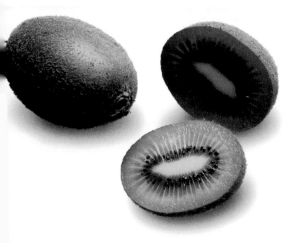

effects can be prevented by poaching the fruit beforehand. Don't overcook the fruit, however; it quickly turns to mush. ❖

KOHLRABI

BENEFITS
- High in vitamin C, potassium, and cancer-preventing antioxidants and bioflavonoids.
- High in dietary fiber.

DRAWBACKS
- May cause gas in some people.

Similar to both cabbages and turnips, kohlrabi comes from the same cruciferous plant family. Because the bulb, which is the edible part of the plant, is not as rich in nutrients as the flowers or leaves, kohlrabi is not in the same nutritional league as broccoli, brussels sprouts, and kale. Still, it is a good source of vitamin C; a one- to

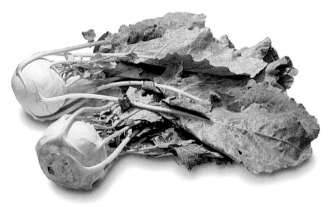

two-cup serving provides 60 percent of the Recommended Dietary Allowance (RDA) for adult women. It also has about 250 mg of potassium, some fiber, and only 25 calories.

This vegetable is high in bioflavonoids, plant pigments that work with vitamin C and other antioxidants to prevent the cell damage that promotes cancer. Kohlrabi is also high in indoles, chemicals that reduce the effects of estrogen, and thus may reduce the risk of breast cancer. Isothiocyanates, another group of compounds in kohlrabi, promote the action of enzymes that may protect against colon cancer.

Kohlrabi should be harvested before it reaches full maturity; otherwise, it becomes woody. It can be sliced and eaten raw, but it is usually steamed until tender. People who get gas after eating other cruciferous vegetables may have the same response to kohlrabi. ❖

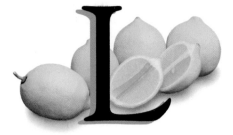

LACTOSE INTOLERANCE

USE

- Lactose-reduced milk, lactase enzyme drops or lactase enzyme tablets if you are unable to digest milk.
- Hard cheese and yogurt, which contain little lactose.

AVOID

- Foods that cause any discomfort.
- Medications containing lactose filler if you are lactose intolerant, provided substitutes are available.

METABOLIC INTOLERANCE

Lactose intolerance, the inability to digest milk sugar, is very common. Lactose is the natural sugar found in milk and milk products. It has to be broken down by an enzyme called lactase into glucose and galactose before it can be absorbed and used by the body. If you don't have enough enzyme to handle the lactose in the food you eat, you will experience a variety of unpleasant symptoms such as gas, bloating, diarrhea, and cramps after the ingestion of lactose-containing foods. This is because the unabsorbed lactose passes into the colon, where it is consumed by bacteria. The by-products of this bacterial activity are gases such as hydrogen and methane, which are responsible for the discomfort. The condition can be diagnosed by measuring the amount of hydrogen exhaled before and after ingesting lactose. An excessive amount of hydrogen confirms lactose intolerance. Except for a few inedible shrubs, milk is the only source of lactose. Once prehistoric humans were weaned, they never had lactose again; hence, they no longer needed lactase, the enzyme that breaks down milk sugar in the digestive tract. With evolutionary thrift, lactase was programmed to disappear as milk was phased out of a child's diet.

Adults who can digest milk are a minority in the world population; 70 percent of people of African and Asian descent are partly or entirely lactose-intolerant after 4 years of age. By contrast, 90 percent of people of Northern European descent continue to produce lactase. This genetic trait probably enabled their forebears to absorb extra calcium in a habitat where there was little sunlight available to develop vitamin D in the skin.

Transient or permanent lactose intolerance may follow an illness that injures the intestinal lining such as gastrointestinal illness, celiac disease, or inflammatory bowel disease. It can also follow treatment with antibiotics or anti-inflammatory drugs. In some cases the intolerance is temporary and will disappear when bowel health returns to normal. In other cases, lactose intolerance is a "threshold intolerance." This means you can handle small amounts of lactose but increasing doses cause a problem.

Lactose is found in dairy products, including milk, yogurt, and cheese. It can also be found as an ingredient or component of various food products such as cookies, breads, processed meats, hot dogs, some artificial sweeteners, and even some medications. Read labels carefully and look for milk, milk solids, cream, whey, cheese flavors, curds, and nonfat milk powder.

Eat small amounts of dairy products. Most lactose-intolerant people can consume some milk without much discomfort. They can also safely eat cultured dairy products such as yogurt because the bacteria used in fermentation use up most of the lactose for fuel. For people with more severe intolerance who still want dairy products, grocery stores sell lactose-reduced dairy products, and pharmacies carry enzyme drops that can be added to milk and enzyme tablets that can be taken before eating dishes containing dairy products.

Warning: Don't confuse lactose intolerance with milk allergy, which is hypersensitivity to the proteins in dairy products. If you are allergic to milk, consuming a lactose-reduced product will not prevent a reaction. ❖

GET REACQUAINTED WITH MILK

Even if you are lactose intolerant, you can include milk products as part of your diet. Just:

- Start very slowly. Try a quarter-cup of milk and gradually work your way up. You'll find, in time, your tolerance will increase. The more you avoid dairy, the more intolerant you will become.
- Drink milk with meals, never on an empty stomach.
- Enjoy yogurt. The active cultures in yogurt make it highly digestible.
- Eat hard cheeses containing only negligible amounts of lactose, like Cheddar, Edam, Gouda.
- Drink lactose-reduced milk.

LAMB

BENEFITS
- An excellent source of protein and B-complex vitamins.
- A rich source of minerals, including iron and phosphorus.

DRAWBACKS
- Some cuts are high in fat.

Lamb is a high-quality, nutritious meat, rich in easily absorbed minerals and B vitamins, particularly B_{12}. Lamb comes from sheep less than one year of age and often as young as 5 to 7 months. Special varieties include baby or hothouse lamb, which is only 6 to 10 weeks old, and the meat of lambs raised in salt marshes, which has an unmistakably briny tang. Mutton comes from sheep older than one year, and it has a more robust taste. Lamb comes in a variety of cuts including legs, shoulder, roast, chops, ground, foreshank, and spareribs.

Lamb is the primary meat in parts of Europe, North Africa, the Middle East, and India. But it has never enjoyed the same popularity in North America. In 2000, for example, per capita consumption of lamb was only 1.12 lb (0.5 kg), while the average North American consumes more than 50 lb (22.7 kg) of beef.

RICH IN NUTRITION

Among red meats, lamb stands out for its high nutritional value. Although some cuts are high in fat, lamb is not marbled like beef. Since much of its fat is on the outside of the meat, it can be trimmed before cooking. In addition, the meat is tender, because it is the relatively little-used muscle of young animals. A 3-oz (85-g) portion of roasted lean lamb contains approximately 200 calories, with about 22 g of protein and less than 10 g of fat.

Lamb is a rich source of protein, B-complex vitamins, as well as iron, phosphorus, calcium, and potassium. Because it is easily digestible and almost never associated with food allergies, it is a good protein food for people of all ages.

Lamb is a source of conjugated linoleic acid (CLA), a group of fatty acids that occur naturally in meat and milk products from ruminant animals. (See Fats.) Animal studies have found that CLA improved cholesterol profiles and delayed the development of atherosclerosis. In addition, CLA may have anticarcinogenic properties. Although it is premature to draw definitive conclusions about the protective benefits of CLAs, there is growing interest and research in this area. ❖

LEEKS

BENEFITS
- Low in calories, with some iron and calcium and folate.

DRAWBACKS
- Like other members of the onion family, may cause bad breath and gas.

Leeks are closely related to onions—as the similarity in flavor shows—and are distant cousins of asparagus. All three are members of the lily family. Although the entire leek is edible, most people prefer to eat the white, fleshy base and tender inner leaves and to discard the bitter dark green leaf tops.

Although leeks probably originated in warm regions of Asia or the Mediterranean, they are now intensively cultivated in temperate to cool climates. In Wales, where leeks are a national symbol, men parade in the streets with leek-bedecked hats on a special holiday.

Low-calorie leeks provide an appreciable amount of minerals and fiber. A half cup of chopped, boiled leeks, served plain, contains only 15 calories with 15 mcg (micrograms) of folate, 0.5 mg of iron, and 16 mg of calcium.

Vegetables in the onion group may have a protective effect against stomach cancer, and like onions, leeks may help to lower cholesterol. On a more negative note, they can cause bad breath and, in some people, gassiness.

Leeks are useful in a range of dishes where their mild oniony flavor is desired. You can boil and sieve them with potatoes for a chilled vichyssoise soup; braise them in fat-free stock to serve hot; or brush them lightly with olive oil and then grill them as part of a mixed vegetable barbecue. To make a reduced-fat quiche, steam chopped leeks and mix them with eggs and low-fat yogurt. ❖

LEEKS HELP TO WARD OFF CANCER

Kaempferol is an anticancer substance found in leeks. It may help to block the development of cancer-causing compounds.

LEGUMES

BENEFITS

- Contain more protein than any other plant-derived food.
- A good source of starch, B-complex vitamins, iron, potassium, zinc, and other essential minerals.
- Most are high in soluble fiber.

DRAWBACKS

- May cause bloating and intestinal gas.
- Can trigger allergies in some people.
- Must be cooked to destroy numerous toxic substances.

The 13,000 different varieties of legumes that are grown worldwide share two major characteristics—they all produce seed-bearing pods, and have nodules on their roots, which harbor bacteria that can convert atmospheric nitrogen to nitrate, a form of nitrogen the plant uses for nutrition. Otherwise, these members of the Leguminosae plant family differ greatly: some are low-growing plants (bush beans, lentils, and soybeans) or vines (many peas and beans); others are trees (carob) or shrubs (mesquite). Although peanuts are often classified as nuts, they are actually legumes; so too are clover and alfalfa, two major hay crops, and fenugreek.

Archeologists have found evidence that beans and peas were cultivated in Southeast Asia some 11,000 years ago, which may mean that they were actually grown before grains. Chickpeas, fava (broad) beans, and lentils have been cultivated in the Middle East since about 8000 B.C., and beans have been grown in the New World since 4000 B.C. The European colonists noted that Native people grew beans between rows of corn. At the time, they believed that this was to reduce weed growth; we now know that most legumes replenish the soil with nitrogen, a nutrient depleted by corn and other grains.

Because legumes may lack certain amino acids (the building blocks of protein), it has been thought that these foods must be eaten at the same time as other foods which contain the missing amino acids to provide a "complete" protein. For example, combining beans and corn to make the popular Indian dish succotash provides complete protein, as does any combination of legumes and grains. These combinations are referred to as complementary proteins. However, it is now known that if there is a mix of amino acids throughout the day, then having complementary proteins at the same meal isn't necessary. Soybeans contain almost all of the essential amino acids that make complete protein; they are also high in calcium. Thus, strict vegetarians whose diets exclude all animal foods can rely on tofu and other soy products for protein and some of their calcium.

NUTRITIONAL WINNERS

Legumes are among our most nutritious plant foods—high in protein, B-complex vitamins, iron, potassium, and other minerals. They provide large amounts of fiber, including the soluble type that is important in controlling blood cholesterol levels. Studies have shown that people who eat more legumes have a lower risk of heart disease.

Legumes contain a range of important phytochemicals that have a number of disease-fighting properties. Some of the important ones include: isoflavones, which are protective against heart disease and cancer; saponins, which help lower cholesterol; and phytosterols, which have anticancer and cholesterol-lowering properties.

Legumes are also a good food for a diabetic diet because their balance of complex carbohydrates and protein provides a slow, steady source of glucose instead of the sudden surge that can occur after eating simple carbohydrates.

Most legumes are low in calories and fat; soybeans and peanuts, however, are high in mostly unsaturated oils.

THE DOWNSIDE

Legumes harbor a number of toxic substances or compounds that interfere with the action or absorption of vitamins. Soybeans, for example, contain substances that interfere with the absorption of beta carotene and vitamins B_{12} and D; beans and peas have an anti-vitamin E compound. Heating and cooking inactivates most of these substances, but to compensate for vitamin loss, balance legume consumption with ample fresh fruits and yellow or dark green vegetables (for beta carotene), lean meat or other animal products (for vitamin B_{12}), and cooked greens, wheat germ, fortified cereals, seeds, nuts, and poultry (for vitamin E).

DID YOU KNOW?

LOSING WEIGHT IS EASIER WHEN YOU EAT LEGUMES

If you are trying to lose weight, a serving of legumes will help you to feel full more quickly. The rich fiber content fills your stomach and causes a slower rise in blood sugar, staving off hunger for longer and giving you a steady supply of energy.

BEANS, BEANS, AND MORE BEANS

There are hundreds of different varieties of beans; the following are among the more popular.

Adzuki. These small red beans are lower in B vitamins but higher in minerals than their larger red cousins, the kidney beans.

Black (turtle) beans. A staple in Latin American dishes, these are somewhat lower in folate than kidney beans but otherwise comparable in nutritional value.

Cannellini. These large white kidney beans are used in minestrone and other Italian dishes; they are usually purchased canned.

Cranberry. These oval-shaped beans with mottled pink skins are used either fresh or dried. Their nutrient content is comparable to that of kidney beans.

Great Northern. The largest white beans, they have a mild flavor that is especially suitable for casseroles and soups. They are somewhat less nutritious than other varieties.

Kidney. These red beans derive their name from their shape and are among the most nutritious of the dried types. They are a favorite for chilies, stews, and soups.

Limas. Used fresh or dried, lima beans are highly nutritious and are one of the most widely available beans. They are often combined with corn to make succotash, a high-quality protein dish.

Navy beans. A small, white version of Great Northerns, these have a milder flavor and slightly more folate and iron than most types.

Pinto. This mottled, multi-colored bean is one of the most nutritious types used in North America.

Red beans. Often combined with rice or used in chili, red beans are similar to kidney beans.

Soybeans. Among the most nutritious of all the legumes, soybeans give rise to many widely consumed products, including bean curd, soy milk, and flour.

People with gout are often advised to forgo dried peas and beans, lentils, and other legumes because of their high purine content. In susceptible people, purines increase levels of uric acid and can precipitate a gout attack. Some people of Mediterranean or Asian descent carry a gene that makes them susceptible to favism, a severe type of anemia contracted from eating fava beans. Anyone with a family history of this disease must not eat this type of bean.

Some legumes, especially peanuts, trigger an allergic reaction or migraine headaches in susceptible people. In such cases the offending foods should be eliminated from the diet.

Dried beans, lentils, and peas are notorious for causing intestinal gas and flatulence. The method of preparation can help reduce gas production. Change the water several times during the soaking and cooking process. (Lentils don't need to be soaked, but rinsing them after cooking lowers their gas-forming potential.) Always rinse canned beans and chickpeas; combining cooked legumes with an acidic food may reduce gas production. Some herbs, especially lemon balm, fennel, and caraway, can help to prevent flatulence. ❖

BEANS, BEANS, THE MAGICAL FRUIT...

The gas-causing culprits in beans are carbohydrates called oligosaccharides. Pre-soaking should help, or take a product called Beano before your meal.

HIGH IN PROTEIN, HIGH IN FIBER, LOW IN FAT. *Legumes are nutritional powerhouses that also help to control cholesterol levels.*

LEMONS

BENEFITS
- An excellent source of vitamin C.
- May relieve dry mouth.

DRAWBACKS
- The peel contains an irritating oil.
- May be sprayed with a fungicide.

Ideal for flavoring everything from fish to vegetables to tea, lemons are one of the most widely used of all citrus fruits. Sweetened, diluted, and chilled, fresh lemon juice is an old-fashioned summer thirst quencher. It's also an excellent source of vitamin C; one cup of lemon juice has about 55 mg of vitamin C, or more than 70 percent of the Recommended Dietary Allowance (RDA) for adult women. To get the most juice, place a lemon in warm water before squeezing.

Many recipes call for fresh lemon zest, which is the grated outer peel. The zest is rich in an antioxidant chemical called rutin, which helps strengthen the walls of veins and capillaries. Because lemons are often sprayed with fungicides to retard mold growth and pesticides to kill insects, wash them thoroughly before grating the peel. Select lemons that have not been waxed (wax may seal in fungicides). Lemon peels contain limonene, an oil that can irritate the skin in susceptible persons. Limonene is being studied for its antitumor activity and may prove useful against breast cancer. ❖

LETTUCE AND OTHER SALAD GREENS

BENEFITS
- Low in calories.
- Some varieties are high in beta carotene, folate, vitamin C, calcium, and potassium.

DRAWBACKS
- Often eaten with large amounts of oily or high-fat creamy dressings.

A green salad is often part of a healthy dinner, and although many vegetables may be used in it, lettuce is by far the most popular ingredient. Lettuce is the second most popular vegetable sold in supermarkets, topped only by potatoes. Two basic reasons account for its popularity: health-conscious people are consuming more fruits and vegetables; and low-cost lettuce and other fresh salad greens are now available year-round, thanks to modern refrigeration and food transportation.

Weight watchers are especially partial to salads—they are low in calories yet filling, since they are high in fiber. Unfortunately, a large green salad that contains only 50 calories can quickly become more fattening than a steak if it's drowned in a creamy high-fat dressing. There are, however, many tasty low-fat alternative dressings—herb vinegar mixed with a little olive oil, a sprinkling of herbs and lemon juice, or low-fat yogurt combined with garlic, chopped parsley, and lemon juice.

GOOD NUTRITION

Some types of lettuce and other salad greens contain high amounts of beta carotene, folate, vitamin C, calcium, iron, and potassium, but the amounts vary considerably from one variety to another. In general, those with dark green or other deeply colored leaves have more beta carotene and vitamin C than the paler varieties. Romaine lettuce, for example, has five times as much vitamin C and more beta carotene and folate than iceberg lettuce.

Such salad greens as arugula, chicory, escarole, mâche, and watercress are all more nutritious than lettuce; many people also find them more flavorful, and they are becoming readily available in restaurants and markets. Some, such as chicory, escarole, and watercress, are slightly bitter, yet they provide an interesting flavor and texture contrast when added to a salad of lettuce and other types of greens.

Arugula, a member of the same plant family as broccoli, cabbage, and other cruciferous vegetables, has a tangy, peppery flavor when grown during the cool spring and fall months, and a stronger, mustardlike taste if harvested during the summer. This is one of the most nutritious of all salad greens: a 2-cup serving has more calcium than most other salad greens and is a source of vitamin C, beta carotene, iron and folate—all for only 12 calories. Watercress, another cruciferous vegetable, is also a nutritional winner: 1 cup contains a mere 5 calories, yet it provides 15 mg of vitamin C and 45 mg of

MIXED SALAD. *The many varieties of lettuces and other salad greens include (clockwise from upper right) romaine, red leaf, watercress, curly endive, mâche, iceberg, radicchio, arugula, Belgian endive, escarole, and spinach.*

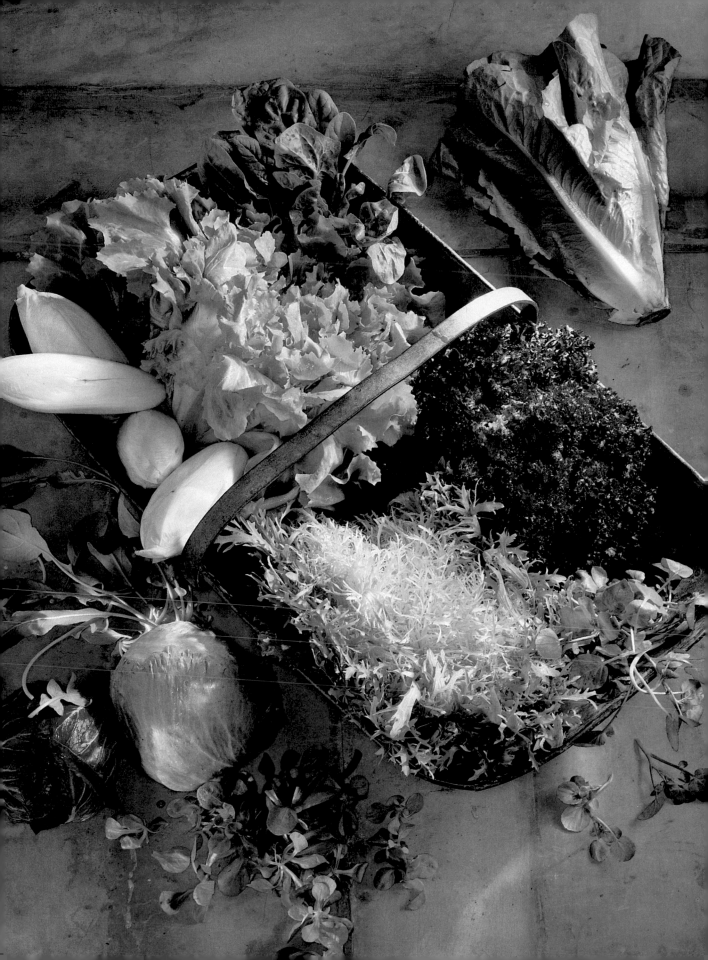

calcium. Deeply colored lettuces and greens are also high in bioflavonoids, plant pigments known to work with vitamin C and other antioxidants to prevent cancer-causing cell damage.

Lettuce and other greens can be mixed or combined with a broad spectrum of raw fruits or vegetables, cold pasta, or chunks of chicken or tuna to make a low-calorie, highly nutritious main dish. Raw spinach is often used as a salad green; although cooking makes some of its nutrients a bit easier to absorb, a spinach salad still provides good amounts of beta carotene, folate, vitamin C, and calcium.

TYPES OF GREENS

There are dozens of different varieties of lettuce; some of the more widely available are listed below. Make your salads with a variety of greens to elevate your fiber intake and antioxidant levels.

Arugula, which resembles dandelion greens, is strongly flavored and tastes best when grown in cool temperatures.

Belgian endive, a slightly bitter relative of chicory, is grown under a soil cover to produce a small head of light yellow or white leaves. It adds an interesting texture and flavor to salads; it can be braised or steamed and served hot.

Butterhead, which includes Boston and bibb lettuces, forms loosely packed heads of tender, mildly flavored leaves.

Chicory and escarole are related greens with a somewhat bitter taste. They are nutritious but are not widely used because of their assertive flavors.

Iceberg, a crisp, tightly packed head lettuce, is the most widely consumed salad ingredient in North America, but it provides less nutrition than most other varieties of lettuce and greens.

Looseleaf includes green and red oak and green and red leaf lettuces, as well as other types that do not form heads.

Mâche, or lamb's lettuce, has small, delicate leaves. This expensive green is most often found in gourmet shops.

Romaine has long, crisp, dark green leaves that form a loose head. Also called cos lettuce, it is used to make Caesar and similar salads.

Watercress grows in cold streambeds in the late winter and early spring; it has a sharp flavor and is used mostly as a garnish or in soups. ❖

DO ONE SIMPLE THING

TOSS YOUR SALAD GREENS WITH OIL

Make your salad with a variety of beta carotene-rich salad greens, like watercress, chicory, and escarole, and a little flavored vinegar, lemon juice, and oil. Oil enhances the absorption of beta carotene, which plays an important role in preventing cancer and vision loss.

LIMES

BENEFITS
- An excellent source of vitamin C.
- Can be used to flavor and tenderize meat, poultry, and fish.

DRAWBACKS
- Peels contain psoralens, which increase sun sensitivity.

In the mid-1700s James Lind, a Scottish naval surgeon, discovered that drinking the juice of limes and lemons prevented scurvy, the scourge of sailors on long voyages. Soon British ships carried ample stores of the fruits, earning their sailors the nickname "limey." It was later learned that vitamin C deficiency causes scurvy, and that limes are very high in this essential nutrient.

Four ounces (115 g) of lime juice has 30 mg of vitamin C, or 40 percent of the Recommended Dietary Allowance (RDA) for adult women. Limes are high in bioflavonoids and other antioxidants, which help protect against cancer and other diseases. Limonene, found mainly in the zest of lemons and limes, may help reduce cancer risk.

Like lemons, limes are useful as flavoring agents. However, unlike lemons, limes do not impart a distinctive taste of their own when used as a cooking ingredient; instead, they tenderize and heighten the flavors of other foods, especially fish and poultry. Lime juice can also be used as a salt substitute for meat and fish dishes. A sprinkling of lime juice over a fruit salad prevents discoloration.

Lime peels contain psoralens, chemicals that make the skin sensitive to the sun; thus, care should be taken to minimize skin contact with lime peels. Cut away the peels before squeezing the fruit so that the citrus oil containing the psoralens doesn't get into the juice. ❖

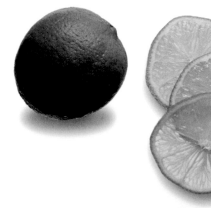

LIVER

See Organ Meats

LIVER DISORDERS

EAT PLENTY OF

- Fatty fish as well as walnuts, soybeans, whole grains, flaxseed and canola oils for omega-3 fatty acids.
- Fresh fruits and vegetables for vitamins, minerals, and phytochemicals.
- Small meals and snacks, if they are more appealing than large meals.

AVOID

- Alcohol in all forms.

The liver, located in the upper right abdomen and protected by the ribs, performs thousands of vital chemical and metabolic functions—among them, the storage of fat-soluble vitamins, iron and other minerals, and glycogen for future needs. It manufactures cholesterol, amino acids, and other essential compounds, removes waste substances from the blood, detoxifies alcohol and environmental chemicals, and metabolizes most medications.

Amazingly, our bodies can still function when only one-quarter of the liver is healthy enough to operate. Unlike most other organs, even after severe damage, the liver can regenerate itself by growing new cells. When severely diseased or subjected to excessive abuse, however, the liver will fail—often with fatal results.

Liver diseases are common, but experts feel that many cases could be prevented by careful attention to diet and hygiene. The most common disorders are hepatitis (usually caused by a virus spread by sewage contamination or direct contact with infected body fluids), cirrhosis, and liver cancer. The risk of liver cancer is higher in those who have cirrhosis or who have had certain types of viral hepatitis; but more often, the liver is the site of secondary (metastatic) cancers spread from other organs. Symptoms are often not felt until the disease is advanced. The most recognized symptom of liver disease is jaundice, the yellowing of the skin and the whites of the eyes, caused by a buildup of bile pigments (bilirubin) in the skin.

People with liver disease are often deficient in the water-soluble vitamins, such as folate, niacin, and thiamine, as well as the fat-soluble vitamins A and D. Vitamin deficiencies are most common among alcoholics, who often substitute alcohol for food. Even when food intake is maintained, alcohol places undue demands on the liver, which must preempt detoxifying it over its other metabolic functions. Liver disease is also linked with problems in metabolizing carbohydrates.

FOOD FOR THE LIVER

Eat small, frequent meals. The diet of a person recovering from a liver disorder should place the least burden on the organ; they should not eat fatty foods that are hard to digest. They often have a poor appetite and find it easier to eat frequent, nutritious snacks rather than meals.

Eat foods rich in fatty acids. Omega-3 fatty acids seem to facilitate the processing of fats in the liver; a diet rich in these nutrients lowers the rate at which the liver manufactures triglycerides, which is beneficial for people with circulatory and heart problems. These fatty acids are in salmon and other fatty fish, walnuts, soybeans, whole grains, flaxseed and canola oils.

Get lots of protein. It is important to include sufficient protein in the diet. Studies have shown that people with liver disease need at least 0.363 g of protein per pound (0.8 g per kilogram) of body weight per day, but the recommended amount is 0.545 to 0.682 g per pound (1.2–1.5 g per kilogram). Some evidence supports the use of vegetable protein foods such as those in soy, peas, and legumes, especially for people who develop mental confusion, a condition called hepatic encephalopathy. A good supply of carbohydrates is needed to meet the body's energy needs.

Consume plenty of vitamin D. Liver disease may cause a thinning of the bones (osteoporosis) if stores of vitamin D, which helps the body absorb calcium, are depleted; such cases may require calcium and vitamin D supplements. For the most part, however, vitamins and minerals should be provided within the diet; supplements can upset the nutritional balance and, in the case of excessive iron, can cause severe liver damage.

Absolutely no alcohol. Alcohol should be avoided until complete recovery; in some cases, however, it must be eliminated for life. ❖

LOBSTER

See Shellfish

LOW-CARB DIETS
▪DO THEY WORK?▪

There's no denying the current popularity of low-carbohydrate diets. Chances are, you, or someone you know, has tried one. Atkins, South Beach, The Zone, Protein Power . . . There is a long list to choose from. But do they work? What are the long-term health consequences of these diets?

How the diet works

The premise behind low-carbohydrate diets is that carbohydrate foods stimulate production of insulin, the hormone that is responsible for transporting glucose into the cells, where it is used for energy, with excess amounts being stored as fat. Since protein-rich foods do not cause the same rise in insulin levels, substituting them for carbohydrate foods promotes the use of stored fat for energy, resulting in weight loss.

Low-carb diets range from extreme to more moderate. Some of the more extreme approaches, like Dr. Atkins or the South Beach diet, recommend a carbohydrate level of 20 or 30 g per day during their initial stages. The current Recommended Dietary Allowance (RDA) for carbohydrate is a minimum of 130 g per day, with most people eating well over 200 g per day. More moderate diets, like The Zone, suggest carbohydrates represent 40 percent of calories (the current recommendation ranges from 45 to 65 percent), balanced with protein and fat at every meal.

Many low-carb diets allow unlimited amounts of meat, poultry, fish, and eggs, some non-starchy vegetables, nuts, seeds, oils and other fats. Some allow small amounts of fruits, dairy, and whole grains. Processed carbohydrates, like breads, pastas, cereals, and sugary foods, are restricted.

Although we don't yet fully understand the implications of low-carb diets, we are beginning to get a better picture of the pros and cons of this weight-loss approach.

Pros

There's good evidence that during the first 6 months, low-carb diets can result in more rapid weight loss than conventional low-calorie, low-fat diets. Studies show that during this time, subjects on low-carb programs lose up to twice the weight as those on conventional diets.

Low-carb diets can initially be easier to follow because the higher levels of protein and fat suppress appetite and keep dieters feeling full longer.

When compared to conventional diets, low-carb diets, in the short term, may have a more beneficial effect on both HDL cholesterol (the "good" cholesterol) and triglyceride levels. Both these factors are important for cardiovascular health. In one 6-month study, participants on a low-carb diet saw their "bad" LDL cholesterol drop by 10 points and their HDL increase by 10 points. Those on a low-fat diet showed a similar reduction in total cholesterol, but some of the loss came from a drop in HDL cholesterol.

Cons

The early weight-loss effect of low-carb diets decreases over time. By about 12 months, there is no significant difference in weight loss using a low-carb diet versus a conventional approach with restricted calories and fat.

Many of the stricter low-carb diets put the body into ketosis. Ketosis is the accumulation in the blood of ketones, which are by-products of fat metabolism. Ketosis is not a normal body state and can result in nausea, dehydration, dizziness, fatigue, and bad breath. The longer-term effects of chronic ketosis on health are unknown.

Because of the low-fiber, high-fat profile of many low-carb diets, constipation is often an unwanted side effect.

The lack of variety of food choices, particularly in the beginning, can make the diet difficult to stick with in the longer term. The lack of variety also means that there is a potential for inadequate intakes of important vitamins and minerals.

There are no studies on the long-term effects of low-carb diets on health. The effects of high protein and high fat intakes on kidney function, bone health, cardiovascular function, and cancer rates are unknown.

The low-carb diets allow far less than the 5 to 10 servings of fruits and vegetables a day associated with good health. In addition, scientific research has linked excessive meat consumption to colon and prostate cancer, and high protein intake with calcium loss from bones.

Bottom line

There is convincing evidence of the short-term effectiveness of low-carb diets. But over longer periods of time, these diets lose their advantage over low-calorie, low-fat diet approaches. In addition, significant concerns over long-term health effects remain.

Whatever your weight-loss goals, remember that good health is an important goal too. Hundreds of studies show that a diet that includes plenty of fruits and vegetables, whole grains, and lean protein sources, which is low in saturated fat, is strongly linked to a decreased incidence of disease.

Recent research highlights

■ Numerous studies have shown that during the first 6 months low-carb diets result in greater weight loss than conventional low-calorie, low-fat diets. However, this gap decreases with time and the difference in weight loss after 12 months is no longer significant.

■ There are no studies assessing the long-term health consequences (particularly kidney health, bone health, and cardiovascular function) of a high-protein, high-fat diet.

■ In the short term, low-carb diets have a stronger positive impact on HDL cholesterol levels and triglyceride levels than conventional diets. There is no difference in the effect on total cholesterol and LDL cholesterol levels between conventional and low-carb diets.

■ Many low-carb diets are also calorie-restricted, either because the program restricts them or because dieters are choosing to eat less food. So we don't know to what extent the weight loss on these diets is a result of simply eating less.

■ Studies of low-carb diets have suffered from high dropout rates by participants, making any findings other than short-term ones difficult to assess.

■ A small, but carefully controlled study presented to the American Association for the Study of Obesity in 2003 introduced intriguing evidence that people on low-carb, high-fat diets can actually eat more than people on standard low-fat diets and still lose more weight.

LUPUS

CONSUME PLENTY OF

- Fruits and vegetables such as grapefruit, broccoli, cabbage, and kale for antioxidants and bioflavonoids.
- Dairy products and fortified soy and rice beverages for calcium and vitamin D.
- Foods rich in essential fatty acids such as fish, nuts, flax, and omega-3 eggs.

LIMIT

- Fats, especially animal fats.

AVOID

- Alfalfa in all forms.
- Celery, parsnips, parsley, lemons, limes, and figs if you are sun sensitive.

Also known as systemic lupus erythematosus (or SLE), lupus is a chronic autoimmune disease. Although arthritic joint pain, skin rashes, debilitating fatigue, and dry mouth are the most common symptoms, it can also damage organs throughout the body, particularly the kidneys. Lupus strikes women about 10 times as often as men. While it is a mild disease for many, lupus can be serious and even life threatening for some people.

Lupus is believed to be caused by a genetic predisposition, triggered by environmental factors, such as a virus; it may be worsened by other factors, such as sun exposure, infection, stress, and certain foods and drugs.

But because lupus is such a variable disease, there is no one treatment regimen that helps everyone. The patient and physician may have to try different approaches to find one that seems to work. Therapy often requires taking a nonsteroidal anti-inflammatory drug (NSAID) to suppress inflammation, and hydroxychloroquine (a drug long used to fight malaria), which can increase resistance to sun exposure and help prevent lupus rashes and joint pain. For more severe problems, steroids or other immunosuppressive drugs may be prescribed.

CAUTION

If you are taking cyclosporine, a powerful immune system suppressor, do not consume grapefruits or grapefruit juice; although generally recommended for most lupus patients, they can dramatically increase the body's ability to absorb cyclosporine, leading to severe toxicity.

HARMFUL FOODS

Alfalfa in any form. Even herbal supplements containing alfalfa worsen lupus symptoms; other legumes may have a similar effect.

Mushrooms and some smoked foods. These may also cause problems for lupus sufferers.

Foods containing psoralens. If you are one of the majority of lupus patients whose disease is worsened by exposure to the sun or unshielded fluorescent light, avoid foods containing psoralens, such as celery, parsnips, parsley, lemons, and limes, which heighten photosensitivity.

Avoid high-protein, high-fat foods. Many lupus patients note an improvement after they decrease the consumption of fatty high-protein foods, especially animal products. Some experts recommend a vegetarian diet that allows eggs, skim milk, and other low-fat dairy products.

HELPFUL FOODS

Cereals, fruits, and vegetables. These foods are high in the antioxidant vitamins and minerals—vitamins C, beta carotene, zinc, and selenium. These are beneficial not only for lupus itself but also protect against heart disease. People with lupus tend to have high blood cholesterol levels, which may be worsened by steroid medications. Some studies have shown that lupus is associated with an increased level of oxidized blood fats and lower levels of circulating vitamin E; preliminary animal studies found that vitamin E may slow the progress of lupus. The best food sources of vitamin E include nuts, seeds, oils, and wheat germ.

Eat lots of cruciferous vegetables, bioflavonoids, and fatty fish. Broccoli and other cruciferous vegetables contain indoles that alter the metabolism of estrogen in a way that has a positive impact on lupus. Fresh citrus fruits, especially grapefruits, are high in bioflavonoids that seem to help lupus patients. Because most lupus patients need to avoid exposure to the sun, they should make sure their diet provides adequate vitamin D. Good sources include fluid milk, fortified soy and rice beverages, as well as salmon and other fatty fish. Researchers have found that fish oils have anti-inflammatory effects and may help relieve the joint pain, soreness, and stiffness associated with lupus.

DRUGS AND DIET

If you take aspirin or other NSAIDs, always take them with meals. If you are taking corticosteroids, cut back on salt; it will increase water retention and contribute to steroid-induced high blood pressure. Because steroids increase your risk of osteoporosis, consume plenty of calcium-rich dairy products, fish with bones, and dark green leafy vegetables. Supplements may be required. ❖

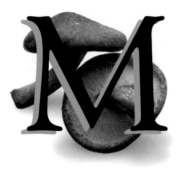

M

MANGOES

BENEFITS

- An excellent source of beta carotene and vitamin C.
- Low in calories, high in fiber.

Mangoes used to be regarded as a somewhat exotic fruit in North America; however, as more of the fruit is grown in Florida, California, and Hawaii, or imported from Mexico and Central America, mangoes are becoming increasing popular. The soft, juicy flesh of a ripe mango makes it difficult to peel and messy to eat, but those who persevere say it's worth the effort (see "How to Eat a Mango," right).

Mangoes are considered a comfort food in many parts of the world. They contain an enzyme with digestive properties similar to papain found in papayas—which also makes them a very good tenderizing agent.

NUTRITIONAL VALUE

Like other orange or deep yellow fruits, mangoes are exceptionally high in beta carotene, which the body converts to vitamin A. One medium-size (8-oz/230-g) mango has 135 calories and 57 mg vitamin C, which is more than 50 percent of the Recommended Dietary Allowance (RDA). It also provides 4 g of fiber and a healthy amount of potassium; mangoes are also high in pectin, a soluble fiber that is important in controlling blood cholesterol.

There are hundreds of different varieties of mangoes, ranging in size from a few ounces (about 100 g) to more than 4 lb (1.8 kg), but most of those sold in North America are 8 to 12 oz (230–340 g). Mangoes are usually picked and shipped while still somewhat green, but the skin should be turning yellow, becoming more orange or red as the fruit ripens.

When buying a mango, look for one with flesh that yields slightly when gently pressed

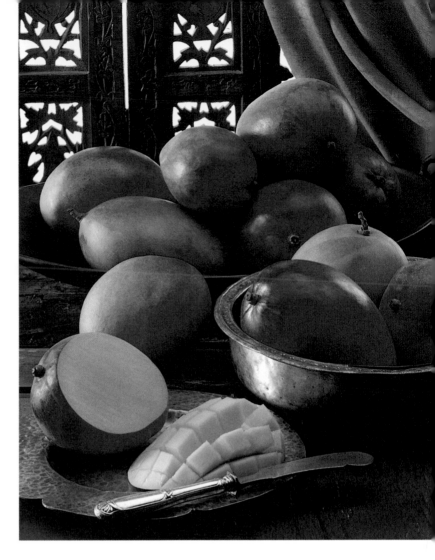

HOW TO EAT A MANGO

Some mango lovers advise eating the ripe fruit in the shower, where you can enjoy it without worrying about the juice running down your chin and onto your clothes. Here's a more practical approach. Make two vertical slices—one on each side of the pit—and use a sharp paring knife to remove one half of the fruit from the large seed. You can then cut the flesh into slices and remove the peel from each slice, one by one. Then cut around the pit of the remaining half, and again, slice and peel the fruit.

THE MANGO IS KNOWN AS THE "KING OF FRUIT" THROUGHOUT THE WORLD. *A favorite fruit in India and other tropical countries, the mango is becoming increasingly popular in North America for its unique flavor.*

---

and with an orange or reddish skin. Large dark spots may mean that the flesh is bruised. (If the skin is completely green, the fruit may not ripen; a fruit past its prime will have shriveled skin.) A flowery fragrance indicates that the mango is ripe and flavorful. If you place an unripe mango in a paper bag in a cool location, it will ripen in 2 or 3 days. (Don't put it in a sunny spot; this can spoil the flavor.) Ripe mangoes should be eaten as soon as possible. ❖

MARGARINE

See Butter and Margarine

MAYONNAISE

BENEFITS

- A good source of vitamin E, depending upon the type of oil used.

DRAWBACKS

- High in fat and calories.
- May trigger an allergic reaction in people sensitive to eggs and molds.
- May contain gluten, which should be avoided by those with celiac disease.
- Raw eggs used in fresh mayonnaise may pose a risk of salmonella.

The rich flavor and creamy texture of mayonnaise accounts for its wide popularity as a sandwich spread and salad dressing. There are several ways to make mayonnaise, but all involve the same basic ingredients—vegetable oil, eggs, and vinegar, lemon juice, or another acidic liquid—whipped together to form a semisolid spread. Egg yolks act as the emulsifying ingredient that allows the oil and vinegar or lemon juice to blend. Mustard, salt, pepper, sugar, and other seasonings may be added.

Most types of mayonnaise are good sources of vitamin E, yielding about 10 percent of the adult Recommended Dietary Allowance (RDA) in one tablespoon. The precise amount varies, however, according to the type of oil used; those made with sunflower, cottonseed, and safflower oils are highest in this antioxidant nutrient. (In general, labels of commercial mayonnaise do not specify the type of oil used.) The eggs do contribute protein and some minerals, but the amounts are negligible considering the number of calories per serving. A tablespoon of mayonnaise provides about 100 calories, about the same amount found in a tablespoon of butter or margarine. The yolks add dietary cholesterol, which should be minimized by anyone with high blood cholesterol, atherosclerosis, or heart disease.

HOMEMADE ENSURES BEST MADE

If you're concerned about the type of oil used, you can make your own mayonnaise at home. Most recipes call for olive oil, which is largely monounsaturated fat, although polyunsaturated oils, such as corn or safflower, can be substituted for a lighter flavor. The raw eggs used in homemade mayonnaise are a potential source of salmonella; this risk can be avoided by using a pasteurized egg substitute. Fresh mayonnaise should be used within 2 or 3 days. Even then, it can become a source of food poisoning if allowed to stand at room temperature for more than an hour. Commercial mayonnaise is safer, because its high vinegar content and antioxidant preservatives discourage the growth of disease-causing organisms.

"LITE" VARIETIES

Mayonnaise-type salad dressings contain less fat and fewer calories than regular mayonnaise. Although similar in texture and appearance, the salad dressings have a more acidic flavor, which can be tempered by adding a small amount of yogurt, whipped nonfat cottage cheese, or nonfat sour cream.

Low-fat, cholesterol-free, and nonfat mayonnaise substitutes are available. The low-fat versions substitute air, water, starches, and other fillers for some of the oil; nonfat varieties may be made with tofu, yogurt, and other such ingredients. A homemade recipe calls for tofu, egg whites, lemon juice, salt, mustard, and a little bit of olive oil. ❖

FIVE WAYS TO HOLD THE MAYO

SIMPLE STRATEGIES TO FIGHT THE FAT

1. If you really can't eat a sandwich made without mayonnaise, cut the amount in half by spreading it on one slice of bread only. And remember that many moist fillings, such as tuna salad, are made with mayonnaise.

2. Try mustard or ketchup in your sandwich instead of mayonnaise. They have much fewer calories, only 15 per level teaspoon, and no fat.

3. Salad dressings made with mayonnaise are laden with calories and fat. Lemon juice sparks up a fresh salad and adds neither fat nor calories. Low-fat yogurt dressings with herbs are also healthier alternatives.

4. When you must have the luxury of mayonnaise, temper the damage by mixing it half and half with low-fat plain yogurt or buttermilk.

5. Substitute half the amount of mayonnaise with nonfat cottage cheese, whipped in a blender for a creamy consistency.

MEDICINE-FOOD INTERACTIONS
■ HIDDEN DANGERS ■

In our body, drugs share the same route of absorption and metabolism as nutrients, which creates the potential for interactions.

When food affects medicine

Foods can affect drug action in many ways. The most common is when foods interfere with absorption, which can make a drug less effective. For example, calcium in milk can bind to the antibiotic tetracycline, interfering with its absorption. Nutrients or other components of food can also interfere with a drug's metabolism, or how it is broken down in the body. Finally, foods can affect the elimination of drugs from the body.

So some drugs should not be taken with food. Other drugs must be taken with food to prevent stomach irritation.

When medicine affects nutrients

Some drugs interfere with the absorption of nutrients. For example, some cholesterol-lowering medications reduce the absorption of fat-soluble vitamins. Others affect the body's use or elimination of nutrients, like diuretics, which can cause a depletion of potassium, and lead to a deficiency.

Dangerous interactions

The following are some of the more serious interactions that can occur between food and medicine (see also "Foods and Drugs That Don't Mix," next page):

MAO inhibitors and foods containing tyramine: Mixing monoamine oxidase (MAO) inhibitors—a class of medications used to treat depression—with foods high in tyramine produces one of the most dramatic and dangerous food-drug interactions. Symptoms include a rapid rise in blood pressure, severe headache, collapse, and even death. Foods high in tyramine include aged cheese, chicken liver, certain red wines, yeast extracts, processed meats, dried or pickled fish, legumes, soy sauce, and beer.

Grapefruit: Grapefruit juice contains a compound that can increase the absorption of certain drugs, which can result in receiving a larger dose than was intended. This effect is not seen with other citrus fruit juices. Examples of drugs that are affected include AIDS medications, cholesterol-lowering "statins," calcium channel blockers, antihypertension drugs, and cyclosporine, an immune system suppressant. As a general rule it is better to stay away from taking any medication with grapefruit juice. Since compounds in grapefruit juice can stay in the blood for 24 hours, effects may be noted even if the medication is not taken directly with the juice.

Foods high in vitamin K: Vitamin K is essential for clotting blood. Foods high in vitamin K, such as Swiss chard, kale, spinach, brussels sprouts, broccoli, and other leafy greens, can interfere with blood thinners.

Alcohol: Alcohol and medications do not mix well. Alcohol can slow down the body's metabolism, so medications stay active longer than they should. In some cases, mixing alcohol with medication can be fatal. Try to avoid it completely when taking prescription or over-the-counter medications.

DID YOU KNOW?

HIGH BLOOD PRESSURE DRUGS DEPLETE POTASSIUM

Many antihypertensive drugs deplete the body's reserves of potassium, an electrolyte that maintains the body's fluid balance and is also essential for nerve and muscle function. People on these medications should eat lots of bananas, citrus and dried fruits, tomatoes, and other potassium-rich foods.

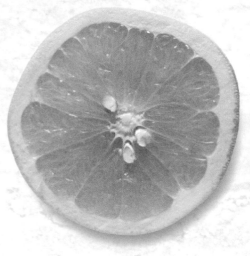

6 tips for taking medicines safely

1. Always carry a list of your medications and doses.
2. When your doctor prescribes a new medicine, tell him about any other drugs you are taking. This includes over-the-counter drugs and vitamin supplements.
3. If you have any side effects from a medication, contact your doctor or pharmacist immediately.
4. It is usually best to take prescription medications with a full glass of water. This can help prevent stomach irritation and improve absorption. Don't take them with soft drinks or grapefruit juice.
5. Don't mix your medications with food or drink unless instructed to by your doctor or pharmacist.
6. Always read and comply with any directions that come with your medication.

FOODS AND DRUGS THAT DON'T MIX

Before taking any medication, always read the package instructions and ask your doctor
or pharmacist about any dietary precautions. In some cases, drugs alter nutritional needs;
in other instances, foods can interfere with how a medication works. The table below details
how particular foods can interact with some of the more commonly used drugs.

DRUGS	EFFECTS AND PRECAUTIONS
ANTIBIOTICS	
Cephalosporins, penicillin	Take on an empty stomach to speed absorption of the drugs.
Ciprofloxacin	Avoid dairy products, caffeine, and supplements, which contain calcium, iron, or zinc, for 2 hours before and after taking the medication.
Erythromycin	Don't take with fruit juice or wine, which decrease the drug's effectiveness.
Sulfa drugs	Increase the risk of vitamin B_{12} deficiency.
Tetracycline	Dairy products decrease the drug's efficacy. Lowers vitamin C absorption.
ANTICOAGULANTS	
Warfarin	Foods high in vitamin K can reduce the drug's effectiveness. Do not increase or decrease the usual intake of broccoli, spinach, kale, brussels sprouts, or cabbage.
ANTICONVULSANTS	
Dilantin, phenobarbital	Increase the risk of anemia and nerve problems due to a deficiency of folate and other B vitamins.
ANTIDEPRESSANTS	
Fluoxetine	Reduces appetite and can lead to excessive weight loss.
Lithium	A low-salt diet increases the risk of lithium toxicity; excessive salt reduces drug's efficacy.
MAO inhibitors	Foods high in tyramine (aged cheeses, processed meats, legumes, wine, beer, among others) can bring on a hypertensive crisis.
Tricyclics	Many foods, especially legumes, meat, fish, and foods high in vitamin C, reduce absorption of the drugs.
ANTIHYPERTENSIVES, HEART MEDICATIONS	
ACE inhibitors	Take on an empty stomach to improve the absorption of the drugs.
Alpha blockers	Take with liquid or food to avoid an excessive drop in blood pressure.
Antiarrhythmic drugs	Avoid caffeine, which increases the risk of an irregular heartbeat.
Beta blockers	Take on an empty stomach; food, especially meat, increases the drugs' effects and can cause dizziness and low blood pressure.
Digitalis	Avoid taking with milk and high-fiber foods, which reduce absorption. Increases potassium loss.
Diuretics	Increase the risk of potassium deficiency.
Potassium-sparing diuretics	Unless a doctor advises otherwise, don't take diuretics with potassium supplements or salt substitutes, which can cause potassium overload.
Thiazide diuretics	Increase the reaction of MSG.

DRUGS	EFFECTS AND PRECAUTIONS
ASTHMA DRUGS	
Pseudo-ephedrine	Avoid caffeine, which increases feelings of anxiety and nervousness.
Theophylline	Charbroiled foods and a high-protein diet reduce absorption. Caffeine increases the risk of drug toxicity.
CHOLESTEROL-LOWERING DRUGS	
Cholestyramine	Increases the excretion of folate and vitamins A, D, E, and K.
Gemfibrozil	Avoid fatty foods, which decrease the drug's efficacy in lowering cholesterol.
HEARTBURN AND ULCER MEDICATIONS	
Antacids	Interfere with the absorption of many minerals; for maximum benefit, take medication 1 hour after eating.
Cimetidine, famotidine, sucralfate	Avoid high-protein foods, caffeine, and other items that increase stomach acidity.
HORMONE PREPARATIONS	
Oral contraceptives	Salty foods increase fluid retention. Drugs reduce the absorption of folate, vitamin B_6, and other nutrients; increase intake of foods high in these nutrients to avoid deficiencies.
Steroids	Salty foods increase fluid retention. Increase intake of foods high in calcium, vitamin K, potassium, and protein to avoid deficiencies.
Thyroid drugs	Iodine-rich foods lower the drugs' efficacy.
LAXATIVES	
Mineral oils	Overuse can cause a deficiency of vitamins A, D, E, and K.
PAINKILLERS	
Aspirin and stronger non-steroidal anti-inflammatory drugs	Always take with food to lower the risk of gastrointestinal irritation; avoid taking with alcohol, which increases the risk of bleeding. Frequent use of these drugs lowers the absorption of folate and vitamin C.
Codeine	Increase fiber and water intake to avoid constipation.
SLEEPING PILLS, TRANQUILIZERS	
Benzodiazepines	Never take with alcohol. Caffeine increases anxiety and reduces the drugs' efficacy.

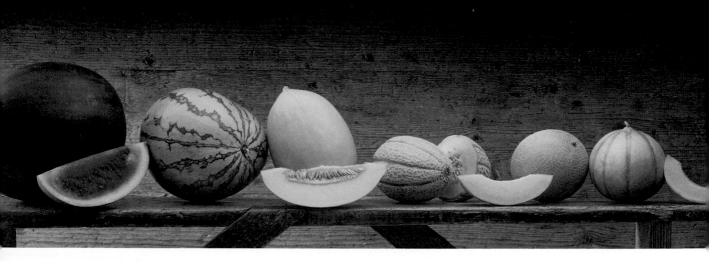

MELONS

BENEFITS

- Sweet and flavorful, yet low in calories.
- Yellow varieties are high in vitamin A.
- Most are good sources of vitamin C and potassium.
- Some are high in pectin, a soluble fiber that helps control blood cholesterol levels.

There are many types of melons; among them, cantaloupe, casaba, crenshaw, honeydew, Persian, and watermelon. Although mostly water, melons are very nutritious, providing vitamin A (in the form of beta carotene), vitamin C, potassium, and other minerals.

Cantaloupes and other yellow varieties are high in beta carotene, which the body converts to vitamin A; one-fourth of a cantaloupe provides about 55 mg of vitamin C, more than 60 percent of the Recommended Dietary Allowance (RDA), more than 600 RE (Retinol Equivalents) of beta carotene, 320 mg of potassium, and only 46 calories. Honeydews are also low in calories, high in vitamin C, and a good source of potassium. Persian melons contain as much beta carotene as cantaloupes. A 1-in.-thick (2.5-cm) slice of watermelon contains about 100 calories, but it is lower in vitamin C and potassium than the others.

Many melon varieties are high in bioflavonoids, carotenoids, and other plant pigments that help protect against cardiovascular disease, cancer, and other diseases.

Because melons are mostly water, they are generally very low in calories. A 4-oz (115-g) serving of any of the varieties contains only 30 to 35 calories. Although melon flesh is free of strings and other sources of insoluble fiber, it does contain pectin, a type of soluble fiber that helps keep blood cholesterol levels in check.

HOW TO BUY A MELON

Because melons do not contain starch that converts to sugar, they don't continue to ripen after they are picked from the vine; therefore, melons that are harvested before they are fully ripe never achieve their peak flavor. In order to select a vine-ripened melon, check the stem area for a smooth, slightly sunken scar; this indicates that the melon was ripe and easily pulled from its vine. In contrast, if part of the stem still adheres to the scar, the melon was picked while it was still green and not fully ripe.

When purchasing melons, don't be shy about sniffing the fruit to see if it is fully ripe; a ripe melon will have a deep, intense fragrance.

A ripe watermelon should rattle when you shake it, because the seeds loosen as the fruit matures; thumping the melon should produce a slightly hollow sound. Watermelons come in several colors, but in all instances the rind should be firm and smooth, with a yellowish undertone.

To best preserve nutrient content, buy melons whole (some stores offer halves or quarters). Certain nutrients, especially vitamin C, are diminished by exposure to the air. ❖

COOL AND REFRESHING—AND PACKED WITH NUTRIENTS. Popular varieties of melon include (from left to right): watermelon, honeydew, and small, sweet cantaloupe, gaylia, and charentais.

DID YOU KNOW?

WATERMELON MAY HELP PREVENT PROSTATE CANCER

Watermelon is a very good source of lycopene, an antioxidant linked with a lower risk of prostate cancer.

MEMORY LOSS

EAT

- Breakfast.
- Lots of fruits and vegetables for vitamin C, beta carotene, and flavonoids.
- Include some vegetable oils, nuts, and wheat germ for vitamin E.

Mild lapses in memory are common with age and simple forgetfulness such as forgetting a name or losing objects is relatively benign.

COFFEE MAY GIVE A
MEMORY BOOST

That afternoon coffee break may do more than you think to get you through the day, especially if you are an older adult. Researchers at the University of Arizona found that memory in older people is often at its best in the morning and declines in the afternoon. When half the seniors in their study drank 12-oz (355-ml) cups of decaffeinated coffee morning and afternoon, their memory performance showed a significant decline from morning to afternoon. The group that drank regular coffee, however, maintained their morning performance levels throughout the afternoon.

Profound memory loss is a universal symptom of dementia or Alzheimer's disease. Benign age-related memory loss may result from shrinkage of the brain's nerves, diminished production of brain chemicals, or restricted blood flow to brain tissue. Genetic factors, head injuries, viruses, and cardiovascular disease may contribute to Alzheimer's disease.

Exercise and a healthy diet can help preserve brain longevity and sustain memory. Protective brain nutrients include complex carbohydrates and B vitamins, which help ensure healthy nerve transmission and sufficient quantities of neurotransmitters.

Eat breakfast. Eating breakfast can do wonders for your memory, according to researchers from the University of Toronto. The study of healthy men and women, aged 61 to 79, showed that taking in calories from either protein, fat, or carbohydrates boosted their performance on memory tests. Previous research has shown that carbohydrates can fuel memory-based performance, possibly due to the rise in blood sugar provided by carbohydrates. The rise in blood sugar could then increase glucose supply to the brain. But this study showed that any food, regardless of source, can help. While it appears that any breakfast is better than no breakfast, the researchers suggest that carbohydrates still generally give longer-term benefits to memory.

Get plenty of beta carotene and vitamin C. There is some evidence that high levels of beta carotene and vitamin C are associated with superior memory performance in people 65 or older. Researchers believe these antioxidants may delay brain aging and enhance mental longevity and fitness by combating free radicals in the brain. Experimental research suggests that flavonoids in blueberries may slow age-related decline in mental function.

Consume lots of vitamin E. Other research is looking at the link between blood levels of vitamin E and memory function in the elderly. In one large study, more than 4,000 people performed tests designed to assess their ability to remember facts. Those classified as having poor memory were more likely than others to have low blood levels of vitamin E. Another study showed an association between past intake of vitamin E and mental acuity in old age, and other studies have found vitamin E helpful in slowing the progression of Alzheimer's disease.

Iron may also be important for memory. Research suggests depressed levels can impair memory function. Studies have shown that when children have an iron deficiency, they score better on tests of memory when this deficiency is corrected.

Try ginkgo biloba. Current research indicates that ginkgo biloba extracts may have a limited effect on improving memory. As with other herbal products, the lack of standardization is a concern, as is the possibility that labels may not reflect contents accurately.

Investigate sage oil. Recently, researchers at Northumbria and Newcastle Universities in England followed up on the recommendation of some old-time herbalists to improve memory with sage oil by giving it to a group of 44 adults in a placebo-controlled study. People who took the sage oil performed significantly better on their memory performance tests.

One more supplement. Phosphatidylserine, a naturally occurring compound in the brain that maintains cell membrane fluidity, is available as a supplement. Limited evidence suggests that it may be of some help in cognitive function but more studies are needed. ❖

MENOPAUSE

EAT PLENTY OF
- Foods high in calcium and vitamin D, such as low-fat dairy products.
- Fresh fruits and vegetables for vitamins and minerals, and bioflavonoids.
- Soy products, such as tofu, soy beverages, and soy nuts.

LIMIT
- Alcohol and caffeine.

Menopause is defined as the end of a woman's monthly menstrual periods. This process usually begins around 45 to 50 years of age, as a result of a progressive decline in levels of the hormone estrogen, and concludes around the age of 55. The beginning of this time of change is referred to as perimenopause, while the period after menopause is called postmenopause.

Menopause used to be viewed as the beginning of old age. Today a majority of women in developed countries can expect to live more than a third of their lives after menopause.

During menopause, fluctuations in estrogen levels can cause symptoms like hot flashes, night sweats, insomnia, vaginal dryness, difficulty concentrating, and weight gain. While some women experience few or no symptoms of menopause, others experience severe symptoms that cause them extreme discomfort.

DO ONE SIMPLE THING

TRY FLAXSEED TO REDUCE HOT FLASHES

Eat one to two tablespoons of ground flaxseed a day. This pleasant, versatile seed is a great source of omega-3 fatty acids, which are important for heart health, as well as the best source of a type of phytoestrogen called lignans, which have been shown to help reduce hot flashes. Grind the seeds and add to cereal or yogurt.

Menopause can also affect a woman's life expectancy and quality of life. Before menopause a woman's hormones protect her from developing heart disease, but with the onset of menopause that protection is lost. By about 55 years of age, women die of heart disease at approximately the same rate as men. In addition, the gradual loss of bone mass that most women experience from the age of 30 onward is drastically accelerated at menopause. Bone loss results in part from the lack of estrogen as well as from inefficient absorption of calcium. A woman may lose 10 to 20 percent of her bone mass in the decade following menopause, with a slower but still significant loss thereafter. This bone thinning, or osteoporosis, increases the risk of fractures, which can lead to disability and pain.

HORMONE REPLACEMENT THERAPY

In the past many women have chosen to counteract the effects of estrogen loss with hormone replacement therapy (HRT), a combination of estrogen and progestin prescribed by their doctors. It was offered not only to treat the symptoms of menopause, but it was also believed that it provided protection against chronic diseases. However, recent findings of a major U.S. study on HRT showing that the risks of taking HRT appear to outweigh the benefits, have caused women, and their doctors, to rethink this strategy.

The Women's Health Initiative Study, which included more than 16,000 women, concluded that, although HRT is effective in relieving symptoms of menopause, its long-term use increases a postmenopausal woman's risk of breast cancer, heart disease, stroke, and blood clots. Combined estrogen-progestin therapy also seems to increase the risk of dementia after age 65. As a result of these unsettling findings, experts are now recommending that HRT be used in the lowest possible dose, for the shortest period of time, when symptoms of menopause are so severe that they are interfering with quality of life.

To treat milder symptoms, and to avoid development of chronic disease, women are encouraged to adopt a healthy lifestyle and to try other approaches, which can include dietary change, exercise, and herbal remedies.

DIET

Although not as simple as swallowing a pill, a healthy diet can help ease the symptoms of menopause and reduce the risk of chronic disease. Here are some helpful dietary strategies:

Eat foods known to reduce menopausal symptoms. Follow a diet high in whole grains, fruits and vegetables, and low in saturated fats. It will provide you with plenty of fiber, vitamins and minerals, phytoestrogens, and bioflavonoids, all important for long-term health and to help minimize menopausal symptoms.

Watch out for trigger foods. These are foods that can worsen symptoms like hot flashes, insomnia, and mood swings. Some common culprits are coffee, tea, chocolate, colas, alcohol, and spicy foods.

Include soy foods. Studies have shown that soy foods not only help protect against heart disease, but they also can help ease hot flashes. Soy foods contain isoflavones, which have a weak estrogenic effect in the body. Soy foods come in many shapes and sizes, including tofu, soybeans, soy beverages, soy nuts, and soy protein. While soy foods are safe enough, the safety and efficacy of isoflavone supplements have not been demonstrated.

REGULAR EXERCISE

Regular exercise may help minimize mood swings and hot flashes. At least 30 minutes of exercise four to five times a week is recommended.

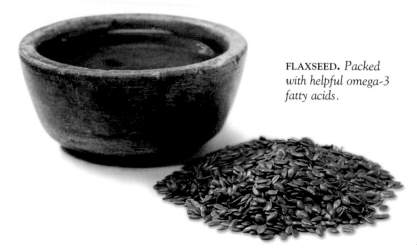

FLAXSEED. *Packed with helpful omega-3 fatty acids.*

FOUR IMPORTANT NUTRIENTS FOR MENOPAUSE

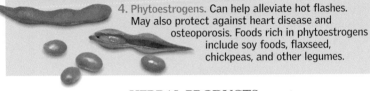

1. Vitamin E. Considered useful in alleviating hot flashes and thought to offer some heart protection although a recent study showed that 400 IU of vitamin E taken twice daily reduced hot flashes just slightly more than the placebo. Although some foods, such as nuts and seeds, egg yolk, and wheat germ contain vitamin E, you'll need to take a supplement to get a therapeutic dose.

2. Calcium. To help prevent the development of osteoporosis. Good sources are milk and milk products, sardines, almonds, broccoli, and spinach. To absorb calcium, the body needs vitamin D, which can be made by the skin after exposure to the sun; dietary sources of this vitamin include fortified milk and margarine, eggs, and fish oils.

3. Magnesium. Works with calcium to maintain bone density. Found in whole grains, milk and milk products, tofu, nuts and seeds, and legumes.

4. Phytoestrogens. Can help alleviate hot flashes. May also protect against heart disease and osteoporosis. Foods rich in phytoestrogens include soy foods, flaxseed, chickpeas, and other legumes.

HERBAL PRODUCTS

Long before hormone replacement therapy, women often sought relief for their menopausal complaints with herbal remedies. Some of the more popular ones—for which there is some evidence of efficacy—are listed below. The evidence, however, is not compelling and the amounts of these substances found in commercial preparations is not standardized, which makes it difficult to assess results.

Black cohosh (*Cimicifuga racemosa*). A number of studies have shown that black cohosh can alleviate many unpleasant symptoms of menopause, including irritability, poor concentration, insomnia, and depression.

Chasteberry (*Vitex agnus-cactus*). This herb has been useful in the management of fluid retention, hot flashes, anxiety, and depression.

St. John's wort (*Hypericum perforatum*). St. John's wort has been shown to be effective in the management of mild to moderate cases of depression. It has a long history of use in the treatment of the melancholy often associated with menopause.

Red clover (*Trifolium pratense*). Extracts of red clover have recently been marketed to help with menopausal symptoms. Chemical analysis does indeed show the presence of estrogenic compounds, but two double-blind studies (both funded by the manufacturer of a major brand) found no difference between red clover and a placebo for treating menopausal symptoms such as hot flashes and vaginal dryness over a period of 12 weeks. Still, many women claim that their symptoms are alleviated by red clover preparations. ❖

MENSTRUAL PROBLEMS

LIMIT
- Alcohol and caffeinated drinks.

AVOID
- Highly salted foods, which promote fluid retention and bloating.

Most women in their reproductive years recognize the mild cramps or slight twinge in the lower back as the normal effects of menstruation. These effects are not symptoms of any sickness and do not usually interfere with normal activities. Many women, however, experience discomfort and even temporary disability from the severe cramps and nausea that can precede their periods, sometimes lasting several days. Some others have to deal with irregular, sparse, or excessive bleeding that can make it difficult to plan and enjoy activities.

PREMENSTRUAL SYNDROME

More than 150 symptoms—notably, bloating, irritability, breast tenderness, food cravings, headache, and constipation—have been linked with premenstrual syndrome (PMS), which seems to be caused by hormonal changes during the latter half of the menstrual cycle. For 10 percent of the women who suffer from PMS, these symptoms can cause serious social problems, disrupting work and family activities.

Eat foods with a low glycemic index. Although no food can prevent PMS, certain substances in food may offer relief from some of the symptoms. To handle symptoms, doctors advise a balanced diet combined with exercise. Women should eat regular, moderate meals, spaced through the day, based on a combination of whole grains, legumes, vegetables, and fruits. Complex carbohydrates can help by increasing production of serotonin, a brain chemical that regulates mood. Foods with a lower glycemic index (see Glycemic Index) are best because they raise blood sugar levels more slowly, helping to control appetite and possibly cravings. Fats, highly refined foods, and caffeinated drinks should be avoided and sodium intake should be reduced. Alcohol can trigger or worsen many symptoms and so should be avoided in the days before menstrual periods.

Get more calcium. Calcium may help reduce mood disturbances, cramping, and bloating resulting from PMS. Some researchers believe PMS symptoms may be the result of low calcium levels, the symptoms of which are very like the symptoms of PMS. Best calcium sources include dairy products, fortified soy beverages, canned salmon or sardines, and leafy greens. Women with PMS often have low magnesium levels, which may predispose them to PMS-induced headaches and depression. Foods rich in magnesium include sunflower seeds, nuts, lentils and legumes, tofu, soybeans, figs, and green vegetables. Some research suggests that foods rich in vitamin B_6 may be useful in alleviating symptoms of PMS. The vitamin B_6 may help stimulate production of serotonin and reduce anxiety and depression caused by PMS. Best food sources are beef, pork, chicken, fish, whole-grain cereals, bananas, avocados, and potatoes.

A caution about vitamin B_6. If you take supplements, do not exceed the upper limit for adults of 100 mg per day. Excess has been associated with nerve damage.

Watch those food cravings. Many women crave sweets—in particular, chocolate—in the days just before their periods start. An occasional piece of chocolate won't do much harm, but eating large amounts of sugary foods only adds empty calories and can worsen the craving for sweets by disrupting normal blood sugar levels. It's much better to satisfy such cravings with complex carbohydrates, such as whole-grain crackers or fresh vegetables, which are metabolized at a slower rate than sweets. These snacks are also packed with fiber, which helps to prevent the constipation that some women experience as part of PMS.

Don't neglect exercise. Women who exercise regularly are less likely to suffer from PMS. The difference may be related to the levels of endorphins, which are released at an increased rate during exercise. Endorphins (chemicals in the brain that are natural mood elevators) can increase the sense of well-being and help the body to deal with stress.

Try evening primrose oil. This oil, available in capsules and in liquid form, contains an essential fatty acid called gamma linolenic acid (GLA). This acid blocks the inflammatory prostaglandins that contribute to cramps and breast tenderness.

PAINFUL PERIODS

Menstrual cramps (dysmenorrhea) are most common among young women who have never been pregnant. In most cases there is no underlying health problem, and symptoms often ease somewhat after pregnancy, or with the use of oral contraceptives.

Herbal teas may help. Raspberry leaf tea contains a substance that is thought to relax the uterus and ease cramping. Chamomile tea also has antispasmodic action and may help. Drink the tea while relaxing in a warm bath or lying down with a heating pad over your abdomen to relieve muscle cramps and tension.

Take an anti-inflammatory. Research has found that prostaglandins, hormonelike substances that cause uterine contractions, play a part in causing menstrual cramps, but the precise mechanism is unknown. Aspirin, ibuprofen, and other nonsteroidal anti-inflammatory drugs (NSAIDs) can block prostaglandin production and alleviate menstrual cramps. Use these drugs with care, because they can cause stomach irritation and bleeding problems.

In some instances, painful periods are related to other conditions, such as fibroid tumors (benign uterine growths) or endometriosis (the growth of uterine tissue outside the uterus). These conditions all require the attention of a gynecologist.

HEAVY PERIODS

Menstrual bleeding tends to be heavy and irregular at the beginning and end of a woman's reproductive years. Heavy periods, caused by hormonal fluctuations, often conclude anovulatory (i.e., no egg is released) cycles in the months following the first period (menarche) and in the year or two preceding menopause.

Eat lots of iron-rich foods. Although it can be inconvenient, heavy bleeding is rarely the signal of a more serious condition. However, excessive blood flow may result in a greater loss of iron, with a risk of anemia. An adult woman needs 18 mg of iron daily. Good sources are red meat, legumes, fortified cereals, leafy green vegetables, and dried fruits. To help the body to better absorb iron, a food rich in vitamin C should be eaten at the same meal.

A woman who experiences persistently heavy or irregular periods should see a gynecologist to determine if she has a problem requiring treatment or, if she is approaching middle age, to obtain information about menopause.

MISSED PERIODS

The most likely reason for a missed period is pregnancy. However, the menstrual cycle may also be interrupted by hormonal imbalances related to obesity or diabetes, thyroid disease, a change in contraceptive pills, or an eating disorder such as anorexia nervosa. Women involved in high-level athletic training are prone to menstrual problems, because they lack the critical amount of body fat to maintain adequate estrogen levels. A systematic meal plan can provide the nutrition essential to maintain top athletic performance while guarding against excess weight. A woman who is not having regular menstrual periods should see a doctor for a thorough checkup. ❖

MIGRAINES AND OTHER HEADACHES

LIMIT
- Coffee, tea, colas, and other beverages containing caffeine.

AVOID
- Alcohol, especially red wine, vermouth, champagne, and beer.
- Any food shown to trigger your attacks.

Headaches afflict about 70 percent of adults at least occasionally and provoke millions of North Americans each year to seek medical relief. Most headaches are transient and due to tension or a temporary condition, such as a cold or the flu, but some reflect a serious underlying problem. Recurrent headaches warrant medical attention to diagnose the type and determine the best treatment.

When you see your doctor, bring a detailed written description of your headaches: their severity, ranging from mild to incapacitating; their frequency; their duration; the exact areas affected by the pain; and any related symptoms, such as nausea.

MIGRAINE HEADACHES
More than 20 million North Americans suffer from migraine, a one-sided, severe, throbbing or pulsating headache often accompanied by sensitivity to light and sound, as well as by nausea and vomiting. Migraines are also called vascular headaches, because they usually involve spasm of the arteries of the head, resulting in a pulsating pain. The headaches may last from a few hours to several days or even longer.

About 10 percent of migraine sufferers experience a warning aura before the headache starts; this early symptom involves a visual disturbance, such as partial or temporary loss of sight or flashes of light and color. An aura may

also cause tingling on one side of the face or body or a disturbance in the sense of smell. Even those who don't experience an aura may have warning signs in the few hours leading up to a migraine, such as feelings of cold, craving for a specific food, mood changes, a sudden burst of energy, or frequent yawning.

Migraines affect women about three times as often as men, and they commonly start between the ages of 18 and 44. Doctors think that they begin when triggers—dietary, hormonal, environmental, emotional, and other factors—cause blood vessels in the brain to constrict and then relax. These distorted blood vessels prompt nerve endings to send out pain signals.

Try relaxation techniques. In addition to using relaxation techniques, some doctors recommend taking a course in biofeedback to learn how to raise the temperature of your hands, thereby diverting some of the blood flow from the head to another part of the body. This technique can be used at the start of an attack.

THE FOOD-MIGRAINE LINK

Many foods, additives, and other dietary components can cause migraines, but the triggers vary greatly from one person to another. The following list covers the more common ones.

- Aged cheeses, sour cream, and certain other milk products.
- Fresh yeast, sourdough, and other yeasty breads.
- Fermented foods, including pickles, soy sauce, and miso.
- Some legumes, especially dried beans, lentils, and soy products.
- Nuts, seeds, and peanut butter.
- Chocolate and cocoa.
- Organ meats and meats that are salted, dried, cured, smoked, or contain nitrites.
- Sardines, anchovies, and pickled herring.
- Many fruits, including avocados, bananas, citrus fruits, figs, grapes, papayas, passion fruits, plantains, pineapples, raspberries, red plums, and raisins.
- Alcohol, especially red wine.
- Chicken livers.
- Seasonings and flavor enhancers, especially artificial sweeteners, ginger, and molasses.
- Sulfites used as preservatives in wine and dried fruits.
- Monosodium glutamate (MSG).

Medications. A number of medications are available to treat migraines. They divide into two broad categories: those that are taken to abort a migraine already under way and those that are taken to prevent an attack. The former include sumatriptan (Imitrex), zolmitriptan (Zomig), ergotamine tartrate (Cafergot), prochlorperazine (Compazine), and Fiorinal (a barbiturate sedative [butalbital] mixed with aspirin and caffeine). Medications taken to prevent a migraine fall into the categories of beta-blockers, calcium channel blockers, serotonin modifiers such as fluoxetine (Prozac), paroxetine (Paxil), or sertraline (Zoloft). Sometimes antiseizure medications such as gabapentin (Neurontin), valproic acid (Depakote), or carbamazepine (Tegretol) are used when other medications fail. Recent research shows that high-dose riboflavin (400 mg) can be effective in preventing migraines.

KNOWN MIGRAINE TRIGGERS

The triggers that can set off a migraine vary widely from one person to another. A number of the following triggers can be avoided entirely; others can at least be minimized.

Environmental triggers. These include glare, bright lights, loud noises, strong odors, cigarette smoke, and changes in temperature, weather, or altitude.

Hormonal triggers. These are experienced by women and are usually related to the menstrual cycle; they can also be caused by the use of estrogen supplements or high-estrogen oral contraceptives.

Activity triggers. These include irregular or no exercise, inadequate or excessive sleep, eyestrain, and motion sickness.

Emotional triggers. These tend to be the negative ones, such as anger, resentment, depression, fatigue, anxiety, and stress.

Dietary triggers. These may be the easiest to control. Keep a food diary, note what foods seem to prompt symptoms (see "The Food-Migraine Link," opposite), and then eliminate them. Eat regular meals, because hunger or a low blood sugar can trigger a headache.

The caffeine in coffee and other beverages—as well as in many over-the-counter analgesic drugs—can play a dual role in migraines. Regular and excessive ingestion can contribute to the frequency of the headaches. On the other hand, once you are completely off caffeine, you may be able to use it to abort an impending attack, because it constricts dilated blood vessels. At the first sign of an aura or a pain, drink

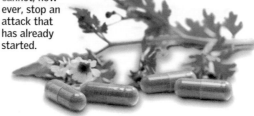
a cup of strong coffee or a cola, take two aspirin, and lie down in a dark, quiet room. The episode may pass within an hour or so.

CLUSTER HEADACHES

The most incapacitating of all vascular headaches, this type lasts from 15 minutes to 3 hours and typically occurs in clusters, coming and going repeatedly over several days or weeks and then disappearing for months or even years. Often starting during sleep, they cause excruciating, stabbing pain on one side of the head, usually behind or around one eye. Some people liken the pain to a hot poker stabbing the eye.

Cluster headaches are far more common in men than in women, especially among those who are heavy smokers and frequent alcohol users. Eliminating these habits may banish the headaches. In addition, keeping a diary of food and lifestyle factors may reveal that some of the factors known to trigger migraines can prompt cluster headaches as well.

TENSION AND OTHER HEADACHES

Tension headaches are the most common type and are caused by muscle contractions or an imbalance of natural chemicals in the brain. The pain causes a bandlike pressure around the head and may be accompanied by a sense of tightness in the head, neck, and shoulder muscles. They often begin in the afternoon or evening and produce a steady pain. Prevention is the best approach; relaxation techniques, such as biofeedback, massage, meditation, and visualization, work for many people. Another recommendation is to eliminate from the diet all foods and drugs that contain caffeine, which can increase tension and anxiety, thus contributing to headaches.

Headaches also may be due to sinusitis, an inflammation of the lining of the sinus cavities. This causes a deep, dull ache around the eyes and sometimes in the forehead and ears. A good diagnostic clue is that the pain tends to worsen when you bend over.

So-called rebound headaches can result from overuse of over-the-counter analgesics, prescription pain medications and sedatives, and caffeine (which is a common ingredient in such drugs), resulting in a vicious cycle of growing tolerance and increasing dependence. These tend to be mild to moderate headaches. Although you may have to go through a painful, headachy period for a week or more to withdraw from dependence on these drugs, you will feel better in the long run.

Dental problems, too, can cause very severe one-sided headaches, which may feel exactly like migraines or clusters, especially if your tooth is abscessed.

The many other factors that can cause headaches include squinting for hours in bright sun, eyestrain, hunger, excessive alcohol consumption, and too little or too much sleep. ❖

MILK AND MILK PRODUCTS

BENEFITS

- An excellent source of calcium.
- A good source of vitamins A, B_{12}, and D, riboflavin, phosphorus, zinc, and magnesium.
- Low-fat dairy products are low in cholesterol and high in protein.

DRAWBACKS

- Whole milk and cream contain saturated fat.
- Some people cannot digest milk sugar.
- Milk protein can trigger allergic reactions in susceptible people.

Milk is an excellent source of dietary calcium, a mineral needed to build healthy bones and teeth and to maintain many of the basic functions of the human body. Calcium helps to prevent osteoporosis, and recent studies indicate that it may also protect against high blood pressure and colon cancer. Milk also provides high-quality protein, vitamins, and other minerals.

DID YOU KNOW?

YOU CAN LOSE WEIGHT BY DRINKING MILK INSTEAD OF SOFT DRINKS

A 2003 study indicates that dairy products may play a role in weight loss. A group of 323 girls in Hawaii lost both weight and abdominal girth when they consumed just 1.5 servings of dairy foods daily. One cup of milk or a small piece of cheese resulted in 0.03 in. (0.9 mm) less abdominal fat and a decrease of as much as 2.2 lb (1 kg) of body weight. The benefits were offset when the girls drank soft drinks. Researchers assume boys would experience similar results.

Two to four servings a day of milk and other dairy foods are recommended. One serving is equal to 1 cup of milk, ¾ cup of yogurt, or two slices (1¾ oz/50 g) of cheese.

Milk has two major solid components: fat, including fat-soluble vitamins; and nonfat solids, which include proteins, carbohydrates, water-soluble vitamins, and minerals. Casein, a protein that is found only in milk, makes up 82 percent of the total protein.

The milk sold in North American markets is fortified with the fat-soluble vitamin D; it is also processed to accommodate preferences and nutritional needs (for example, to remove fat) as well as to improve its keeping qualities. Homogenized milk is pressure-treated to break up the fat globules and disperse them evenly.

Widely available milks include regular whole milk (not less than 3.25 percent fat), low-fat and skim milk (with fat from 2 percent to less than 0.5 percent), and cultured buttermilk (less than 1 percent fat). Another type of milk known as UHT (ultra-high temperature) is processed at high temperatures so that it can be stored without refrigeration for long periods.

Many North Americans have some degree of intolerance to milk because they lack the enzyme that is needed to digest milk sugar (lactose). (See Lactose Intolerance.) The alternative is lactose-reduced milk or even small amounts of regular milk. In general, lactose-reduced milks taste sweeter than traditional milks. Cow's milk can be allergenic in children and should be kept out of the diet during the first year of life. In some cases milk can cause nasal and sinus congestion, which in turn can facilitate ear infections.

Warm milk is a cold-weather treat, but children may be put off by the skin that forms on the surface when water evaporates and calcium and protein combine. If the skin is removed, valuable nutrients are lost. Instead, cover the pan to reduce evaporation.

PASTEURIZATION

Claims made for the superiority of raw milk should not be trusted. Disease-causing organisms often find their way into unpasteurized milk because of contamination from the cow, its human handlers, or from the milking and processing equipment. In the pasteurization process, milk is heated hot enough and long enough to kill most microorganisms without compromising the taste or the nutritional content of the milk. The sale of unpasteurized milk is illegal in North America and health regulatory bodies urge pregnant women, and people with weakened immune systems, to avoid raw-milk cheese.

STORAGE

When buying milk, pay attention to the date on the carton, which indicates the last day on which the milk can be sold. Look for milk dated several days in the future. Even pasteurized milk contains bacteria and will quickly spoil unless refrigerated. (Putting milk in the microwave oven for 60 to 90 seconds before refrigerating extends its shelf life another 4 or 5 days.) Place milk toward the back of the refrigerator, where it is colder than on the door. A temperature just above freezing is ideal; however, milk should not be frozen. Milk is very sensitive to light, which rapidly breaks down the riboflavin and causes unpleasant changes in taste. Cardboard containers preserve their content better than clear plastic or glass bottles; milk stored in bottles should be kept in the dark.

GOAT'S MILK

Although it has a more pungent taste than cow's milk, goat's milk is a pleasant alternative to soy- or rice-based milk substitutes. It is similar in composition to cow's milk, but its fat is much more easily digested. Goat's milk may or may not contain vitamin D, so read the label carefully. Goat's milk is no better tolerated by people with lactose intolerance or milk allergies than cow's milk.

CHOCOLATE MILK

Made from white milk with added sugar and cocoa powder, most store-bought brands of chocolate milk contain about 1 percent fat. The amount of sugar in chocolate milk is about the same as is contained in unsweetened orange juice. ❖

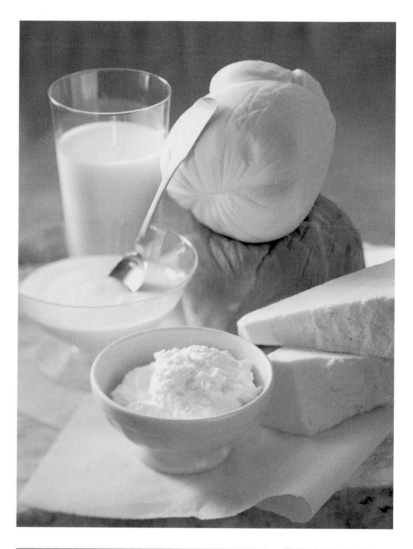

THE MANY FACES OF MILK. *Whether as beverage, yogurt, or one of the many varieties of cheese, milk packs a powerful nutritional punch.*

THE "GOT MILK?" CONTROVERSY

There is an ongoing rancorous debate among health professionals regarding the most popular source of dietary calcium—milk and other dairy products—and how much we should consume. There are those who believe that the currently recommended three to four servings of dairy per day will help prevent osteoporosis. Others believe that our need for dairy foods is greatly overstated and that too much dairy may actually cause harm. What is clear is that an adequate intake of dietary calcium is necessary to reduce the risk of osteoporosis, and milk is a convenient source. Milk is a good source of protein and is fortified with vitamin D. Also, consumption of calcium in dairy products has been shown to have benefits beyond the health of your bones. It may lower the risk of high blood pressure as well as colon cancer. You can reap most of the benefits by drinking just one glass of milk per day.

MINERALS
■ ALL YOU NEED TO KNOW ■

Minerals are those elements that remain largely as ash when animal or plant tissues are burned. They constitute about 4 percent of our body weight and perform a variety of functions. They are essential to maintain good health and promote proper metabolism and various other bodily functions in humans. Minerals are generally classified according to daily dietary requirement. Calcium, phosphorus, and magnesium are classified as macrominerals since you need and can store larger amounts. Iron, fluoride, manganese, iodine, selenium, zinc, molybdenum, chromium, and copper are classified as trace, or micro, because the requirements are much smaller and they are stored in extremely small amounts in the body. The electrolytes, sodium, potassium, and chloride are involved in generating electrical impulses to transport nerve messages; they also maintain the proper balances of fluids and body chemicals. All these minerals are vital to health and since the body is unable to make them on its own, they must be provided from food.

A varied and balanced diet provides all the essential minerals; supplements are generally not recommended, because many are highly toxic if consumed in large amounts. There are a few exceptions—for example, during pregnancy, when extra iron is needed. Also, the mineral content of foods varies according to the composition of the soil where the plants are grown or animals are grazed. Therefore, people may need dietary supplements in areas where the soil is deficient in a particular mineral.

A number of factors influence the body's ability to absorb and metabolize minerals. In general, the body is more efficient in absorbing a mineral during periods of increased need; thus, a person who is anemic will absorb more iron from the diet than an individual who has a normal reserve of the mineral. Bran and other types of dietary fiber bind with some minerals to reduce absorption; in contrast, vitamin C increases the uptake of iron and some other minerals.

The macrominerals

Minerals make up about 3 to 5 percent of normal body weight; most of this comes from the macrominerals that are stored in the bones. But minerals also circulate in the blood.

Calcium. The most abundant mineral in the body, calcium weighs in at roughly 980 to 1,260 g in the typical adult male, compared to only 760 to 900 g for women. Because calcium is essential for building and maintaining strong bones and teeth, it's not surprising that these structures hold 99 percent of the body's calcium. This mineral also ensures proper nerve and muscle function as it moves in and out of bone tissue and circulates through the body. It helps prevent osteoporosis, regulate blood pressure, and may reduce risk of colon cancer.

Milk, cheese, yogurt, and other milk products are the best sources of calcium; the mineral is also found in fortified soy and rice beverages, canned sardines and salmon (if the bones are eaten), tofu (soybean curd), broccoli, and a variety of other vegetables and fruits. In general, the calcium in milk or soft bones is easier to absorb than that in plant foods. Both vitamin D and lactose-containing foods enhance calcium absorption. Phytates found

DID YOU KNOW?

YOU ALSO NEED TRACE MINERALS— EVEN ARSENIC—TO MAINTAIN HEALTH

There is evidence from animal studies that minerals, such as nickel, silicon, boron, vanadium, and arsenic, play a beneficial role in some physiological processes. However, the available data has not been as extensive as for other minerals studied and their effects on human health have not been consistently observed. Therefore, neither an RDA (Recommended Dietary Allowance) nor an AI (Adequate Intake) has been established for these minerals.

in cereals and oxalates found in vegetables such as spinach and beets can interfere with absorption.

Calcium deficiency can cause rickets in children and osteoporosis (a disorder characterized by brittle, porous bones) in adults. In some cases, calcium deficiency is due to a lack of vitamin D, which the body requires to absorb the mineral. The deficiency may also be a result of physical inactivity, especially complete bed rest, which increases calcium loss.

Magnesium. The body contains only about 28 g of magnesium, 60 percent of which is stored in the bones; the rest circulates in the blood or is stored in muscle tissue. Magnesium is essential to build bones and is needed for proper muscle function, energy metabolism, to transmit nerve impulses, and to make genetic material and protein.

Magnesium is found in green leafy vegetables, whole grains, legumes, nuts, beans, and milk—deficiency is rare. There is some evidence to suggest that many North Americans are not reaching the Recommended Dietary Allowance (RDA) for magnesium, which is 400 mg for men 19 to 30 and 420 mg for men 31 and over; women 19 to 30 should get 310 mg daily and women over 30 should have 320 mg. Reserves can be depleted, however, by alcoholism, prolonged diarrhea, liver or kidney disease, severe diabetes, and a poor diet.

Phosphorus. The second most plentiful mineral in the body, phosphorus works in conjunction with calcium and fluoride to give bones and teeth their strength and hardness. On average, it makes up 1 percent of normal body weight; 85 percent of this is in the bones, and the remainder is found in soft tissue. Phosphorus is essential for many metabolic processes and the storage and release of energy, as well as the activation of the B-complex vitamins and many enzymes.

Foods that are high in calcium (see "All About Minerals," next page) also tend to be high in phosphorus; other good sources include meat, fish, eggs, and nuts.

The trace minerals

Only very small, or trace, amounts of the following minerals are required to meet normal body requirements.

Chromium. Insulin and chromium appear to act together to metabolize glucose, the body's major fuel. Brewer's yeast is very high in chromium; other good sources include wheat germ, whole-grain products, liver, cheese, chicken, mushrooms, peas, and molasses.

Copper. A component of many enzymes, copper is essential for making red blood cells, skin pigment, connective tissue, and nerve fibers; it also stimulates absorption of iron. Excessive zinc appears to reduce the body's ability to absorb and store copper. Copper deficiency results in anemia, deterioration of the heart muscle, inelastic blood vessels, various skeletal defects, nerve degeneration, skin and hair abnormalities, and infertility.

Liver is the richest source of copper, but the mineral is also found in seafood, legumes, nuts and seeds, prunes, and barley. Using unlined copper pans can result in copper toxicity. Excessive copper can cause severe liver disease and mental deterioration; several metabolic disorders can cause a buildup of copper in the liver and other tissues. Patients suffering from

(continued on page 258)

Minerals are necessary for building bones and for proper nerve and muscle function.

ALL ABOUT MINERALS

MINERAL	BEST FOOD SOURCES	ROLE IN HEALTH
MACROMINERALS		
Calcium	Milk and milk products; fortified soy and rice beverages; canned sardines and salmon (including bones); dark green vegetables; tofu.	Builds strong bones and teeth; vital to muscle and nerve function, blood clotting, and metabolism; helps regulate blood pressure.
Magnesium	Leafy green vegetables; legumes and whole-grain cereals and breads; meats, poultry, fish, and eggs; nuts, milk.	Stimulates bone growth; necessary for muscle function and metabolism.
Phosphorus	Meat, poultry, fish, egg yolks, legumes, dairy products, soft drinks.	Helps maintains strong bones and teeth; component of some enzymes; essential for proper metabolism.
MICROMINERALS		
Chromium	Brewer's yeast, whole-grain products, liver, cheese, chicken, mushrooms, molasses.	Works with insulin to metabolize glucose.
Copper	Liver, shellfish, legumes, nuts, prunes.	Promotes iron absorption; essential to red blood cells, connective tissue, nerve fibers, and skin pigment. Component of several enzymes.
Fluoride	Fluoridated water; tea.	Helps maintain strong bones and teeth.
Iodine	Iodized salt, seafood, foods grown in iodine-rich soil.	Necessary to make thyroid hormones.
Iron	Liver, meat, seafood, eggs, legumes, fortified cereals, dried fruits, whole grains, leafy greens, nuts and seeds.	Needed to produce hemoglobin, which transports oxygen throughout the body.
Manganese	Tea, nuts, legumes, bran, leafy greens, whole grains, egg yolks.	Component of many enzymes needed for metabolism; necessary for bone and tendon formation.
Molybdenum	Liver and other organ meats; dark green leafy vegetables; whole-grain products, legumes, nuts.	Component of enzymes needed for metabolism; instrumental in iron storage.
Selenium	Brazil nuts, poultry, seafood, whole-grain products, onions, garlic, mushrooms, nuts, brown rice, organ meats.	Antioxydant that works with vitamin E to protect cell membranes fron oxidative damage.
Zinc	Oysters, meat, yogurt, milk, eggs, wheat germ, nuts.	Instrumental in metabolic action of enzymes; essential for growth and reproduction; supports immune function.
ELECTROLYTES		
Chloride	Table salt, seafood, milk, eggs, meat.	Maintains proper body chemistry. Used to make digestive juices.
Potassium	Avocados, bananas, citrus and dried fruits; legumes and many vegetables; whole-grain products.	Along with sodium, helps to maintain fluid balance; promotes proper metabolism and muscle function.
Sodium	Table salt, dairy products, seafood, seasonings, most processed foods.	With potassium, regulates the body's fluid balance; promotes proper muscle function.

DAILY RECOMMENDED DIETARY ALLOWANCE (RDA) FOR ADULTS OVER 19		DAILY TOLERABLE UPPER INTAKE LEVELS (UL) FOR ADULTS OVER 19
MALES	**FEMALES**	
1,000 mg* 19–50 years 1,200 mg* 51+	1,000 mg* 19–50 years 1,200 mg* 51+	2,500 mg
400 mg 19–30 years 420 mg 31+	310 mg 19–30 years 320 mg 31+	350 mg**
700 mg	700 mg	4,000 mg
35 mcg* 19–50 years 30 mcg* 51+	25 mcg* 19–50 years 20 mcg* 51+	Not established
900 mcg	900 mcg	10,000 mcg
4 mg*	3 mg*	10 mg
150 mcg	150 mcg	1,100 mcg
8 mg	18 mg 19–50 years 8 mg 51+	45 mg
2.3 mg*	1.8 mg*	11 mg
45 mcg	45 mcg	2,000 mcg
55 mcg	55 mcg	400 mcg
11 mg	8 mg	40 mg
Not established	Not established	Not established
Not established	Not established	Not established
Not established	Not established	Not established

This table presents daily Recommended Dietary Allowances (RDAs), except where there is an asterisk. The values with an asterisk (*) represent daily Adequate Intake (AI). The RDAs are set to meet the known needs of practically all healthy people. The term Adequate Intake is used rather than RDA when scientific evidence is insufficient to estimate an average requirement.

Source: Institute of Medicine, Food and Nutrition Board. National Academy Press, Washington, D.C.

**The UL for magnesium represents intake from a pharmacological agent only and does not include intake from food and water.

MYTH BUSTER

Myth: Chromium supplements build muscle and burn fat.

Reality: Found in trace amounts in most foods, chromium acts like a key to unlock insulin. Without it, insulin has a hard time controlling blood sugar and building proteins. Studies indicate that most North Americans don't get enough in their diets. Many people have turned to chromium supplements, but not because they want to control blood sugar. They believe the claims that there is "scientific evidence" to prove that this mineral, often sold as chromium picolinate, helps bulk up muscles while reducing body fat. Researchers have spent 20 years studying chromium and now believe it does not have any effect on weight loss, though there is still no consensus on whether supplements have any effect on the muscles.

Wilson's disease, for example, must take medication to eliminate the copper from their bodies.

Fluoride. Best known for preventing cavities and other dental disorders, fluoride is also needed to maintain strong bones. Fluoride occurs naturally in some areas; in fact, it was in these regions that the relationship between decreased incidence of tooth decay and fluoride was first noted. Some groups oppose adding fluoride to drinking water, claiming it is a carcinogen. The prevailing scientific opinion, however, is that fluoridating drinking water is an appropriate health measure.

Iodine. This mineral has only one known function in humans: it is necessary to make thyroid hormones. An iodine deficiency can result in an overgrown thyroid gland, or goiter; in severe cases, it can lead to hypothyroidism. In addition, a baby borne by a woman with iodine deficiency may develop cretinism, a devastating type of mental retardation. Seafood, kelp, and vegetables grown in iodine-rich soil are good sources of the mineral. Iodized salt is advisable in areas where the soil lacks iodine.

Iron. The body has only 3 to 5 g of iron, 75 percent of which is in hemoglobin, the pigment in red blood cells that carries oxygen. Iron-deficiency anemia is the most common nutritional deficiency in developed countries. There are two types of iron: Heme is found in red meat, pork, lamb, poultry, fish, and eggs; nonheme is also found in animal products, as well as in vegetables, fruits, juices, grains, and fortified cereals. About 20 to 30 percent of heme iron is absorbed; lesser amounts of nonheme iron are absorbed, depending upon need and other dietary factors. Consuming nonheme iron with vitamin C or meat increases its absorption; bran, the tannins in tea, phytates in grains, and oxalates in many foods reduce its absorption.

As the body breaks down old red blood cells, it recycles most of their iron. A healthy adult man loses about 1 mg of iron per day; compared to 1.5 mg per day in a woman who is still menstruating. People most likely to develop an iron deficiency are teenagers, menstruating women, pregnant women, preschool children, some athletes, and people on very restricted diets.

Manganese. A component of numerous enzymes, manganese is important for metabolism and is needed to build bones and tendons. Manganese deficiency is unknown in humans, largely because most plant foods contain small amounts. Legumes, nuts, seeds, peas, leafy greens, whole grains, egg yolks, and some fruits are good sources.

Molybdenum. Another component of many enzymes, molybdenum helps regulate iron storage and is instrumental in the production of uric acid. A deficiency of this mineral almost never occurs.

Selenium. An important antioxidant, selenium interacts with vitamin E to prevent the free radicals produced during oxygen metabolism from damaging body fat and other tissues. Research is looking at the role of selenium in lowering risk of lung, prostate, stomach, and colorectal cancers. Human selenium deficiency is rare except in areas where the soil contains little of the mineral.

Foods that are high in selenium include Brazil nuts, seafood, some meats and fish, whole-grain products, oats, and brown rice. Plant foods, especially wheat, provide much of the selenium in the North American diet, although dietary intake from these foods will vary according to the selenium content of the soil in which it is grown. Selenium toxicity is uncommon but there have been cases among people taking high doses. Symptoms include nausea, diarrhea, fatigue, skin and nerve damage, and loss of hair and nails.

Zinc. An essential component of many enzymes, zinc is necessary for some metabolic processes, normal growth and sexual development, and proper immune system function. It is also needed to make genetic materials and for proper wound healing. Deficiencies result in increased susceptibility to infection, fatigue, appetite loss, balding, and taste abnormalities.

Zinc is found in many foods; especially good sources include beef and other meats, oysters and other seafood, eggs, milk, yogurt, wheat germ, and nuts. The phytates in whole-grain products and other plant products, however, bind with zinc and prevent absorption. For this reason, vegetarians may need as much as 50 percent more zinc than nonvegetarians.

The zinc in food cannot hurt you but excess zinc supplements can be toxic and can depress the immune system, increasing the susceptibility to infection. Taking large doses can interfere with your body's absorption of copper, can reduce HDL cholesterol, and impair red blood cell formation.

The electrolytes

Three essential minerals are classified as electrolytes, substances that dissociate into ions when placed in water or other fluids. In the human body electrolytes conduct electrical charges and are instrumental in nerve and muscle function; they also help maintain the proper balance of body fluids.

Chloride. A component of table salt, chloride is needed for nerve conduction and to make hydrochloric acid, which the stomach uses to digest food. A diet that includes a moderate amount of salt provides adequate chloride; deficiencies are rare but may occur during periods of excessive sweating or prolonged vomiting or diarrhea.

Potassium. Along with sodium, potassium helps regulate the body's balance of fluids. Potassium is essential for many metabolic processes; it is also instrumental in the transmission of nerve impulses, proper muscle function, and maintaining normal blood pressure. Most plant foods contribute varying amounts of potassium; especially rich sources include dried fruits, bananas, tomatoes, citrus fruits, avocados, potatoes, milk, and melons.

Prolonged diarrhea or the use of diuretics to treat high blood pressure can lead to a potassium deficiency; typical symptoms include an irregular heartbeat, muscle weakness, and irritability. Caution is necessary when taking potassium supplements, however; an overdose can cause nausea, diarrhea, and serious cardiac arrhythmias that can result in sudden death.

Sodium. Table salt is composed of sodium and chloride, and the terms salt and sodium are often used interchangeably. Sodium is found in all body fluids and is largely responsible for determining the body's total water content. Like potassium, sodium ions help regulate nerves and muscles. These two electrolytes maintain the fluid balance inside and outside of body cells. Sodium maintains the acid-base balance, sends nerve impulses, and helps muscle contraction. Sodium deficiency is very rare; overconsumption is much more common. In susceptible people excessive salt is linked to high blood pressure; it can also cause swollen ankles and fingers and other signs of a buildup of body fluids. Sodium occurs naturally in many foods but much of what we consume is added in processing or food preparation.

DO ONE SIMPLE THING

WATCH YOUR IRON INTAKE

The effect of too much iron on heart disease has been debated by researchers for years. Many studies have shown that people with very high levels of iron in their blood are at increased risk for heart problems. In one study healthy men were given megadoses of iron and then had their blood flow measured. Researchers found that the normal blood vessel dilation was reduced by as much as one-third. Doctors recommend controlling your consumption of iron supplements. Postmenopausal women, whose iron levels are no longer being depleted by menstruation, should consult their doctors before taking a multivitamin that contains iron.

MONONUCLEOSIS

CONSUME PLENTY OF

- Fruit and vegetable juices for vitamins and minerals.
- Milk shakes for calories, minerals, and vitamin D.
- Soups for energy and fiber.
- Soft foods to soothe a sore throat.

AVOID

- Alcohol.

A common disease, mononucleosis is caused by the Epstein-Barr virus, which infects at least half of all North American children by the age of 5. The majority of these infections pass unrecognized, because the symptoms of mild fever and slight fatigue last only a short time and resolve spontaneously. The Epstein-Barr virus is transmitted in the saliva by coughing, sneezing, or kissing. Otherwise, most people who have only casual contact with an infected person do not get the disease.

Mononucleosis causes more debilitating illness in adolescents and adults, who generally have fatigue, fever, severe sore throat, and swollen lymph nodes. Patients usually lose their appetite and complain of headaches and general achiness. Often, the fever and sore throat are misdiagnosed as tonsillitis. If the sore throat is treated with ampicillin, an antibiotic similar to penicillin, the patient with mononucleosis develops a rash. The spleen—and, less often, the liver—may become enlarged. In very severe cases the patient may develop jaundice.

The symptoms typically last for a week or two, and most people are able to return to work at that time. In a few cases, however, recovery may take several months, as a low-grade fever, poor appetite, and fatigue persist for weeks after the other symptoms have disappeared. When this happens, mononucleosis may be mistaken for chronic fatigue syndrome. In the past, chronic fatigue syndrome was at times referred to as chronic Epstein-Barr infection, but it is now known that they are unrelated.

THE ROLE OF DIET

Consume lots of immune-boosting nutrients. A well-balanced diet can aid in recovery and boost the strength of the immune system to fight mononucleosis. Stimulate a poor appetite with several light, appetizing meals rather than a few larger ones, which may be daunting.

Drink at least eight glasses of water or juice daily. During the acute phase, when fever may be high, it's important to drink plenty of liquids in order to prevent dehydration. During recuperation, juices have the added benefit of providing vitamins and other immune-boosting nutrients.

Milk shakes and fruit nectars diluted with water soothe a sore throat and provide calories for energy, along with minerals and vitamins.

Try soft foods and foods with fiber. Applesauce and other stewed fruits supply soluble fiber, which helps prevent constipation. Soups are nutritious and easy to eat. Soft foods, such as puddings, scrambled eggs, cottage cheese, and yogurt, are easily swallowed, even by someone with a sore throat. Fruits and vegetables can be pureed to make them easier to swallow; serve vegetables as a sauce over complex carbohydrates, such as rice or soft noodles. Herbal teas are soothing, and gargling with tepid salt water can relieve a sore throat. Avoid alcohol, which weakens the immune system and can further damage the liver.

TREATMENT

See a physician if you think you have mononucleosis, since blood tests are necessary for a definitive diagnosis. Rest is an important part of recovery. Take aspirin or some other nonsteroidal anti-inflammatory drug (NSAID) to ease symptoms. However, since the disease is a viral and not a bacterial infection, it should not be treated with antibiotics. People with mononucleosis just have to wait it out. Long-term complications are rare, but activity should be limited until you feel strength returning. Don't engage in vigorous activity until the doctor says the spleen has returned to its normal size; abrupt force can rupture an enlarged spleen and cause serious problems. ❖

MOOD DISORDERS

CONSUME

- Small, meals/snacks through the day; don't skip meals.

AVOID

- Cut down on caffeine and alcohol, which can cause sleeplessness and feelings of anxiety.

Our thoughts, emotions, moods, and attitudes, as well as nerve and muscle functions, are all centered in the brain. While diet affects the health of all the organ systems, the links between diet and emotional health appear to be mostly negative ones. Deficiencies of some of the B vitamins, for example, can result in memory loss and various other mental and emotional changes. Now rare, thanks to the abundance of food and the fortification of grain products in the industrialized countries, these disorders are generally only experienced by people with special nutritional problems, such as alcoholics.

Positive links—foods that lift the mood—are harder to find. The brain's neurons communicate with one another by means of chemicals called neurotransmitters. These compounds are synthesized as needed from amino acids and other components of the diet.

Consume more tryptophan. The amino acid tryptophan, found in complete proteins, such as meat, milk, and eggs, is used by the brain to produce serotonin. This neurotransmitter regulates sleep, pituitary hormone secretion, and pain perception. Brain levels of serotonin are affected by the intake of tryptophan. After a high-protein meal, little tryptophan reaches the brain because of competition from other amino acids. Following a carbohydrate meal, on the other hand, insulin causes the competing amino acids to be absorbed into muscle tissue, thereby shunting tryptophan to the brain, where it is converted to serotonin. A typical effect of serotonin is the drowsiness that follows a sugary snack or a high-carbohydrate lunch.

MOODS AND JUNK FOODS

There is no evidence that food allergies, including the much-disputed "yeast sensitivity," cause emotional or behavioral changes. Likewise, there is no evidence that food additives or junk foods influence mood or behavior, even though some courts have allowed defendants to enter the "Twinkie defense" as a justification for their misdeeds. In some rare cases, children do have intolerances to certain food additives and these can be manifested as behavioral problems. Many parents maintain that their children become hyperactive after eating sugary foods. A number of scientific studies have shown, however, that the opposite is actually the case. Sugar enhances serotonin formation and therefore tends to calm active children.

DIETARY MOOD CHANGERS

The best-known mood-altering dietary item is caffeine, a stimulant found in coffee, tea, colas, and chocolate. While a cup of coffee may be a welcome eye-opener, too much caffeine causes palpitations, sleeplessness, and anxiety.

Be careful how much you drink. Alcohol is the next most often used mood-altering substance. Alcohol is a depressant that slows down certain physiological processes, including respiration, which decreases the supply of oxygen to the central nervous system. Alcohol can actually cause depression. People who awake depressed and short-tempered might benefit from taking a critical count of the previous evening's drinks. In addition, alcohol interferes with sleep, which can cause irritability, anxiety, and depression.

Don't skip meals. Besides the types of food you eat, when and how much you eat can also affect your mood. Eating small amounts of food frequently through the day can keep your energy levels and mood more constant. Skipping meals can have a negative effect on your mood and energy, and eating very large meals can make you feel sleepy or less energetic. Some researchers feel that there is more that affects the food/mood connection than just chemistry. The learned associations and familiar feelings you have when you eat a certain food can also be strong determinants of mood. ❖

A CALMING MEAL.
A pepper stuffed with rice and beans provides the amino acids and carbohydrates used to make soothing brain chemicals.

MOUTH ULCERS

CONSUME PLENTY OF

- Lean meat, legumes, dried fruits, fortified cereals, and other high-iron foods.
- Dark green leafy vegetables, wheat germ, and legumes for folate.
- Lean animal products for vitamin B$_{12}$.
- During an attack, soft, bland foods.

AVOID

- Salty, spicy, and acidic foods, or any other food that worsens symptoms.
- Alcohol and very hot beverages.

Commonly referred to as canker sores, mouth ulcers (or aphthous stomatitis) appear as several painful white or yellowish raised spots. In severe cases, a dozen or more may arise, either as sores scattered through the mouth or as large clusters. They tend to be acutely painful for the first few days, last about 1 to 2 weeks, and then heal without consequence. Larger ulcers may last weeks or months and may also be accompanied by fatigue, fever, and swollen lymph nodes.

Although the cause of mouth ulcers is unknown, physicians believe that an abnormal immune response or a viral infection may be the problem. Stress or local trauma, such as from ill-fitting dentures, may precipitate an attack. In unusual cases, mouth ulcers may be a symptom of a systemic disorder, like allergic reactions to foods, anemia, celiac disease, Crohn's disease, or lupus. Deficiencies of iron, vitamin B$_{12}$, and folate have been associated with an increased risk of mouth ulcers; eating foods high in these nutrients may help to prevent occurrences.

DO ONE SIMPLE THING

CHEW AN ANTACID TABLET TO RELIEVE THE PAIN

Any over-the-counter antacid tablet will do. Or you could hold the tablet on the sore and let it dissolve. It will ease pain by neutralizing acids that eat into the sore. A damp tea bag will have the same effect.

MOUTH ULCERS AND NUTRITION

During attacks, avoid any food or beverage that may irritate the sores. The most common offenders are hot beverages, alcohol, salty or spicy foods, and anything acidic.

Try a diet of bland soft foods. If painful ulcers interfere with eating, try sipping liquid or pureed foods through a straw. Foods that cause the least pain include jello, yogurt, custard, rice, and poached chicken.

For recurrent or severe ulcers, a dentist may prescribe a protective paste to speed healing. ❖

MULTIPLE SCLEROSIS

CONSUME PLENTY OF

- Fiber-rich foods to prevent constipation.
- Cranberry juice to ward off cystitis.
- Pureed foods to ease swallowing.

LIMIT

- Caffeine to avoid bladder irritation.

AVOID

- Foods that can cause choking.

A chronic, often disabling disease of the central nervous system that most often strikes people between the ages of 20 and 40. MS is characterized by the gradual destruction of the myelin sheaths that insulate the nerve fibers, thus robbing nerves of the ability to transmit impulses. Although the symptoms vary depending on the sites where myelin is destroyed in the brain and spinal cord, most people suffer abnormal fatigue, impaired vision, slurred speech, loss of balance and muscle coordination, difficulty chewing and swallowing, tremors, bladder and bowel problems, and, in severe cases, paralysis.

MS AND NUTRITION

A low-fat, high-fiber diet that contains fruits, vegetables, and whole grains can be helpful in managing MS by providing energy and nutrients to maintain and repair tissues, to fight infections, and to keep the risk of constipation low.

The Swank diet. Some physicians, as well as MS support groups, advocate the Swank diet (named for the professor who proposed it in 1950), which eliminates most animal fats. This diet was evaluated for many years in a large number of MS patients, with inconclusive results. While a low-fat diet carries no significant risks, and indeed is beneficial for healthy and infirm people alike, the Swank diet has not been shown effective in preventing the progression of MS. Other diets that have been proposed for treating MS are riskier, because they may lead to unbalanced or inadequate nutrition. Among them are liquid diets, crash diets that can lead to potassium deficiency, raw food diets, diets that restrict intake of pectin and fructose, and gluten-free regimens. None of these have been proved effective.

Vitamin therapy. Vitamin therapy has been promoted as helpful for people with MS, but there is no evidence that MS is caused by a vitamin deficiency.

Antioxidants. Some scientists believe that free radical damage can promote the progression of MS. Antioxidants are believed to counter the effect of these free radicals, so it is prudent to include antioxidant-rich foods in your daily diet. These include fruits and vegetables for vitamin C and beta carotene; vegetable oils, nuts, and seeds for vitamin E; and whole grains, nuts, and seafood for selenium.

Vitamin D. Some studies suggest that vitamin D might prevent progression of the disease or may play other protective roles. In addition, people with MS are at risk for osteoporosis, and vitamin D plays an important role in lowering this risk. Good food sources include fluid milk, fortified soy and rice beverages, fatty fish, and margarine.

The main role of diet in MS is to help people control symptoms, such as fatigue, constipation, urinary tract infections, and problems with chewing and swallowing. A balance between healthy diet, exercise, and rest can help to minimize fatigue. Eating more frequent but smaller meals also helps to provide a constant source of energy. A nutritious breakfast is very important; it provides an energy boost to start the day.

MANAGING COMPLICATIONS

Watch your weight. It is especially important to maintain an appropriate weight related to height. Excess weight can add to mobility problems and fatigue and strain the respiratory and circulatory systems. Skin becomes irritated and breaks down more easily in overweight, relatively inactive people. Being underweight is also undesirable, because it may decrease resistance to infection and increase the risk of developing pressure sores and other skin ulcers.

Fluid intake. Urinary tract infections are often a problem for people with MS, particularly when they have to undergo frequent catheterizations. Drinking cranberry juice increases urinary acidity and creates an environment hostile to bacteria. If urinary incontinence is a problem, people with MS should avoid caffeinated drinks, such as coffee, tea, and colas, and save chocolate (it also contains caffeine) for an occasional treat. Caffeine has a diuretic effect and irritates the bladder.

Fiber intake. Constipation is aggravated by an inadequate fluid intake. Plenty of water and fiber-rich foods, such as fruits, vegetables, and whole-grain products, encourage smooth bowel function. Prune juice and bran cereal are good breakfast choices. Cut down on refined foods that promote constipation.

Avoid problem foods. Some people with MS have problems with bowel incontinence, which may be worsened by diet. Try eliminating suspect items—for example, coffee, alcohol, and spicy foods—from the diet for a few days; then reintroduce them one at a time to see if the problem recurs. Because nicotine can (among many other health effects) stimulate the bowel, it is important not to smoke.

Be careful with food textures. Difficulties with chewing and swallowing can be helped by modifying food preparation but adhering to recommended guidelines. For example, substitute shakes, yogurt, fruit and vegetable purees, thick soups, and puddings for firm or dry dishes. Serve chopped spinach in place of salad, or diced, stewed fruit instead of a fresh apple or pear. Use a blender or food processor to achieve an acceptable texture, and serve smaller but more frequent meals. Your doctor might recommend a speech pathologist for advice about positioning food in the mouth or changing breathing patterns to relieve swallowing difficulties. ❖

MUSCLE CRAMPS

CONSUME PLENTY OF

- Low-fat dairy products for calcium to regulate muscle contractions.
- Potassium-rich foods, such as bananas, citrus fruits, dried fruits, tomato juice, cantaloupe, squash, greens, potatoes, milk, and avocado.
- Complex carbohydrates, such as rice, legumes, and pasta, for energy.
- Fortified whole-grain breads and cereals for iron and B-complex vitamins needed for energy conversion.
- Water to maintain the circulation and help flush lactic acid and other waste products from the muscles.

LIMIT

- Caffeine in coffee, tea, and cola, which can decrease the circulation to muscles.

AVOID

- Highly salted foods, which can cause fluid retention.
- Smoking, which restricts the blood supply to the muscles.

Cramps are painful spasms that mainly affect muscles in the legs and feet. A cramp generally lasts a few minutes and then ends on its own, although massage and stretching can hasten the process, and certain foods may help to prevent its recurrence.

The human body is made up of about 600 groups of muscles, which constitute 40 percent of an average person's weight. Each muscle is made up of many thousands of long fibers bound together with connective tissue. The bundled fibers can shrink or lengthen, allowing muscles to contract or relax.

HOW MUSCLES GET ENERGY

Most of the fuel necessary for muscular activity comes from glucose, the end-product of carbohydrate metabolism, which is stored as glycogen in the liver and muscles.

Vitamins. The vitamins in the B group are crucial to the process by which energy is derived from carbohydrates, proteins, and fats. In fact, our need for thiamine is directly related to the amount of energy we expend.

Minerals. We need iron to form hemoglobin, the blood pigment that supplies muscles with oxygen for energy conversion. Also critically important to muscle function are sodium, potassium, and chloride; these minerals are called electrolytes, because their electrically charged particles (ions) relay nerve impulses from the brain to the muscles, instructing them when to contract and relax. Calcium is the trigger for muscle contraction. And to come full circle, potassium is stored in the muscles with glycogen and—like glycogen—it is rapidly depleted whenever the muscles undergo a vigorous workout.

CRAMP CONTROL. *Certain foods can help to reduce muscle cramps, including yogurt, pasta, bananas, tomato juice, milk, water, oranges, and whole-grain bread.*

When muscles burn glycogen for energy, lactic acid forms as a waste product and remains in the muscle tissue until circulating blood clears it away. During periods of intense exercise, a buildup of lactic acid can cause severe muscle pain and fatigue. The pain, which is similar to muscle cramps, dissipates with rest, which allows the blood to remove the extra lactic acid.

The correct fluid balance is important in muscle function. The spasms of true cramps may be caused by an inadequate supply of blood to the muscle, overstretching, or an injury. If the fluid volume is too low, the electrolyte balance is thrown off kilter, the kidneys respond by conserving sodium at a high rate, fluid is retained in the tissues, and there is not enough circulating fluid to flush out waste products and keep the muscle contraction mechanism working smoothly. There should be enough water to keep electrolytes in the proper concentration for relaying impulses from the nerves to the muscles, but not too much water, which dilutes the blood and lowers the electrolyte concentration.

Electrolyte depletion is not often a problem, because these minerals are amply supplied by a properly balanced diet. Although the electrolytes are excreted in sweat, the amounts lost are very small, even with profuse perspiration during vigorous activity. The exception is potassium, which is drawn out of body stores along with glycogen.

MANAGING MUSCLE CRAMPS

People who may suffer from leg cramps include athletes, who can deplete their glycogen reserves through very intense activity and lose potassium and salt in heavy perspiration; those being treated for hypertension with beta-blocking drugs or certain diuretics, which increase the amount of potassium excreted in the urine; and women in the later months of pregnancy, who also lose larger quantities of potassium in the urine.

Eat lots of high-potassium foods. A daily serving of a high-potassium food—for example, a handful of dried fruits; a glass of tomato juice, citrus juice, or milk; a slice of melon, an orange, or a banana—can help to banish leg cramps and prevent their recurrence. Caffeine and nicotine constrict blood vessels, decreasing the circulation to the muscles and contributing to cramps. If cramps are a problem and you smoke, make every effort to quit; also switch to decaffeinated beverages if you haven't already done so.

People confined to bed rest or chair rest for extended periods often suffer leg cramps. Apart from dietary measures, the best remedy is regular exercise to tone the muscles and improve the circulation. Try curling and uncurling the toes a dozen times in quick succession; alternatively, straighten the leg, bend the foot upward, and then extend the foot and point the toes a dozen times in quick succession. Repeat these exercises throughout the day.

Occasional cramps that abate within a few minutes are no cause for concern. Frequent or prolonged cramps or spasms accompanied by other symptoms, particularly in older adults, should be evaluated by a doctor. Quinine can sometimes bring relief from muscle cramps, but the amount in tonic water is insufficient.

RESTLESS LEGS

Some people are awakened during the night by a jerking of their leg muscles; others suffer an aching, uneasy sensation that doctors call "restless legs syndrome." Certain medications that affect the nervous system may cause these conditions; often, they occur with no apparent cause. Doctors may detect iron, folate, or magnesium deficiencies and recommend supplements. In some cases, drugs may help; getting out of bed and walking, or frequently changing positions, may give some relief. ❖

MUSHROOMS AND TRUFFLES

BENEFITS

- Fat-free and very low in calories.
- Rich in minerals.
- Some are rich in plant chemicals, which may boost immune function.

DRAWBACKS

- Wild mushrooms may be poisonous.
- Truffles are expensive because they can't be cultivated as crops.

All types of mushrooms, as well as truffles, are classified as fungi. They are primitive plants that cannot obtain energy through photosynthesis and therefore draw their nutrients from humus, the partially decomposed tissues of more complex vegetation. Many varieties of fungi live symbiotically with trees. The fungus draws sugars from the tree roots, while at the same time supplying the tree with minerals, such as phosphorus, which it gets from the soil more efficiently than the tree.

Mushrooms and truffles have another unique feature. Their cell walls are made of chitin, the same material that forms the external skeleton of insects. By contrast, higher plants' cell walls are composed of cellulose, which we value not as a nutrient (humans can't digest cellulose) but as fiber that promotes the elimination of digestive waste.

Used in every age and culture as food, mushrooms have also served as medicines and as stimulants or hallucinogens. Evidence that Stone Age humans used dried mushrooms as tinder was provided by 5,000-year-old Oetzi, the Iceman, whose body was discovered in the Tyrolean Alps.

MANY VARIETIES

The common white mushroom, *Agaricus bisporus* (see next page), was first cultivated by the French more than 300 years ago in abandoned gypsum quarries near Paris. Today, mushrooms are cultivated on beds of manure, straw, and soil in darkened buildings controlled for temperature and humidity. Only recently has it become possible to cultivate a number of other species on a commercial scale. Thanks to this development, a wide range of mushrooms is now offered by many supermarkets, including brown varieties such as the small crimini and the larger, flatter portobellos, the delicate brown or grey oyster, orange chanterelles, the chewy shiitakes with their dark brown caps and white gills, the crisp white enokis with their long, thin stems and tiny caps, and the ominously black but perfectly safe trumpets of death. Although they are cultivated, many varieties, especially the popular portobello mushroom, preserve much of the rich, earthy flavor of field mushrooms. With its firm, meaty texture, the portobello is especially suitable for barbecuing and can take the place of meat in a meal. Many other mushroom varieties, including cèpes and tree-ears, are available dried.

Because of their high concentration of glutamic acid—

DID YOU KNOW?

MUSHROOMS GROW LIKE MAGIC

If not picked, a white button mushroom will double in size every 24 hours. First it becomes a closed cup mushroom, then the cup opens to show the brown gills. If left undisturbed, it grows on to become a large flat mushroom with open gills. As the mushroom increases in size, its flavor increases.

the naturally occurring form of monosodium glutamate (MSG)—mushrooms are natural flavor enhancers in many dishes.

Warning: Many common species of wild mushrooms produce toxins that are quickly lethal whether eaten raw or cooked. Because there is no feature that distinguishes dangerous mushrooms, and poisonous varieties often closely resemble edible ones, never gather or eat wild mushrooms unless a mushroom expert has identified them as safe.

CAUTION

Some wild mushrooms, although safe to eat on their own, can be deadly when consumed with alcohol.

NUTRITIONAL VALUE

A good substitute for meat in many recipes, mushrooms can be combined with grains to make a meatless "meat" loaf. They are also appetizing and nutritious on their own. Extremely low in calories (a half cup contains only 10), mushrooms are virtualy fat-free and a valuable source of dietary fiber. They provide good amounts of potassium, selenium, riboflavin, thiamin, folate, B$_6$, and zinc. They are also one of the best plant-based sources of niacin. Three ounces (85 g) of portobello mushrooms provide almost 20 percent of the daily niacin requirement. The same-size serving of white mushrooms provides 17 percent, while shiitakes yield 6 percent.

Mushrooms are a long-time staple of many Asian diets, and Japanese scientists have taken the lead in investigating their possible health benefits. Japanese studies have shown that certain mushrooms may favorably influence the immune system, with potential benefits in fighting cancer, infections, and such autoimmune diseases as rheumatoid arthritis and lupus. This effect may be related to the high content of glutamic acid, an amino acid that seems to be instrumental in fighting infections, among other immune functions. Shiitake mushrooms contain lentinan, a phytochemical that may help boost immune activity, as well as eritadenine, which helps lower cholesterol by promoting cholesterol excretion. Other compounds in shiitakes are being studied for their role in lowering heart disease and cancer risk as well as high blood pressure. All mushrooms contain good amounts of potassium, which can have a positive effect in lowering blood pressure. In addition, tree-ear mushrooms, used in many Chinese dishes, inhibit blood clotting and are thought to lower cholesterol. This may prove valuable in treating some heart diseases.

Portobello and white mushrooms are good sources of selenium. Selenium may help prevent prostate cancer as it is known to work with vitamin E to clean up the free radicals that damage cells. The Baltimore Longitudinal Study on Aging found that men with the lowest levels of selenium in their blood were four to five times more likely to have prostate cancer than men with high selenium levels.

Researchers at Beckman Research Institute in California have early laboratory findings that suggest substances in the common white mushroom (*Agaricus bisporus*) slow an enzyme used in the production of estrogen, which may promote cancer in postmenopausal women. The results have not yet been replicated, however.

TOXINS

Although it is also true that mushrooms contain toxins, the good news is that cooking reduces these substances. The common white button mushroom contains trace amounts of the carcinogen agaritine, but cooking decreases the effect considerably. In any case, scientists have found that most naturally occurring carcinogens cause cancer only when very high doses are given to lab animals over a lifetime and that they do not pose a risk to humans. ❖

A MUSHROOM PRIMER

- When buying mushrooms, look for firm buttons with no bruises. All mushrooms are handpicked, but bruise easily. Handle them carefully.

- Flavor develops as the mushrooms grow, so the largest of any variety have the most flavor.

- Don't store mushrooms in cling wrap or plastic. Place them in paper bags and store in the vegetable crisper of the refrigerator.

- Five days should be the maximum storage time in the refrigerator.

- Rinse mushrooms just before using them, but do not peel them or remove the stalks. The nutrition of mushrooms is just under the skin and will be lost by peeling. Just slice, quarter, or chop with the skins intact.

- Cook mushrooms quickly. If using them in a slow dish such as a casserole, add the mushrooms for the last 20 minutes.

ALL SHAPES AND SIZES. *Varieties of mushrooms include the giant portobello (center and far right) as well as (clockwise from upper right) the shiitake, morel, oyster, and button.*

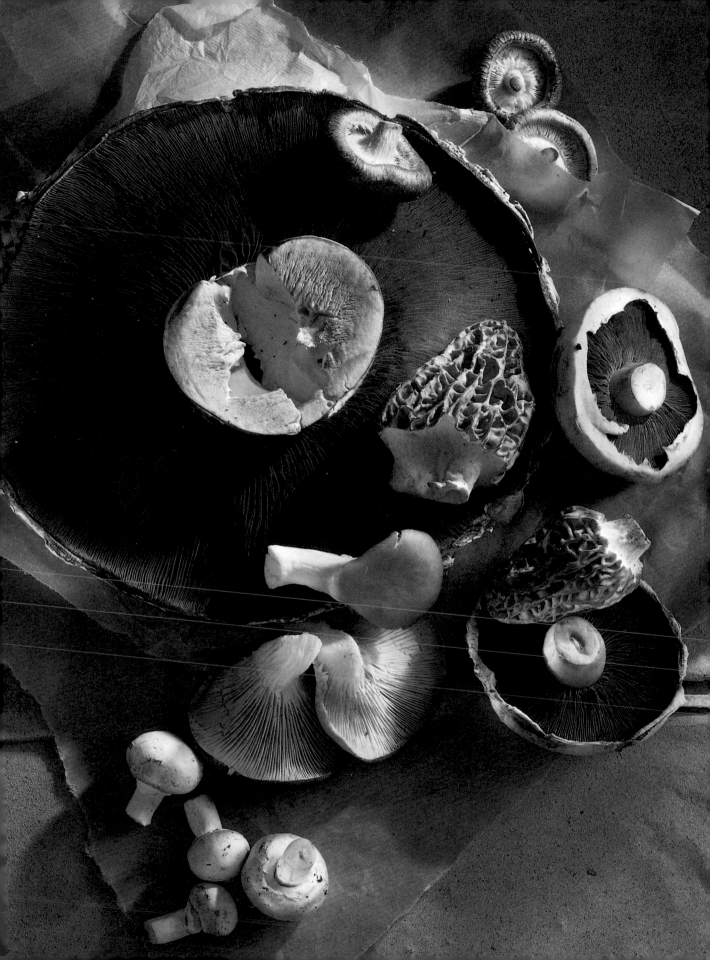

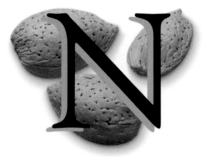

NAIL PROBLEMS

CONSUME PLENTY OF

- Lean meat, poultry, and fish for iron and high-quality protein.
- Citrus fruits for vitamin C.
- Dark green leafy vegetables, whole-grain products, legumes, and fruit juices for folate and other B vitamins.

AVOID

- Overuse of polish removers and other harsh chemicals.

Most nail problems stem from abuse—everything from picking and biting to overuse of polish removers, glues, and other harmful chemicals. In some instances, however, unhealthy nails actually reflect a nutritional deficiency or an underlying medical problem.

Normally, nails grow about ⅛ in. (3 mm) a month, although illness, age, and even cold weather slow the rate of growth. Nails are composed of keratin, the same hard protein that forms the outer layer of skin (the epidermis) and hair. The visible portion, called the nail plate, rests over the tips of the fingers and toes and grows out of the lunula, the pale half-moon at its base. The cuticle acts as a protective seal between skin and nail. Only the lunula is living tissue; the rest is made of dead cells.

Even though nails are mostly dead tissue, they are an important indicator of a person's state of health; this is the reason a doctor carefully examines them for clues to many diseases. Soft spoon-shaped nails that curve upward, for example, point to iron-deficiency anemia. Rounded, club-shaped nails indicate either impaired circulation or a serious lung disorder; thickened, discolored nails may be due to a fungal infection; psoriasis can cause pitting; and horizontal ridges may indicate a systemic infection or debilitating illness.

Healthy nails are strong and smooth, with a pinkish cast. Like hair, they need moisture for flexibility; without it, they become yellowish and break or chip easily. In order to maintain healthy growth and strength, nails require a steady supply of oxygen and other nutrients. But because the body is very efficient in delivering nutrients to its areas of greatest need, and the nails are not vital organs, they are one of the first parts to be short-circuited if there is greater demand elsewhere in the body.

Many of the nail problems that reflect diseases and nutritional deficiencies disappear when the underlying condition is corrected. In order to make keratin, the body needs high-quality protein from lean meat, poultry, fish, seafood, and other animal products; a combination of grain products and legumes will also supply complete protein.

You may need iron-rich foods. A more common nutrition-related problem involves iron-deficiency or other anemias, in which the blood does not deliver adequate nutrients to the nails. Increasing the consumption of iron-rich foods—lean, poultry, fish, seafood, dried apricots, and enriched cereals and breads—may be enough to cure mild iron-deficiency anemia. A doctor should be consulted, however, to determine whether the anemia is due to other nutritional deficiencies or to chronic hidden

---

MYTH BUSTER

Myth: Gelatin, calcium, or zinc supplements aid nail health.

Reality: These nutritional supplements, promoted as nail builders, hardeners, and healers, have little if anything to do with nail health. In reality, gelatin is an incomplete protein and lacks the amino acids to give nails strength. Nails contain very little calcium, so taking supplements will not enhance their growth or strength. And the same is true of zinc. In the past, the white spots that sometimes develop in nails have been attributed to a zinc deficiency. Those spots, however, are usually caused by an injury, and taking zinc will not get rid of them.

NAIL CONDITIONERS

Brittle and splitting nails are usually caused by excessive dryness, which increases with aging and is exacerbated by exposure to detergents and chemicals. Soaking the fingers in water and then applying a moisturizing hand cream or a conditioner formulated for the nails can restore lost moisture and prevent moisture loss. Application of nail hardeners may also help seal in moisture and provide a protective hard surface over the nails. Dermatologists generally recommend protein hardeners or products that contain nylon rather than ones made with formaldehyde, which causes reactions in some people. Contrary to some promotional claims, however, protein and other substances applied to the surfaces do not sink into or "feed" the nails.

bleeding. (Never self-treat with iron supplements; they can lead to toxicity and many other serious problems.) Vitamin C helps the human body absorb iron from plant sources; thus, a balanced diet should include citrus fruits and a variety of other fresh fruits and vegetables.

Try folate. Some types of anemia that affect the nails are caused by a deficiency of folate, an essential B vitamin. Whole grains, legumes, dark green leafy vegetables, peas, nuts, and orange juice are good sources of folate and other important B vitamins. ❖

NECTARINES

BENEFITS

- A fairly rich source of beta carotene and potassium.
- Provide moderate amounts of vitamin C.
- High in pectin, a soluble fiber.

DRAWBACKS

- The flesh darkens when exposed to air.
- The pits contain cyanide.

Sweeter and more nutritious than peaches, their genetic cousin, nectarines were named after the Greek god Nekter; their juice was later called the drink of the gods. This juicy fruit, which is often described as being like a peach without the fuzz, is especially high in beta carotene, an antioxidant that the body converts to vitamin A. One medium-size nectarine has 65 calories and provides more than 800 IU of vitamin A, 250 mg of potassium, and some vitamin E. With only 7 mg of vitamin C, a nectarine is not nearly as high in this nutrient as many other fruits.

The flesh of nectarines is rich in antioxidants—especially carotenoids—that help to protect against cancer and other diseases by reducing the cellular damage that occurs when the body burns carbohydrates, fats, or proteins. Nectarines are also high in pectin, a soluble fiber that helps control blood cholesterol levels. The skins contribute insoluble fiber, which helps prevent constipation.

Cutting or peeling a nectarine releases an enzyme that causes a darkening of the flesh. The fruit may look less appetizing, but the browning doesn't alter its flavor or nutritional value. The discoloring can be slowed by immediately dipping the fruit in an acidic solution (for example, a teaspoon of vinegar diluted in a cup of water) or tossing sliced nectarines with a little lemon or lime juice.

Warning: Nectarine pits contain amygdalin, a compound that releases cyanide in the stomach. Although accidentally swallowing an occasional pit is not harmful, consuming several of them at a time can cause cyanide poisoning.

SELECTING THE BEST

Purchase fruit that is moderately firm but brightly colored. The fruit is ready to eat when the flesh yields to gentle pressure and has a sweet, fruity fragrance. To ripen firm nectarines, place them in a paper bag at room temperature; they should achieve full ripeness in 2 or 3 days. Reject nectarines that are hard or have a greenish skin. These were harvested too early; even though they will soften, they will never achieve peak sweetness and flavor. ❖

MYTH BUSTER

Myth: A nectarine is a cross between a peach and a plum.

Reality: Nectarines originated as a genetic variant of a peach. When peach trees are crossed or even self-pollinated they may produce some fruit whose seeds will grow into nectarine trees and others that will be peach trees. Amazingly, nectarines will sometimes grow on peach trees, and peaches on nectarine trees!

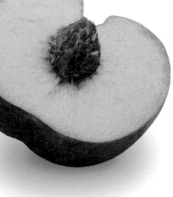

SUCCULENT SWEETNESS. *Worldwide, there are more than 150 varieties of nectarines.*

NEURALGIA

EAT PLENTY OF

- Lean meat, poultry, eggs, and low-fat dairy products for vitamin B_{12}, and enriched breads and cereals for thiamine; also eat spinach, potatoes, and melons for vitamin B_6.
- Vegetable oils, nuts, seeds, wheat germ, avocado, and whole-grain foods for vitamin E.

AVOID

- Alcohol in all forms.

Neuralgia is an umbrella term for any type of throbbing, or paroxysmal, pain that extends along the course of one or more of the peripheral nerves. Neuralgia is classified by both the part of the body affected and the cause. In some cases, doctors can't find a cause; in others, the cause is an infection or underlying disease, such as arthritis, diabetes, or syphilis. Tumors, both cancerous and benign, can cause neuralgia, as do structural problems in which nerves become compressed or pinched. Sciatica, the throbbing pain that can extend from the lower back and buttocks to the feet, is one of the most common examples. Various medications, as well as arsenic and other toxins, can also produce neuralgia.

Keep up vitamin B_6 levels. The long-term use of hydralazine (a powerful antihypertensive medication) or isoniazid (used to treat tuberculosis) can result in vitamin B_6 deficiency, manifested by sensory loss and neuralgia. Anyone taking these drugs should follow a diet that provides extra B_6; good sources include lean meat, poultry, fish, spinach, sweet and white potatoes, watermelon, bananas, and prunes. A doctor may prescribe B_6 supplements; self-treating with high doses, however, can also damage sensory nerves.

Don't neglect vitamin B_{12}. A deficiency of vitamin B_{12}, found in all animal products, can lead to degeneration of the spinal cord and widespread neuralgia, as well as pernicious anemia. Most B_{12} deficiencies are due to a lack of intrinsic factor, a substance made by the stomach that is necessary to absorb the vitamin. Less often, a strict vegetarian diet can result in vitamin B_{12} deficiency.

In rare cases, malabsorption problems resulting in low vitamin E levels can cause a type of neuralgia. Doctors usually give supplements of 30 mg to 100 mg a day; good dietary sources include nuts, seeds, wheat germ, vegetable oils, fortified cereals, eggs, poultry, and seafood. ❖

ALCOHOLICS ARE AT RISK FOR NEURALGIA

Deficiencies of the B-complex vitamins can result in neuralgia involving numerous nerves throughout the body, a condition known as polyneuralgia or polyneuropathy. This condition often occurs in alcoholics, whose diets are generally poor. A deficiency of thiamine—a B-complex vitamin found in various animal products and fortified cereals, breads, and other grain products—is especially common among alcoholics, who may suffer from nerve pain as well as muscle weakness. Their treatment starts with detoxification, to rid the body of alcohol, and high-dose thiamine supplements. As recovery progresses and the diet improves, the supplements can gradually be decreased.

NUTS AND SEEDS

BENEFITS

- Rich in vitamin E and potassium.
- Most are high in minerals, including calcium, iron, magnesium, and zinc.
- Many are good sources of folate, niacin, and other B vitamins.
- A good source of protein, especially when combined with legumes.

DRAWBACKS

- High in fat and calories.
- Oils quickly turn rancid when exposed to oxygen.
- Common allergy triggers.
- May cause choking in children and people with swallowing problems.
- The molds in peanuts and other nuts may produce cancer-causing aflatoxins.

The embryos of various trees, bushes, and other plants, nuts and seeds are packed with all the nutrients needed to grow an entire new plant and have been valued for their nutritional content since prehistoric times. Nut- and seed-bearing plants have been cultivated as early as 10,000 B.C.

Coconuts are the world's leading nut crop, followed by peanuts, which are actually legumes but often classified and consumed as nuts. Nuts are emerging as nutritional superstars as scientists continue to find positive health benefits from consuming them.

NUTRITIONAL VALUE

Most nuts and seeds are a rich source of vitamins, especially folate, B vitamins, and vitamin E; minerals such as iron, calcium, selenium, magnesium, manganese, phosphorus, zinc, and potassium; fiber; essential fatty acids; plant compounds such as flavonoids; and plant sterols.

Certain nuts are higher in certain nutrients. A half-cup serving of almonds, peanuts, pine nuts, pistachios, or sunflower seeds, for instance, provides more than 500 mg of potassium, more than is in a whole banana.

A 1-oz (30-g) serving of almonds provides almost 50 percent of the Recommended Dietary Allowance (RDA) of vitamin E and a similar serving of hazelnuts, about 30 percent. Nuts and seeds are one of the best food sources of vitamin E, an important antioxidant that enhances the immune system, protects cell membranes, and helps make red blood cells. A half cup of almonds contains 3 mg of iron; pistachios have 2 mg. Pumpkin, sesame seeds, and flax are also good sources. A cup of almonds has 400 mg of calcium, more than is found in a cup of milk.

Most nuts and seeds contain magnesium, phosphorus, and zinc, as well as B vitamins such as niacin, thiamin, and folate. Just a half cup of peanuts contains 100 mcg, 25 percent of the RDA; 1/3 cup of sunflower seeds contains 95 mcg.

Brazil nuts are high in the antioxidant selenium. One-quarter ounce (7 g) provides more than twice the RDA for this mineral.

Walnuts are especially rich in ellagic acid, an antioxidant that may inhibit the growth of cancer cells. Walnuts are also rich in omega-3 fatty acids. In one study men and women with high cholesterol levels added walnuts to a healthy Mediterranean diet. Their LDL cholesterol and heart disease risk both dropped.

Hazelnuts are rich in vitamin E, fiber, and copper and contain the same amount of potassium as half a banana. One ounce (30 g) of sunflower seed kernels contains about 75 percent of the RDA of vitamin E. Sunflower seeds are also rich in selenium, copper, fiber, iron, zinc, folate, and vitamin B_6.

Most nuts provide good amounts of protein. With the exception of peanuts, however, they lack lysine, an essential amino acid necessary to make a complete protein. This amino acid can easily be obtained by combining nuts with legumes. Nuts can provide a good source of protein in a vegetarian diet.

Finally, most nuts and seeds are a good source of dietary fiber. A cup of almonds, for example, provides about 15 g.

Researchers have been looking at the health benefits of nuts, including their cholesterol-lowering effects, their association with a lower risk of stroke, and even weight management. Their healthy qualities may be attributed to their fatty acid profile along with their protein, fiber, vitamin E, and magnesium content.

Nuts also contain plant sterols that can lower cholesterol and may offer some protection against cancer.

Several large studies have found that a regular intake of nuts protects against heart disease. The Nurses' Health Study found that women who ate more than 5 oz (140 g) of nuts per week had a 35 percent lower risk of heart attack and death from heart disease compared with those who never ate nuts or ate them less than once a month. The Physician's Health Study found that men who ate nuts two or three times per week had a 47 percent reduced risk of sudden death from cardiac arrest compared with those who rarely or never ate nuts. And a third study showed that almonds significantly lowered LDL cholesterol in those who already had elevated cholesterol levels.

THE ISSUE OF FATS

Nuts have two major drawbacks: they are high in calories and fats. But with the exception of coconuts and palm nuts, their fat is mostly mono- or polyunsaturated. These are considered heart-friendly fats, especially when they replace saturated fats. In most research, nuts and seeds have had the best effect when used as a substitute for, not an addition to, highly saturated fats. Still, nuts should be consumed in moderation. Macadamia nuts have more than 1,000 calories per cup; Brazil nuts are a close second. Other nuts and seeds contain about 700 to 850 calories per cup.

Refrigerate or freeze shelled nuts; their oil quickly turns rancid. Never use nuts that are moldy or have an "off" taste; molds, especially on peanuts, create aflatoxins, substances that cause liver cancer.

OTHER PROBLEMS

Some nuts, especially peanuts (although technically these are not nuts but legumes), provoke allergic reactions in many people. Symptoms range from a tingling sensation in the mouth to hives and, in extreme cases, to anaphylaxis, a life-threatening emergency. But because the different varieties are not closely related, a person who is allergic to walnuts, for example, may be able to eat another type of nut or seed. ❖

A NUT PRIMER

• Gathered from trees in the Amazon basin, Brazil nuts are rarely cultivated.

• There are two varieties of almonds—the edible type is sweet; the inedible, or bitter, almond contains a form of cyanide.

• All pistachios are tan, but imported ones are usually dyed red, and some domestic varieties are bleached white.

• By weight, both pumpkin and sesame seeds have more iron than liver does.

• Cashew shells contain urushiol, the same irritating oil that is in poison ivy. Heating inactivates urushiol, so toasted cashews are safe to eat; the raw nuts, however, should never be eaten.

• Betel nuts are frequently chewed by many Asians despite the high probability that they contain a carcinogen and are likely responsible for numerous cases of oral cancer.

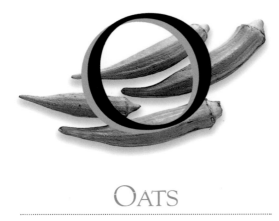

OATS

BENEFITS

- An excellent source of soluble fiber.
- A source of calcium, iron, manganese, folacin, and vitamin E, thiamin, niacin, riboflavin, and other B vitamins.

Oatmeal and other whole-grain oat products such as oat bran and oat flakes are a tasty, convenient, versatile, and economical source of nutrients and phytochemicals. Commonly used as a breakfast cereal and in baking, oats can be added to many dishes, including meat loaf, burgers, and fish cakes, and can be used to thicken soups and sauces or as a topping for fruit crisps. They have beneficial effects on cholesterol, blood pressure, blood sugar, satiety, and gastrointestinal health.

On a weight for weight basis, oats contain a higher concentration of protein, fat, calcium, iron, manganese, thiamin, folacin, and vitamin E than other unfortified whole grains. Oats also contain polyphenols and saponins, powerful antioxidants with disease-fighting properties.

HEALTH BENEFITS

Oat bran is high in beta-glucan, a soluble fiber that can help lower blood cholesterol levels, thus possibly reducing the risk of heart attacks. To reduce blood cholesterol by roughly 5 percent and lower heart attack risk by about 10 percent, a person needs to eat 3 g of beta-glucan a day. This amount of beta-glucan is found in one cup of cooked oat bran, one and a half cups of cooked oatmeal or three pouches of instant oatmeal. The U.S. Food and Drug Administration granted the first food-specific health claim for use on oatmeal labels, stating, "Soluble fiber from oatmeal, as part of a diet low in saturated fat and cholesterol, may reduce the risk of heart disease." Some studies have shown that oats not only lower LDL cholesterol but may also boost levels of the protective HDL cholesterol.

Regular consumption of oatmeal may reduce the risk of heart disease in women in other ways than through cholesterol reduction. The Nurses' Health Study found that those who ate oatmeal five or more times per week had a heart disease risk reduction of 29 percent. The authors suggest that there is more to this effect than just the soluble fiber. Antioxidants found in oats may also play a role. Oats contain a unique blend of antioxidants, including the avenanthramides that prevent LDL cholesterol (the "bad" cholesterol) from being converted to the oxidized form that damages arteries. And Yale researchers have found that eating a large bowl of oatmeal may improve the harmful reduction in blood flow that may happen after eating a high-fat meal.

Oats have a high satiety value, meaning they take a long time to digest and therefore keep you feeling full longer. It is thought that both the protein and fiber in oats contribute to this effect. In one study comparing oatmeal to a sugared flaked cereal for breakfast, researchers found that subjects who ate oatmeal at breakfast consumed one-third fewer calories for lunch, thus helping with weight management.

Oats can reduce blood pressure. A study in Minnesota looked at a group of people who were taking medication for high blood pressure. Half of them were asked to consume about 5 g of soluble fiber per day in the form of one and a half cups of oatmeal and an oat-based snack, while the other half ate cereals and snacks with little soluble fiber. The people who were consuming the oats showed a significant reduction in blood pressure.

Oats also have been shown to reduce both blood sugar and insulin levels, an important asset in controlling diabetes. Human studies confirm that oat-soluble fiber reduces after-meal blood sugar and insulin in both healthy and diabetic people.

There are many varieties of oats:

- Oat groat, or whole-oat groats, or whole oats are minimally processed—only the outer hull is removed. They are very nutritious but they are chewy and must be soaked and cooked a long time. They can be used as a substitute for barley or rice.

- Rolled oats, also called oatmeal, rolled oatmeal, or old-fashioned oats, are oat groats that are steamed, rolled, and flaked so they cook quickly.

- Instant oatmeal consists of very thin, precooked oat flakes that need only to be mixed with a hot liquid. They often have flavorings and salt added.

- Steel-cut oats, also called Irish oats, Irish oatmeal, Scotch oats, or Scotch oatmeal, are groats that have been chopped into small pieces but not rolled into flakes. They are chewier than rolled oats and are often used for hot oatmeal cereals and muesli. ❖

OBESITY

EAT MODERATE AMOUNTS OF

- Complex carbohydrates, such as pasta, potatoes, rice, legumes, and whole-grain products, for energy, vitamins, and fiber.
- Fresh vegetables and fruits for vitamins and minerals.
- Fish, skinless poultry, and lean meat for high-quality protein and minerals.
- Low-fat dairy products for vitamins and calcium.

AVOID

- High-calorie items, such as candy, pastries, fatty meats, alcohol, and potato chips.

Being overweight is the most common nutrition-related health problem in North America, affecting more than 60 percent of all adults. Of these, more than 20 percent are considered obese and are consequently at increased risk for an early death.

Many experts believe that it is not just the amount of fat but also its distribution that is a key factor in the risk to health. For example, excess abdominal fat has been linked to more

---

ASSESSING BODY WEIGHT

The most widely accepted methods to assess weight and body fat are body mass index (BMI) and waist circumference.

Body mass index

This method is used by many health experts to assess whether your weight is putting you at risk. The measurement is based on a mathematical formula that includes both height and weight.

To calculate your BMI:

1. Divide your weight in pounds by 2.2 to get your weight in kilograms (kg).
2. Multiply your height in inches by 2.54 to get your height in centimeters (cm).
3. Divide your height in centimeters by 100 to get your height in meters.
4. Square your height in meters.
5. Your BMI is your weight in kilograms divided by your height in meters squared (BMI = kg/m²).

BMI categories

- Underweight = less than 18.5
- Normal weight = 18.5 to 24.9
- Overweight = 25 to 29.9
- Obesity = 30 or greater

Waist circumference

This measures where fat is accumulated on the body. An accumulation of fat around the abdomen is closely related to increased health risk.

An increased risk of developing health problems comes with a waist circumference greater than 35 in. (88 cm) for women, and greater than 40 in. (102 cm) for men.

---

serious health problems, including heart disease, stroke, and type 2 diabetes, than has fat in the hips and thighs. The reason is that the liver converts more of the abdominal fat into forms that circulate in the bloodstream.

Few people are truly "fat and happy"; obesity can have devastating effects on health. Because slimness is highly valued in our culture, people who are overweight often have a poor self-image and are subjected to discrimination.

Obesity can also cause such physical problems as shortness of breath, skin chafing, and difficulty moving around, making it hard to enjoy a normal life. Obese people have an increased risk of coronary heart disease, high blood pressure, stroke, diabetes, and certain types of cancer. Other health consequences include damage to the weight-bearing joints. This leads to osteoarthritis and disability, which perpetuate the vicious circle by restricting movement, leading to further weight gain.

Obesity is frustrating and often difficult to overcome. Newspaper and magazine articles and advertisements attest to the constant demand for safe, sure, and rapid weight loss. It is estimated that North Americans spend more than $33 billion a year on commercial weight-loss programs and diet aids.

CAUSES OF OBESITY

If we eat more than we need, the surplus food is converted into, and stored as, fat. For reasons that are not understood, but may have a genetic basis, some people gain weight more readily than others. In fact, researchers have discovered a gene that appears to promote obesity. Hormones may also play a role.

Invariably, eating too much food and exercising too little are the key factors. One theory holds that each person has a biological set point for his or her "ideal" weight, and that the body adjusts its metabolism to maintain this set point whenever the person eats more or less than is expended. This set-point theory may be valid; nevertheless, research shows that we can reset our set point through gradual weight loss and increased physical activity.

Set a good example. While obesity often seems to run in families, the truth may be that parents who overeat encourage overeating in their children. It is true that fat cells are laid down in childhood and remain for a lifetime. They may grow larger or smaller to accommodate fat stores, but the number remains the same. That's why a person who was obese as a child may always store fat more readily than a person who started life thin.

Because metabolism slows with age, some put on weight as they approach middle age. Older people also may be less active; in either case, calorie needs decline with age, and a person's food intake should be scaled back accordingly.

CONTROLLING OBESITY

The biggest challenge is not losing weight but keeping it off. Most dieters regain all the weight they've lost within 1 to 5 years. The only successful route to permanent weight loss is a combination of exercise and diet. However, anyone who is 20 percent or more above their ideal weight should see a doctor before embarking on any exercise program or restrictive diet.

Very low calorie diets or fad diets tend to lead to the yo-yo phenomenon, in which people lose weight, then quickly regain all they've lost and more. The additional weight is often even harder to shed.

Limit calories. A diet providing about 1,500 calories a day for a woman and 2,000 for a man is a reasonable approach. Combined with a moderate exercise program, it should allow a loss of 1 to 2 lb (0.45–0.90 kg) a week. Since the aim is to find a diet you can live with in order to keep weight off permanently, it's better to shed weight gradually by eating moderate amounts of lean meat and other high-protein foods, pasta and other starchy foods, and ample vegetables and fruits. Skim milk and low-fat dairy products supply calcium and other nutrients.

Watch empty calories. No foods need to be totally forbidden, but empty calories in alcohol, sugary desserts, and high-fat, high-salt snack foods should be avoided. Weight loss is its own reward. As weight is shed, the urge to lose more will grow and the desire for fatty, sugary foods will fade. A dietitian can help get you started on a sensible weight-loss diet and monitor your progress as you gain control of your weight. ❖

OILS

BENEFITS
- Provide essential fatty acids needed for hormone production.
- Make possible the absorption of fat-soluble vitamins A, D, E, and K.
- Improve the texture and flavor of food.

DRAWBACKS
- High in calories.
- Saturated types may raise blood cholesterol levels.

Throughout history, various plant oils have served as an essential source of concentrated energy and nutrients during times of need. Before refrigeration, preserving foods with oil was critical to survival. Today, even with a limitless supply of healthy foods, oils are an important diet component. They add an appetizing flavor, aroma, and texture to foods, and because they take longer to digest than the other main food groups, they satisfy hunger.

Oils and fats belong to the lipid family and differ only in their melting points. Oils are liquid at room temperature; fats are solid. The two kinds of lipids are otherwise interchangeable and are needed in moderate amounts for several essential body functions. All fats and oils have a practically identical calorie content: 9 calories per gram, or 240 to 250 per ounce. They provide a concentrated source of energy and fatty acids that are essential to build and maintain cell walls. Fats are also necessary to make growth and sex hormones and prostaglandins

FLAVORED OILS. *The range of oils now available include: sesame, olive, virgin olive, cold-pressed extra virgin olive, peanut, walnut, sunflower, hazelnut, garlic, chili oil, and more.*

(the hormonelike substances that regulate many body processes), as well as to absorb and use fat-soluble vitamins A, D, E, and K. Vegetable oils contain no cholesterol; it is found only in animal products.

Among the oldest crops for oil are olives—which have been cultivated for both oil and fruit in the Mediterranean region of Europe for at least 6,000 years—and sesame, grown from Africa to India. Coconut palms and oil palms flourished untended in the tropics, where foragers gathered the nuts to extract oils. As techniques for extracting and preserving oils have improved, many more plants have been introduced to cultivation. Currently, the main oil crops are coconut, corn, cottonseed, olive, palm, peanut, rapeseed (marketed as canola), soybean, and sunflower.

Most vegetable oils are concentrated in seeds or fruits, which are broken down by pressing or grinding. For some oils the tissues that remain after pressing are further treated with solvents and heat to remove the last of the oil. "Virgin" oils are those extracted by pressing alone. Most oils are refined by lye treatment, centrifugation and filtration to remove undesirable solids, and steam deodorization; some go through "winterization" to remove substances that crystallize and make the oil cloudy when it is chilled.

HEALTH PROFILE

Oils contain varying amounts of saturated, monounsaturated, and polyunsaturated fatty acids. Saturated fats tend to raise levels of artery-clogging LDL (low-density lipoprotein) cholesterol. Polyunsaturated and monounsaturated fats tend to lower LDL cholesterol, especially when they replace saturated fats in the diet. This is the reason people who are concerned about cholesterol are encouraged to avoid most saturated fats and replace them with mono- and polyunsaturates. The saturated fatty acids mostly responsible for raising cholesterol are lauric, myristic, and palmitic acids. Coconut, cottonseed, palm, and palm kernel oils all contain high levels of these damaging fatty acids. Palm, palm kernel, and coconut oils, like animal fats, are solid at room temperature and are highly saturated. The best all-purpose dietary oils are canola, corn, olive, peanut, safflower, soybean, and sunflower oils, which contain predominantly mono- and/or polyunsaturated fats with very low levels of saturated fats. (See Fats.)

Oils used to make margarines and shortenings are often hydrogenated to give them a solid consistency and increase their shelf life. The hydrogenation process creates trans fatty acids, which act similarly to saturated fats by raising detrimental LDL cholesterol levels and lowering HDL levels. Many margarines are now nonhydrogenated and are better for cholesterol watchers than butter. About 20 percent of the fat in hard margarine and 13 percent of the fat in soft margarine is saturated; both of these products have much less than the 68 percent saturated fat content of butter, which is also high in cholesterol.

CAUTION

If you like to make flavored oils by adding herbs, garlic, or other ingredients, keep them refrigerated, and throw them out after 2 days. Oil can support the growth of the bacterium that causes botulism, which is potentially fatal. Commercially prepared flavored oils usually contain additives that prevent bacteria from growing.

USING OILS

Monitor your oil consumption by buying single-source oils, such as pure canola or pure olive, rather than blended oils. Read labels: A blended oil often has an overwhelming proportion of the cheapest and probably least healthful oil mentioned, with only a token amount of the more expensive, better-quality oil. Check labels, too, for the oil content of processed commercial foods, especially baked goods. If a label states "Contains one or more of the following oils: corn, safflower, or coconut," the product is probably made only with coconut oil because it's the least expensive of the three listed oils.

Oils add a distinctive flavor and texture to salads and sauces. Along with margarines, they can replace dairy fats in many baking recipes. Oils are almost indispensable in the preparation of foods for grilling, broiling, and roasting. When frying, keep oil absorption low by making sure the oil is at the correct temperature before you add raw foods. Use an oil thermometer if you find it hard to judge the temperature. Before serving fried foods, drain off any excess oil on paper towels or bags.

OMEGA-3 FATTY ACIDS

Fish oils contain omega-3 fatty acids, which protect against heart disease and may help people with certain inflammatory conditions such as rheumatoid arthritis. The full benefit of the oils can be obtained from eating fish two or three times a week. Similar protective fatty acids are also found in several plant oils, including canola, flaxseed, and walnut.

Fish oil supplements should be taken with care. High doses can cause nausea and diarrhea. Because fish oils have a blood-thinning effect, the supplements are not advised for anyone taking blood-thinning medications such as heparin or warfarin. It is best to avoid fish liver oil supplements, which are concentrated sources of vitamins A and D and can be toxic when taken in large amounts for a long time.

DO ONE SIMPLE THING

USE OIL INSTEAD OF BUTTER ON YOUR BREAD

Dip your bread in olive oil instead of using butter. You'll consume about 50 fewer calories—and very little saturated fat.

POWERFUL PODS. *Use okra to thicken your soup; it will lower your cholesterol.*

MINERAL OILS

Oils that have been extracted from petroleum and other forms of nondigestible hydrocarbons are sometimes used as laxatives, particularly by people who are trying to lose weight rapidly by purging. This is a dangerous practice that interferes with the absorption of many nutrients, especially fat-soluble vitamins. It may also cause embarrassing bowel leakage. ❖

OKRA

BENEFITS
- A good source of folate and fiber.
- Contains vitamins C and B_6, thiamin, magnesium, and potassium.
- Low in fat and calories.
- A thickener of soups and stews.

DRAWBACKS
- Glutinous consistency is displeasing to some people.

A relative of the hibiscus, okra was brought to the Americas from Africa in the 1600s. The dark green pods are the main ingredient in spicy Creole stews or gumbos. In fact, okra is nicknamed gumbo in many parts of the world.

This low-calorie, starchy vegetable is high in folate; a half-cup serving contains about 30 percent of the Recommended Dietary Allowance (RDA). It is also a source of the antioxidant vitamins A and C and of potassium, an electrolyte that maintains proper fluid balance, helps to transmit nerve impulses, and is needed for proper muscle function and metabolism.

Okra's unique flavor and thickening properties make it a wonderful addition to stews and soups. As it cooks, it releases sticky juices that thicken any liquid to which it is added. This is due in part to the high content of pectin and other soluble fibers. Pectin helps lower blood cholesterol levels by interfering with bile absorption in the intestines and forcing the liver to use circulating cholesterol to make more bile.

The large amount of soluble fibers also helps prevent constipation by absorbing water and adding bulk to the stool.

Those who are put off by its gummy consistency should try steaming or blanching the pods until they are just tender. Don't slice the okra before cooking—less juice will be released if the inner capsule remains intact. Prepare okra along with an acidic vegetable, such as tomatoes, to reduce its gelatinous consistency. Some people prefer eating okra raw with dips, as part of a fresh vegetable tray, or in a salad. ❖

OLIVES AND OLIVE OIL

BENEFITS
- High in monounsaturated fats, which benefit blood cholesterol levels.

DRAWBACKS
- Some varieties are high in sodium.

The all-purpose crop of the Mediterranean area, olives are indispensable in this region in the preparation of traditional dishes, such as braised duck and lamb stew. In contrast, North Americans tend to use them as a relish or garnish for salads and pizzas. Once a staple for cooking, lighting, cosmetics, and high-quality soap, olive oil is now used mainly in salad dressings, as a cooking oil, and for canning fish.

A medium-size olive contains approximately 5 calories if green and 9 calories if ripe. High in monounsaturated fats, which may raise levels of the beneficial high-density lipoprotein (HDL) cholesterol, and very low in saturates, olives and their oil are thought to contribute to the low rate of heart disease in the Mediterranean countries. Olives provide some calcium and iron. Those pickled in brine or dry salt cured, however, are high in sodium, which may raise blood pressure in some people.

The three main commercial methods of processing are the Spanish method, which ferments unripe green olives; the American method, which soaks half-ripe olives in an iron solution to achieve a black color; and the Greek method, which preserves the fully ripe, almost black fruit. Most methods involve soaking the olives in a lye solution to neutralize their natural bitterness.

OLIVE OIL
Olive oil, the primary source of fat in the healthy Mediterranean diet, is rich in unique disease-fighting phytochemicals, vitamin E, and monounsaturated fat, which all help to clear cholesterol from arteries. The antioxidant

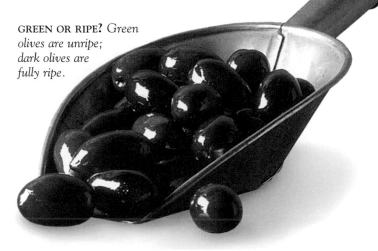

GREEN OR RIPE? *Green olives are unripe; dark olives are fully ripe.*

phytochemicals hydroxytyrosol and oleuropein may work together, according to laboratory studies, to help protect against breast cancer, high blood pressure, infection-causing bacteria, and heart disease. Lignans, present in extra virgin olive oil may protect against cancer by suppressing early cancer changes in cells. Olive oil contains 120 calories per tablespoon.

The classification of olive oil is the same worldwide and is governed by the International Olive Oil Council. The acidity of the oil, which can be affected by the quality of the olives and harvesting techniques, determines the classification and whether any refining is needed. Since the heat and chemicals used in processing olive oil can diminish nutrient content, it is best to choose oils that are minimally processed, such as extra-virgin or cold-pressed oil.

Virgin olive oil is the oily juice pressed from the olive. It is unrefined. The term virgin refers to oils that are slightly more acidic than the extra-virgin ones; they must contain no more than 3 g of free oleic acid per 100 g.

Extra virgin olive oil is the least acidic and has a maximum acid level of 1 g of free oleic acid per 100 g of oil. It is highly regarded as it offers the widest variety of flavors and aromas with a "fruity" flavor. The flavor differences are due to the regions where the olives are cultivated, the climate, the variety of olive, and to some degree the manner in which the olives are harvested. Extra light and light olive oils are the most refined. They are no lower in calories or fat and lack the taste and many of the benefits of the other olive oils.

To preserve flavor, store olive oil in an airtight container in the refrigerator or other dark, cool place. Refrigerated olive oil will solidify, so you will have to let it reach room temperature before it is pourable. ❖

OMEGA-3S AND OMEGA-6S
■ ESSENTIAL FATTY ACIDS ■

Omega-3 fatty acids are called essential fatty acids because they are needed for human health but the body can't make them itself. That is why we need to get them from the foods that we eat. These fats can be found in fatty fish and certain types of plant oils.

It is important to maintain a good balance of omega-3s and omega-6s (another essential fatty acid found in many seeds, nuts, and vegetable oils) in the diet as these two substances work together to promote health. Omega-3 fatty acids help reduce inflammation and most omega-6 fatty acids tend to promote inflammation. So an imbalance of these essential fatty acids contributes to the development of disease. A healthy diet should only contain approximately one to four times more omega-6s than omega-3s, but the typical North American diet contains 11 to 30 times more. So most of us need to pay special attention to good food sources of omega-3s. (In contrast, the Mediterranean diet has a much better balance between omega-6 and omega-3 fatty acids, perhaps because there is less meat, which is high in omega-6s.)

Different types

There are three main types of omega-3 fatty acids: alpha-linolenic acid (ALA), eicosapentaenoic acid (EPA), and docosahexaenoic acid (DHA). The body has enzymes that can convert ALA to EPA and DHA, the two types of omega-3 fatty acids more readily used by the body. You get the EPA and DHA directly and more efficiently by eating oily fish.

EPA and DHA are found primarily in oily cold-water fish such as salmon, tuna, mackerel, herring, and sardines. ALA is found primarily in flaxseed and flaxseed oils, walnuts, and smaller amounts in dark green leafy vegetables.

Health benefits

Scientists originally made the connection between omega-3s and health while studying the Inuit people of Greenland. As a group they suffered far less from certain diseases, including heart disease, rheumatoid arthritis, and psoriasis than other populations. Yet their diet was high in fat from eating whale, seal, and salmon. Researchers determined that these foods were rich in omega-3 fatty acids, providing real disease-fighting benefits.

Researchers are continuing to explore the benefits of these essential fatty acids. At this time the evidence is strongest for heart disease and related concerns, but there are now a wide range of other possible therapeutic uses.

Heart disease

Evidence suggests that EPA and DHA found in fish oil help reduce risk factors for heart disease, including high blood pressure and high cholesterol. Research has also shown that these fatty acids can inhibit the development of plaque and blood clots, lower triglycerides, reduce cardiac arrhythmia, and offer protection from sudden cardiac death. Studies of heart-attack

Best food sources of omega-3 fatty acids

✔ **Oily fish:** Salmon, sardines, herring, tuna, or mackerel. Eat these fish several times a week.

✔ **Ground flaxseed:** Grind these sweet, nutty-tasting seeds in a coffee grinder and sprinkle on your cereal, salad, or soup. Use 1 or 2 tablespoons every day.

✔ **Walnuts:** Enjoy fresh, flavorful walnuts in your salad or eat an occasional handful. Walnut oil is delicious on salads too.

NEW FISH OIL RECOMMENDATIONS

The American Heart Association has, in the past, recommended fish and fish oils to reduce risk of developing heart disease. But they are now also suggesting that people who already have heart disease or high triglyceride levels could benefit from them as well. Here are their recommendations:

DISEASE	WHAT TO EAT
To decrease heart disease risk	At least two fish meals a week (mostly fish known to be low in mercury).
If you've had a heart attack or other heart disease "event"	About 1,000 mg of fish oil daily, from a combination of fatty fish (if possible) and supplements.
If you have high triglycerides	2,000 to 4,000 mg of supplemental fish oil daily under a physician's care.

survivors have found that daily omega-3 supplements can reduce the risk of death, subsequent heart attacks, and stroke. (See "New Fish Oil Recommendations," above.)

Diabetes

People with diabetes often have high triglyceride and low HDL levels. Omega-3 fatty acids from fish oil (EPA or DHA) can help lower triglycerides and raise HDL. ALA may not be as effective for diabetics as they may lack the ability to efficiently convert ALA to the more usable EPA or DHA.

Arthritis

Several studies have concluded that omega-3 supplements can reduce tenderness in joints, decrease morning stiffness, and allow a reduction in the amount of medication needed to relieve the pain experienced by people with rheumatoid arthritis.

Depression

People who are deficient in omega-3s in their diet may be at increased risk for depression. These fatty acids are important components of nerve cell membranes. They help nerve cells communicate with each other, which is important in maintaining good mental health.

Attention deficit/hyperactivity disorder (ADHD)

Children with ADHD may have low levels of essential fatty acids in their bodies. Research has shown that those children with lower levels of omega-3 fatty acids demonstrate more learning and behavioral problems than those with normal levels. There are at this time no well-controlled studies that look at the effect of omega-3 fatty acid supplements on these symptoms, but a diet high in these fats remains a reasonable approach.

Breast cancer

The balance between omega-3 and omega-6 fatty acids appears to be an important factor in the development and growth of breast cancer. More research is needed, however, before we can understand this relationship. Some researchers have speculated that omega-3s in combination with other nutrients such as vitamin C, vitamin E, and selenium may prove to have value in the prevention and treatment of breast cancer.

CAUTION

Because fish oil can reduce the time it takes blood to clot, use supplements only under the supervision of your doctor, especially if you are also taking a blood-thinning medication such as warfarin (Coumadin).

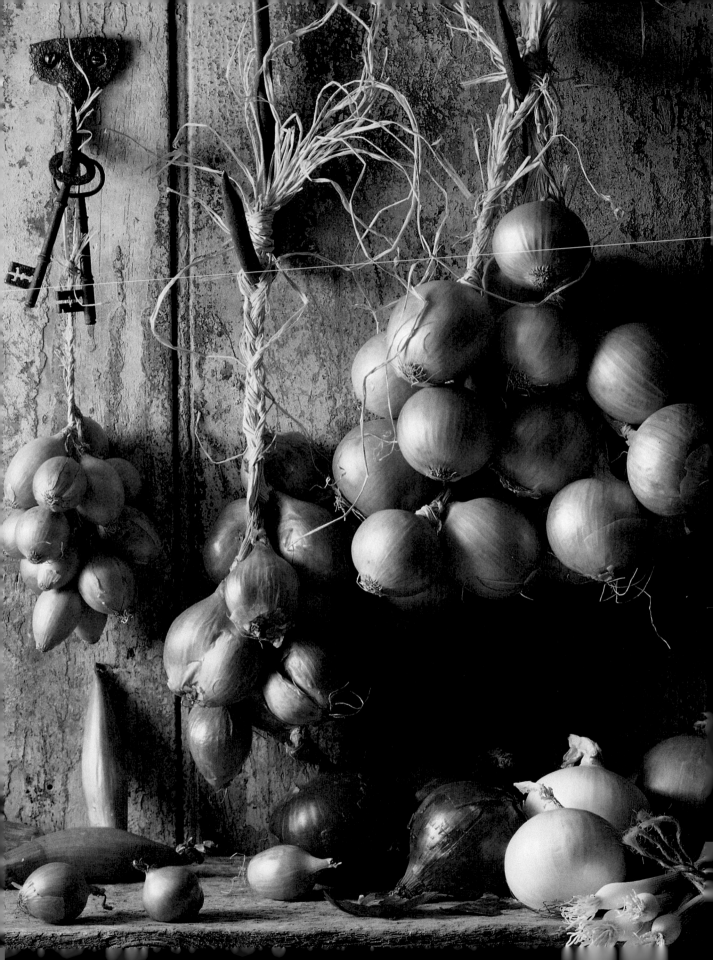

ONIONS

BENEFITS

- The green tops are a good source of vitamin C and beta carotene.
- May lower elevated blood cholesterol.
- Reduce the ability of the blood to clot.
- May help lower blood pressure.
- Mild antibacterial effect may help prevent superficial infections.
- Sulfur compounds block carcinogens.

DRAWBACKS

- Low in most nutrients.
- Can cause bloating and gassiness.
- Raw onions produce unpleasant breath and skin odors.

Folklore is filled with fascinating facts about the onion—among them that Alexander the Great fed huge quantities to his troops to strengthen them for battle. The Egyptian tomb paintings abound with onions; in fact, they are depicted more often than any other plant. Early Hebrew writings reveal that it was one of the foods that the Jews longed for after their flight from Egypt. And throughout history, healers have accorded onions near-magical powers to cure everything from baldness to infections.

Onions are members of the allium plant family, which also includes garlic, leeks, and shallots. There are scores of different varieties of onions, with new ones constantly emerging. In general, however, onions are divided into two categories: spring onions, which have a mild flavor and whose green tops and bulbs are eaten; and globe onions, which have a more pungent flavor and dry outer skins that are discarded. Shallots possess features of onions and garlic, but are milder.

With so many sizes, shapes, and flavors, and so many varieties of spring and globe onions available year-round, choosing an onion can be somewhat tricky. Scallions should have crisp, dark green tops and firm white bottoms.

PUNGENT OR SWEET. *Onions come in many sizes, colors, and flavors. Common varieties include (hanging, left to right) small yellow onions, shallots, yellow field onions, and (on board, left to right) banana shallots, more small yellow onions, red onions, white onions, large sweet onions, and scallions.*

Although they will keep for a few days in the refrigerator, scallions should be used before they begin to soften. Globe onions should be firm, with crackly, dry skin. Reject any that feel soft, have black spots (indicating mold), or have green sprouts showing at the top (these are well past their prime). They should have a mild odor—a strong, oniony smell points to decay. Globe onions should be stored in a cool, dry place away from direct light, which can give them a bitter taste. They should not be stored near potatoes, which give off moisture and a gas that causes onions to spoil more quickly.

Red onions have a mild, somewhat sweet flavor, which makes them a favorite for salads and sandwiches. Stronger white and yellow varieties are ideal for cooking, because they become milder and sweeter upon heating and they also impart a pleasant flavor to other foods. There are a number of new sweet varieties of yellow onions, which are often named for the areas where they were originally developed.

THE MANY USES OF ONIONS

The versatility of onions is evidenced by the numerous ways they are used: sliced raw in salads and sandwiches; cooked into stews, soups, and omelets; and baked, boiled, sautéed, or creamed and served as a side dish. Spring onions can be included in a raw vegetable tray, chopped into salads or dressings, or braised and served hot. Build a light meal around a bowl of French onion soup. To reduce the calorie content, use a defatted broth stock and just a sprinkling of low-fat cheese.

HEALTH BENEFITS

Cooks value onions more for the flavor they impart to other foods than for their nutritional content. Although onions are not high on the nutritional scale, the green tops of spring onions are a good source of vitamin C and beta carotene. A cup of boiled onions provides about 225 mg of potassium.

Recent research has verified some of the centuries-old beliefs about onions. For example, folk healers have long recommended onions as a heart tonic; researchers have now documented that adenosine, a substance in onions, hinders clot formation, which may help prevent heart attacks. Studies also indicate that onions may protect against the artery-clogging damage of cholesterol by raising the levels of the protective high-density lipoproteins (HDLs). Still other studies suggest that eating ample amounts of onions may help prevent high blood pressure.

LUNG CANCER PROTECTION

A study published in the *Journal of the National Cancer Institute* reported on the significant correlation between the high intake of dietary flavonoids and a reduced risk of lung cancer. Food sources of the flavonoids that offer the best protection include onions, as well as apples and white grapefruit.

BETTER RAW THAN COOKED

Cooking onions at a high heat significantly reduces the benefits of diallyl sulfide, their cancer-protective phytochemical. Fresh raw onion offers the most health benefits, and mincing (or even chewing) the onion helps to release its phytochemical power.

Sulfur compounds in onions can cause bad breath and an unpleasant skin odor; however, they also block the cancer-causing potential of some carcinogens. In addition, onions contain substances that have a mild antibacterial effect, which may validate the old folk remedy of rubbing a raw onion on a cut to prevent infection.

Cutting an onion allows its sulfur compounds to combine with enzymes and release volatile molecules that react with moisture in the eyes to form sulfuric acid. Tearing is a natural reaction of the eyes to eliminate the irritant. This effect may help clear any congested nasal passages during a cold. A syrup made from onions and honey is an old cough remedy. But consuming raw onions can cause bloating and gas in some people. ❖

ORANGES

BENEFITS

- An excellent source of vitamin C.
- A good source of folate, thiamine, and potassium.

DRAWBACKS

- May produce allergic reactions in some susceptible people.

One of our most popular fruits, oranges are usually associated with vitamin C, and with good reason. One medium-size orange provides about 70 mg, more than 90 percent of the Recommended Dietary Allowance (RDA) for women. As an antioxidant, vitamin C protects against cell damage by the free radicals produced

DO ONE SIMPLE THING

EAT THE PITHY PART

Eat the orange with the pith (the spongy white layer between the zest and the pulp). A good amount of the fruit's fiber and antioxidant plant chemicals are found there.

when oxygen is used by the human body, and it may reduce the risk of certain cancers, heart attacks, strokes, and other diseases. Oranges also contain rutin, hesperidin, and other bioflavonoids, plant pigments that may help to prevent or retard tumor growth. Beta-cryptoxanthin is a carotenoid in oranges and tangerines that may help prevent colon cancer. Nobiletin, a flavonoid found in the flesh of oranges, may have anti-inflammatory actions and tangeretin, the flavonoid found in tangerines, has been linked in experimental studies to a reduced growth of tumor cells. They also have smaller amounts of other vitamins and minerals; these include thiamine, folate, and potassium.

Oranges are low in calories (one orange contains approximately 60). An additional benefit is that the membranes between the segments of the fresh fruit provide a good amount of pectin, a soluble dietary fiber that helps control blood cholesterol levels.

Fresh oranges are a delicious snack or dessert and a flavorful ingredient in salads and some meat dishes. A half cup of freshly squeezed juice has roughly the same amount of nutrients found in the fresh fruit; much of the pulp and membranes are strained out of most commercial brands. Canned oranges lose most of their vitamin C and some minerals during processing, and are usually packed in high-sugar syrups.

The peel of the orange is sometimes dried to make candied orange peel or flavorings. Caution is needed, however, because the peel may be treated with sulfites, which can trigger serious allergic reactions in susceptible people. Also, orange peels contain limonene, an oil that is a common allergen. Many people who are allergic to commercial orange juice, which becomes infused with limonene during processing, find they can tolerate peeled oranges.

TYPES OF ORANGES

The following are the most common.
- Hamlins are grown mostly in Florida. These oranges are seedless and pulpy; they are used mainly for juicing.

- Jaffas are imported from Israel and other sunny regions. They are slightly sweeter than Valencias.
- Maltese, or blood, oranges are sweet, deep red oranges originating in Italy.
- Navel oranges are sweet and seedless; they are the second most common type in North America.
- Sevilles are sour oranges that are used mostly for marmalades.
- Temples are sweet, juicy, full of seeds, and are a cross between tangerines and oranges.
- Valencias, the most common North American variety, are used for eating and juicing. ❖

ORGAN MEATS

BENEFITS
- An inexpensive source of protein.
- Liver and kidneys are excellent sources of vitamins A and B_{12}, folate, niacin, iron, and other minerals.
- Most are good sources of potassium.

DRAWBACKS
- Most are very high in cholesterol.
- The liver may harbor toxins.

Despite their high nutritional value, organ meats have never achieved in North America the popularity that they enjoy in Europe. In recent years they have fallen even further out of favor because some, especially liver and brains, are very high in cholesterol. The furor over "mad cow disease" (bovine spongiform encephalitis) has led to fear of contracting a similarly fatal new human variant of the brain disease, Creutzfeldt-Jakob disease (vCJD). It is unclear whether vCJD is linked to beef from cattle infected with mad cow disease, and dishes such as calf's liver, kidneys, sweetbreads (calf thymus and pancreas), and tripe (stomach) still appear regularly on the menus of many restaurants. Pâtés and popular luncheon meats, such as liverwurst, are often made from organ meats and perhaps other variety cuts, such as the feet.

LIVER

Because the liver is a storehouse for vitamin A, iron, and many other nutrients, it follows that it is also a highly nutritious meat source. A 4-oz (115-g) serving of beef liver provides more than 10 times the Recommended Dietary Allowance (RDA) of vitamin A, 50 times the RDA of vitamin B_{12}, and 50 percent or more of the RDAs for folate, niacin, iron, and zinc.

The 200 calories in a 4-oz (115-g) serving of liver is less than in most other cuts of beef, but liver's major drawback is its high cholesterol content of approximately 400 mg in 4 oz (115 g) of braised beef liver. However, an occasional serving of liver in an otherwise low-fat, low-cholesterol diet probably is not harmful unless you already have heart disease or high blood cholesterol; then it may be advisable to forgo this meat.

One of the liver's main functions is to metabolize and detoxify various chemical compounds. Thus, the liver may harbor residues of antibiotics and other drugs fed to meat animals, as well as environmental toxins. For this reason, some doctors advise against eating liver on a regular basis.

Liver is one of the richest dietary sources of vitamin A. When a person consumes more vitamin A than is needed, the excess is stored in the body. Over time a buildup of vitamin A can result in liver damage, fatigue, and other problems. Studies show, for example, that consuming 5 to 10 times the RDA of vitamin A before and during early pregnancy can increase the risk of birth defects. Normally, it's difficult if not impossible to consume toxic amounts of vitamin A from an ordinary diet. But because liver is so high in this nutrient, an individual who regularly consumes it several times a week may develop a toxicity.

OTHER ORGAN MEATS

Liver is probably the most popular of the organ meats in North America. Here are a few others:
- Brains are higher in cholesterol than any other food; a 4-oz (115-g) serving of beef brains has more than 2,000 mg, and pork brains contain an even larger amount. However they are an excellent source of vitamin B_{12}.
- Heart is also high in vitamin B_{12}, iron, and potassium; in addition, it provides high-quality protein and less fat and cholesterol than other organ meats.
- Kidneys are low in fat and high in protein. They provide large amounts of vitamin B_{12}, riboflavin, and iron, and useful amounts of B_6, folate, and niacin.
- Sweetbreads are high in fat, but they provide useful amounts of potassium.
- Tongue, also high in fat, contains useful amounts of the B vitamins, especially B_{12}.
- Tripe provides high-quality protein, a fair amount of potassium, and small amounts of some minerals. ❖

ORGANIC FOODS
■ ARE THEY WORTH THE COST? ■

I f you are concerned about pesticide residues in foods today, you can turn to organic products—but don't expect them to be nutritionally superior.

Only a few years ago, organic foods were found solely in health-food stores or at farmers' markets. Today many supermarkets stock organic fruits and vegetables, meats, milk, eggs, cereals, cookies, snack foods, frozen dinners, even wines, along with their conventionally produced counterparts. The organic industry is growing between 20 to 25 percent annually, and has been for the last several years. More than $5 billion worth of organic products are now sold in North America each year.

Consumers are clearly willing to spend more money for organic foods, which have improved in quality and variety in recent years. But what are shoppers getting for the money?

The meaning of "organic"

Organic food is produced by farmers who protect the environment for future generations by rotating crops (which promotes biological diversity), conserving and renewing the soil, and protecting sources of water. These crops are grown, handled, and processed without synthetic fertilizers, pesticides, or herbicides; artificial ingredients, or preservatives. By law, organic food is not irradiated, and, if the product is labeled "100 percent organic," doesn't contain genetically engineered ingredients (see Genetically Modified Organisms). Organic meat, poultry, eggs, and dairy products come from animals that are given no antibiotics or growth hormones.

Organic food crops can, however, be grown with pesticides—just not synthetic ones. One popular organic pesticide is *Bacillus thuringiensis*, a naturally occurring soil bacterium that is toxic to the larvae of several species of insects but harmless to wildlife and people. Not all of these organic pesticides are harmless, however—pyrethrins, natural insecticides isolated from flowers, can cause allergic reactions, for example. Naturally occurring copper compounds can also be used in organic agriculture, even though they are potentially toxic.

Organic foods can also be contaminated with synthetic agricultural chemicals that are carried by the wind from other fields, or persist in the soil. Still, the pesticide levels are much lower than in conventional foods. In one study of 94,000 food samples from more than 20 major food crops, sponsored by the nonprofit Consumers Union, organically grown foods had about one-third the residues of conventionally grown foods, which were also more likely to contain residues from several pesticides.

Is organic food more nutritious?

There have been a handful of studies suggesting a difference in nutritional value, but they are far from conclusive. One study published in the January 2003 *Journal of Agricultural and Food Chemistry* found that frozen organic corn had 52 percent more vitamin C than conventional corn, but corn doesn't have much vitamin C anyway. An August 2002 Italian study in the same journal found that organic peaches and pears have higher levels of health-protective polyphenols, and a smidgen more vitamin C (8 percent). Another found that organic soup had more salicylic acid—an

Organic labeling

Is it organic? In the United States it's now easy to tell—read the label, and look for the organic seal. Since October 2002, all foods that are sold as organic in the United States—wherever they're grown—have to be certified in accordance with federal standards. (In Canada, the certification program is voluntary—although it's mandatory in the province of Quebec—but standards are similar to those in the United States.) Here's what the USDA labels mean:

✔ "100 percent organic." All ingredients are organic. May carry the USDA Organic seal.

✔ "Organic." At least 95 percent of ingredients are organic. May carry the USDA Organic seal.

✔ "Made with organic [ingredients]." If the product contains at least 70 percent organic ingredients, it can list up to three of them on the label. For example, a macaroni-and-cheese box might say it's made with organic wheat flour, cheese, and milk. But it can't carry the USDA Organic seal.

✔ "Organic [ingredients]." If the total is less than 70 percent, a product can't call itself organic on the front panel or carry the seal, but it can list organic ingredients on the side panel. If a cereal has organic raisins, for example, it can list that.

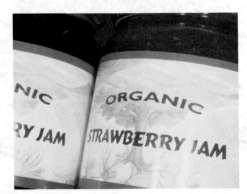

anti-inflammatory compound found in food that might have health significance—than nonorganic soup. All of these studies had methodological problems. And even if the differences are real, they are small. You'd get a lot more vitamin C eating an extra orange than in choosing organic corn for dinner.

The label "Certified Organic" is not meant to be a nutrition claim. Nor does it mean that the food is any less likely to be contaminated with pathogens that cause food-borne illness: Organic chickens can be contaminated with salmonella and other food-borne pathogens, just like conventional chickens. Nor is it safer to eat raw organic eggs than raw conventional eggs.

The safety factor

Is organic food safer to eat than conventionally produced food? That's the big debate, of course. Synthetic pesticides, herbicides, fungicides, insecticides, and other agricultural chemicals can certainly have adverse health effects on the farm workers who use them. But the evidence is not conclusive about their effect on consumer health. Part of the difficulty is that, when it comes to consumers, what needs to be determined is the effect of lower levels of intake over a lifetime, which is more difficult for researchers to establish.

There may be a greater benefit in shielding children from pesticide residues since their bodies are smaller and they eat a less-varied diet. In a University of Washington study, Seattle preschoolers whose families ate primarily organic foods had much lower urine levels of organophosphate pesticides. In large amounts, these are toxic to the nervous system. While the researchers found that children who ate conventional foods were more likely to be exposed to these pesticides at levels above those recommended by the United States government, such guidelines have a wide margin of safety. So there's no clear evidence that there is a risk to eating conventional food, or a benefit to eating organic ones.

Environmental benefits are more established. Agriculture that relies on organic methods helps prevent soil erosion (which is a serious problem in North America), protects groundwater, and preserves wildlife.

The bottom line

North Americans are privileged to enjoy an abundant and safe food supply. It does not, however, come without a price. Scientists are concerned that modern agricultural methods and our liberal use of pesticides will eventually upset the delicate ecological balance and create major problems. We have seen indications of this in the past—for example, the decimation of bird populations that led to the banning of DDT. There are also many questions being raised about the link between pesticide use and cancer rates. Due to the increasing availability of organic foods, consumers who are concerned about chemical residues can now purchase organic alternatives.

What's best to buy?

Since organic food is typically more expensive, it makes sense to shop selectively. One way to save money is to buy organic produce instead of nonorganic only for those foods where the nonorganic examples have been documented to have the highest pesticide residues by nonprofit research groups such as Consumers Union and the Environmental Working Group. Although there is no evidence that fruits and vegetables with higher residues pose a hazard, selecting the organic versions of these is a logical place to start:

✔ Choose these organic fruits: peaches, nectarines, apples, grapes, pears, cherries, raspberries, and strawberries.

✔ Choose the following organic vegetables: green beans, spinach, bell peppers, celery, and potatoes.

✔ Consider organic meat. While most people worry about produce, animals actually accumulate more residues, especially in their fat. So you may want to buy organic hamburger, steak, pork chops, and lamb.

✔ Save money with nonorganic low-residue foods. These include asparagus, avocados, bananas, broccoli, cauliflower, sweet corn, kiwi, mangos, onions, papaya, pineapples, and sweet peas.

✔ Skip the organic OJ and milk. Surprisingly, processed foods tend to have much lower residue levels than whole fruits and vegetables. Levels in orange juice, apple juice, canned peaches, and canned or frozen peas and corn are quite low. Milk tends to have few residues, too.

OSTEOPOROSIS

GET PLENTY OF

- Low-fat milk, yogurt, canned fish with bones, and other foods rich in calcium.
- Foods rich in vitamin D, such as oily fish and fortified milk, and soy or rice beverages.
- Legumes for phosphorus.
- Weight-bearing exercise.

LIMIT

- Alcohol.
- Coffee, tea, colas, and other beverages containing caffeine.

AVOID

- Smoking.

Throughout life, our bones are in a state of constant renewal, called remodeling. While some bone cells are breaking down and being resorbed, others are forming to take their place. When resorption occurs faster than formation, the bones become weak and extremely porous. Fractures can occur with little or no pressure. This condition is called osteoporosis. Lack of estrogen appears to be its key contributing factor, but a falling off of androgens—the male hormones—is also involved, coupled with an inadequate intake of calcium and vitamin D.

Throughout childhood, bones grow in length and density. In adolescence bones build density and finish growing in length (usually ages 11 to 14). Peak bone mass is usually reached in your 20s. The denser your bones, the lower risk of osteoporosis later. Once peak bone mass is achieved, you can't improve it; it is determined by genetics and nutrition.

Both men and women begin to lose some mass with increasing age. In women, the loss is greatly accelerated with the decline in estrogen production at menopause. Osteoporosis affects both women and men, but women of Northern European and Asian ancestry have the highest risk. Women of Mediterranean and African descent are less affected, perhaps because they tend to have more bone mass and typically get the sun needed to make vitamin D.

DID YOU KNOW?

STRONG BONES ARE DEVELOPED IN ADOLESCENCE

Adolescence is the critical window for developing strong bones to last a lifetime. One recent study found that women over 50 who drank less than a glass of milk a day as girls had significantly lower bone density and twice the risk of fractures compared with those who drank a glass or more. The difference existed no matter how much milk the women drank as adults or how much calcium they took.

Moderate weight-bearing exercise can help the bones at any age; in fact, exercise is one factor that is known to improve bone strength in later life. However, a very high level of athletic training in adolescent girls robs their bodies of the fat they need to produce and store estrogen. Highly trained teenage athletes and ballet dancers, who often have menstrual irregularities, may be more at risk for developing early, severe osteoporosis. Anorexic girls who starve themselves in order to get rid of the normal subcutaneous layer of fat are at high risk as well.

Smoking greatly increases the risk of severe osteoporosis. Women smokers have lower levels of estrogen at all ages, and may enter menopause up to 5 years earlier than nonsmokers. In addition, nicotine is known to interfere with the ability of the body to use calcium.

Women whose ovaries are surgically removed experience an abrupt withdrawal of estrogen production rather than a gradual decline. They may suffer more severe osteoporosis than those who have normal menopause. Kidney diseases and the use of steroid drugs also are risk factors.

PREVENTION

Osteoporosis prevention should begin in childhood, with a healthy diet and regular exercise. Plenty of calcium, the building block of bone, and vitamin D are needed. The recommendation for calcium is 1,300 mg per day for 9 to 18 year olds, 1,000 mg per day for adults up to 50, and 1,200 mg per day after 50. Phosphorus, also essential to bone formation, is found in most foods that contain calcium as well as meat, poultry, and eggs.

Calcium. Foods especially rich in calcium and phosphorus include milk and dairy products, fortified soy and rice beverages, dried beans and peas, tofu, canned fish eaten with the bones, nuts, and dark green leafy vegetables. The darker the greens, the more calcium they contain. An exception is spinach; it is high in oxalic acid, which inhibits calcium absorption.

Those who shun whole milk because of its fat content can drink skim milk, which has even more calcium volume for volume. Low-fat cheese, yogurt, and lactose-free milk are excellent calcium sources for people who have a milk intolerance. Strict vegetarians can get calcium from fortified soy and rice beverages and tofu, beans, lentils, nuts, and green vegetables.

If the doctor recommends a calcium supplement, read the label carefully to find out how much elemental calcium is in each pill and what form it's in. Calcium citrate is the most easily absorbed form; calcium carbonate is less well absorbed, especially by people over 50 and may in rare cases cause constipation, bloating, and gas. Calcium gluconate is well absorbed but infrequently can cause diarrhea. Taking supplements along with meals helps absorption. Some physicians suggest that women obtain extra calcium from over-the-counter indigestion remedies; the active ingredient in these is calcium carbonate. Bone meal and dolomite supplements are not recommended because they may be contaminated with heavy metals.

Vitamin D. Just as important as calcium is vitamin D; the body needs it in order to absorb calcium. The RDA for adults up to 50 is 200 IU (5 mcg); for adults 51 to 70, 400 IU (10 mcg); and over 70, 600 IU (15 mcg). The main source is sunlight, but it can also be obtained from fluid milk, fortified soy and rice beverages, oily fish, egg yolks, butter, and margarine.

Vitamin K. New research suggests that vitamin K may help to increase bone density and also reduce fracture rates. Both the Nurses' Health Study and the Framingham Heart Study found that people who consume the most vitamin K have a lower risk of hip fractures than those who consume less. Friendly bacteria that live in your intestines help to make a large percentage of the vitamin K you need, and the rest can be found in leafy green vegetables, green peas, broccoli, spinach, brussels sprouts, romaine lettuce, cabbage, kale, and beef liver. There is some in egg yolks, dairy products, and plant oils such as canola, soybean, and olive.

Soy. Studies suggest that soy may play a role in prevention of osteoporosis as it contains isoflavones, a type of plant estrogen that may help conserve bone mass, particularly during perimenopause and menopause.

Flaxseed. A study of postmenopausal women suggests that flaxseed, which is high in lignans, may retain bone mass, elevate antioxidant status, and help prevent urinary loss of calcium.

Vitamin C. Studies have linked higher intakes of vitamin C with higher bone density. Vitamin C also helps to form the connective tissue that holds bones together. Some of the best food sources are fruits and vegetables, especially citrus fruits, berries, melons, and peppers.

Regular weight-bearing exercise. Walking, jogging, aerobics, tennis, and dancing are all excellent in helping to maintain bones. This type of activity stimulates the remodeling process and improves the circulation, which brings vitamins and minerals to the bones.

WHAT TO AVOID

Evidence indicates that the following should be avoided.

Caffeine. Drinking coffee, tea, or colas increases the amount of calcium you excrete.

Sodium. It also can cause the kidneys to excrete calcium. Minimize salt used in cooking and at the table; cut back on processed and canned foods.

High levels of dietary protein. This too can cause calcium to be excreted. Eating more plant proteins in place of animal proteins is a strategy to keep your protein intake more moderate.

Medications can affect the levels of calcium in the body. Antacids containing aluminum can promote calcium excretion. Calcium is also lost during long-term use of other drugs, including certain antibiotics, diuretics, and steroids.

BEYOND DIET

Many doctors recommend a baseline bone density scan for women when menstrual periods become irregular. Depending on the results, the doctor may recommend calcium and vitamin D supplements or other therapy.

ESTROGEN REPLACEMENT

For women, treatment for osteoporosis has often been hormone replacement therapy (HRT) to replace estrogen lost at menopause. Estrogen does decrease bone loss; however, newer research suggests that HRT may work only in women who have osteoporosis when they begin taking the hormone. In addition, HRT has been under scrutiny (see Menopause).

Newer nonhormonal drugs offer men and women an alternative. These include bisphosphonates, such as etidronate (Didrocal) and alendronate (Fosamax). They decrease bone resorption and shift the balance toward the formation of healthy tissue. Calcitonin (Miacalcin), a hormonal preparation taken by injection or as a nasal spray, works in a similar fashion.

Yet another new medication is raloxifene (Evista), which helps prevent osteoporosis by modulating the body's estrogen receptors. This drug, while not a hormone, offers many of the same benefits as estrogen without increasing the risk of breast and uterine cancers. ❖

MYTH BUSTER

Myth: Black cohosh, red clover, and chasteberry can help osteoporosis.

Reality: While many women try these herbal remedies to relieve menopausal symptoms, there is no evidence that black cohosh, red clover, chasteberry, or any other herbal preparation has any effect on calcium metabolism related to bone loss.

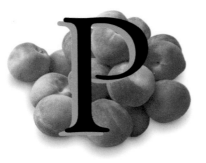

PAPAYAS

BENEFITS
- An excellent source of vitamin C and potassium.
- High in folate and beta carotene.
- An extract is used to tenderize meat.

DRAWBACKS
- Can cause dermatitis in some people.

Native to Central America, papayas are now grown in tropical climates around the world. They should not be confused with the North American pawpaw—although often called by the same name, the two are unrelated.

Like most yellow-orange fruits, papayas are high in vitamin C and beta carotene, the plant form of vitamin A. One medium-size papaya supplies more than twice the adult Recommended Dietary Allowance (RDA) of vitamin C, almost 30 percent of the RDA of folate, and 800 mg of potassium.

Papayas contain papain, an enzyme that is similar to the digestive juice pepsin. Because this enzyme breaks down protein, papain extract from papayas is marketed as a meat tenderizer. It has also been used medically to treat ruptured spinal disks, but this treatment has fallen out of favor in most places. Topical ointments containing

THE SEEDS OF A PAPAYA ARE EDIBLE TOO. *Just rinse them and add to a salad for a nutty and slightly peppery taste.*

papain are sometimes applied to promote the shedding of dead tissue. Papain causes the dermatitis that some people experience when handling papayas; this irritation is not necessarily an allergic reaction.

Usually eaten raw, the fruit should be washed, split open, and the black seeds scooped out. These seeds are normally thrown away, but they can be dried and used like peppercorns.

You can also use papayas in cooking; they impart a sweet Caribbean flavor to chicken or fish dishes. A few pieces of papaya added to a stew tenderizes the meat, while its pectin serves as a natural thickener.

Papaya nectar is a popular beverage, but many bottled varieties are mostly water and sugar. A product that contains only 33 percent papaya juice can still be sold as papaya nectar. ❖

PARKINSON'S DISEASE

CONSUME PLENTY OF
- Fresh vegetables, fruits, and whole-grain products.
- Fluids to promote good digestion.
- Soft or pureed foods to ease swallowing.

LIMIT
- High-protein foods if taking levodopa.

AVOID
- Excessive weight gain.

About 150 people out of every 100,000 North Americans are afflicted with Parkinson's disease, a chronic and progressive nerve disorder that causes uncontrollable shaking or trembling (tremors), a fixed staring expression, muscle rigidity, stooped posture, and an abnormal gait. The disease varies from one person to another; some people develop speech problems and difficulty swallowing, while others suffer progressive dementia. Parkinson's affects men and women equally and generally develops only after the age of 50.

The symptoms of Parkinson's disease are due to progressive destruction of a part of the brain, the substantia nigra, where cells make dopamine, a chemical necessary for proper neuromuscular function. The underlying cause of the disease is usually unknown. In some cases, however, cocaine use and head injuries, such as those suffered by boxers, have resulted in a type of parkinsonism. In a few cases, the use of a street "designer drug" (an altered version of demerol) induced parkinsonism in drug addicts. Some studies have shown a higher incidence of Parkinson's among agricultural workers suggesting that the use of pesticides may be linked to the disease.

There is no cure for Parkinson's, but various medications, especially levodopa, can reduce symptoms and slow the progression. Preliminary research indicates that coenzyme Q_{10}, a dietary supplement, may be beneficial. There are also surgical treatments, but these are usually reserved for severe advanced disease.

THE ROLE OF DIET

Although there are no nutritional treatments for Parkinson's disease, diet helps to increase the effectiveness of treatment with levodopa and manage such problems as constipation and difficulty in chewing and swallowing.

Makes treatment more effective. To be its most effective, levodopa should be absorbed from the small intestine as soon as possible after it is taken. Some physicians advise taking the drug 20 to 30 minutes before meals, but if this provokes nausea, it can be taken with a carbohydrate snack, such as crackers or bread. Protein delays the absorption of levodopa, so the medicine should not be taken with animal products. There have been some reports that a reduced intake of protein may be beneficial. Some doctors advise consuming the day's protein allowance in the evening, when it's less likely to create problems.

A proper diet helps to control other symptoms. Constipation can be minimized by consuming ample fresh fruits and vegetables, whole-grain cereals and breads, and other high-fiber foods, as well as drinking six to eight glasses of water or other fluids daily. Exercise promotes healthy bowel function and is advised for anyone with Parkinson's disease, because it preserves muscle tone and strength. It is also important to avoid becoming overweight, as this makes mobility even more difficult.

PROBLEM SOLVING

Patients with advanced Parkinson's often have trouble chewing and swallowing food, because the tongue and facial muscles are affected.

Excessive drooling and shaky hands. These are common problems. Medications can help reduce drooling, and meals should emphasize foods that are easy to chew and swallow. These include cooked cereals or well-moistened dry cereals, poached or scrambled eggs, soups, mashed potatoes, rice, soft-cooked pasta, tender chicken or turkey, well-cooked boneless fish, pureed or mashed vegetables and fruits, custard, yogurt, and juices. If eating is tiring, try smaller but more frequent meals.

To avoid choking. Sit up straight and tilt your head slightly forward when swallowing. Take small bites, chew thoroughly, and swallow everything before taking another bite. Concentrate on moving food backward in your mouth with your tongue, and swallow again if you feel that food did not go down completely. Sip a liquid between bites to help wash food down. If you do cough or choke, lean forward and tuck your chin down while coughing. ❖

PARSNIPS

BENEFITS
- Low in calories and high in fiber.
- A flavorful alternative to potatoes.
- A useful source of vitamin C, folate, and potassium.

Parsnips have a sweet, nutty flavor that goes well with other vegetables in soups or stews. They can also be served as a side dish or instead of potatoes or other starchy foods. This winter root vegetable tastes best after the first frost; exposure to cold begins to convert its starch into sugar. Because parsnips are too fibrous to be eaten raw, they are served cooked.

Parsnips are a low-calorie, nutritious starchy food. A half-cup serving has only 60 calories and is high in fiber; it also provides 300 mg of potassium, 10 mg of vitamin C, and 45 mcg (micrograms) of folate.

When buying parsnips, select ones about the size of a medium carrot; reject any that are covered with roots or are soft and shrunken. If the tops are still attached, cut them off before storing them so they don't draw moisture from the roots. They can be kept for a few weeks in the refrigerator. Parsnips can effectively liven up any soup. ❖

PASTA

BENEFITS

- A useful source of protein, B vitamins, iron, and other minerals.
- Low in fat and sodium.
- Versatile and inexpensive.

DRAWBACKS

- Often topped with high-fat sauces.

First introduced to North America by Thomas Jefferson, pasta has become a staple in many homes. Most of us fondly remember dinners of macaroni and cheese, spaghetti and meatballs, or baked ziti. But with the advent of the low-carbohydrate diet came a new status for pasta: dietary evil. Is pasta really bad for you?

Ordinary white pasta is made from refined flour. Because refined flour is digested quickly, a large plate of pasta can send your blood sugar levels soaring, only to crash several hours afterward, and trigger renewed hunger.

Such blood-sugar swings are linked with weight gain, which is why some nutrition experts have begun to recommend that people limit the amount of white bread and white pasta they consume. Whole-grain pasta, on the other hand, which contains about three times the fiber of white pasta, won't cause dramatic blood-sugar swings, and a diet rich in whole grains has been shown to lower the risk of diabetes, heart disease, and several forms of cancer.

A growing number of supermarkets also carry pastas made from corn, quinoa, Jerusalem artichokes, buckwheat, and other types of flours, as well as varieties flavored with spinach and tomato, which have minimally more nutrition.

THE CALORIE QUESTION

Pasta is not especially high in calories. One cup of cooked pasta contains 210 calories. The trouble is that people tend to eat more than one cup of pasta at a sitting—especially if they are eating out at a restaurant. And all too often pasta is turned into a fattening dish with butter, cheese, and rich sauces. Fettuccine Alfredo, for instance, is sometimes called "a heart attack on a plate" because one serving can contain more than 700 calories and as many as 50 g of fat. But there are many ways to avoid extra calories. The 400 to 500 calories in a 6-oz (170-g) serving of a traditional meat-and-cheese lasagna, for example, can be cut almost in half by substituting vegetables for the ground meat and using low-fat or skim ricotta and mozzarella.

NUTRITION

Pastas are a good source of iron (about 2 mg in a 1-cup serving) and potassium; many are also enriched with thiamine, niacin, and other B vitamins. Although the protein in pasta (about 5 to 7 g in a 1-cup serving) lacks some essential amino acids, these can easily be obtained from

DID YOU KNOW?

PASTA IS A "MOOD FOOD"

The brain uses the chemical serotonin to make us feel good. When you eat carbohydrates such as pasta, there's a rapid increase in blood sugar and serotonin levels. The good feelings arrive within about 30 minutes and last for several hours. Eating protein with the pasta, however, can negate the effect, while whole-grain pastas, which take longer to break down, prolong it.

A MEDLEY OF PASTA. *Not all pastas are equal. Egg noodles contain protein, but also fat. White pastas may be enriched, but whole-grain pastas are the most healthy.*

DO ONE SIMPLE THING

MEASURE THE PORTION YOU PUT ON YOUR PLATE

While a 1-cup serving of cooked pasta has only about 210 calories, if your portion size is large, the calories will add up. Keep your serving size in check by visualizing a portion that should be approximately the size of a baseball.

HEALTHY PASTA SAUCES

Pasta dishes can be transformed by the addition of sauces. Traditional ingredients include olive oil, garlic, onions, mushrooms, tomatoes, and fresh basil. Many classic sauces, such as cheese, pesto, and bolognese, are high in fat and calories. The following are ideas for creating tasty low-calorie dishes.

- Toss pasta with fresh, diced tomatoes and herbs.
- Use half of the oil, cheese, and nuts in a pesto recipe, while increasing the basil and garlic. Add white wine if the sauce is too dry.
- Puree vegetables in a blender or food processor, simmer them with herbs and spices, and toss with spaghetti or another pasta.
- When making a cream sauce, substitute low-fat milk or evaporated skim milk for the cream.
- Toss a pasta salad with a dressing made from nonfat yogurt or sour cream instead of regular sour cream or mayonnaise.
- Combine pasta with beans, lentils, or other legumes to create a high-protein vegetarian meal.
- Instead of a buttery cheese sauce, toss pasta with a broth and sprinkle it lightly with grated Parmesan or Romano cheese.
- Add vegetables instead of meat to a light tomato sauce.

a sprinkling of Parmesan cheese as a low-calorie (25 calories per tablespoon) topping. Egg noodles provide complete protein, but they also contain a modest amount of fat and about 50 mg of cholesterol per serving. There are also high-protein pastas that are enriched with soy flour and milk solids.

A VERSATILE FOOD

Pasta is most nutritious when used as a "vehicle" for healthful foods such as vegetables and fish. For lunch, toss some cooked pasta with vegetables, tuna, or thinly sliced chicken. Sauté or stir-fry fresh vegetables and toss them with pasta to make a primavera dish for an appetizer, a side dish, or an entrée. For a special occasion, top linguine or angel hair pasta with a seafood medley of clams, mussels, shrimp, and scallops. Remember, when cooking pasta, adding salt to the water is optional and just a small amount of oil (1 teaspoon) may help prevent spillovers and keep pasta from sticking. Tortellini, bow-shaped farfalle, and ziti are a few of the interestingly shaped pastas that are ideal as beginner foods for toddlers. ❖

PEACHES

BENEFITS
- A good source of beta carotene, with useful amounts of vitamin C and potassium.
- A good source of dietary fiber.

DRAWBACKS
- May provoke allergic reactions in susceptible people.

Nutritious and versatile, peaches can be enjoyed fresh, added to fruit salads, or cooked with meat and poultry dishes. They can also be baked, grilled, broiled, or poached to create pies, cobblers, and other desserts.

While there are hundreds of varieties, peaches are usually classified into one of two categories: freestone, with a loose, easily removed pit, or cling, in which the stone is enmeshed in the fruit's flesh. Freestones are mostly sold fresh, while clingstones are reserved for canning, freezing, and preserves.

Fresh peaches are a low-calorie source of beta carotene and some vitamin C. They contain fiber, especially pectin, a soluble fiber that is instrumental in lowering high blood cholesterol. A medium-size peach contains only 35 calories. Canned and frozen peaches are higher in calories than the fresh; a cup of sweetened frozen peaches contains 235 calories, compared to 190 in those canned in heavy syrup, and 110 in juice-packed brands.

Volume for volume, dried peaches contain the most calories, because it takes 6 to 7 lb (2.7–3.2 kg) to produce just 1 lb (0.45 kg) of the dried. Ten dried peach halves provide 310 calories; on the plus side, they are also a more concentrated source of various essential nutrients. Those 10 halves provide 1,295 mg of potassium, and 5 mg of iron. After eating dried peaches, brush your teeth to remove their sticky residue; it can create dental problems.

Dried peaches often contain sulfites, a preservative that produces an allergic reaction in susceptible people.

Peaches may produce an allergic reaction in people with allergies to such related fruits as apricots, plums, and cherries, as well as almonds. They also contain salicylates, which may provoke a reaction in aspirin-sensitive people.

In North America, the season for peaches runs from April through mid-October, peaking in July and August. Peaches do not increase in sweetness after picking, so when choosing fruits

PEACH-PICKING TIPS
- Look for peaches that are yellow or creamy with a rosy blush on their cheeks. Avoid peaches with green undertones, they were picked too early.
- Select peaches with unwrinkled skin and no bruises.
- Sniff the stem end of the peach. You should be able to smell the peachy fragrance.
- Watch out for peaches with tan circles. It's an early sign of decay.

avoid those that are rock hard. A peach should feel heavy, indicating that it is juicy, and it should have a sweet odor. The skin should be smooth and have a warm yellow or reddish color. Avoid any peaches that are bruised.

In terms of texture, it is best to choose relatively soft peaches if they are to be eaten right away. If you buy firm peaches, placing them in a paper bag at room temperature will hasten the ripening process. Unless they are going to be eaten within the day, store ripe peaches in the refrigerator; they will keep for 3 to 5 days. ❖

PEANUT BUTTER

See Jams and Spreads

PEANUTS

BENEFITS

- A good source of monounsaturated fats.
- Contain potassium, thiamine, niacin, vitamin E, phosphorus, magnesium, copper, selenium, and zinc.

DRAWBACKS

- Common allergy triggers.
- Molds can contaminate peanuts and produce cancer-causing aflatoxins.

Despite its name, the peanut is not actually a nut. It is a pulse and belongs to the legume family along with lentils and beans. The peanut, while grown in tropical and subtropical regions throughout the world, is native to the Western Hemisphere. It is believed that the first peanut plants were found in the Andean lowlands of South America. Today peanuts are found in a wide variety of products and are part of many cuisines around the world.

Peanuts have a number of health benefits. They are an economical source of protein and are rich in monounsaturated fats, which help lower LDL cholesterol. A 1-oz (30-g) serving of peanuts (a small handful) contains 40 mcg (micrograms) of folate, or 10 percent of the Recommended Dietary Allowance (RDA), as well as useful amounts of potassium, thiamine, niacin, vitamin E, phosphorus, magnesium, copper, selenium, and zinc. Peanuts also contain resveratrol (the substance found in red wine) as well as other flavonoids and antioxidants. A 1-oz (30-g) serving of peanuts contains about 160 calories, so

CAUTION

Refrigerate or freeze shelled nuts; their oil quickly turns rancid. Never use peanuts that are moldy or have an "off" taste; molds that grow on peanuts create aflatoxins, substances that cause liver cancer.

despite their health benefits, they still should be used moderately. A growing number of studies indicate that the beneficial effect of peanuts and nuts may not only be due to their fatty acid composition but other key nutrients, especially when they replace less-healthful foods in the diet.

NUTS HAVE SUPERFOOD STATUS

Research has shown that peanuts may reduce the risk of heart disease when consumed regularly. A recent study found regular consumption of foods rich in monounsaturated fats such as peanuts, peanut butter, and olive oil (along with a diet low in saturated fat) decreased total cholesterol by 10 percent, LDL cholesterol by 14 percent, and overall risk for heart disease by 21 percent. Large-population studies, such as the Physicians Health Study and the Iowa Women's Health Study have shown a relationship between cardioprotective benefits and peanut and nut consumption.

A study published in the *Journal of the American Medical Association* found that eating nuts and peanuts may lower the risk of type 2 diabetes in women. Reduced risk was greatest in people who ate the most nuts. Those who never or almost never ate nuts had no change in risk, and those who consumed nuts five or more times a week had a 27 percent lower risk. Women who consumed peanut butter five or more times per week had a 21 percent lower risk compared to women who never or almost never ate peanut butter.

Peanuts may also help with weight management. Peanuts and peanut butter are known to have high satiety values, which means they will keep you feeling full longer than carbohydrate-based foods. A recent study showed that participants' hunger was reduced for 2 hours following a snack of peanuts or peanut butter, versus only 30 minutes after eating various other snack foods (like pickles and rice cakes).

The <u>participants who ate peanuts and peanut butter also consumed fewer total calories throughout the day.</u>

Research has also shown that people who followed a moderate-fat, Mediterranean-style diet lost more weight and kept it off for a longer period of time than those who followed a low-fat diet. The moderate-fat diet encouraged the consumption of monounsaturated fats such as peanuts, peanut butter, olive oil, and other nuts.

Peanuts may provoke allergic reactions in certain people. Symptoms can range from a tingling sensation in the mouth to hives and, in extreme cases, to anaphylaxis, a life-threatening emergency.

Warning: Choking deaths are often traced to nuts. Young children and those who have difficulty chewing or swallowing should not be given nuts unless they are finely chopped. ❖

PEARS

BENEFITS
- A good source of dietary fiber.
- Contain vitamin C and folate.

DRAWBACKS
- Dried pears often contain sulfites, which provoke asthma attacks or allergic reactions in susceptible people.

Called the "butter fruit" by many Europeans in reference to its smooth texture, a pear makes an ideal snack, dessert, or even a sweet or spicy side dish. Pears are a delicious treat when served fresh, but they can also be baked, poached, or sautéed.

One medium-size (6-oz/170-g) pear has about 100 calories and provides about 5 g of fiber. The fiber in pears is pectin, a soluble fiber that helps control blood cholesterol levels and cellulose, an insoluble fiber that promotes normal bowel function. Pears also have useful amounts of vitamin C, folate, and potassium. Dried pears provide a more concentrated form of calories and nutrients than fresh pears;

however, their high sugar content and sticky texture may promote tooth decay. Most dried pears also contain sulfites, which can provoke asthma or an allergic response in susceptible individuals.

Canned pears lose most of their vitamin C due to the combined effect of peeling and heating. They are also higher in calories, especially if they are packed in heavy syrup.

TYPES OF PEARS

While there are hundreds of varieties of pears in North America, four types predominate: Anjou, a juicy, oval-shaped winter pear that has a yellowish green skin; Bartlett, a summer pear that is eaten fresh or canned; Bosc, which has a slender neck and a firm, crunchy texture that makes it ideal for baking and poaching; and Comice, a green-skinned variety that is considered the sweetest and tastiest winter pear. ❖

PEAS AND PEA PODS

BENEFITS
- A source of vitamins C and B$_6$, folate, thiamine, and potassium.
- High in pectin and other types of fiber.
- Provide complete protein when served with grain products.

DRAWBACKS
- High in purines, which can precipitate a flare-up of gout symptoms in people with this disorder.

Throughout history the pea has been a plant of significance. It is mentioned in the Bible, and dried peas have even been found in Egyptian tombs. In more recent times pea plants provided data for Gregor Johann Mendel, the founder of modern genetics. Peas are classified as legumes, and as such, they form a complete protein when combined with grains. Fresh green peas are more convenient than dried legumes, because they do not require a long cooking time and can even be eaten raw.

Besides being high in protein, fresh green peas are a good source of pectin and other soluble fibers, which help control blood cholesterol levels. (There is no truth to the notion that eating three dried peas a day lowers blood cholesterol). The pods are high in insoluble fiber, which helps prevent constipation. Green peas are lower in calories and fat than other high-protein foods; a half-cup serving contains about 60 calories and 4 g of protein. A half-cup of cooked green peas provides about 20 percent of the Recommended Dietary Allowance (RDA) of vitamin C for women, and 10 to 15 percent of the RDAs of thiamine and folate, as well as 1 mg of iron and 215 mg of potassium.

Peas contain lutein, a plant chemical linked to lowered risk of macular degeneration, the leading cause of blindness in older adults.

The younger green peas are, the sweeter and more tender they are; very young peas can be eaten in their pods. Once picked, peas should be eaten or refrigerated, because their sugar quickly converts to starch. After shelling, green peas can be eaten raw or cooked. To minimize the loss of vitamins, peas should be cooked in as little water as possible until just tender. Cooking some of the pods with the peas or with soup stock adds flavor and nutrition; discard them before serving. Peas are also sold frozen or canned. Of the two, frozen peas are better than canned, which have fewer nutrients, added salt and sugar, and less color and flavor.

Snow, or sugar, peas are often used in Chinese stir-fried dishes and are available fresh or frozen. They are eaten in their flat pod, because they are harvested while still immature; consequently, they contain less protein than green peas. However, they are higher in vitamin C (a half cup supplies about 40 mg, or 50 percent of the RDA for women) and have slightly more iron.

Eaten in their fibrous pods, a serving of snow peas has about 35 calories per cup.

Like other legumes, peas are high in purines, which can precipitate an attack of gout in people with this disease. ❖

PEPPERS

....

BENEFITS

- An excellent low-calorie source of beta carotene and vitamin C.

Sweet peppers are related to chilies, or hot peppers. Both are native to the Western Hemisphere and were named by Spanish explorers who confused them with the unrelated peppercorn.

The four-lobed bell peppers are the most common of the sweet varieties in North America. Depending on the degree of ripeness, bell peppers range in color from green to yellow to red. Those picked while green will not become red, because peppers ripen only on the vine. Peppers grow sweeter as they ripen, which is the reason red ones are sweeter than yellow ones, which are sweeter than green ones. Other varieties of peppers include banana peppers, which derive their name from their yellow color and elongated shape; cubanelles, which are tapered, about 4 in. (10 cm) long, and range from green to red in color; and orange-red pimientos, which are heart shaped.

NUTRITIONAL VALUE

One medium pepper contains only 32 calories, but the vitamin content varies according to color. Volume for volume, peppers are a better source of vitamin C than citrus fruits. One medium green pepper provides more than 100 percent of the adult Recommended Dietary Allowance (RDA) for vitamin C, whereas red peppers provide 50 percent more of this antioxidant. In contrast, a green pepper supplies only about 45 RE (Retanol Equivalents) of beta carotene, compared to 438 RE of beta carotene in red peppers. In addition, peppers supply smaller amounts of vitamin B_6 and folate.

Deeply colored peppers are high in bioflavonoids, plant pigments that help prevent cancer; phenolic acids, which inhibit the formation of cancer-causing nitrosamines; and plant sterols, precursors of vitamin D that are believed to protect against cancer. Peppers also supply lutein and zeaxanthin, antioxidants linked to a reduced risk of macular degeneration, the leading cause of blindness in older adults.

Peppers can be steamed, roasted, or stuffed and baked, or served raw in a salad, or along with other vegetables and a delicious low-fat dip. Steaming, stir-frying, and other fast cooking methods do not significantly lower their nutritional value. ❖

PESTICIDES AND POLLUTANTS
■ HOW SAFE ARE OUR FOODS? ■

Antibiotics in the food supply

Sometimes a substance that's added to food affects human health, but only indirectly. That's the case with antibiotics given to beef cattle, pigs, poultry, and other livestock. There is little if any direct effect on people who eat the meat from these animals. But the widespread use of these antibiotics—many of which are very similar to the ones used to treat human illness—may be helping to weaken some of medicine's strongest weapons.

Antibiotics can treat bacterial infections in animals as well as humans. And many years ago agricultural scientists discovered that when healthy animals are given very small ("subtherapeutic") doses of antibiotics, they often grow faster and fatter. Unfortunately, bacteria develop resistance to those antibiotics, and that resistance is often passed on to humans. As a result, many antibiotics used in modern medicine are becoming less effective.

North American governments haven't banned subtherapeutic use of antibiotics, but McDonald's is pressuring the market to limit them. In June of 2003, they directed their chicken suppliers to stop using antibiotic growth promoters altogether, and they are encouraging beef and pork producers to do the same.

Pesticides help assure an abundant food supply, but there is some concern that their overuse may adversely affect human health and the environment. Eating a variety of foods helps minimize exposure. Certain foods, especially colorful fruits and vegetables, may boost the body's ability to detoxify potentially toxic compounds.

The remarkable productivity of modern agriculture depends to a large degree on a wide array of complex compounds synthesized by the agricultural chemicals industry. These include fertilizers and pesticides applied to crops, antibiotics and hormones given to livestock, and additives included in animal feed. In North America, the system provides an abundance of food at a very low cost.

Inevitably, though, most crops retain traces of pesticides, and animal products may contain somewhat larger amounts. Potentially harmful chemicals can enter the food supply during growing, processing, and packing. Environmental pollutants—heavy metals such as mercury, persistent toxic compounds such as PCBs and dioxins—in the air, water, and soil may also make their way into the food supply.

Just because a tiny trace is there, however, doesn't mean it's harmful. The risk to your health depends not only on the toxicity of a substance, but on the extent and type of exposure you receive. As the famed alchemist Paracelsus stated in the 16th century, "Only the dose makes the poison."

Workers exposed to pesticides during manufacture face much higher risks than people who consume foods with trace residues of the same chemicals. Similarly, pesticides that are harmful in large doses in animal tests may pose little danger to human health when consumed in tiny amounts as part of a varied and balanced diet. However, some toxic compounds persist for years in the environment, and they can become more and more concentrated as they move up the food chain, making certain foods—such as mercury-contaminated fish—a risk to human health.

Are pesticides safe?

The question is a little like asking if medicines are safe. It depends on which medication, in what dose, how it is taken, by whom it is taken, and for what reason it is taken. Two aspirin may take an adult's headache away but may result in a child contracting a disease called Reye's syndrome—and a bottle-full can kill just about anyone.

So it is with pesticides. It depends on how they are used—there is no universal guarantee of safety. After all, pesticides are designed to kill their targets, whether insects, weeds, or fungi. The best we can do is to evaluate the risks and the benefits of each substance and make appropriate judgments.

Because high doses of certain pesticides have been linked to health problems in animals, it is not surprising that North Americans are

Mercury in the food chain

Mercury, a heavy metal that enters the atmosphere primarily from coal-burning electric utilities, becomes more toxic when bacteria in lakes and oceans convert it into methylmercury, which fish then absorb into their fat tissues. The bigger a predatory fish—like swordfish—the more methylmercury it's likely to harbor.

Methylmercury is particularly toxic to pregnant women, nursing mothers, and young children. Even low-level exposure can affect the developing brain and have neurological and behavioral effects. In adults, dietary methylmercury may also increase the risk of heart disease.

Seafood is nutritious—a low-saturated-fat source of high-quality protein rich in heart-healthy omega-3 fatty acids—so public health experts are eager to determine the level of mercury in seafood that can be safely consumed. In the United States, the Food and Drug Administration (FDA) considers a safe limit to be one part per million (ppm) of methylmercury. However, the U.S. Environmental Protection Agency (EPA), which doesn't regulate food, uses a more stringent limit of 0.25 ppm, and in April 2003, the FDA's Food Advisory Committee recommended that the FDA adopt that limit. Health Canada's guidelines are in the middle: 0.5 ppm.

Based on the current FDA standard, women of childbearing age (especially if they are already pregnant) should avoid shark, swordfish, king mackerel, and tilefish, and limit themselves to 12 oz (340 g) of any other fish or seafood per week. Health Canada advises all adults to limit consumption of swordfish, shark, and fresh or frozen tuna to one meal a week—and for pregnant women, to one meal a month.

concerned that residues of them in foods we eat could cause birth defects, neurological diseases, and even cancer. Several agricultural pesticides are indeed classified as "possible" or "suspected" human carcinogens. Because there is no known threshold for carcinogens—levels at which they pose absolutely no risk—scientists believe that the greater the overall residue consumption, the higher the statistical risk of developing cancer.

Fortunately, food surveys find that North Americans actually have very low overall exposure to pesticide residues. And the level of that exposure has been declining in the last few years and will likely decline further. One reason is that newer pesticides tend to break down more quickly in the environment, often before food crops are harvested. And new agricultural approaches such as integrated pest management (IPM) can reduce pesticide use even more. IPM refers to the appropriate use of insect traps, genetically modified crops, crop rotation, natural insect predators, and more specific and powerful pesticides when needed to control pests. The small but growing market for organically grown foods also, by definition, lowers the use of synthetic pesticides.

Protecting infants, children, and women

Certain populations may be more susceptible to pesticide residues in food. Infants and children, in particular, tend to consume large amounts of single foods such as apples and bananas, and they take in more food per body weight than adults—after all, their bodies are small and they're growing rapidly. A child who eats potatoes can get, in theory, sick from pesticide residues, even if the level is safe for adults. In 1996, a U.S. law, the Food Quality Protection Act, required that pesticides be regulated to ensure that they are safe for infants and children. To date, the U.S. EPA has evaluated about a third of the more than 9,000 pesticide rules to make sure kids are protected, a process that will be completed by 2006. Similarly, Canada passed a new Pest Control Products Act in 2002, and this new legislation strengthens protection for Canadians' health—especially children—and improves the post-registration controls on pesticides. Under this modernized system, Canada's Pest Management Regulatory Agency will continue its re-evaluation of pesticides that were registered prior to 1995 to ensure that they meet current scientific standards. The target is to re-evaluate 405 older pesticide active ingredients by 2006–07. To date, 64 of these ingredients have been addressed. Still, scientists admit there are many gaps in our knowledge of how pesticides affect the growth, development, and health of children.

Another population group about which too little is known: pregnant and breast-feeding women. When women nurse their infants, studies show, they pass along small amounts of potentially toxic compounds such as PCBs (polychlorinated biphenyls) to their infants, although scientists emphasize that the many benefits of breast-feeding still far outweigh any risks.

There is also concern that certain pesticides that mimic the major female hormone estrogen can disrupt endocrine systems, damaging reproductive health. Some critics of the pesticides believe these so-called estrogen disruptors are behind a worldwide drop in sperm production. Other experts contend that the amounts in food are minute and safe.

How pesticides are regulated

In both the United States and Canada, pesticides are among the most strictly regulated chemical products. Federal agencies, along with state and provincial counterparts, monitor the levels of pesticides in animals, people, and the environment. They approve them only if the levels of residues in the resulting food crops are a fraction of the level—as little as one one-hundredth—that is safe for laboratory animals.

Before a pesticide is officially "registered," scientists must agree that its risk profile is acceptable. It must be tested for the potential to cause cancer, birth defects, hormonal changes, and damage to the nervous system, as well as for possible effects on children, pregnant women, seniors, pesticide applicators, and agricultural workers. As new science emerges, risk assessments are refined. It's a slow, cumbersome process—it can take decades to get a pesticide off the market—but as a result, pesticides, such as methyl parathion and chlorpyrifos, have been severely restricted. In the light of current knowledge, today's pesticides have a positive risk-benefit ratio.

Does that mean that we know that all the pesticides and other chemicals used in agriculture have no health consequences for food consumers? Absolutely not. There may be subtle effects in humans that show up only after years of exposure and may never be linked to pesticides. The cumulative effects of the many different pesticides in our food supply may combine to do more damage than we can know from studying them individually. Regulations in many foreign countries are less strict than in North America, too. While imported produce is supposed to meet the same safety requirements as domestic products, only a minority of these food products are tested. Still, studies show that pesticide levels in imported produce tend to be quite low, too—often lower than in North American foods.

Levels of mercury in seafood

If we accept a standard of 0.25 ppm of mercury in our food supply, even tuna might look iffy. (White tuna averages 0.32 ppm.) In any case, it makes sense to choose seafood sources that are lowest in mercury. Among the lowest in mercury are catfish, flounder, salmon, shrimp, haddock, pollock (used in frozen fish products), sardines, crab, and scallops. When choosing canned tuna, select "light" over "white" varieties. If you fish, check local advisories. Trim the fat from swordfish and other high-fat predator fish. Here is how some popular seafoods stack up:

Seafood	Mean levels of mercury (parts per million)
Tilefish	1.45 ppm
Swordfish	1.00 ppm
Shark	0.96 ppm
King mackerel	0.73 ppm
Tuna (fresh or frozen)	0.32 ppm
Lobster	0.31 ppm
Grouper	0.27 ppm
Halibut	0.23 ppm
Pollock	0.20 ppm
Tuna (canned)	0.17 ppm
Catfish	0.07 ppm
Scallop	0.05 ppm

Source: United States Food and Drug Administration (FDA database FY 85–99)

What you can do to lower your risk

Eating a well-balanced diet rich in fruits and vegetables protects against possible risks from agricultural residues. It's true that the fruits and vegetables themselves may contain pesticide residues, but scientists agree that the protection offered by the beneficial compounds in these foods greatly outweighs the risks posed by the residues. And remember that for contaminants we can't avoid, our bodies are remarkably well equipped with preventive mechanisms to detoxify them.

Here are five ways to minimize your risk:

1. Eat a wide variety of foods. Doing so helps protect you from overeating any one type of food that may have high levels of pollutants or pesticides.

2. Trim the animal fat. Whether a contaminant is harmful or not depends on how long it lingers in the body or the environment. A substance that resists chemical or biological breakdown accumulates as it is ingested by one species after another, steadily building up as the food chain progresses from small, weak species to the large and dominant. The highest levels of pollutants, therefore, are ingested by large animals. Many of these persistent pollutants are stored in an animal's fat, which is why choosing lower-fat foods and trimming fat from meat can help to reduce the amount of pollutants you consume.

3. Consider buying organically grown foods. You may want to purchase just those foods, such as apples and potatoes, that tend to have the highest pesticide residues. (See Organic Foods.)

4. Eat plenty of fresh fruits and vegetables, whole grains, nuts, and seeds. They're rich in fiber and antioxidants that may help protect the body from carcinogens.

5. Eat your broccoli . . . and cauliflower, cabbage, watercress, and brussels sprouts. They contain compounds that release isothiocyanates, which in turn stimulate the liver to produce enzymes that can detoxify carcinogens before they can cause harm. Phenolic compounds (in apples and other fruits) and bioflavonoids (high in citrus fruits) protect in similar ways.

Other elements of a healthy diet may help counter any carcinogenic pesticide residues. The same omega-3 fatty acids that help to prevent heart disease suppress tumor development. Sulfur compounds in onions and garlic may also have cancer-protective activities—they bind to carcinogens, neutralizing them. And calcium, abundant in dairy products as well as in dark green leafy vegetables, may help guard against colon cancer.

A low-fat diet that provides ample vegetables and fruits will be naturally rich in detoxifying compounds. But many other factors, such as heredity, lifestyle, and exposure to environmental pollutants, affect your susceptibility to disease. Our food supply has low and declining levels of pesticide residues, but there are always risks, and a healthy lifestyle is the best protection.

PICKLES AND OTHER CONDIMENTS

BENEFITS
- Sauerkraut is a good source of vitamin C, iron, potassium, and other nutrients.
- Pickles are low-calorie snacks.

DRAWBACKS
- Most pickles and condiments are extremely high in sodium.
- Sweet pickles, ketchups, and chutneys are high in sugar.
- In large amounts, pickled foods may increase the risk of cancer.

Pickling was once essential for keeping sufficient food stores over the winter. Long before vitamin C and other essential nutrients were identified, sauerkraut—pickled cabbage—was used to prevent scurvy during extended sea voyages. Today, however, popular pickled foods are consumed mostly for their taste.

In pickling, food is preserved by saturating it with acid, which prevents most microorganisms from growing. Two basic methods are used: soaking in acid, usually a vinegar-based solution; and brining, a fermentation process that takes place through the action of acid-producing bacteria.

In the first method, vegetables are presoaked in brine to draw off moisture that would dilute the vinegar. They are then sealed in jars to mature, usually with pickling spices. This method is used for sweet and sour pickles. Chutney and ketchup are cooked, pulped variations on the basic vinegar pickle. Bacteria rarely grow in these mixtures, but molds and yeasts may flourish on imperfectly sealed surfaces.

Fermented pickles, such as dill pickles, are vegetables that are immersed in a brine that is strong enough to inhibit the growth of unwanted bacteria but mild enough to nourish several species that produce lactic acid. This and other compounds contribute to the characteristic flavor. (Dill pickles are also flavored with dill seeds and fronds.) No bacteria are inoculated into the brine; instead, they are attracted to the mixture from the surrounding air.

Fermented pickles are more difficult to make than vinegar pickles because, given the wrong temperature or salt concentration, hostile bacteria will thrive and make them unpalatable.

SAUERKRAUT
One of the few pickled dishes served as a vegetable, sauerkraut has only 20 calories in a half-cup serving. It provides 17 mg of vitamin C, almost 2 mg of iron, and useful amounts of the B vitamins, calcium, potassium, and fiber. Sauerkraut is high in sodium (800 mg per half cup), and the salt content may be increased by foods often served with it, such as frankfurters.

KETCHUP AND OTHER SAUCES
Most ketchup is made from tomatoes, although plums and other soft fruits, and even green walnuts, can be used. The huge variety of commercial barbecue sauces are variants on the basic ketchup recipe of tomatoes, brown sugar, vinegar, salt, pepper, and spices. These sauces are condiments, with negligible nutritional value, although tomato ketchup does contain a fair amount of the antioxidant lycopene. The high salt content in most may be harmful to people with high blood pressure or on a low-salt diet.

Soy sauce, basic to Asian cooking, is very high in sodium—1,000 mg per tablespoon compared with 200 mg in mustard and ketchup.

Mustard is a spice obtained from the seeds of a plant in the cabbage family. Its pungent smell and flavor develop only after the seed is crushed and moistened, allowing enzymes to react with isothiocyanates to form mustard oils. Most mustards are sold premixed, and many specialty varieties, which are mixed with white wine or herb-flavored vinegars, are marketed both as fine pastes and as coarser blends that contain unground seeds. The addition of turmeric gives some types their brilliant yellow color and extra tanginess. In making prepared mustard, the dry powder is usually blended with wheat flour to improve its mixing qualities; people with celiac disease, who are gluten sensitive, should look for mustards that don't contain wheat.

CANCER RISK
A diet that is high in pickled or salt-cured foods and condiments has been linked to an increased risk of stomach and

esophageal cancers. This is thought to stem from their high levels of nitrates, which are converted to cancer-causing nitrosamines during digestion. Nitrates are often used in the pickling solution to impart flavor and prevent the growth of undesirable microorganisms. Vitamins A and C, beta carotene, and other antioxidants are thought to inhibit the cancer-causing potential of nitrosamines; eating ample fresh vegetables and fruits may counteract any risk from pickled foods. ❖

PINEAPPLES

BENEFITS

- A good source of vitamin C, with useful amounts of vitamin B$_6$, folate, thiamine, iron, and manganese.

DRAWBACKS

- May cause dermatitis in individuals sensitive to bromelain, an enzyme in pineapple juice.

Native to South America, pineapples are now grown in tropical areas worldwide. They are available in frozen and dried forms, but the majority of the crop is reserved for canned varieties, juices, or fresh fruit. Although pineapples are available year-round, their peak season takes place during June and July.

The sweet and tangy flavor makes fresh pineapple a delicious choice; it can be added to fruit salads and grilled or baked with sea-food, ham, poultry, or other meats. As pineapple is cooked, its texture softens due to the breakdown of cellulose, a type of fiber in its walls.

HEALING PROPERTIES

Fresh pineapple contains bromelain, an enzyme that is similar to the papain in papayas that dissolves proteins. Consequently, fresh pineapple is a natural meat and poultry tenderizer when it is added to stews or marinades. If pineapple is to be used in a gelatin mold, however, the fruit should be canned or boiled beforehand in order to deactivate the bromelain; otherwise, the gelatin (a form of protein) will not set properly and will become soupy.

Bromelain is an anti-inflammatory enzyme, and preliminary research

DID YOU KNOW?

PINEAPPLE CONTAINS AN ANTI-INFLAMMATORY ENZYME

Pineapple contains bromelain, which some claim helps control inflammation associated with arthritis and many other conditions. Preliminary research suggests that bromelain's anti-inflammatory property may also reduce blood clots, which may lower the risk for heart attack and stroke.

suggests that it may reduce the risk of blood clots, thereby lowering the risk for heart attack and stroke. This is difficult to explain, since bromelain is a protein and such proteins are readily broken down in the digestive tract. Topically applied, bromelain may help control tissue swelling and inflammation associated with arthritis, strains, and sprains, but it can also cause skin irritation or allergic dermatitis in susceptible people.

One cup of fresh pineapple chunks contains 75 calories and provides 25 mg of vitamin C. It also offers useful amounts of other nutrients, including 0.17 mg of thiamine, 16 mcg (micrograms) of folate, 0.15 mg of vitamin B$_6$, 0.6 mg of iron, and 2.6 mg of manganese. Pineapple is high in soluble fiber, which helps in controlling high blood cholesterol. Pineapple is a good source of ferulic acid, a plant chemical that helps prevent the formation of cancer-causing substances.

Canning does not significantly lower pineapple's vitamin C; a cup of juice-packed fruit retains all of its vitamin C, while a cup packed in heavy syrup provides about 20 mg. However, canning heats the fruit enough to destroy its bromelain, so such products can be used to make gelatin-type desserts. Pineapple is often canned in syrup, which can add calories. A cup of juice-packed chunks contains 150 calories, compared to 200 in a cup packed in heavy syrup.

After picking, a pineapple will not ripen further. When buying a pineapple, look for one that exudes a fragrant odor and has light yellow or white flesh. Brown patches indicate spoilage. If you are buying the fruit whole, make sure that it seems dense and heavy for its size and that the leaves are green. ❖

PIZZA

See Fast Foods

PLUMS

BENEFITS

- A useful source of vitamin C and potassium.

DRAWBACKS

- May cause allergic reactions in susceptible people.

Whether they are eaten whole, added to fruit salads, baked goods, compotes, puddings, or meat dishes, or made into butters, jams, purees, or sauces, plums are a nutritious low-calorie food. One medium-size fresh plum contains only 36 calories and is a good source of such dietary fibers as cellulose and pectin. It also supplies useful amounts of several nutrients, including 6 mg of vitamin C and 113 mg of potassium. Canned plums contain comparable amounts of riboflavin and potassium but are significantly lower in vitamin C (one canned plum provides only 1 mg). Fruits canned in heavy syrup are higher in calories than fresh—for example, one canned plum packed in a sugary syrup yields 60 calories. In their dried form some plums become prunes, which are a more concentrated source of calories and nutrients.

Plums contain anthocyanins, the reddish blue pigments that lend them their intense color. These antioxidant pigments may help protect against cancer and heart disease by mopping up free radicals, unstable molecules that damage cells.

VARIETIES OF PLUMS

More than 140 varieties of plums are available in North America—the season extends from May to October—so it's not surprising that they vary in shape, color, and flavor. Despite this wide array of choice, there are five main types:

American plums. These include the DeSoto, Golden Beauty, and Pottawattomi varieties. These native plums are available locally, but they generally are not produced commercially.

Damson plums. They have dark flesh and skins, and resemble European plums but are slightly smaller in size and more tart in flavor. They are often used to make jams and preserves.

European plums. These are also referred to as common plums, have blue or purple skins and a golden yellow flesh. These plums are denser, smaller, and less juicy than the Japanese varieties. Some varieties are sold fresh, others are dried. The ones that are more tart in flavor are ideal for cooking or making preserves.

Japanese plums. These are consumed fresh, cooked, or canned, but they are never dried to make prunes. Most have a juicy reddish or yellow flesh and skin ranging from deep crimson to black-red.

Ornamental plums. These are used mostly for jellies and jams.

Fresh plums do not ripen after they have been picked; before buying one, look for brightly colored fruit that yields slightly to the touch. Color, which varies from one variety to another, may not be a good indicator of ripeness. Overripe plums tend to be soft, with a bruised or discolored skin, and they are sometimes leaky. Firm plums can be stored for a day or two at room temperature to soften them.

Plums may produce an allergic reaction in individuals with confirmed allergies to apricots, almonds, peaches, and cherries, which come from the same family. Similarly, people who are allergic to aspirin may also encounter problems after they have eaten plums. In addition, like peaches and apricots, the pits of plums contain amygdalin, a compound that breaks down into hydrogen cyanide in the stomach, and can cause cyanide poisoning if consumed in large amounts. ❖

POMEGRANATES

BENEFITS

- A good source of fiber, vitamin C, and niacin.
- Rich in plant chemicals.

The word pomegranate is old French for "seeded apple," a fitting name for this apple-sized fruit filled with jewel-like clusters of red seeds. There are many types of pomegranates cultivated around the world. One of the most popular in North America is called Wonderful. It is perhaps the best pomegranate for juicing. The fruit is available from fall to early winter.

Pomegranates have a leathery, deep red to purplish rind. The interior is bursting with hundred of tiny, edible seeds packed into compartments called arils and separated by bitter, cream-colored membranes. The fruit can be eaten out of hand by deeply scoring vertically and then breaking it apart. The clusters of juice sacs are then lifted out and eaten.

Pomegranate fruits are most often consumed as juice and can be juiced in several ways. The sacs can be removed and put through a basket press or the juice can be extracted by reaming the halved fruits on an ordinary juice squeezer.

Another approach is to make a cut in the stem end and place it over a glass to let the juice run out, squeezing the fruit from time to time. One fruit yields about ⅓ cup of juice. The juice can be used to make jellies, sorbets, or sauces, as well as to flavor cakes and baked apples.

Pomegranates are a good source of potassium. One fruit contains about 400 mg, more than in most oranges. They also contain vitamin C and fiber. Pomegranates and their juice are rich in anthocyanins and ellagic acid, both of which have antioxidant properties. Research has shown that pomegranate juice has two to three times the antioxidant capacity of equal amounts of red wine or green tea, and anthocyanins make an important contribution to the pomegranate's antioxidant power. A recent study suggests that drinking as little as one-quarter cup of pomegranate juice daily may improve cardiovascular health by significantly reducing oxidation of LDL cholesterol. ❖

PORK

BENEFITS

- Fresh, lean pork is a good source of high-quality protein, B vitamins, and zinc.

DRAWBACKS

- Ham, bacon, and other cured pork products are high in salt and may also be high in fat.

Thrifty cooks used to boast that when it came to pigs, they could use everything but the squeal. A pig yields chops and other cuts of fresh meat; cured or processed products, such as ham and bacon; and skin for gelatin.

Globally, pork continues to be the world's most eaten meat, with consumption continuing to grow. The latest data shows that of the world's meat consumption, 41 percent is pork (versus 29 percent poultry and 25 percent beef). Over the last 20 years, the volume of pork consumption has increased by 73 percent worldwide. The hog industry is involved in activities that serve to protect its excellent swine herd health status. These include traceability initia-tives as well as quality assurance programs that include protocols for barn sanitation, feed mixing, medication use, and injection techniques.

Although some pork products are high in saturated fat, trimmed, lean pork is close to skinless poultry in its fat and calorie content. A 3-oz (85-g) serving of lean roast pork has 185 calories, with substantial amounts of high-quality protein and the B vitamins thiamine, riboflavin, niacin, B_6, and B_{12}; it also has about 45 percent of the Recommended Dietary Allowance (RDA) of thiamine, 25 percent of the RDA for niacin, and 20 percent of the RDA for B_{12}. Lean pork provides important minerals such as phosphorus, magnesium, iron, and zinc. About half the iron in pork is heme iron, the most readily absorbed and digested type of dietary iron. The tenderloin, center-cut leg, and loin chops are the most lean. Pork cooked to an internal temperature of 160°F (70°C)—or medium doneness—will remain moist and tender. This temperature also ensures the destruction of the parasites that cause trichinosis.

While pork has a higher proportion of unsaturated fats than other meats, its cholesterol content is also higher: 75 mg in a 3-oz (85-g) pork chop and 100 mg in 3 oz (85 g) of spare ribs. The role of dietary cholesterol is still unclear; recent studies indicate it has less effect on blood cholesterol than saturated fats do. Still, some experts recommend limiting dietary cholesterol intake to 300 mg a day. Salt-cured pork products are high in sodium.

Some pork products such as sausages and bacon are also high in fat and should be eaten in moderation. Two slices of pork bacon, for instance, contain 6 g of fat, 2.2 of them from saturated fat, and 73 calories. Two slices of turkey bacon contain 5 g of fat, 2 g of it saturated, and 70 calories. Bacon also contains nitrates, which can lead to the formation of carcinogenic nitrosamines. (See Smoked, Cured, and Pickled Meats.) ❖

DID YOU KNOW?

MODERATE PORK CONSUMPTION MAY NOT RAISE CHOLESTEROL LEVELS

Although pork is high in saturated fat, about 30 percent of that fat comes from stearic acid, a type of saturated fat that does not appear to have the same heart-damaging effects of most saturated fat. In fact, some studies suggest it can actually lower cholesterol.

POTATOES

BENEFITS
- A good source of vitamins C and B$_6$, and potassium and other minerals.
- An inexpensive, filling, and nutritious starchy food.
- The skin is a good source of fiber.

DRAWBACKS
- Green and sprouted potatoes may contain solanine, a potentially toxic substance.

Although they are often associated with Ireland, potatoes are native to the Andes Mountains and were first cultivated by Peruvian Indians at least 4,000 years ago. Spanish explorers introduced potatoes to Europe in the 1500s, where they became a staple food source for the poor. Potatoes are now cultivated worldwide; in fact, they are the world's largest and most economically important vegetable crop. For most North Americans, potatoes are a major component of the diet—usually in processed forms that are high in fat and salt.

There are many varieties of potato, but yams and sweet potatoes are not among them; they are not even related to the white potato, which is a member of the nightshade family, and is related to peppers and tomatoes.

Potatoes are surprisingly nutritious and low in calories. When eaten with the skin, they are high in complex carbohydrates and fiber; one medium-size baked potato (with the skin) provides 25 mg of vitamin C, which is more than 25 percent of the adult Recommended Dietary Allowance (RDA), along with a good supply of vitamin B$_6$, thiamine, niacin, and magnesium, 800 mg of potassium, and a moderate amount of zinc. The skins are rich in chlorogenic acid, a phytochemical that has anti-cancer properties.

Potatoes have a relatively high glycemic index (GI), which may be an issue for diabetics or people trying to lose weight by following a low-GI diet. The way a potato is prepared plays a large role in determining its GI; a boiled potato has a GI of 58; a baked potato has a GI of 60; and a mashed potato's GI is 74. New potatoes are digested more slowly than mature white potatoes or Russets.

Many people think potatoes are fattening, but this is true only when they are fried or served with butter and rich sauces. A medium-size baked or boiled potato has between 120 and 150 calories, a small amount of protein, and almost no fat. The same potato turned into potato chips has 450 to 500 calories and up to 35 g of fat; 4 oz (115 g) of French fries contain about 300 calories and 15 to 20 g of fat. One-half cup of mashed potatoes with milk provides about 120 calories, compared to 355 calories in a cup of scalloped and au gratin potatoes. French fries and other processed potatoes are almost always high in salt.

When preparing potatoes, it is best not to remove the skin because the fiber is in the skin and many of the nutrients are near the surface; instead, scrub them under water with a vegetable brush. If you do peel them, try to remove as thin a layer as possible. Once sliced or peeled, raw potatoes will discolor when exposed to oxygen, so cook them immediately or place them in water with vinegar or lemon juice added. Baking, steaming, or microwaving preserves the maximum amount of nutrients. Pierce a potato's skin with a fork before baking or microwaving to avoid having it explode. If

DO ONE SIMPLE THING

EAT MORE SWEET POTATOES
Sweet potatoes are higher in fiber and nutrients and have a lower glycemic index than white potatoes. These roots may help to prevent cancer, macular degeneration, and heart disease.

WHY POTATOES SOMETIMES TURN BLACK
Potatoes contain small amounts of iron from the soil, in an ionic form known as ferrous iron. When a potato is cut, or cooked, the ferrous ion reacts with oxygen and converts to a form called ferric iron. The ferric iron-chlorogenic acid complex is black. This can often be seen as harmless black-blue spots in cooked potatoes.

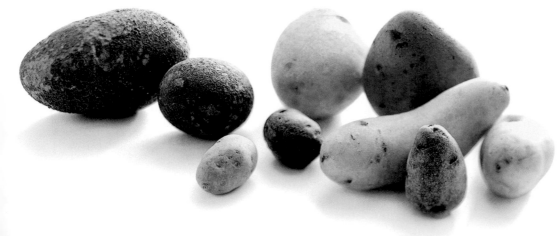

MANY SHAPES, SIZES, AND COLORS. *Just a few of the hundreds of varieties of potatoes grown worldwide.*

you boil potatoes, leave the skin on, use as little water as possible, and cook in a covered pot. Some nutrients, particularly vitamin C, are lost during boiling. To salvage some lost nutrients, add the potato water to soups or stews.

When shopping, look for potatoes with few eyes and no black spots. Avoid those with a green tint to the skin, and remove any sprouts; they will taste bitter and may contain solanine, a toxic substance that can cause diarrhea, cramps, and fatigue.

Store potatoes in a dark, cool place, but not in the refrigerator. Temperatures below 45°F (7°C) convert the starch to sugar, giving the potato a strange taste. Don't store potatoes and onions together; the acids in onions aid the decomposition of potatoes, and vice versa. ❖

POULTRY

BENEFITS
- An excellent source of protein.
- A good source of vitamin A, the B vitamins, and minerals.

DRAWBACKS
- Susceptible to bacterial contamination.

Higher in protein and lower in saturated fat than red meats, poultry—including chicken, turkey, Rock Cornish game hen, duck, goose, guinea fowl, squab, pheasant, and quail—is an excellent source of high-quality protein, with all the essential amino acids, as well as calcium, copper, iron, phosphorus, potassium, and zinc.

All poultry has a similar range of nutrients; the main difference, apart from flavor, is in the fat content. A 3-oz (85-g) portion of roasted, skinless light turkey is the lowest in calories and fat, with 135 calories, 3 g of fat, and 25 g of protein, compared to 170 calories, 9 g of fat, and 20 g of protein in a comparable portion of skinless roasted duck. A 3-oz (85-g) serving of roasted chicken breast without skin has 26 g of protein, 142 calories, and 3 g of fat compared to the same serving with skin at 195 calories and 8 g of fat.

Most poultry fat is under the skin; removing the skin before eating the meat greatly reduces fat content. The fattiness of duck can be reduced by pricking the skin all over

POULTRY DONENESS CHART	
	Temperature
● Whole chicken (stuffed or unstuffed)	180°F (82°C)
● Chicken pieces	170°F (77°C)
● Whole turkey (stuffed)	180°F (82°C)
● Whole turkey (unstuffed)	170°F (77°C)
● Turkey pieces	170°F (77°C)
● Ground chicken or turkey	175°F (80°C)

before roasting it to allow the fat to drain off. You can roast, broil, or grill poultry with the skin on to preserve moisture, but it's best to remove it before eating.

Poultry meat is a good source of vitamin A and many B vitamins. Chicken and duck contain the same amounts of cholesterol—75 mg in a 3-oz (85-g) portion of skinless roasted meat—whereas a similar serving of turkey contains 60 mg.

Duck and dark-meat turkey are good sources of heme iron, the most absorbable form of this important mineral. A 3-oz (85-g) serving of cooked skinless chicken breast supplies nearly 12 mg of niacin, over half of the Recommended Dietary Allowance (RDA). Duck and turkey are also excellent sources of this vitamin, which is important for energy metabolism, healthy skin, and healthy digestive and nervous systems. Dark turkey is particularly high in selenium. A 3-oz (85-g) serving contains 35 mcg or more than 50 percent of the RDA. Poultry contains tryptophan, an essential amino acid that may help ease depression and insomnia. Though all poultry has vitamin B_6, light-meat chicken and turkey are the best sources with 3 oz (85 g) providing 0.5 mg or 40 percent of the RDA. Turkey, duck and dark-meat chicken also provide generous amounts of zinc.

Dark poultry meat comes from muscles that get more exercise. That's why drumsticks are darker than breast meat, and why game birds, which spend much of their life on the wing, often have breast meat that is dark.

POULTRY SAFETY

Because most poultry is sold with its skin intact, it is susceptible to spoilage from bacteria that remain on the skin and in the cavity after processing. Kept at 40°F (4°C), the average refrigerator temperature, chicken skin will become slimy in about 6 days, indicating a 10,000-fold increase in bacteria. All raw poultry should be washed under running water. You should wash your hands often during preparation, and scrub knives and cutting boards in hot, soapy water.

Poultry is thoroughly cooked when the leg joints move easily and the juices run clear if the thigh is pierced with a knife. Chickens that come with plastic meat thermometers often require an additional 10 or 15 minutes of roasting after the thermometer pops up to get rid of bloody streaks around the joints. The best way to judge doneness is to use a meat thermometer. Put the thermometer into the breast of a whole chicken, thigh of a whole turkey, or into the thickest part of cut-up poultry. Stuffing in poultry or cooked separately should reach 165°F (74°C) before serving.

Never refrigerate a stuffed bird before cooking it. Stuffed poultry should be cooked at 325°F (160°C); lower temperatures may allow bacteria in the stuffing to multiply, while higher temperatures may cook the meat but leave the stuffing undone. Use the leftovers within a day or two, or freeze them.

Packaged poultry is seldom wrapped appropriately for freezing. Wrap meat tightly in plastic or freezer paper. Freezing promotes oxidation of unsaturated fats, which causes a rancid taste and limits freezer life of raw poultry to a few months. Thaw poultry in the refrigerator, allowing 12 to 15 hours per pound (26–33 hours per kilogram). ❖

PREGNANCY

CONSUME PLENTY OF
- Lean meat, poultry, fish, dried beans, lentils, and eggs for protein and iron.
- Milk and dairy products, canned sardines and salmon (with bones included), and other high-calcium foods.
- Citrus fruits, dark green vegetables, legumes, whole grains, and fortified cereals for folate.

LIMIT
- High-fat foods.
- Sugary desserts and candy.
- Coffee and other caffeinated drinks.

AVOID
- Alcohol use and smoking.
- All drugs unless prescribed by a doctor.

At no other time in a woman's life is good nutrition more essential than during pregnancy. While the need for calories increases only about 15 percent, the requirements for some nutrients more than doubles, and a woman needs to plan her diet carefully to meet these needs. She should work with her doctor or other health professional providing prenatal care to design an eating program that supplies optimal nutrition for her and her baby. Any woman planning a pregnancy should also evaluate her eating habits. Even before trying to conceive, she should eat well to achieve ideal nutritional status as well as a healthy weight. Women who are too thin often have low-birth-weight babies, while those who are overweight have a greater risk of gestational diabetes and giving birth to an oversized baby. Infants who are either too small or too large at birth often suffer serious problems, including respiratory disorders.

This is also the time to abstain from alcohol consumption, because alcohol causes the most harm to a fetus during the first few weeks of a pregnancy, and the woman may not know that she has conceived. Studies show that women who have one to two drinks a day tend to have undersized babies. A greater danger is incurred by alcoholics during early pregnancy; these women have a high risk of giving birth to a baby with fetal alcohol syndrome, a constellation of congenital defects that may include mental deficiency, facial and heart malformations, an undersized head, and retarded growth.

The use of vitamin supplements also should be evaluated. In particular, high doses of vitamin A should be stopped several months before attempting pregnancy, because large stores of this vitamin can cause severe birth defects. Women planning a pregnancy are encouraged to take 400 mcg (micrograms) of synthetic folic acid daily from fortified foods and/or a supplement.

NUTRITIONAL GUIDANCE
During pregnancy, the recommended weight gain for a woman of average weight experiencing an average pregnancy is approximately 25 to 35 lb (11–16 kg). Women who are underweight at conception may need to gain as much as 40 lb (18 kg), however, and women who are overweight may be advised to gain no more than 15 to 25 lb (6.8–11 kg). Obese woman should not try to lose weight during pregnancy; to do so exposes her fetus to numerous hazards.

FOOD CRAVINGS

From pickles to ice cream, stories abound about the food cravings of pregnant women. The cravings are certainly real, but they rarely reflect any true nutritional problem. The one exception is craving ice, which may be a sign of iron-deficiency anemia. Some women, however, inexplicably develop pica, a craving for bizarre, inedible substances, such as clay, soil, paint, coffee grounds, and laundry starch. Some studies have linked such cravings to iron deficiency, even though in reality, eating soil, clay, or starch lowers iron absorption.

will certainly gain excessive weight. Appropriate foods that add up to 300 extra calories include 2½ cups of low-fat milk; a sandwich made with 3 oz (85 g) of lean chicken; or an egg and two slices of toast.

Protein. A pregnant woman needs to consume an extra 25 g of protein daily—the amount found in 1½ cups of milk (12 g of protein) and 2 oz (60 g) of cooked meat (14 g of protein). Because North Americans tend to eat more protein than necessary, no specific effort to increase protein consumption should be made during pregnancy. Some studies suggest that excessive protein may be detrimental to the fetus, causing delayed growth or premature birth.

When selecting protein-rich foods, include lean meats, poultry, and fish, which are also good sources of B vitamins and iron and other trace minerals. Other foods high in protein include eggs, cheese, and a combination of grains and legumes. Lacto-ovo vegetarians can obtain protein from milk and eggs; vegans, who eat only plant foods, should consult a dietitian on how to plan an adequate diet.

Vitamin supplements. Experts agree that women should take folate and iron supplements during pregnancy, but there are differing views about whether other supplements are necessary. Many doctors believe that a balanced diet that includes a variety of foods in the recommended amounts will meet most needs, while others prescribe a multivitamin supplement as added insurance against deficiencies.

Calcium. A pregnant woman needs 1,000 mg of calcium a day. Because many North American women do not get enough calcium, it's a good idea to increase consumption of calcium-rich foods before becoming pregnant. This is especially important for women under 30, whose bones are still increasing in density. Low-fat milk and dairy products are the best dietary sources of calcium; other good sources include fortified soy and rice beverages, tofu, canned sardines and salmon with the bones included, nuts and seeds, and leafy green vegetables. One cup of milk has about 300 mg of calcium per day—almost a third of the way toward the recommended 1,000 mg. One ounce (30 g) of cheddar cheese contains

The pattern of weight gain is just as important as the amount gained. It is normal for most women to gain no weight during the first trimester. After that, a healthy woman at ideal weight before conceiving should gain an average of 1 lb (0.45 kg) a week; underweight women should gain slightly more each week; overweight women should gain more slowly.

Most women need to add approximately 300 calories to their daily diet to support normal fetal growth, especially during the last two trimesters. This is a relatively small amount, despite the saying about "eating for two." A woman who doubles what she normally eats

EATING FOR TWO. *Being pregnant should not mean eating double portions; however, a healthful balance of nutritious food will help the baby get off to a good start.*

204 mg, 1 oz (30 g) of low-fat mozzarella contains 207 mg, and ½ cup of yogurt contains about 230 mg. If you're not a milk drinker, you can get about the same amount of calcium as a cup of milk from one cup of fortified soy or rice beverage, 2 cups of baked beans, 4 oz (115 g) of canned salmon, with the bones, 7 sardines, 3 cups of cooked broccoli, ⅔ cup of tofu, ¾ cup of almonds, or 2¼ cups of soy beans. Calcium is also present in kale, Swiss chard, and other greens. If a doctor recommends calcium supplements, they should be consumed with meals to increase absorption and reduce intestinal upsets.

Iron. A woman's iron requirement almost doubles during pregnancy, going from 18 mg to 27 mg daily. This is because the woman's blood volume doubles and because the fetus must store enough iron to last through the first few months of life. Iron-rich foods include red meat, fish, poultry, enriched breads and cereals, legumes, eggs, dried fruits, and leafy green vegetables. However, the heme iron in animal products is absorbed more efficiently than the nonheme iron in plants and eggs. Absorption of nonheme iron can be increased by eating the iron-rich food together with one that is high in vitamin C, such as orange juice.

Even a well-balanced diet provides only about 12 mg to 15 mg of iron a day, and if a woman's iron stores are low when pregnancy begins, she risks developing anemia. Most women need to take an iron supplement during pregnancy. These supplements are absorbed best if they are taken between meals with liquids other than coffee, tea, and milk, which decrease the absorption of iron.

Folate. Adequate folate, or folic acid, can help prevent birth defects, especially those involving the brain and spinal cord, such as spina bifida—a condition in which the spine does not form normally. It is estimated that 50 to 70 percent of such defects could be prevented if all women of childbearing age consumed folate. The Recommended Dietary Allowance (RDA) calls for 400 mcg (micrograms) of folate for women who are not pregnant; this increases to 600 mcg during pregnancy and then changes to 500 mcg during breast-feeding.

Many women, particularly those who have been taking birth control pills, have low levels of folate. Because the most critical period for folate consumption is during the first 4 to 6 weeks of pregnancy, when the fetal central nervous system is being formed, women planning to become pregnant are generally advised by their doctors to take a supplement before conceiving. Good dietary sources include green leafy vegetables, orange juice, lentils, peas, beans, asparagus, liver, fortified flour, and pasta.

Sodium. In the past, pregnant women were routinely advised to cut down on salt because it was thought to increase the risk of toxemia, a potentially life-threatening condition. There is no evidence, however, that salt restriction prevents or alleviates toxemia; on the contrary, a woman's sodium requirement actually increases during pregnancy. In most cases, though, it is not necessary to consume additional salt.

Artificial sweeteners. Controversy has swirled around the use of artificial sweeteners. Extensive studies on aspartame suggest that it is safe to use during pregnancy, unless the woman has phenylketonuria (PKU). Saccharin can cross the placenta, but there is no proof that it harms the fetus. Acesulfame-K and sucralose pass through the digestive tract and are excreted unchanged, and no toxic effect has been shown. Most experts believe that sweeteners used moderately are not harmful during pregnancy. (See Artificial Sweeteners.)

Caffeine. A recent study found an increased risk of spontaneous abortion and low birth weight in pregnant women who consumed more than 150 mg of caffeine per day. Some evidence suggest high levels of caffeine may delay conception. And yet other studies have failed to find any association between caffeine consumption and birth defects or premature birth. Since adverse effects on pregnancy outcomes have been linked to high caffeine intake, a position paper from the American Dietetic Association states that it would be prudent to limit caffeine intake to under 300 mg per day. One cup of filter drip coffee has about 200 mg of caffeine and 1 cup of black tea has about 100 mg.

Mercury is an established environmental pollutant with known toxicity in humans. Pregnant women and women who may become pregnant should avoid king mackerel, tilefish, shark, swordfish, and fresh tuna. (See Pesticides and Pollutants.) ❖

CAUTION

Food safety is an important consideration during pregnancy. For example, foods contaminated by *Listeria monocytogenes,* bacteria which are widespread in our environment, can cause listeriosis, which is especially dangerous for pregnant women and may even cause abortion. To prevent listeriosis, the following steps should be taken: Avoid hot dogs, luncheon or deli meats unless they are reheated until steaming hot; avoid soft cheeses such as feta, Brie, and Camembert, blue-veined cheeses, and Mexican-style cheeses such as "queso blanco fresco" (hard cheese, semi-soft cheeses such as mozzarella, pasteurized processed cheese slices, and cottage and cream cheese can be safely consumed); avoid pâté or meat spreads, smoked seafood unless it is an ingredient in a cooked dish; do not drink raw or unpasteurized milk or eat foods that contain unpasteurized milk. It is also wise to avoid raw meats, raw fish (e.g. sushi), raw poultry or eggs, as well as unpasteurized cider.

PROBIOTICS
■ BENEFICIAL BACTERIA ■

The term probiotic means "for life." Probiotics are organisms that contribute to the health and balance of the intestinal tract and are commonly referred to as the "friendly," "beneficial," or "good" bacteria, which when ingested act to maintain a healthy intestinal tract and help fight disease.

The concept of probiotics is in contrast to antibiotics, which are compounds that suppress or destroy bacteria. Probiotics combat "bad" bacteria and also help maintain the health of the cells that line the gastrointestinal tract. There are many different probiotics with *Lactobacillus acidophilus*, *L. rhamnosus* GG, and bifidobacteria, among those more commonly studied.

Probiotics have a number of modes of activity, including affecting inflammatory processes, secreting compounds that regulate cell function, and protecting the intestine against invasive "bad" bacteria. They inhibit the growth of disease-causing bacteria by preventing their attachment to the intestine and by producing substances that suppress their growth.

A large body of scientific research has examined the role of probiotics in the treatment of gastrointestinal diseases such as diarrhea; inflammatory bowel diseases such as Crohn's and ulcerative colitis; as well as urinary tract infections, vaginal infections, asthma, and some cancers. While exactly how they do so is not understood completely, probiotics appear to affect the body's immune system.

These beneficial bacteria can be obtained through consumption of fermented foods such as yogurt as long as these are produced using live cultures of lactobacillus or bifidobacteria. Probiotics are also available as a dietary supplement in pill or powder form. Like many items sold in health-food stores, commercial probiotics vary considerably in their effectiveness.

The science of probiotics is an exciting field and while the research looks promising, more research is still needed. If you do choose to buy a probiotic supplement, do your homework before you decide on which product to purchase, and consider these points:

■ All probiotics products are not the same. Some contain a single type of organism and others contain many.

■ The health effects are species and strain specific and cannot be generalized to other bacteria. For example, lactobacillus GG has been shown to be helpful for childhood diarrhea but not for Crohn's disease, while other products have been shown to be helpful in Crohn's disease. Find out which probiotics have been studied for the condition you want treated.

■ Look for a product with billions of bacteria in it. You need this many to effectively colonize your intestine. The bacteria should be available at time of consumption, not at time of preparation, so look on the label for the viable count at time of use. Also, look for the specific strains of bacteria in the product. If they are not listed on the label, they may not be there.

■ Store probiotic supplements in a cool, dry place, such as the refrigerator.

■ Yogurt or any fermented milk product must contain 100 million bacteria per dose to be effective. Look for live cultures of acidophilus or bifidobacteria, or both. Products which are pasteurized or have been sitting in the refrigerator for a long time will have very few active bacteria.

DID YOU KNOW?

YOUR INTESTINE IS HOME TO MANY VARIETIES OF BACTERIA

You are born with none, but your digestive tract is quickly colonized and by 2 weeks of age, you will have a large population of bacteria that will stay with you for your entire life. There are times when some bacteria may be destroyed, such as during a course of antibiotics, but the bacteria in your intestine will eventually return. It is important to have a proper balance of different bacteria. If the normal bacteria become depleted or the balance is disturbed, potentially harmful bacteria can multiply and become established, causing digestive and other health problems.

PROSTATE PROBLEMS

CONSUME PLENTY OF

- Tomatoes and tomato products, red grape-fruits, and watermelons for lycopene.
- Nuts, seafood, fish, bread, wheat bran, wheat germ, oats, and brown rice for selenium.
- Vegetable oils, nuts and seeds, and wheat germ for vitamin E.
- Fruits, vegetables, and whole grains for antioxidants.
- Fluids to flush the bladder.

LIMIT

- Fatty foods, especially animal products.

AVOID

- Alcohol, caffeine, spicy foods, and other substances that irritate the urinary tract.
- Excessive weight gain.

The prostate, a walnut-size gland located just below the bladder, is the source of many male urinary problems, including cancer, benign enlargement, and inflammation (prostatitis). Urinary tract infections, lifestyle habits, and a high-fat diet seem to predispose a man to some of these problems. But often, factors that are beyond our control are more instrumental.

As men age, the prostate tends to enlarge, a condition called benign prostatic hypertrophy (BPH). About one-third of all men over 50 experience this noncancerous enlargement that can cause severe obstruction of urinary flow.

Prostate cancer, with an estimated 18,000 new cases a year, is the most common male malignancy. If treated in an early stage, it is highly curable. In many cases, however, it may have spread to other organs by the time of diagnosis. For this reason, the American and Canadian Cancer societies urge all men over 40 to undergo annual or biannual screening, starting with a digital rectal examination. A blood test to measure prostate-specific antigen (PSA), a possible indicator, is also recommended, starting at the age of 50.

THE ROLE OF DIET

Diet may play a role in maintaining prostate health, and may help ward off cancer.

Lycopene. A recent study of nearly 48,000 men found that this substance, found in such foods as tomatoes, tomato products, red grape-fruits, and watermelons appears to reduce the

DID YOU KNOW?

TAKING A ZINC SUPPLEMENT MAY BE DANGEROUS FOR MEN

According to research led by the National Institutes of Health, zinc takers had twice the risk of prostate cancer. Researchers examined zinc intake and prostate cancer risk in nearly 47,000 men. Compared with men who did not take supplements, men who took more than 100 mg of zinc a day had more than twice the risk of advanced prostate cancer.

risk of prostate cancer. These findings support the recommendations to increase consumption of fruits and vegetables, which are high in other antioxidants and bioflavonoid pigments that protect against various cancers. Cooking appears to release more of the lycopene in tomatoes, so tomato-based pasta sauces and soups may be especially beneficial. Lycopene is fat soluble so is better absorbed when eaten with a little fat.

Vitamin E. It is known to reduce inflammation and may protect against prostate cancer. Men, especially smokers, who have low levels of vitamin E appear to be at increased risk. Good sources include margarine, vegetable oils, nuts and seeds, wheat germ, and whole grains.

Selenium. It may protect against prostate cancer. This antioxidant is found in nuts, especially Brazil nuts, seafood, some meats, fish, wheat bran, wheat germ, oats, and brown rice.

Isoflavones. Soy products can help prevent prostate enlargement, may help protect against prostate cancer, and may slow tumor growth. This effect is attributed to isoflavones, plant chemicals that help lower dihydrotestosterone (DHT), a male hormone that stimulates the overgrowth of prostate tissue.

Eat lots of cruciferous vegetables, omega-3s, and other foods that protect the prostate. Fish and vegetable oils high in omega-3 fats seem to reduce the risk of prostate cancer. A diet that is high in saturated animal fats has been linked to an increased incidence. Vegetables from the cruciferous family such as broccoli, cabbage, and cauliflower contain isothiocyanates, phytochemicals that appear to be protective. Whole grains offer fiber, selenium, vitamin E, and phytochemicals, all of which play a role in the prevention of cancer.

Drink plenty of fluids. Anyone with an enlarged prostate should drink plenty of water and other nonalcoholic fluids and reduce intake of caffeine. ❖

HERBAL HELP FOR PROSTATE PROBLEMS

The herb saw palmetto can help relieve the symptoms of an enlarged prostate, but there are no herbal products that can be recommended for the treatment of prostate cancer. Initial optimism about PC-SPES, a blend of herbs, has waned. The benefits originally attributed to it appear to have been due to undeclared prescription drug ingredients.

PROTEIN
■ A BODY-BUILDING NUTRIENT ■

Protein is the quintessential nutrient that every cell in the human body requires for growth or repair. Also, the antibodies that protect us from disease, the enzymes needed for digestion and metabolism, as well as hormones like insulin are all proteins. Cholesterol travels through the bloodstream attached to lipoproteins (fat-carrying proteins). Connective tissue made from protein forms the matrix of bones; chromoproteins are a combination of protein and pigments that form hemoglobin; keratin, still another type of protein, is used by the body to make hair and nails. The neurotransmitters that deliver messages to the brain are made from amino acids derived from dietary protein.

With so many essential functions allotted to protein, you might assume that it should make up the bulk of the diet, but this is not the case. In an ideal balanced diet, only 10 to 12 percent of daily calories should come from protein. Healthy adults only need 0.36 g per pound (0.8 g per kilogram) of body weight of protein every day. Thus, a person weighing 154 lb (70 kg) requires 56 g of protein per day. A 3-oz (85-g) serving of meat, fish, or poultry contains about 21 g of protein, one egg contains 6 g, one cup of milk contains 8 g, and one-half cup cooked lentils contains 8 g.

Amino acids

Proteins are exceedingly complex and diverse structures built of amino acids that are linked together into long chains by peptide bonds. There are many thousands of different proteins, but they all have a backbone of carbon atoms interlaced with nitrogen atoms. Various groupings of atoms can be attached to this backbone.

The human body requires 20 different amino acids to build all the proteins it needs. Of these, 11 can be made in the body, but the other 9, referred to as essential amino acids, must come from the diet. Just as the various letters in the alphabet are joined to make words, so too are amino acids arranged in an almost infinite number of different ways to form the more than 50,000 different proteins in the body. Proteins are made up of hundreds of amino acids. DNA (deoxyribonucleic acid), the genetic material that is found in the nucleus of each body cell, provides the blueprint for how amino acids are arranged to form individual proteins.

Dietary protein

The body is constantly building protein from amino acids, some of which are recycled from the body tissue that is being rebuilt. Even so, a certain amount of protein is lost through normal wear and tear and must be replaced from the diet. But to use this protein, the body must first break it down into its individual amino acids and then reassemble them according to instructions found in the genetic code.

With the exception of oils and pure sugar, all foods contain at least some protein, but its quality varies according to the variety of amino acids it provides. Animal protein (with the exception of gelatin) provides all nine essential amino acids in the proportions required by the body and is therefore

DID YOU KNOW?

HIGH-PROTEIN MEALS ARE A PICK-ME-UP

Most of the 35 or more neurotransmitters that tell the brain to make us feel high, low, sleepy, or alert are made from amino acids that come from dietary protein. A high-protein meal provides tyrosine and can increase norepinephrine levels that stimulate the brain. On the other hand, a high-carbohydrate meal provides the brain with tryptophan and has a calming effect.

referred to as complete, or high-quality, protein. In contrast, plant proteins (with the exception of soy, which is almost as complete as animal food) lack one or more of the essential amino acids. Because not all plant foods lack the same amino acids, the body can build a complete protein if these foods are combined in such a way that they complement each other. For example, grains are high in the essential amino acid methionine, but they lack lysine. This essential amino acid is plentiful in dried beans and other legumes, which are deficient in methionine. By combining a grain with a legume, you can obtain the complete range of amino acids.

Interestingly, low-meat ethnic diets all have dishes that provide complementary proteins: the refried beans and corn tortillas of Mexico; the rice and dahl of India; the tofu, rice, and vegetable combinations in Asian cuisine; and the chickpeas and bulgur wheat in Middle Eastern dishes. Even strict vegetarian diets can supply ample protein by combining complementary grains and legumes. However, if an essential amino acid is missing from the diet, the body breaks down lean tissue to get it.

Moderate cooking makes protein easier to digest because heat breaks down some of the bonds that join amino acids together. Overcooking, however, can cement some amino acids together, making the protein more difficult to digest and to break down into individual amino acids.

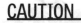

In the stomach, long chains of amino acids are broken into shorter chains called polypeptides. Digestion continues in the small intestine, where pancreatic and other enzymes complete the process. The individual amino acids are absorbed into the bloodstream and transported to the liver, where some are used to make lipoproteins and new enzymes. Others are returned to the bloodstream, which carries them to cells.

Because amino acids are not stored as such, those that are not used in a relatively short time are returned to the liver, where the nitrogen is removed and passed on to the kidneys to be excreted as urea. The remaining protein molecules are stored as fat or may be converted to glucose for energy.

High-protein weight-loss diets

High-protein, low-carbohydrate diets (see Low-Carb Diets) are a very popular weight-loss regime. While people do lose weight on these diets, there is concern about the effects of high protein and high fat intakes on kidney function, bone health, cardiovascular function, and cancer rates. A diet that is high in protein is likely to be low in fruits and consequently low in the numerous beneficial compounds that fruits provide.

Protein deficiency

People in affluent countries generally consume more than enough protein, but deficiencies are common, especially among children, in Africa. Kwashiorkor, the medical term for severe protein deficiency, is marked by poor growth and mental impairment in children, edema, anemia, muscle wasting, decreased immunity, and metabolic abnormalities.

Excessive protein

The typical North American diet provides more protein than the human body needs. This does not pose a serious threat for healthy persons, but too much protein adds to the workload of the kidneys and liver. Thus, people with diseases affecting these organs are often put on a low-protein diet.

CAUTION

Purified protein and amino acid powders or pills are often promoted as high-energy, muscle-bulking supplements for athletes and body-builders, as well as weight-loss aids for dieters. There is no evidence that athletes benefit from high protein intakes. A balanced diet provides all the needed protein; any excess is just excreted. Taking individual amino acid supplements can have some unforeseen consequences. Studies have also shown that amino acid supplements can upset normal protein synthesis, setting the stage for nutritional imbalances. Some researchers also maintain that taking protein supplements increases calcium excretion and may increase the risk of osteoporosis. Excessive intake of dietary protein may also cause the same problem.

PRUNES

BENEFITS
- A rich source of fiber.
- High in vitamin A, potassium, and iron.
- Help to relieve constipation.

DRAWBACKS
- Leave a sticky residue on the teeth that can lead to cavities.

Although all prunes are plums, not all plums are prunes. Prunes are the dried fruit from a few particular species of plum trees whose fruit has firm flesh and is naturally high in sugar and acidity. These traits allow the fruit to dry without fermenting if the pit is left in.

Like all dried fruits, prunes contain very little water and are a more concentrated source of energy and nutrients than their fresh fruit counterparts. They are also higher in calories and sugar (a half cup of the stewed fruit or five large pitted prunes contain approximately 115 calories), and they leave a sticky residue on the teeth that can cause cavities. On the plus side, prunes are rich in fiber: 5 prunes contain 3 g of fiber as well as good amounts of vitamin A, iron, and potassium.

Prunes are popular as a remedy for preventing or treating constipation. This effect can be attributed to prunes' high dietary fiber content; they also contain isatin, a natural laxative.

Unlike other types of juice, prune juice retains most of the fruits' nutrients because it is made by pulverizing the dried prunes and then dissolving them in hot water. One cup of prune juice contains between 16 and 35 percent of the adult RDA of iron and about 700 mg of potassium. However, it is also very high in calories, about 200 per cup. Because prune juice is naturally high in sugar, it does not need any additional sweeteners. Although prune juice is not as good a source of fiber as whole prunes, it still helps to relieve constipation because it, too, contains isatin. ❖

PUMPKINS

BENEFITS
- A rich source of beta carotene.
- A good low-calorie source of iron and potassium.
- High in fiber.
- The seeds are a good source of protein, iron, zinc, B vitamins, vitamin E, and fiber.
- Can be stored for long periods of time.

To most North Americans, pumpkins (a type of winter squash) are a symbol of Halloween and Thanksgiving. In fact, they have more uses than just as traditional jack-o'-lanterns and pie filling—the strong-flavored flesh of pumpkins can be cooked and enjoyed in many ways.

Like all orange-pigmented vegetables, pumpkins are rich in beta carotene, the plant form of vitamin A; one cup of canned or baked pumpkin provides about 1,260 RE of beta carotene, more than a carrot. Studies have shown that this antioxidant may help prevent some forms of cancer. One cup of cooked pumpkin contains 80 calories, 4 g of fiber (similar to two slices of whole-wheat bread), and 3.4 mg of iron, which is almost 20 percent of the Recommended Dietary Allowance (RDA) for women. Pumpkins are a rich source of potassium, important for good blood pressure control. Because pumpkins absorb water, they lose some nutrients and have fewer calories when they are boiled. Sugar pumpkins, which are smaller and sweeter than the large deep-orange pumpkins, are the best choice for cooking.

Although the seeds are often thrown away, they are a rich source of protein. One ounce (30 g) of pumpkin seeds provides 7 g of protein—almost as much as an equal serving of peanuts—as well as 3 mg of iron (20 to 30 percent of the adult RDA). They are high in unsaturated vegetable oil, a source of vitamin E, and rich in B vitamins. When the coverings are consumed too, the seeds are high in fiber. Pumpkin seeds are easy to prepare: scoop out the seeds, wash them and let dry, then bake them on an oiled baking sheet at 250°F (120°C) for an hour. Commercial varieties are often salted.

Because pumpkins have hard shells, they are ideal for storing. Pumpkins last about a month in a cool, dry place. ❖

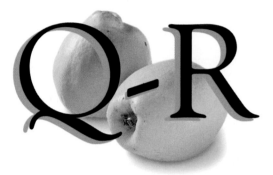

Q-R

QUINCE

BENEFITS
- A source of vitamin C, iron, and potassium.
- High in pectin, a soluble fiber.

DRAWBACKS
- Often cooked with large amounts of sugar to offset tartness.
- Seeds contain a cyanide compound.

A member of the same rose family as apples and pears, the quince has an acidic tartness; so it is rarely eaten raw. Cooking cuts the acids, and the fruit takes on a mellow flavor similar to that of an apple, with the texture of a pear.

Raw quinces are high in vitamin C; a medium-size fruit provides more than 20 mg, or 25 percent of the adult Recommended Dietary Allowance (RDA) for women. Much of the vitamin C is lost when the fruit is cooked. The same-size quince provides 1 mg of iron and 275 mg of potassium.

There are 90 calories in a medium-size quince; it is also high in pectin, a soluble fiber that helps control blood cholesterol levels and promotes smooth digestive function. Because pectin forms a semisolid gel when cooked, quinces are ideal for making jams and jellies.

Quinces may be round or somewhat pear-shaped. Look for fruit that is firm, with pale yellow skin covered with fuzz; reject any that are small, irregularly shaped, or bruised. Poaching and baking are the most nutritious methods of preparing the fruit. Don't be misled by the tartness of raw quince; the fruit becomes sweeter as it cooks. Cooking also changes the color of the flesh from yellow to pink or red.

Warning: Remove the seeds before cooking. As with apples and similar fruits, the seeds contain amygdalin, a compound that can break down to release hydrogen cyanide. Eating large amounts can result in cyanide poisoning. ❖

QUINOA

BENEFITS
- An excellent source of iron, magnesium, potassium, phosphorus, zinc, and other minerals.
- A good source of B-complex vitamins.
- High in protein.

DRAWBACKS
- Not widely available and more expensive than most grains.

Although it is often classified as a grain, quinoa is actually a member of the same plant family as spinach. While the green leafy quinoa (pronounced ki-NOH-wah) tops are edible, it's the seeds that are served most frequently.

For more than 5,000 years, quinoa has been the staple food of peoples of the Andes, where it is one of the few crops that grows well in the dry mountainous climate and poor soil.

A NUTRIENT POWERHOUSE

The tiny quinoa seeds are packed with important nutrients; a 1-cup serving (made from ¼ cup of dry quinoa) provides about 4 mg of iron, more than any unfortified grain product. One cup also contributes large amounts of several other essential minerals, including 90 mg of magnesium, 175 mg of phosphorus, 315 mg of potassium, and 1.5 mg of zinc, as well as numerous B vitamins, especially B_6, folate, niacin, and thiamine.

Most of the 160 calories in 1 cup of cooked quinoa come from complex carbohydrates. However, it also provides 7 g of protein, which is of a higher quality than similar products because it provides lysine, an amino acid missing in corn, wheat, and other grains. Quinoa is a good source of saponins, phytochemicals that help to prevent cancer and heart disease.

A VERSATILE FOOD

Quinoa cooks quickly into a fluffy, delicately flavored grainlike dish that lends itself to many uses. It can be served as a substitute for rice, potatoes, and other starchy foods; combined with vegetables, poultry, or seafood to make a pilaf; and added to soups and stews. ❖

DID YOU KNOW?

QUINOA IS A COMPLETE PROTEIN

It provides an essential amino acid balance close to the ideal set by the United Nations Food and Agriculture Organization (FAO). And the National Academy of Science calls it "one of the best sources of protein in the vegetable kingdom."

RADISHES

BENEFITS
- A fair source of vitamin C.
- Low in calories and high in fiber.

DRAWBACKS
- Can produce gas in some people.
- Salicylate content may provoke an allergic reaction in people sensitive to aspirin.

A member of the cruciferous family, the radish is closely related to cabbage, kale, turnips, and cauliflower. While not especially high in most essential nutrients, radishes are tasty, as well as low in calories, making them ideal for snacking and as a spicy addition to salads, soups, and vegetable side dishes.

A fair source of vitamin C, radishes also contain small amounts of iron, potassium, and folate. Five medium-size raw radishes provide 5 mg of vitamin C and they yield only 5 calories. They also supply sulfurous compounds that may protect against cancer.

Like other cruciferous vegetables, radishes can cause bloating and gas in some people. Also, radishes contain salicylates—compounds similar to the active ingredient in aspirin; many people sensitive to aspirin may suffer an allergic reaction to radishes.

The peak season for radishes spans from April to July, but most varieties are available year-round. Summer radishes have a more intense peppery flavor than those cultivated during spring or fall. Although the bright red globe variety is the best-known in North America, other types include black radishes, daikons, and white icicles.

When selecting red globe radishes, avoid the larger ones if possible, as they may be pithy. A bright color indicates freshness. If there are leaves on the stems, make sure they are green and crisp. Regardless of which variety of radish you are buying, the vegetables should feel solid and have an unblemished surface. Unless the radishes are going to be served the same day, you should remove any leaves and tops; the radishes will stay fresh longer without the tops. If they are not already packaged, store radishes in plastic bags. ❖

RAISINS

See Grapes

RASPBERRIES

BENEFITS
- An excellent source of vitamin C.
- Contain useful amounts of folate, iron, and potassium.
- Provide bioflavonoids, which may protect against cancer.
- High in fiber.

DRAWBACKS
- Contain a natural salicylate, which can cause an allergic reaction in aspirin-sensitive people.
- Contain oxalic acid, which can aggravate kidney and bladder stones in susceptible persons.

There is no sweeter surprise on a summer day than to stumble across a wild raspberry patch. Raspberries—both wild and cultivated—are low in calories and a rich source of vitamin C.

A 1-cup serving of raspberries contains 60 calories and 30 mg of vitamin C (40 percent of the Recommended Dietary Allowance, or RDA, for women). It also provides 30 mcg (micrograms) of folate, 190 mg of potassium, and some iron. The vitamin C content increases the iron's absorption, although this may be offset by the oxalic acid in raspberries, which binds with this mineral.

There are 7 g of fiber in 1 cup of raw raspberries. The seeds in raspberries provide insoluble fiber that helps prevent constipation. The fruit is also high in pectin, a form of soluble fiber that helps control blood cholesterol levels. In addition, raspberries contain anthocyanins, antioxidant plant pigments that have been shown to prevent cancer and heart disease as well as ellagic acid, another cancer-fighting substance. Cooking does not destroy ellagic acid.

Raspberries spoil faster than most berries because of their delicate structure and hollow core. Once picked, they should be eaten as soon as possible. Freezing, however, will preserve them for up to a year.

Cultivated raspberries can be found year-round in gourmet and specialty stores, and

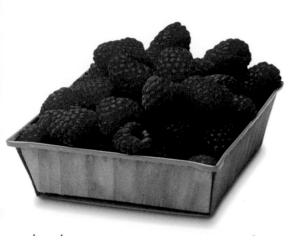

when they are in season, at many supermarkets. Before buying raspberries, check that all of them, not just the ones on top, are in good condition; even then, they mold quickly and should be used within 24 hours.

Berries often produce allergic reactions, and raspberries are no exception. Those who are sensitive to aspirin may also react to raspberries, which contain a natural salicylate, similar to the major ingredient in aspirin. Oxalic acid can precipitate kidney and bladder stones in susceptible people; however, it would take a very large amount of raspberries to create problems. ❖

RESPIRATORY DISORDERS

CONSUME PLENTY OF
- Nonalcoholic fluids to help thin mucus.
- Fresh fruits and vegetables for beta carotene, vitamin C, and other antioxidants.
- Lean meat, oysters, yogurt, and whole-grain products for zinc.

LIMIT
- Foods that cause bloating and gas.

AVOID
- Smoking and exposure to secondhand smoke and other air pollutants.
- Alcohol.

Among our leading causes of sickness, disability, and death, respiratory disorders range from colds and flu, which are usually minor infections, to chronic diseases, such as asthma, which are much more problematic. Any condition that affects the passage of air to and from the lungs should always be taken seriously. The onset of respiratory symptoms is sufficient cause to see your doctor. The following are some of the more common respiratory disorders.

BRONCHITIS

Difficulty breathing, a relentless cough, and production of thick mucus, or phlegm, are the characteristic symptoms of bronchitis—an inflammation of the bronchi, or branching tubes, that carry air to and from the lungs. There may also be a low-grade fever and a burning sensation in the chest. Acute bronchitis, often a complication of a severe cold, flu, or other infection of the upper respiratory tract, may require antibiotic treatment, but it usually goes away in a week or two.

Chronic bronchitis is an extremely serious problem that develops when the bronchial tubes are irritated over a long period of time. Cigarette smoking is by far the most common cause, although exposure to air pollution and occupational dusts and chemicals may also be involved. Whatever the cause, the tubes become thickened, a mucus-producing cough is present almost all of the time, and air flow to the lungs is often greatly impaired. This creates an ideal breeding ground for infection and sets the stage for progressive lung damage.

EMPHYSEMA

Also known as chronic obstructive pulmonary disease (COPD), emphysema afflicts more than 1 million North Americans. It takes years to develop, often as a consequence of smoking or chronic bronchitis. As the disease worsens, the air sacs, or alveoli, lose their elasticity and fill with stale air, leading to an increased shortness of breath and a distended, barrel-shaped chest.

PNEUMONIA

There are many different types of pneumonia, but the symptoms generally include a cough with a great deal of sputum, fever, chills, and chest pain. Pneumonia's causes include viruses, bacteria, fungi, parasites, and exposure of lung tissue to toxic substances. AIDS patients often develop *Pneumocystis carinii*, a rare type that strikes people with weakened immunity. One common bacterial type, pneumococcal pneumonia, can be prevented by a vaccine, which is recommended for everyone over 65 and for anyone over the age of 2 who has a chronic disease

DO ONE SIMPLE THING

TRY AROMATHERAPY TO RELIEVE SYMPTOMS

A soothing means of relieving lung problems is to inhale the steam from a bowl of hot water that contains a few drops of highly concentrated essential oils. A combination of eucalyptus, thyme, pine, and lavender oils is often recommended to ease bronchitis. Eucalyptus oil is particularly good for relieving the feeling of congestion and may be helpful to people with emphysema. Peppermint oil may also be added to hot water to relieve bronchial symptoms.

that increases their risk for pneumonia.

HELPFUL FOODS

A nutritious and well-balanced diet can help prevent or reduce the severity of bronchitis, pneumonia, and other lung infections because people who are in good health are more likely to fight off the underlying causes.

Fluids. During any respiratory infection, adequate fluid intake is especially important because it helps to thin mucus and make breathing easier. Physicians generally recommend that their patients drink at least six to eight glasses of nonalcoholic fluids a day. Although chicken broth and other warm fluids are particularly helpful in thinning mucus, cold fluids are also beneficial.

Antioxidants. These help protect lung tissue from the cellular damage caused by free radicals, unstable molecules that are released when the body uses oxygen. Important antioxidants are vitamins A, C, and beta carotene, which the human body converts to vitamin A.

Vitamins A and C. They are also necessary to build and repair epithelial tissues, which line the lungs, bronchi, and other parts of the respiratory system; the tissues act as a barrier against bacteria. In addition, these vitamins are essential to building an immunity against lung disease. A balanced diet that provides ample fresh fruits and vegetables, particularly those that are yellow, orange, and dark green, will provide reasonable amounts of vitamins A and C.

Zinc. Important for boosting immunity, especially against upper respiratory infections, zinc is found in many foods, especially lean meat, oysters, yogurt, and whole-grain products. While zinc helps your immune system, excess can do the opposite. Consuming more than 40 mg per day can depress your immune system, making you more susceptible to infection.

EATING APPROACHES

People with emphysema generally feel better if they eat smaller, more frequent meals. Consuming too much at one time can increase the volume in the stomach and crowd the already distended lungs. Cut down on fried and other fatty foods. Fats remain in the stomach longer because they require more time to digest; thus, the stomach may crowd the lungs longer than when filled with other foods. Anything that causes gas and bloating should also be avoided; common offenders include beans and other legumes, cabbage, brussels sprouts, broccoli, and onions. The volume of food in the stomach can be reduced by taking liquids an hour before eating and an hour afterward, rather than with your meals.

Some of the medications used to treat respiratory disorders can cause a loss of appetite. Ask your doctor about taking medicines right after eating. Make your meals enticing and don't rush; have small servings and eat slowly. Sharing a meal with a friend can also help improve your appetite. If you simply can't eat enough solid foods, juicing or high-calorie liquids may be a solution.

LIFESTYLE HABITS

Smoking is by far the leading cause of chronic respiratory disorders, including chronic bronchitis, emphysema, and lung cancer. If you smoke, make every effort to stop. Also try to avoid secondhand smoke and air pollutants. If your job exposes you to harmful dusts or chemical gases, be sure to wear the proper protective masks.

Alcohol lowers immunity and should be avoided during any infection. Because chronic bronchitis and emphysema predispose a person to develop lung infections, it's a good idea to abstain from all alcoholic beverages. ❖

RHUBARB

BENEFITS
- Contains vitamin C, potassium, and fiber.

DRAWBACKS
- Usually prepared with substantial amounts of sugar or other sweeteners.
- Contains oxalic acid, which inhibits calcium and iron absorption.
- Leaves are highly poisonous.

Although rhubarb is generally regarded as a fruit, botanically it is a vegetable. It is available in frozen and canned forms, but most people prefer to cook the fresh stalks themselves. One cup of fresh diced rhubarb yields a mere 26 calories and provides 10 mg of vitamin C, as well as

350 mg of potassium. This same serving size also contains more than 100 mg of calcium; however, rhubarb is not considered a good source of this mineral, since it also contains oxalic acid, which not only blocks the absorption of its calcium, but also that from any other dietary sources. Because it has a high oxalic acid content, large amounts of rhubarb should be avoided by anyone with a tendency to develop oxalate-containing kidney or gall stones.

Only the rhubarb stalks are eaten—the leaves are highly poisonous. Because raw rhubarb stalks are stringy in texture and tart in flavor, most people will consume them only when cooked with large amounts of sugar or honey, thus inflating the calorie count. One cup of cooked sweetened rhubarb yields 280 calories. To avoid extra calories, cook the stalks with sweet fruits, such as strawberries or apples.

A favorite springtime pie filling, rhubarb can also be made into preserves, or it can be stewed to make a compote or sauces to complement poultry, other meat dishes, and desserts.

When cooked and sweetened, rhubarb will turn brownish in color. It should not be prepared in aluminum or cast iron pots, which will interact with the acid in the vegetable and darken both the pot and the rhubarb. ❖

RICE

BENEFITS

- Enriched varieties provide B vitamins and iron.
- Makes a complete protein when combined with beans and other legumes.
- Gluten-free and suitable for people with celiac disease.
- Easy to digest and useful in restoring bowel function after a bout of diarrhea.
- Rarely, if ever, causes food allergies.

For thousands of years, rice has been the staple food for more than half the world's population. In some Asian countries per capita consumption exceeds 300 lb (135 kg) a year, and survival still depends on the rice crop. In contrast, the average North American eats just over 25 lb (11 kg) of rice a year, which includes all types of rice, as well as breakfast cereals.

Like barley and oats, rice grows in a protective husk that has to be removed if the grain is to be used as food. (Wheat and corn require less processing.) Many nutrients are lost with the bran and germ that are removed in milling to make white rice. Brown rice—intact kernels that retain their bran layers—is somewhat more nutritious than white rice, but it also contains phytic acid, a substance that interferes with the absorption of iron and calcium.

Since it is a refined carbohydrate, white rice is digested quickly, elevates blood sugar levels, and provides energy, but with less nutritional value and fiber content than brown rice. The glycemic index (GI) is a standard used to assess the impact of carbohydrates on the body; the lower the load, the better. Five ounces (140 g) of cooked white rice can have a GI as high as 72. The same amount of brown rice has a GI of 50, which is in the low to medium range. (See Glycemic Index.) While it is true that some of the white rice processed and sold in North America is enriched or fortified with iron and B vitamins after it is refined, many of the nutrients are lost forever. Furthermore, enrichment is typically applied to the outside of the grain. Rinsing the grain before cooking washes away these nutrients. Rice should be cooked in just twice its volume of water, which will be completely absorbed by the grain and will preserve the nutritional content.

Converted rice is processed by a 2,000-year-old method; this involves parboiling the whole grain, which makes milling easier by loosening the husk. Conversion improves the nutritional quality of the grain by causing the B vitamins in the bran and germ to permeate the endosperm. It also gelatinizes the fat- and nutrient-bearing aleurone layer, which then adheres to the grain instead of being lost with the bran. Thanks to this technique, the thiamine deficiency known as beriberi was never a serious threat to people in India and Pakistan, although it ravaged Asian people who subsisted on unconverted white rice. Instant rice should not be confused with converted rice, which takes at least as long to cook as other types. Much of the rice sold in North America is also polished in special machines to make it shiny. An extra sheen is achieved by coating the grains with talc and glucose. This is a cosmetic process with no nutritional impact.

NUTRITIONAL VALUE

Ninety percent of the calories in rice come from carbohydrates. A half cup of white rice contains about 80 to 100 calories, while brown rice may have 105 to 110. Brown rice is significantly higher in fiber, with 1.6 g per half cup compared to 0.03 g in the same volume of white rice.

SOME FACTS ABOUT RICE

- Although the United States produces only one percent of the world rice crop, it is one of the largest exporters of rice.
- Wild rice grows in marshlands and waterways from Manitoba to the Atlantic Ocean. It is one of the few wild plant foods harvested and marketed in Canada.
- The outer, most nutritious parts of the rice kernel are removed and fed to livestock when rice is milled.
- Broken grains of rice are used for brewing beer.
- We commemorate an ancient Asian fertility symbol when we shower bridal couples with rice.

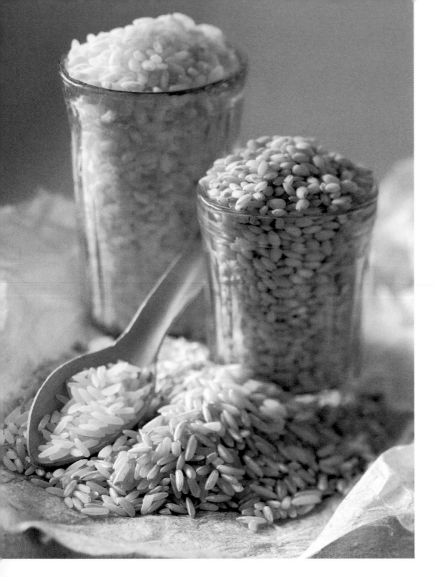

carbohydrate, it provides a slow, steady supply of glucose, and not the rapid rise that occurs after eating sugars or refined white rice.

Along with lamb and a few other foods, rice rarely if ever provokes an allergic reaction. This quality makes rice ideal as the basis of the strict elimination diet that is sometimes used to identify food allergens.

A VERSATILE STAPLE

Rice is a true staple in menu planning. Risotto, made with fat-free broth and vegetables, and pilaf, based on fat-free broth, chopped nuts, and dried fruits, are economical, nutritious, low-fat entrées. Rice is an ingredient of hot and cold breakfast cereals, an excellent base for salads, and a natural companion to vegetables, fish, meats, and cheese. Rice bran also adds bulk to baked goods.

RICE VARIETIES

Rice is classified by size and shape (long, medium, and short grain). Long-grain rice remains dry and separate when cooked; short-grain rice, which is wetter and stickier, is more often used in Asian and Caribbean cooking.

Arborio rice is a creamy-textured, medium-grain Italian rice that is used in making risotto because it remains firm at the center through very long cooking.

Basmati is an aromatic rice native to Pakistan and India. When cooked, the grain swells only lengthwise. Basmati grains stay dry and separate and are especially suitable for pilafs.

Jasmine is an aromatic rice with origins in Thailand. It has a soft, moist texture and grains that cling together.

Wild rice, a very distant relative of common rice, is a grass native to the lakes and marshes of the Great Lakes region. Once gathered by hand in the wild by Chippewa Indians, wild rice is now cultivated commercially and harvested by machine. Wild rice contains more protein than common rice does and is richer in lysine, the amino acid lacking in most grains. ❖

RICE—EASY TO DIGEST AND HYPOALLERGENIC. *That is why rice is an important component of many commercially produced baby foods.*

Brown rice also contains more selenium, vitamin E, magnesium, phosphorus, and manganese. The protein content of rice, ranging from 2.0 to 2.5 mg per half cup, is less than that of other cereals, but the amino acid balance is superior to that of other grains. Processed rice contains only a trace of fat and no sodium.

HEALTH BENEFITS

Rice has a binding effect in diarrhea, and as such, is part of the BRAT (for banana, rice, applesauce, and toast) diet. It helps restore normal bowel function and provides needed energy for someone recovering from diarrhea. Rice pudding made with low-fat milk and flavored with cinnamon is a soothing, easy-to-digest dish for convalescents.

Several studies have shown that rice bran helps to reduce cholesterol and may reduce the risk of bowel cancer. Some studies also show that brown rice helps regulate glucose metabolism in people with diabetes. As an unrefined complex

DID YOU KNOW?

SAKE IS ACTUALLY A TYPE OF BEER

Rice wine, or sake, is a kind of beer that is fermented with a mold that secretes starch-digesting enzymes as it grows on rice. Sake's alcohol content is high. Unlike Western beers, which are drunk chilled, sake is flat and served warm.

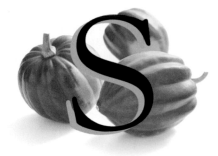

SALAD DRESSINGS

BENEFITS

- Add flavor and interest to lettuce and other salad greens.
- A good source of vitamin E.

DRAWBACKS

- Cheese, creamy, and oil dressings, as well as mayonnaise, are high in fat.
- Those made from raw eggs may harbor salmonella bacteria.
- Additives can cause allergic or adverse reactions in susceptible people.

Various dressings give flavor and zip to lettuce and other greens; they are even more important in potato, egg, tuna, and similar salads because they help hold the ingredients together. The olive, corn, canola, and other vegetable oils used in most salad dressings provide vitamin E and because their fats are unsaturated, they do not tend to raise blood cholesterol levels. But traditional salad dressings also add lots of calories, and those made with eggs, cheese, or sour cream contain saturated fats and cholesterol. Fortunately, there is an increasing number of low-fat alternatives, although these are not necessarily low in calories.

The classic vinaigrette dressing is a mixture of vinegar and oil. The standard recipe calls for 3 to 4 parts oil to 1 part vinegar, but you can reduce the amount of oil in several ways. For instance, you don't need as much oil if you mix it with a mild balsamic, wine, or rice vinegar. Another option is to dilute with water, defatted broth, wine, or juice, depending upon the desired taste. You can also reduce the amount of oil by selecting one with an assertive flavor, such as walnut or olive oil.

For a creamy texture and appearance without the saturated fat, add nonfat yogurt to the vinaigrette dressing. Or replace some of the oil with buttermilk. Experiment with herbs and spices. When eating at a restaurant, mix your own low-fat dressing by asking for oil and vinegar or a fresh lemon. If you select a house dressing, ask that it be served on the side.

Blue cheese dressings rank near the top in fat and calories, and their distinctive flavor is hard to duplicate with low-fat alternatives. Try blending equal amounts of low-fat cottage cheese and yogurt with a little vinegar to make a creamy dressing; then crumble in a small amount of blue cheese for flavor.

If a recipe calls for a mayonnaise dressing, start with a low-fat type. Then blend the mayonnaise with an equal part of low-fat yogurt.

SAFETY ISSUES

Although some dressing recipes, such as mayonnaise and Caesar salad dressing, call for raw eggs, they should not be used because they may harbor salmonella bacteria. Instead, use imitation egg products; these contain egg whites that have been treated to kill bacteria. Commercial salad dressings are pasteurized to kill any microorganisms, and their high vinegar content discourages the growth of new ones. Commercial dressings often contain wheat or corn starches, soy, and perhaps eggs. Anyone with food allergies, celiac disease, and other food intolerances should check the labels carefully. Products made according to a standard recipe do not list all the ingredients. In such cases, call the manufacturer for a list of ingredients. ❖

SALT AND SODIUM

BENEFITS

- Sodium helps to maintain fluid balance, regulate blood pressure, and transmit nerve impulses.
- Salt improves the flavor of many foods.
- Salt is a useful food preservative.

DRAWBACKS

- Sodium promotes fluid retention and may contribute to high blood pressure.

While the terms are often used interchangeably, salt and sodium are not the same. Sodium is an element that joins with chlorine to form sodium chloride, or table salt. Sodium occurs naturally in most foods, and salt is the most common source of sodium in the diet. Sodium works to maintain the body's acid-alkaline balance and helps maintain the body's fluid

DON'T OVERDRESS

A salad that's drenched in dressing is high in unnecessary calories and becomes soggy quickly, because vinegar wilts lettuce and other greens. Use a very light sprinkling of oil to coat the greens, and mix the other ingredients—such as raw vegetables or artichoke hearts—with a small amount of vinegar. Then toss the two together just before serving.

As a general rule, 1 to 2 tablespoons of dressing should be ample for 4 cups of salad greens, and 1/4 cup of a mayonnaise-type dressing should be enough for 4 cups of potato, tuna, or chicken salad.

balance. It also helps control nerve function and muscle movement.

Scientifically speaking, the term "salt" actually refers to a class of substances composed of ions held together by virtue of their opposite charges. Calcium carbonate (chalk) is a salt, as is sodium bicarbonate (baking soda). Sodium chloride is the most abundant salt occurring naturally in food. The amount of sodium the body needs daily is far less than what is usually consumed. Circumstances and climate will dictate the amount needed, but in general, the human body needs less than 500 mg of sodium per day to maintain health. Because salt is so abundant in our food supply, a dietary deficiency is unlikely. A typical North American diet can have 4,000 to 7,000 mg per day. One teaspoon of salt supplies over 2,000 mg of sodium. There is no health risk to moderating the amount of salt in your diet.

Sodium finds its way into food in several ways; it is naturally present in foods, added during processing or cooking, or added at the table. The major sources in the diet are processed and preserved foods. Salty foods, such as potato chips and salted crackers and nuts, are easy to identify, but hidden sodium has to be tracked down on package labels. Cereals, cold cuts, canned soups, canned vegetables, prepackaged meals, and commercial baked goods are usually high in sodium. Sodium is also found in MSG (monosodium glutamate), garlic salt or other seasoned salts, sea salt, meat tenderizers, commercially prepared sauces and condiments like ketchup, soy sauce, chili sauce, and steak sauce, in soups, cured or smoked foods, olives, and pickles. In general, the more processed a food is, the higher the sodium content.

THE CONNECTION BETWEEN BLOOD PRESSURE AND SALT

People with high blood pressure are typically advised to cut back on salt, because sodium affects the kidneys' ability to rid the body of wastes and fluid. When the body's sodium level is low, the kidneys retrieve the chemical from the urine and return it to the circulating blood. Some individuals, however, have a genetic tendency to conserve sodium, which may predispose them to high blood pressure. As the kidneys retain more salt than necessary, they excrete less urine so that fluid is available to maintain the sodium at the correct concentration. As a result, the heart is forced to pump harder to keep this extra fluid in circulation, and the blood pressure increases to maintain

the blood flow. Restricting salt intake may correct this form of high blood pressure.

The most controversial issue around salt is the extent of its impact on blood pressure. While no one disputes the low-sodium diet for people with high blood pressure, experts disagree when it comes to making recommendations for the public at large. Some say that asking everyone to try to reduce their salt intake is not based on science. But many people have undiagnosed high blood pressure and would benefit from reduced salt intake.

Studies have shown that as salt in the diet is increased, blood pressure goes up. Populations with low salt intake have lower blood pressure. The Yanomami Indians of Brazil add no salt to their food and hypertension is unknown. By contrast, North Americans, with their penchant for salty foods, such as hot dogs, chips, and pizza, are in the midst of a hypertension epidemic. Whether a reduced-salt diet lowers blood pressure in people who do not have high pressure to start with is not critical. Eating fewer salty processed foods automatically leads to a healthier diet, and limiting salt intake can cause no harm.

Some people are more salt-sensitive than others, and they will get the biggest payoff from cutting back on salt. African-Americans and people with diabetes tend to be more sensitive to salt, as are older people.

The increase in blood volume that occurs during pregnancy temporarily increases the body's need for salt, but the amount required is normally supplied in a varied, balanced diet. Pregnant women should prepare meals with only a little salt and not add salt to food at the table.

MYTH BUSTER

Myth: Sea salt is a healthier product than table salt.

Reality: There are no documented health advantages to sea salt, and the sodium content is similar.

FIVE WAYS TO CUT SALT

1. **Use spices that don't contain sodium,** like fresh herbs, garlic powder or fresh garlic, onion flakes (instead of onion salt), dry mustard, coriander, lemon, mint, cumin, chili, curry, rosemary, thyme, basil, bay leaves, ginger, hot peppers, pepper, chives, and parsley.

2. **Make your own salad dressing** rather than using the bottled ones. Use flavored vinegars instead of salt for extra taste.

3. **Eat more fresh or frozen fruits and vegetables.** If you use canned vegetables, buy them sodium reduced. Use fresh potatoes rather than instant, fresh cucumbers instead of pickles. Add spices and herbs instead of salt to the water in which you cook vegetables.

4. **Eat fresh or frozen fish** instead of canned or dried varieties, choose sliced roast beef or chicken instead of bologna, salami, or other processed meat.

5. **Re-educate your taste buds.** Taste food before adding salt. Cook from scratch instead of packages. Adapt your favorite recipes by using half the amount of salt called for.

REDUCING SALT INTAKE

Preparing most dishes from scratch and avoiding processed foods helps to cut down on salt intake. Supermarkets and food stores now stock a growing variety of salt-free or low-salt versions of processed foods, including canned broths. All food labels now list the amount of sodium in a serving; however, the serving specified on the label—and therefore the sodium content—may be much less than the amount you eat. Also check the label for code terms, such as brine, broth, corned, cured, pickled, soy sauce, and teriyaki sauce, that indicate other high-sodium ingredients have been added.

For many people, adding salt to food at the table is a reflex response to seeing the salt shaker; remove the shaker and you may not miss the salt. The amount of salt and other sodium-containing seasonings in most recipes can be cut by half or even more without a noticeable change in taste. Herbs and spices, fresh garlic, or lemon juice are healthful alternatives. Adding these ingredients shortly before serving keeps flavors from being lost during prolonged cooking.

Warning: Most commercial salt substitutes contain potassium. These may be dangerous for people with kidney disorders or those taking potassium-sparing diuretics or supplements. Before using a salt substitute, especially if you're taking a diuretic or potassium supplements, first check with a doctor.

Pickles and condiments, such as mustard, ketchup, salad dressings, and sauces, are high in sodium. When eating in restaurants, ask for dressings and sauces to be served on the side. In restaurants where the food is made to order, ask that it be prepared without salt.

The use of a home water softener may add a substantial amount of sodium to your drinking water. The company that installed the water softener should tell you how much sodium is in the system; you may prefer to drink bottled water instead.

Many over-the-counter medications contain sodium. If you are on a sodium-restricted diet, check with your physician or pharmacist before using antacids, painkillers, or laxatives. ❖

SAUCES AND GRAVIES

BENEFITS

- Used sparingly, sauces complement flavors and enhance appearance.
- Salsa-style garnishes supply fiber and antioxidant vitamins, provided they are carefully prepared.
- Pasta sauces based on fresh vegetables and olive oil are good sources of vitamins, fiber, complex carbohydrates, and unsaturated fat.

DRAWBACKS

- Traditional sauces made from butter, flour, cream, and egg yolks are very high in fat, saturated fat, and cholesterol.
- Asian-style sauces are high in salt and should be avoided by people on low-sodium diets.

An 18th-century Italian unfavorably compared England and France: "England has 60 religions," he wrote, "and one sauce, whereas France has 60 sauces and one religion." Like so many exaggerations, this one had a grain of truth. French cuisine has always been renowned for its sauces, while British cuisine still has a reputation for favoring brown gravy. Italian cooks are famous for vegetable-based mixtures that are often enlivened with fresh herbs and a sprinkling of grated cheese.

Whatever the type of cuisine—French, Italian, Asian, Indian, or Mexican—contemporary sauce style is continually evolving. Today's chefs can draw from an international medley of delicious and exciting sauces that can transform an ordinary dish into a culinary delight.

The word *sauce*, like *salsa*, comes from the root meaning "salty." Early sauces were heavily salted and spiced to preserve food and mask the flavors of any tainted meats. Sauces today are added to enhance or complement the flavors of foods.

Fresh-made sauces are limitless in variety and taste, from a world-renowned chef's classic concoctions to the home cook's on-the-spot invention. Commercially prepared sauces, such as barbecue sauces and hot pepper sauces, are made to patented formulas of ingredients.

Traditional sauce-making techniques are based on four main methods: the reduction of stock or vegetable pulp; the roux, in which similar quantities of fat and flour are cooked together, blended with milk or other liquid to a velvety consistency, and flavored; hot egg-based sauces (such as hollandaise), in which egg yolks and butter are blended to make an emulsion with concentrated wine or vinegar and seasonings; and cold egg sauces (such as mayonnaise), where oil is blended into an emulsion with egg yolks and vinegar or lemon juice.

These traditional sauces generally contain only moderate amounts of vitamins A and D from their milk, cream, butter, and egg yolk components. Considering the small portions in which they are meant to be served, however, the vitamin quotient is negligible and is far outweighed by the negative impact of saturated fats and calories. Two tablespoons of a homemade white sauce contain about 50 calories; the addition of grated cheese to make a Mornay sauce typically increases the calorie count to 125.

Sauces made from commercial mixes are somewhat lower in calories than homemade ones, but are high in sodium, however, and offer few nutrients.

The trend away from flour-based sauces got its first big push from the calorie-conscious nouvelle and spa cuisines that emerged in the 1970s. Professional chefs and home cooks alike began to spurn flour thickeners and butter enrichment in favor of the pure, intense flavors obtained by concentrating fat-free stocks and vegetable purees. While traditional sauces were typically laden with saturated fat and cholesterol, the new garnishes manage to add piquancy in a low-fat, low-calorie form.

SALSA

Fresh salsas are mixtures of fine-chopped vegetables or fruits, highly seasoned with garlic, scallions, citrus juice, and fresh herbs, such as cilantro and basil. In contrast to the traditional sauces, salsa homemade from fresh fruits or vegetables is virtually fat-free if made without oil, high in fiber, very low in calories, and rich in such antioxidants as vitamin C and beta carotene. Commercial salsas, however, are usually modified vinegar pickles cooked and thickened with starch.

PASTA SAUCES

Pasta sauces, such as Alfredo, that are made with cream, butter, egg yolk, and cheese, are very high in fat and cholesterol. They should be used only sparingly, and people with high cholesterol levels should avoid them altogether.

The variety of low-fat pasta sauces is limited only by a cook's imagination and the ingredients available. Excellent sauces can be made with fresh tomatoes chopped with herbs and garlic and blended with other ingredients. All tomato-based sauces provide some fiber, beta carotene, vitamins C and E, lycopene, and a small amount of unsaturated fat.

HEALTHY TOPPING. *Salsa is a more healthful approach to garnish than a butter- and cream-based sauce.*

THANKSGIVING TURKEY GRAVY

Nobody expects you to do without the gravy that glazes the Thanksgiving turkey. You can, however, reduce the fat and calorie content and improve the nutritional quality by using a stock-based method. Here's how:

Brown the turkey giblets and trimmings in a hot oven or under the broiler, drain off the fat, and simmer the browned scraps with vegetables and herbs (an unpeeled onion stuck with a clove, a celery stalk, carrot, leek, and turnip; thyme, parsley stems, peppercorns, and a bay leaf) to make a rich stock. Drain the stock, discard the vegetables, then chill the stock, which will make it easier to remove the congealed fat from the surface. Next, concentrate the skimmed stock by boiling it down to a half or third of its volume. When the turkey is done, drain the fat from the roasting pan and pour in the hot stock to dissolve the clinging browned bits of meat. Boil the liquid to blend the flavors together, season, and serve hot with the turkey.

GRAVIES

Gravies are variations on the roux. Flour is cooked in fat drippings from dry-cooked meat, then blended with a liquid to make a sauce. Canned gravies are also available. Two tablespoons of canned beef or mushroom gravy contain approximately 15 calories, compared to 25 in the same amount of canned chicken gravy. Individuals on low-sodium diets should avoid commercial gravies, which are extremely high in salt. Gravies have fairly substantial amounts of fat and, whether canned or homemade, they have only a negligible amount of nutrition.

ASIAN SAUCES

Many of the sauces used in Asian cooking are extremely high in sodium. Those most familiar are soy, fish or oyster sauce (*nuoc mam* or *nam pla*), hoisin and other bean-based sauces, and stir-fry sauce (a mixture of other sauces). Some of these may be thickened with wheat gluten and should be avoided by people with celiac disease.

DESSERT SAUCES

Dessert sauces, such as hot fudge, elevate the fat and calorie content of an ice cream sundae to dizzying heights. Fat-free versions of many of the classic dessert sauces are available, but the calorie content is still high, and the nutritional value is low or nonexistent. More healthful alternatives include nonfat frozen yogurt topped with chopped fresh fruit and nuts, or frozen berries. ❖

SAUSAGES

See Smoked, Cured, and Pickled Meats

SEAWEEDS

BENEFITS

- An excellent source of iodine.
- Provides a wide spectrum of minerals, including calcium, copper, iron, magnesium, and potassium.
- Some types are rich in the B vitamins, vitamin C, and beta carotene.
- Some are a good source of protein.

DRAWBACKS

- Some are very high in sodium.

There are more than 2,500 varieties of seaweed, which include everything from the algae that forms on ponds to kelp and other marine plants. In general, seaweed is classified according to its color—brown, red, green, and blue-green.

A remarkably versatile and tasty vegetable, seaweed can be used in a broad spectrum of ways. In Japan, for example, seaweed makes up 25 percent of all food in the diet; it is also used to enhance flavors in a variety of dishes, from salads and soups to meat and seafood dishes. Kombu, a type of kelp (a brown plant that is one of the most common seaweeds), is used to flavor soup stocks. Wakame, another type of kelp, is used in Japan in soups and stir-fries.

Seaweeds are found in the diets of other cultures. For example, laver, a red algae called nori by the Japanese, is used by the Irish and Welsh to make flat cakes. The Scots use a seaweed called dulse to make soup. Irish moss, a red algae that is a major source of carrageenan, is used in the industrialized world as a thickening agent in such products as salad dressings.

An excellent source of many essential nutrients, including protein, most seaweeds are a rich source of iodine. The thyroid gland needs iodine to make the hormones that regulate body metabolism.

The mineral content of the various types of seaweed differ, but most provide calcium, copper, iron, potassium, and magnesium. Some supply beta carotene, a precursor of vitamin A; the levels vary with the cooking method.

Seaweed also tends to be low in calories; a ½-cup serving of kelp contains about

SEAWEED SEASONING

Dried sheets or strips of seaweed, or nori, impart a distinctive salty flavor due to their high sodium content. Sold at Asian groceries and health-food stores, nori is used to season salads, soups, and noodles and is soaked to use as wrappers for rice cakes and sushi.

MYTH BUSTER

Myth: Kelp tablets, spirulina, chlorella, and other seaweed supplements are energy boosters. Some alternative practitioners also claim that they boost the immune system.

Reality: None of these claims has ever been proved. In fact, some seaweed supplements can cause health problems. High doses of kelp tablets can set off an outbreak of acne. The high iodine content can cause thyroid disorders; and varieties containing iron can provoke iron overload.

50 calories. The same serving also provides 2 g of protein, almost 200 mcg (micrograms) of folate (50 percent of the adult Recommended Dietary Allowance, or RDA), 120 mg of magnesium (about 30 percent of the RDA), and useful amounts of iron and calcium. In comparison, a ½-cup serving of raw laver contains only 40 calories, and provides 6 g of protein, 5,200 IU of vitamin A as beta carotene, and 2 mg of iron. This type, however, contains less magnesium and calcium than kelp does.

The major drawback to seaweed is that many types are high in sodium. A ½-cup portion of raw wakame contains approximately 900 mg of sodium; an equivalent amount of dried spirulina yields more than 1,100 mg. (A recommended daily sodium intake for a healthy person should not exceed 2,400 mg.) The same amounts of kelp and laver are lower in sodium, containing 250 mg and 60 mg, respectively. However, anyone on a low-salt diet should avoid foods containing seaweed. ❖

SEX DRIVE

EAT PLENTY OF

- Fruits and vegetables for vitamin C.
- Oils, nuts and seeds, green vegetables, and wheat germ for a good supply of vitamin E.
- Meat, fish, legumes, nuts and seeds, and enriched or fortified cereals for iron.
- Oysters, meat, poultry, eggs, milk, beans, nuts, and whole grains for zinc.

LIMIT

- Saturated fats and alcohol.

AVOID

- Smoking.

Some people vouch for the effect of foods on their sex drive, but extravagant claims for aphrodisiacs are not borne out by scientific studies. While sexual function may be our physical response to a cascade of hormones, sexual drive is basically maintained by an active mind in a healthy body.

A healthy sex life depends on good nutrition. Good nerve function, healthy hormone levels, and an unobstructed blood flow to the pelvic area are essential to sexual performance. To keep these systems in working order, a diet should be based on legumes, grain products, and other complex carbohydrates, with plenty of fruits and vegetables and modest levels of protein; this diet provides plenty of vitamins and minerals. Particularly important are citrus fruits for vitamin C to strengthen blood vessel walls, and low-fat dairy products, enriched or fortified cereals, whole grains, and green vegetables for riboflavin to maintain the mucous membranes that line the female reproductive tract.

Vitamin E and sexual function. Although there are no confirming clinical studies, many experts believe that without a good supply of this vitamin from oils, margarine, nuts, seeds, green vegetables, and wheat germ, sexual function is likely to suffer.

Fatigue and depression are common culprits in sexual complaints. These conditions are often linked, and both may be helped by a program of regular exercise, which stimulates the production of endorphins (mood-elevating brain chemicals). In some cases, iron-deficiency anemia may be responsible for fatigue. A diet that includes meat, fish and shellfish, nuts and seeds, legumes, enriched or fortified grains and cereals, leafy greens, and dried fruits helps to replenish iron stores.

THE TRUTH ABOUT APHRODISIACS

- Herbalists recommend saffron as a sexual stimulant, but there is no evidence of its aphrodisiac effect. Some also recommend summer savory as a sexual stimulant and tonic, and winter savory to dampen sexual desire. Neither claim has ever been proved.

- Both the Food and Drug Administration (FDA) and Health Canada classify the herb ginseng as safe, but neither regulatory agency will allow claims for aphrodisiac or medicinal qualities. Studies show that ginseng boosts stamina and mating behavior in mice and rats. It's not a safe bet, however, that effects in mice and men are similar.

- Yohimbe, a tropical tree, is valued as an aphrodisiac in some countries. It has no effect on the mind but may dilate blood vessels and help with impotence. There are conflicting studies about its effectiveness.

- Spanish fly, an extract of dried cantharide beetles, causes irritation in the urinary tract and genitals, which some misinterpret as sexual stimulus. In reality, cantharidin, the active component, is a potentially lethal drug.

Consume more zinc. It is known that zinc is tied to sexual function, although its importance to the sex drive has yet to be explained. Without enough zinc, sexual development in children is delayed, and men, too, need zinc to make sperm. Zinc is found abundantly in foods of animal origin, including seafood (especially oysters), meat, poultry and liver, as well as eggs, milk, beans, nuts, and whole grains.

Eat a diet low in saturated fats. People readily accept the link between a high intake of saturated fats, elevated blood cholesterol levels, and a buildup of atherosclerotic fatty plaques on the blood vessels around the heart. It's less well understood, however, that similar plaques develop on the myriad tiny vessels in the penis. Without free-flowing circulation, the penis cannot physically respond to messages from the sex drive.

Curb alcohol consumption. Alcohol's effect on sexual function was neatly stated by William Shakespeare, who noted that wine "provokes the desire, but takes away the performance." Excessive alcohol lifts behavioral inhibitions, but this liberating effect may be canceled out by its depressant effect. Alcohol also has an action similar to the female hormone estrogen. This can have a devastating effect on masculinity, causing impotence and shrinking of the testes in men who drink heavily.

Stop smoking. Nicotine is an enemy of the arteries. Nicotine not only promotes the formation of atherosclerotic plaque in the penile blood vessels but also constricts them. ❖

SHELLFISH

BENEFITS

- A low-fat source of high-quality protein.
- A rich source of minerals, including calcium, fluoride, iodine, iron, and zinc.
- A good source of B-group vitamins.

DRAWBACKS

- Some are high in cholesterol.
- Susceptible to spoilage and environmental contamination.
- Can provoke allergic reactions in some people.

Shellfish is the catchall term applied to mollusks and crustaceans—water-dwelling creatures that wear their skeletons on the outside. Mollusks, such as oysters and mussels, lead a sedentary life inside rigid shells, which they affix with threadlike excretions to rocks or pilings. But octopus and squid, which are free swimming and have no shells (squid have a transparent internal quill, or beak), are also mollusks. Another exception is snails, which are mollusks that live on dry land or in water and move about, carrying their shells.

The soft bodies of crustaceans, such as lobster, shrimp, and crab, are covered by hinged plates of chitin, like suits of armor, that allow mobility but shield them from predators. Soft-shell crabs are taken in the molting season, when they have discarded their old shells but before the new shells have hardened.

NUTRITIONAL VALUE

Shellfish are among our most valuable sources of high-quality protein. In contrast to protein from warm-blooded animals, shellfish protein is very low in actual fat. Some varieties such as squid and shrimp contain fairly high levels of cholesterol. The warnings about the cholesterol content of shellfish have been tempered recently with the realization that dietary cholesterol appears to have relatively little effect on blood levels of cholesterol. Shellfish are very low in saturated fat, the lipid most likely to raise blood cholesterol levels. Shellfish also contain vitamin B_{12} and fewer calories, weight for weight, than other sources of animal protein do.

Shellfish are especially rich in minerals, including calcium and phosphorus needed for healthy bones and teeth; copper to help in the production of blood cells, connective tissue, and nerve fibers; iodine for thyroid gland function; iron for healthy red blood cells; magnesium for metabolism, bone growth, and production of genetic material; potassium for nerve and muscle function and general metabolism; selenium, an important antioxidant linked to lower cancer risk; and zinc for the immune system and reproductive health.

POTENTIAL DANGERS

If grown in polluted waters, shellfish may be contaminated with bacteria and carry a particular risk for hepatitis. Don't gather shellfish at the seashore or near wharf pilings or built-up areas. Instead, buy them from fish markets and food stores that keep shellfish well covered with ice or, in the

TALK OF TOXINS

Mussels accumulate toxins more quickly than other types of shellfish. In fact, scientists who monitor waters for poisons use them as an indicator species. Scallops, on the other hand, pose less risk than other bivalves because we don't eat the animal itself but the muscle that holds the shell halves together.

CAUTION

Many people are allergic to shellfish, and an allergic reaction to one type often means that the others should be avoided too. A severe reaction, with widespread hives, swelling, and difficulty breathing, indicates possible anaphylaxis, a life-threatening emergency. People allergic to shellfish may react to the iodine used in many of the dyes administered for contrast X-rays. Tell your doctor if you have ever experienced an allergic reaction to shellfish.

Nutrients in Different Shellfish

Low in saturated fat and high in protein, shellfish are rich
in B vitamins and are useful sources of trace minerals.
However, they are prone to contamination, so extra care should
be taken when buying, preparing, and cooking shellfish.
All values below are for 3½ oz (100 g) except where noted.

SHELL-FISH	PROTEIN (g)	FAT (g)	SODIUM (mg)	VITAMINS	MINERALS
Abalone (canned)	16	0.3	250	Good source of thiamine. Contains some riboflavin and niacin.	Good source of iron and magnesium.
Clams (raw)	12.6	1.6	60	Useful source of riboflavin and vitamins A and C.	Excellent source of iron, potassium, and zinc. Contain some calcium.
Crabs, Alaskan king (steamed)	19.3	1.5	180	Useful source of vitamin A, folate, and pantothenic acid. Some vitamin B_6.	Good source of zinc. Contain some iron, and magnesium.
Crabs, blue, Dungeness (steamed)	17.3	1.9	250	Useful source of pantothenic acid, niacin, and vitamins A and B_6.	Good source of zinc. Contain some iron, potassium, magnesium, and calcium.
Crabs, soft-shell (1 medium)	12	1.3	300	Fair source of niacin. Contain some vitamin B_6, riboflavin, and thiamine.	Good source of iron. Contain some calcium and magnesium.
Lobster (boiled)	18.7	1.5	350	Excellent source of vitamin B_{12}. Contains some folate.	Good source of zinc. Some magnesium, potassium, and calcium.
Mussels, blue (steamed)	22	4.2	570	Contain some vitamins A and E, riboflavin, thiamine, and niacin.	Good source of iron. Contain zinc and magnesium.
Oysters (meat only, raw)	14	5.1	205	Contains some thiamine, riboflavin, and vitamins A and C.	Rich in zinc. Excellent source of iron. Contain some magnesium.
Scallops, bay, sea (steamed)	23.2	1.4	160	Good source of vitamin B_{12}.	Contain some magnesium and zinc.
Shrimps (boiled)	20.8	1.1	222	Contain some niacin, vitamin B_6, and folate.	Fair source of iron. Some zinc and magnesium.
Squid (raw)	16.1	0.7	310	Contains some riboflavin.	Good source of iron. Contains some zinc.

case of lobsters, in tanks with circulating water aerated with oxygen. Shallow-water shellfish, such as clams and mussels, are the most susceptible to pollution; sea scallops and other deep-water varieties are less likely to be exposed to waste. Fresh shellfish may be covered with ice chips and stored for several hours at 32°F (0°C). Eat them on the day they are purchased.

Oysters are available year-round, and cooked oysters can be safely eaten at any time. Raw oysters, particularly those harvested in the Gulf states, can present a problem because of contamination with the *Vibrio vulnificus* bacterium. Contamination is more likely in the warm months because the bacteria do not tolerate cold water well. Diabetics, people with liver disease, and those with compromised immune systems have to be especially careful.

From time to time, swarming plankton cause the phenomenon known as "red tide" in coastal waters. Shellfish exposed to the red tide ingest the microorganisms, which produce a toxin that can survive cooking. The symptoms of red tide poisoning usually appear within 30 minutes of consuming contaminated fish; they include facial numbness, breathing difficulty, and muscle weakness. Never take shellfish from red-tide areas. ("Red tide" doesn't necessarily mean there is a red tinge to the water.) Mussels tainted with domoic acid, another toxin derived from algae, are undetectable by consumers.

Because of their susceptibility to spoilage, shellfish should be kept alive until they are ready to be cooked or served. Buy clams, mussels, and oysters only if the shells close tightly when tapped. An open shell indicates that the shellfish has died and is therefore not safe to eat. Conversely, when steaming or boiling mollusks in the shell, discard any that have failed to open by the end of the specified cooking time.

Fresh shellfish, whether in the shell or shucked, should smell briny, without any hint of iodine or fishiness. Oysters and clams show their freshness by "flinching" when you squeeze lemon juice on them.

Shrimp and crabmeat are exceptions to the live-shellfish rule. Most shrimp are trimmed and frozen in bulk at sea, then thawed for sale. Shrimp processed in this way should be labeled "previously frozen." Most crabmeat is cooked in the shell, or extracted and pasteurized, then frozen. Shellfish that is frozen or canned is usually ready to eat as purchased. Because crabmeat is separated from the shell by being passed through rubber rollers, however, it should be picked over to remove shell fragments.

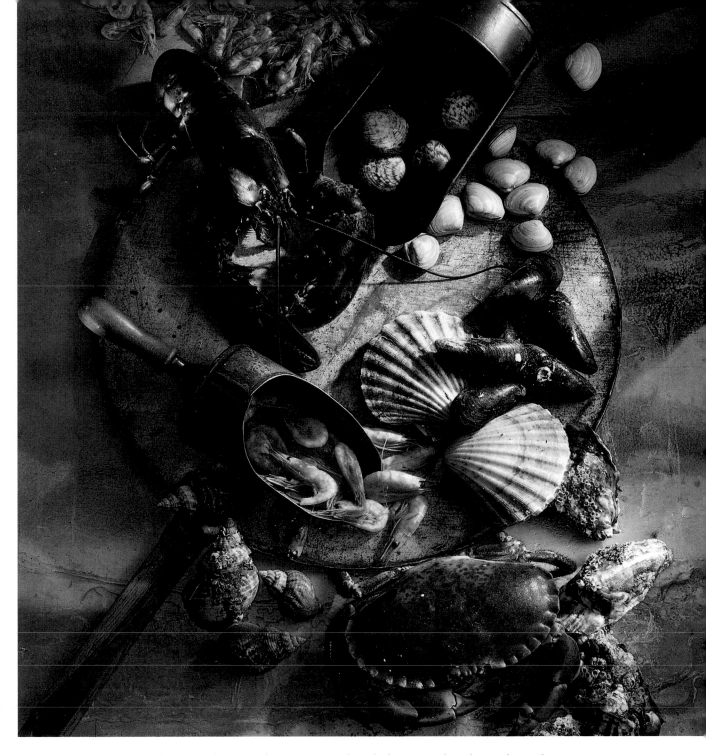

Don't eat lobster tomalley or crab mustard, soft organs that filter impurities and may have high levels of toxins.

PREPARING SHELLFISH

Like finned fish, shellfish have fragile flesh that should be cooked just to the point where its protein coagulates. Cooked too long, the tissues toughen or dry out and fall apart.

Commercially prepared shellfish are often needlessly high in calories and fat because they are coated with batter or bread crumbs and intended for frying.

The dips and sauces often served with shellfish add calories and saturated fat. Cocktail sauce is lower in calories and fats than tartar sauce. Minced shallots blended with lemon juice and herbs complement clams, lobsters, and other shellfish. To make a calcium-rich sauce, you can pound the shells of shrimp and lobster smooth, then boil them down with clam juice, lemon juice, white wine, and herbs. ❖

SEAFOOD PLATTER. *Shellfish are low in saturated fat and rich in heart-healthy omega-3 fatty acids.*

SHINGLES

EAT PLENTY OF

- Olive and other vegetable oils, nuts, seeds, and wheat germ for vitamin E.
- Fresh fruits and vegetables for antioxidants and bioflavonoids.

Herpes zoster, the medical term for shingles, is a reactivation of the varicella-zoster virus that causes chicken pox. What causes a reactivation of the virus is unknown, but it often develops when the immune system is suppressed.

An attack typically starts with a localized tingling and burning sensation of the skin. A few days later blisters similar to those of chicken pox develop. These blisters follow the path of a nerve. Serious complications can develop if the virus infects an eye or migrates to the brain.

Some doctors believe that good nutrition may help prevent postherpetic neuralgia, a long-term complication marked by nerve pain even after symptoms of shingles disappear.

Beneficial nutrients. Vitamin E, an antioxidant found in nuts, seeds, wheat germ, and vegetable oils, and the bioflavonoids found in fruits and vegetables that are high in vitamin C may also help prevent the inflammation associated with postherpetic neuralgia. Vitamin C supports your body's immune system, as do zinc-rich foods like seafood, meat, poultry, milk, yogurt, beans, nuts, and whole grains. If neuralgia does develop, however, the pain may be eased with applications of an ointment that contains capsaicin. ❖

SINUSITIS

CONSUME PLENTY OF

- Fluids such as water and juice.
- Fresh fruits and vegetables for vitamin C and bioflavonoids.
- Garlic, onions, and chilies to alleviate sinus congestion.

AVOID

- Smoking.
- Dry, overheated rooms.

Sinusitis is a painful inflammation of the membranes lining the sinus cavities in the skull. It occurs most often after a cold or in people who suffer from hay fever or other allergies involving the nasal passages. Normally, mucus produced by these membranes drains through narrow ducts into the nasal cavity. Acute sinusitis is usually the result of a viral, bacterial, or fungal infection. Chronic sinusitis is more apt to be caused by allergic reactions or dental infections.

Regardless of the cause, the sinus lining swells and blocks the passages, resulting in a stuffed-up feeling, and possibly swelling, and a deep, dull headache. A good clue in the diagnosis of sinusitis is that the pain tends to worsen whenever you bend over. There may also be a thick yellow or green nasal discharge. Depending upon the cause, a doctor may prescribe antihistamines, decongestants, antibiotics, or steroids.

DIETARY AND OTHER APPROACHES

Although nutrition does not play a direct role in sinusitis, some dietary measures may help. In one study, patients with chronic sinusitis reported improvement after eliminating milk products from their diets. People trying this approach should ask their doctor about supplements or increase their consumption of non-dairy calcium.

Fluids can help dilute secretions and promote drainage. Drink at least 8 to 10 cups daily of water, juice, tea, and even soup.

Eat plenty of fresh fruits and vegetables for vitamin C. Citrus fruits (rather than just the juice), grapes, and blackberries are useful because they also contain bioflavonoids, plant pigments that have anti-inflammatory properties. Vitamin E, too, has anti-inflammatory benefits. Dietary zinc is also an important immune booster and may have anti-inflammatory properties. Zinc-rich foods include seafood, meat, poultry, milk, yogurt, beans, nuts, and whole grains.

Some foods are natural decongestants. These include garlic, onions, chilies, and horseradish. Decongestant herbs and spices include ginger, thyme, cumin, cloves, and cinnamon.

If you smoke, make every effort to stop. Smoking causes nasal and sinus inflammation, as can secondhand smoke. Heat and dry air can produce swollen, dry nasal membranes that are predisposed to sinusitis; a humidifier may be a simple solution.

For fast relief, cover the face with hot, wet towels to promote drainage and increase blood flow to the area. Steam inhalation also promotes drainage. Hot tea may help reduce congestion; it contains theophylline, a compound believed to ease breathing by relaxing the smooth muscles in the walls of the airways. ❖

AN ALL-TOO-COMMON AILMENT

More than 40 million North Americans have at least one episode of sinusitis every year, making it one of the most common ailments. Researchers speculate that the dramatic rise in the incidence of sinusitis in the last 10 years may be due to increased pollution and increased resistance to antibiotics.

SLEEP AND DIET
■ EATING TO SLEEP WELL ■

The quality of sleep has an enormous impact on daily life, since poor or disordered sleep can affect your work, concentration, and ability to interact with others. During sleep, both physical and mental restoration take place, allowing you to feel fresh and alert in the morning.

Sleep needs vary from one person to another; the optimal average is 7 to 9 hours. You can judge whether or not you're getting the right amount by how you feel the next day—too much or too little sleep leave a person feeling tired and irritable. Because growth hormones are released during sleep, babies, children, and adolescents require more sleep than adults do.

Sleep researchers discount the common myth that older people require less sleep; instead, the amount of sleep that an adult needs remains fairly constant. With advancing age, however, the nature of sleep changes and the incidence of sleep disorders rises. The degree of time spent in the deeper stages of sleep often lessens with age, and an older person is likely to awaken more frequently during the night.

What makes us sleep?

This is still not fully understood, but scientists know that a person's circadian rhythm is established shortly after birth and is then maintained as a "body clock." Some natural chemicals in the body enhance sleep, and diet plays a part. Here are some things that are known to affect sleep:

■ **Eating too much or too little can disrupt sleep.** A light snack at bedtime can promote sleep, but too much food can cause digestive discomfort that leads to wakefulness.

■ **Alcohol is a double-edged sword.** Small amounts of alcohol can help you fall asleep. However, as the body metabolizes the alcohol, sleep may become fragmented. Alcohol can worsen insomnia and also impair rapid eye movement (REM) sleep, the time when the body is in its restorative phase. It can also dehydrate you, leaving you tired the next day.

■ **Caffeine can disturb sleep.** Any food or beverage that contains caffeine can disturb sleep, although this is not true for everyone. Research has shown that older adults who suffer from insomnia report higher caffeine intakes. If you are sensitive to caffeine, avoid it in the afternoon and evening.

■ **Forget the fat.** If you consume a high-fat meal in the evening or eat foods that you have found cause you indigestion and heartburn, your sleep can be disturbed and restless.

■ **Do not eat late at night.** People who suffer from heartburn or acid reflux should avoid late, heavy meals that delay the emptying of the stomach. Lying down with a full stomach puts you at a gravitational disadvantage, encouraging acids and gastric juices to flow up into the esophagus, causing uncomfortable heartburn that will make sleep more challenging.

■ **Drinking fluids too close to bedtime can cause problems.** Avoid fluids after dinner to reduce the need to go to the bathroom during the night.

A good night's sleep problem solver

■ Keep a sleep log for several weeks to help identify activities and behavior that may interfere with your sleep. Each day, write down the times you wake up and go to bed, and when you drink caffeinated beverages, exercise, and take naps.

■ Exercise regularly, preferably in the late afternoon. Do not exercise strenuously within 2 or 3 hours of bedtime, as this may impair your ability to fall asleep.

■ Don't take a long nap during the day; this may make it more difficult to fall asleep at night.

■ Eat at regular times during the day, and avoid a heavy meal close to bedtime.

■ After lunch, stay away from anything that contains caffeine.

■ Don't smoke; if you can't quit, at least try not to smoke for an hour or two before bedtime.

■ Avoid excessive mental stimulation before bedtime.

■ Establish a schedule to help regulate your body's inner clock. Go to bed and get up at about the same times every day, and follow the same bedtime preparations each night to create a sleep ritual.

■ A warm bath or a few minutes of reading in bed, listening to soothing music, or meditating are all useful sleep rituals. Try each one to see what works for you.

■ Keep your bedroom dark and quiet. If you can't block outside noise, mask it with an inside noise, such as the hum of a fan.

■ Use your bedroom only for sleeping, not for working or watching TV.

■ Wear nightclothes that are loose-fitting and comfortable.

■ If your worries keep you awake at night, deal with them some other time. Devote 30 minutes after dinner to writing down problems and possible solutions, and then try to set them aside.

■ If you can't sleep, don't stay in bed fretting for more than 15 minutes or so. Get up, go to another room, and read or watch TV until you are sleepy. Be sure to get up at your regular time the next day.

■ **Milk and honey promote sleep.** Milk contains tryptophan, an essential amino acid that is among the natural dietary sleep inducers. Tryptophan works by increasing the amount of serotonin, a natural sedative, in the brain. This is why so many folk remedies include warm milk with a teaspoonful of honey, a simple sugar. (Carbohydrates facilitate the entry of tryptophan into the brain.) A turkey sandwich provides another sleep-inducing combination of tryptophan and carbohydrates. A banana with milk gives you vitamin B_6, which helps convert tryptophan to serotonin.

Helpful herbs

Many herbs are said to be useful for inducing sleep; one of the most popular and reliable is valerian. Its qualifications as a sedative have been supported by research demonstrating that active ingredients in the valerian root depress the central nervous system and relax smooth muscle tissue. Valerian that is brewed into a tea or taken as a capsule or tincture can lessen the time it takes to fall asleep and produce a deep, satisfying rest. It does not result in dependency or cause a "hungover" feeling. Valerian is not recommended for use during pregnancy or breast-feeding, since it has not been studied for these conditions. Other herbal remedies that have been suggested for sleep problems include teas made of chamomile, hops, lemon balm, and peppermint, but there is not much evidence that they work.

The role of melatonin

A hormone produced by the brain, melatonin is instrumental in regulating the body's sleep-wake cycle. Researchers think that it may control the onset of puberty, a woman's menstrual cycle, mood, and the release of growth hormones. Melatonin can alleviate insomnia, although in some cases it has caused disturbed sleep (melatonin supplements are available in the United States, but their sale is not allowed in Canada). When taken correctly, it can prevent jet lag, but the many other claims for melatonin—for example, that it can prevent cancer, boost immunity, and forestall aging—are unproved.

Melatonin appears to be safe when it's taken in small amounts to overcome a temporary bout of insomnia. But experts caution against taking large doses or long-term use because of melatonin's potential side effects, which include grogginess, depression, and sexual dysfunction. Melatonin should not be taken by women who are attempting to conceive, pregnant, or breast-feeding; nor should it be administered to children or used by anyone with severe allergies, mental illness, rheumatoid arthritis or other autoimmune diseases, and lymphoma and certain other types of cancers.

Sleep disorders

Insomnia can be one of the symptoms of anxiety, depression, or stress, or it can be caused by a medical problem. Overcoming the underlying cause of these disorders is essential to improving the quality of sleep, but attention to nutrition and other aspects of sleep hygiene can also help.

Obesity may interfere with sleep if it affects breathing. Sleep apnea is a potentially serious sleep disorder in which a pattern of loud snoring builds to a crescendo, after which the person stops breathing and awakens briefly. It is more common in overweight people, especially middle-aged men. People with obstructive apnea can stop breathing for 10 seconds or longer a hundred or more times a night. Muscle cramps and restless legs, a vague discomfort relieved only by moving the legs, can also interfere with sleep.

SMOKED, CURED, AND PICKLED MEATS

BENEFITS

- Used sparingly, add flavor without excessive fat or calories.

DRAWBACKS

- Nitrites in preserved meats may form cancer-causing nitrosamines.
- High sodium content makes most unsuitable for people on low-salt diets.
- Preserved meats must be carefully handled to prevent food poisoning.
- Sausages made with corn solids or syrup or cereal fillers may cause symptoms in people sensitive to these grains.
- Cured meats may contain high levels of tyramine, which triggers migraine in susceptible people and causes serious reactions in those taking certain drugs.

Before the development of refrigeration, people the world over used similar methods for preserving meat: salting, smoking, and air drying. Although curing is no longer essential in industrialized countries, our taste for salty, smoky flavors persists.

Cancers of the esophagus and stomach are common where people eat large quantities of smoked and salt-cured foods. In North America, however, deaths due to stomach cancer have decreased in recent decades, even though consumption of smoked and processed meat has increased. In part, the reason for this may be that foods cured in North America are less heavily treated with preservatives than in countries where refrigeration is not widely available. Also, most foods sold as "smoked" are not smoke-cured but are flavored with liquid smoke, a smoke extract that does not have the same carcinogenic potential.

Warning: Tyramine, a metabolic product of the amino acid tyrosine, is found at high concentrations in cured meats. It can trigger migraine attacks in susceptible people. More seriously, it can cause an abrupt rise in blood pressure, headache, and even fatal collapse in persons taking monoamine oxidase (MAO) inhibitors to treat depression.

SMOKE CURING

Smoking preserves meat and fish both by slow cooking at a low temperature and by treatment with chemicals in the smoke. More than 200 components have so far been identified in smoke, including alcohols, acids, phenols, and several toxic—and possibly cancer-causing—substances. These chemicals inhibit the growth of microorganisms that cause meat spoilage, and the phenolic compounds slow the oxidation of fat and prevent it from becoming rancid. Smoking is now used primarily for flavor—for example, the distinctive hickory or oak aroma associated with smoked bacon, and mesquite and other aromatic wood chips that are used to enhance the taste of grilled foods.

AIR CURING

Air curing, or preserving by dehydration, has been used for thousands of years. Drying generally concentrates some nutrients, especially minerals, but the vitamin content of dried meat is much less than that of fresh. Native peoples dried venison, buffalo meat, and fish—sometimes mixing them with fat and dried berries—to make a nutritious and long-keeping food. Chipped beef is an air-dried throwback to pioneer preserving methods. Prosciutto is air-cured ham. As with other preservation techniques, air curing has been superseded by refrigeration and is now used mainly to give flavor and texture, although dried meats keep well.

SALT CURING

Whether in a brine solution or a dry salt bed, salt curing draws water from the meat and from bacteria and molds through the process of osmosis. While the meat remains wholesome, the microorganisms shrivel and die. We no longer need to salt meat to store it over the winter, but the method is still used because people like the taste of salty meats, such as ham and bacon.

The more salt used in curing, the better the meat's keeping qualities but the greater the loss of nutrients. When heavily salted meat is soaked to make it palatable, even more vitamins and minerals are lost. Today's curing solutions, however, are much weaker than those formerly used, and salted meat seldom needs to be soaked before cooking.

DID YOU KNOW?

HOW CORNED BEEF GOT ITS NAME

Years ago in England, when ice was the only refrigeration available, butchers faced a problem every Friday. They had to close for the weekend, but the ice would melt over two days and meat would spoil. To preserve the meat, butchers soaked it in strong brine or covered it with grains of coarse salt, called "corns." The name has stuck ever since.

SAUSAGES

Link sausages are usually made from pork with cereal fillers, herbs and spices, and preservatives.

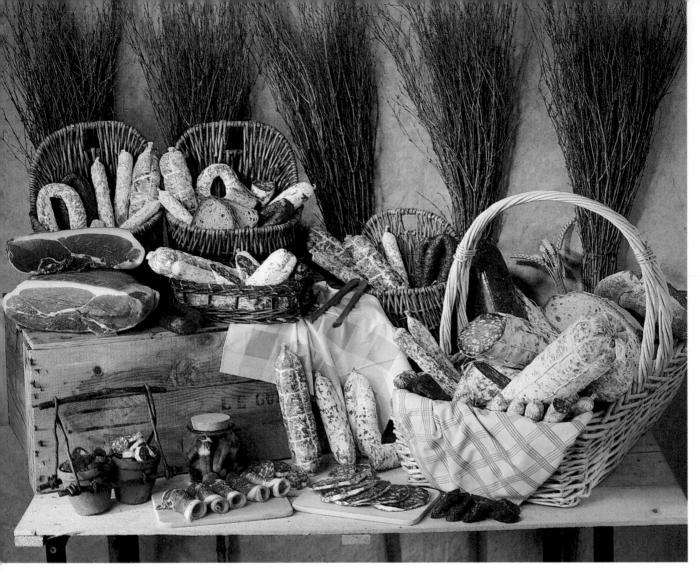

DELI DELIGHTS.
Smoked and cured meats such as salamis and prosciutto are tempting and tasty favorites, but their high saturated fat content means that they should be consumed in moderation.

People with celiac disease or who are allergic to corn or wheat should avoid sausages made with corn syrup or solids or cereal fillers.

Because sausages, like ground meat, go through several stages of handling, they are more susceptible to contamination than fresh meat and should be cooked very thoroughly before consumption.

Sausages in the wurst family vary in their meat, filler, and additive content. Kosher frankfurters and bologna generally contain less filler. In addition, kosher products must be made only with approved cuts of meat; they do not contain scraps and certain organ meats.

All pork and beef sausages are high in salt and saturated fat. Reduced-fat franks, knockwurst, and other sausages are available, but the benefits of lower fat may be offset by the higher amounts of salt added to boost flavor.

Liverwurst varies in ingredients according to the brand. While high in minerals, vitamins A and C, and the B vitamins, liverwurst is also high in saturated fat; several brands are flavored with bacon, which substantially raises the sodium content.

Dry salami and other sausages made by traditional methods are air cured, and sometimes smoked as well. Salami is the single exception to rules about discarding moldy meat; salami with a small amount of mold, or "bloom," may be eaten, provided that 1 in. (2.5 cm) of the meat surrounding the mold is cut away. Salami and other dried sausages contain high levels of saturated fat and sodium.

POTTED MEATS

Rarely eaten in North America, potted meats are popular in Europe. They are made by cooking pork, duck, or goose very slowly to render the fat. The well-cooked meat is then shredded (although small joints of poultry may be left whole), mixed with some of the fat, packed in earthenware or glass jars, and sealed with the remaining fat to keep out air. The shredded meats are usually spread on bread, while the whole joints are used in hearty, long-baked legume dishes. Potted meats conserve most of the nutrients of fresh meat, but they are extremely high in saturated fat and should be consumed only occasionally and in very small amounts.

NITRITES AND NITRATES

The reddish-pink color of cured meats, including the cold cuts at the deli counter, is due to the presence of nitrites, chemicals that enhance the effect of salt by inhibiting bacterial growth and slowing fat oxidation.

Critics claim that nitrites should be banned because they combine with amino acids during cooking and digestion to form cancer-causing nitrosamines. What's more, nitrite itself can cause tumors in laboratory animals that consume it in very high doses. But the meat industry and the government insist that nitrite should be retained because it is extremely effective against *Clostridium botulinum*, the microorganism that causes botulin poisoning, or botulism. They also point out that only about a fifth of the nitrites that form nitrosamines come from meats—the rest are formed in the body from nitrates in various plant foods.

C. botulinum thrives in oxygen-free surroundings (such as sealed cans, jars, and plastic packaging), and its spores survive long boiling. If vacuum-packed or canned meats are allowed to reach 50°F (10°C), any spores present may develop into active bacteria and produce the lethal toxin. Botulin toxin is destroyed at temperatures of about 160°F (70°C), but cold cuts are not usually cooked before eating, and even a baked or boiled ham may not be cooked long enough to reach a high enough temperature in the center.

Not only does nitrite suppress active bacteria, but it also weakens the heat-resistant *C. botulinum* spores. This means that the spores can be destroyed without the need for pressure cooking and reduces the risk that spores will develop if the meat is carelessly handled.

The risk of cancer from nitrites in the doses currently used in North America is much less than the risk of contracting botulism from tainted meat. However, even these risks are smaller than the risk of coronary disease from excessive consumption of the saturated fats that are, in general, plentiful in nitrite-preserved foods. If you enjoy smoked and salted meats, make sure you consume them only occasionally and in moderate amounts. ❖

SMOOTHIES

BENEFITS

- An excellent source of calcium.
- Fruits and vegetables add vitamins, minerals, and phytochemicals.
- A fast, tasty, nutritious breakfast or snack food.

Though often high in calories, smoothies have become popular with North Americans as a way to get high-quality nutrition in a glass. They are quick to make and a great way to give calcium to the kids; they can be breakfast made in a couple of minutes or a beneficial drink before or after a strenuous workout. All you need is a blender or food processor, fruits or vegetables, and yogurt or milk and you have a drink rich with vitamins, minerals, antioxidants, and great taste. A smoothie can also be a meal replacement for people on the go. Ideally it should contain a variety of foods and nutrients: vegetables and fruits, milk and milk products, a protein source, and grains.

You can make smoothies out of any combination of things, but typically they include milk and/or yogurt, fruits or vegetables, either fresh, canned, or frozen, and sometimes juice. The milk provides calcium, vitamin D, riboflavin, potassium, and more. One cup of milk contains 300 mg of calcium, 30 percent of the daily requirement, as well as 100 IU of vitamin D and 380 mg of potassium. If you are allergic to cow's milk or prefer not to drink it, you can use a fortified soy or rice beverage or even goat's milk. The fruits or vegetables provide vitamin C, folate, beta carotene, bioflavonoids, and other antioxidants.

The healthfulness of your smoothie can be boosted even further by adding a bit of wheat germ, flax, bran cereal, tofu, skim milk powder, some peanut butter, or even molasses. Making smoothies does not have to be complicated; check your refrigerator for any usable leftovers such as last night's fruit cocktail. Experiment with different flavors—sweet, tart, or a combination. If you are making an eggnog-style smoothie, don't use raw eggs because of the risk of salmonella poisoning. Use a pasteurized egg substitute instead. ❖

SUPER SMOOTHIE

For a nutrition-packed drink that will appeal to children, try a combination of banana and mango. Bananas are loaded with potassium and mangoes are rich in vitamin C. Dice half a ripe mango and blend it with a small banana, $2/3$ cup of low-fat milk, $1/2$ cup of orange juice, a teaspoon of sugar, and 2 tablespoons of frozen vanilla yogurt. On busy days this can serve as a quick breakfast.

SNACK FOODS

BENEFITS

- Snacks can help meet nutritional recommendations.
- Fruit and vegetable snacks are fat-free and high in vitamins and minerals.
- Well-timed, low-calorie snacks can take the edge off hunger and help to prevent overeating at mealtimes.

DRAWBACKS

- Snacking on candy bars and high-fat foods adds empty calories and fats.
- Many commercially prepared snacks and dips are high in sodium.

The human body is programmed to send out hunger signals whenever it needs an energy boost, which is usually between meals. The stores of carbohydrate (glycogen) in the liver and muscles, which help maintain a normal level of blood sugar, are used up in 4 to 6 hours. Food replenishes them, and snacks help.

Properly handled, snacking can be a healthy response to hunger. It can even help you lose weight by keeping your blood sugar levels steady so that you never get overly hungry. The trouble is that many people reach for a snack even when they're not hungry—while watching TV, attending a ball game, or simply out of boredom. And often the snacks they consume are poor nutritional choices—potato chips, candies, chocolate, nachos—foods often referred to as "junk" foods. Entire grocery store aisles are devoted to these fat-laden, calorie extravaganzas, and it's easy to fall into the trap of reaching for them. Weight gain can result.

Snacks don't have to be fattening. Eating a low-calorie snack during a long stretch between meals can take the edge off hunger and prevent overeating at the next meal. If snacks are well timed, they won't spoil the appetite for meals and may help to boost flagging energy, especially in children. Some people intentionally blunt their appetites with a low-calorie snack before an event where calorie-laden foods are served.

For many people, snacking or having frequent small meals is an alternative to the usual three large ones. This is a good solution for young children whose small stomachs can't consume enough at one sitting to sustain their need for energy. Older adults often can eat only small portions; supplemental snacks can help them to maintain a balanced diet. The same is true for people who are convalescing.

Fast-growing adolescents should snack to fuel their growth and compensate for lapses in their eating patterns. Athletes of all ages typically have an increased demand for energy, especially from carbohydrates, which the body converts to glucose, its major fuel. Pregnant women often suffer bouts of nausea during the early months, and heartburn or a feeling of constant fullness toward the end of pregnancy. Many are more comfortable snacking than eating a large amount at one time.

SMART SNACKING

If you are among those who snack regularly, it is important to consider snacks in your overall nutrition plan. Choose those that will provide balanced nutrition as well as energy.

Snacks can be the same as small meals, so a sandwich, a bowl of hearty vegetable soup, cheese and crackers, yogurt with fruit, or a low-fat muffin all make the nutritional grade. If you are looking for salty, crunchy taste, choose pretzels, bread sticks, low-fat pita crisps, or air-popped popcorn. Combine them with a low-fat yogurt-based dip or a bean dip to up the nutritional ante. Other healthy snacks include a bowl of cereal with low-fat milk and fresh fruit, or mini-pizzas made from English muffins or pitas topped with pizza sauce and part-skim mozzarella cheese.

Snacks can provide several of the recommended daily servings of starchy foods or the 5 to 10 servings of fruits and vegetables. Half a bagel with an apple, or a pita pocket filled with chopped raw vegetables, makes a filling, nutritious snack that can be worked into the day's meal plan. Other quick, low-fat foods, such as bags of fresh raw vegetables and dips such as hummus or other bean dips, or a mixture of low-fat yogurt or sour cream blended with herbs are good after-school snacks. For a satisfying beverage, make a latte (½ regular or soy milk and ½ decaffeinated coffee) or a smoothie out of yogurt, fruit, and juice.

PROOF POSITIVE

Some studies show that eating frequent small meals is a better weight-management strategy than eating one or two large meals. It's also an effective way to lower cholesterol and regulate blood sugar levels.

A study in England showed that middle-aged and older adults who ate frequently throughout the day had lower LDL cholesterol compared with those who tended to eat one or two large meals a day. In fact, many experts think that eating 5 or 6 small meals daily is best for overall health.

One strategy is to divide your food evenly over your waking hours, eating something small but nutritious every few hours.

DO ONE SIMPLE THING

TRY TO AVOID FOODS THAT CONTAIN TRANS FATS

Trans fats are in the same category as saturated fats as far as health risks are concerned. Try to reduce consumption of foods that list "hydrogenated" fats or oils as ingredients. The hydrogenation process, used by manufacturers to extend shelf life, leads to the production of trans fats.

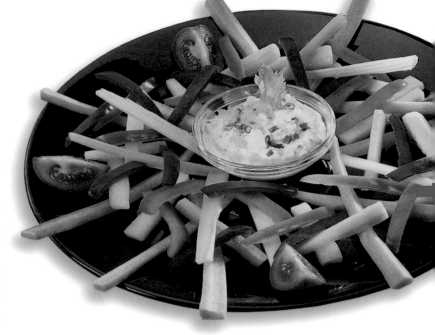

SNACK TRAPS

Everybody knows that a raw carrot is healthier than a frosted doughnut, but some snack foods that sound nutritious are not much better than a doughnut. Read labels carefully to find hidden sugar and fats.

Beware of granola bars; they are often loaded with sugar and fat. Fruit drinks may contain very little fruit juice but have large amounts of added sugar, such as high-fructose corn syrup. Microwave popcorn is often high in fat, as are trail mixes and other packaged combinations of nuts and seeds. Most commercial fruit rolls and pastes contain very little fruit and provide large amounts of added sugar and starch thickeners. Unsweetened apricot and other fruit leathers are usually made from pure fruit, but snackers should be careful to brush their teeth after eating them to remove clinging remnants that can promote cavities.

TWENTY 100-CALORIE SNACKS

SNACK	AMOUNT
Air-popped popcorn	3 cups
Almonds	16 to 20
Apple	1
Baked tortilla chips	10
Banana	1
Fig bars	2
Fruit-juice popsicle	1
Ginger snap cookies	2 2-in. (5-cm) cookies
Grapes	3/4 cup
Hard-cooked egg	1
Low-fat or nonfat yogurt, plain or artificially sweetened	1 cup
Low-fat string cheese	1 piece
Nonfat frozen yogurt	1/2 cup
Orange	1
Peanut butter	1 tablespoon
Pistachios (in shells)	1 handful
Pretzels	40 thin sticks
Pumpkin or sunflower seeds (in shells)	1 handful
Raisins	3 tablespoons
Sorbet	1/2 cup

COPING WITH HUNGER

If you look for a snack once hunger pangs have hit, you're likely to find yourself at the mercy of a vending machine. Instead, anticipate snack attacks with nutritious, low-calorie foods that require little preparation. Take snacks to work or buy them when you buy lunch.

Any number of simple and speedy solutions can fill in the gaps after school, work, or play. Canned, juice-packed mandarin orange slices, for example, mixed with a sliced banana, chopped apple, and a few frozen blueberries or other fruit make an instant fruit salad. For a quick dessert, cut a banana lengthwise, add nonfat frozen yogurt, and top with berries.

On cold days a cup of soup is a warming snack. Many canned and dried soups contain high levels of sodium, however, and may not be suitable for people on low-salt diets. Another hearty cold-weather snack is half a baked potato topped with low-fat cottage cheese and a sprinkling of chives.

Add several healthy snacking foods to your weekly shopping list. When you have the right foods on hand, it's easy to prepare snacks to take on trips, to school, or to work. Stay away from prepackaged high-fat items, such as potato and tortilla chips. If you can't resist cookies, you can sample the low-fat ones now on the market, but it's better to control fat and sugar content by making them at home.

Don't forget dental hygiene. Remind children to brush after snacking or to rinse their mouths vigorously with plain water. ❖

HEALTHY SNACK.
Snacking on healthy foods like vegetables and low-fat dip helps prevent overeating at mealtime.

THE SOFT DRINK-
FAST FOOD LINK

One reason that soft drinks are linked to obesity may be because they are often consumed with fast foods that are loaded with fat. The sugar in the soft drink activates the pancreas to produce insulin, but insulin also tells the body to store fat. So, as the pancreas is feeling the effects of the soda, the hamburger and fries arrive, and since the body has more insulin than it needs for the meal, it stores the fat instead of burning it.

SOFT DRINKS

BENEFITS

- Carbonated drinks are refreshing and may provide a quick energy boost from their sugar or caffeine.
- Sipping ginger ale or cola can help to quell nausea and provide energy for people unable to take solid food.

DRAWBACKS

- Contain large amounts of sugar and acids that can lead to weight gain and dental decay.
- High phosphorus content may interfere with calcium absorption.
- Caffeine may cause health problems in adults or behavior and development problems in children.

Carbonated waters were originally invented to cash in on an 18th-century fad for naturally sparkling mineral water. The taste for carbonated drinks (originally hangover cures) has never faltered; indeed, the average North American consumes about 48 gallons (182 liters) a year.

Soft drinks are broadly defined as nonalcoholic beverages, and carbonated soft drinks are classified as soda pop, or in some areas simply sodas or pop. They consist mostly of carbonated water mixed with sugar or an artificial sweetener, plus various patented natural or artificial flavorings, and coloring agents. Many of them also contain caffeine.

Apart from a quick energy boost from the caffeine or sugar, most soft drinks and soda pop offer little or no nutritional value. An 8-oz (240-ml) cola contains about 100 calories; a diet soft drink, because it is artificially sweetened, is less than 10 calories, although it may have caffeine.

HEALTH IMPLICATIONS

An occasional soft drink is fine, but drinking them regularly contributes empty calories that can add to weight problems. These drinks are also bad for the teeth. Their sugar encourages the growth of cavity-causing bacteria, and many contain acids that can erode tooth enamel.

Consumers should read labels carefully to determine what's actually in various soft drinks and mineral waters. Colas for example,

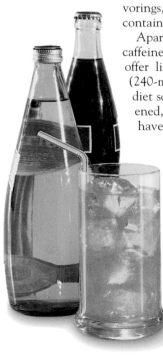

MEDICAL PROOF THAT SOFT DRINKS AND OBESITY ARE LINKED

A U.S. study published in *The Lancet* medical journal suggests that a soft drink a day gives a child a 60 percent greater chance of becoming obese. The study, from the Children's Hospital in Boston, Massachusetts, followed 548 children aged 11 and 12 for two school years. The researchers found that for every can or glass of sugar-sweetened beverage a child drank during that time, their body mass index inched up and their chances of becoming obese increased 60 percent. This held true regardless of initial body mass, diet, television viewing habits, and physical activity. One possible explanation for this link might be that while people tend to eat less at a meal if they have consumed excess calories at a previous one, they don't tend to do that if those extra calories come from beverages. It is not likely that a child would eat less food to compensate for the extra soft drink calories. The overall result would be that more calories are taken in than are burned off.

contain large amounts of phosphates, which may impair calcium absorption. A greater concern is that soft drinks cause a decrease in calcium intake by displacing milk from the diet. Children and adolescents who drink soft drinks instead of milk are missing the calcium critical to the growth of their bones. Some soft drinks and mineral waters may contain high levels of sodium. Also consider that when a 60-lb (27-kg) child drinks a 12-oz (355-ml) cola containing 50 mg of caffeine, he's getting the equivalent of a couple of cups of coffee in a 175-lb (80-kg) man. A child who is restless or sleepless may be experiencing the effects of too much soda pop. In adults, excessive caffeine may raise blood pressure and cause irregular heartbeats. People who react to caffeine should choose one of the decaffeinated soft drinks.

When patients can't take other foods and liquids, soft drinks can provide energy during the illness. Some people find that sipping flat ginger ale or cola quells the nausea associated with migraine and morning sickness.

Don't be misled by fruit-flavored drinks. On close reading, labels will disclose that noncarbonated fruit drinks often contain less than 10 percent fruit juice while harboring large amounts of sweeteners and dyes.

Soft drinks and soda pop need not be harmful if consumed in moderation. The danger is that if taken regularly in large amounts, they may satisfy hunger and take the place of essential nutrients in the diet. Children who fill up on sugary drinks shortly before and during meals may spoil their appetites for more healthful and nutritious foods.

HEALTHY DRINKS

You can make refreshing and economical drinks at home by mixing sodium-free seltzer or fruit-flavored sparkling waters with fruit juice, a mixture of chopped fresh fruit, or any of the wide variety of fruit nectars and syrups now sold in food stores and supermarkets. ❖

SORE THROAT

CONSUME PLENTY OF

- Fruits and vegetables for vitamin C.
- Yellow and orange fruits and vegetables and green vegetables for beta carotene.
- Seafood, lean meat, yogurt, and grains for zinc.
- Nonalcoholic and caffeine-free fluids.

AVOID

- Alcohol and tobacco smoke.

A raw, stinging throat can often be the first sign of a viral upper respiratory infection, such as a cold or flu, or less commonly, a bacterial infection, such as a strep throat. In children, swollen and infected tonsils can cause a sore throat; among adults, smoking is a common cause of mild, chronic throat pain. Respiratory viruses and strep organisms spread easily from one person to another, but attention to hygiene and good nutrition helps prevent many episodes.

DIETARY FACTORS

Get lots of vitamin C. Although scientific evidence is lacking, many people are convinced that high doses of vitamin C help to reduce the duration and severity of a sore throat and other symptoms of viral respiratory infections. Like other antioxidants, vitamin C is instrumental in immune function, so adequate amounts can protect against viruses, bacteria, and other infectious agents. What constitutes "adequate," however, remains unresolved. A recent study indicates that 200 mg of vitamin C a day may be a more optimal amount than the present Recommended Dietary Allowance (RDA) of 75 to 90 mg. This same study found that doses above 200 mg are of no added benefit, because body tissues are unable to absorb more than that amount. Indeed, for many people, higher amounts may be detrimental because they can lead to iron overload and other problems.

Eat plenty of fruits and vegetables. It is recommended that we eat 5 to 10 servings of fruits and vegetables a day, and such a diet can easily provide 200 mg of vitamin C, as well as other essential vitamins and minerals. Especially rich sources of vitamin C include citrus and other fruits, berries, red peppers, melons, and dark green vegetables. One cup of orange juice or 1 cup of strawberries contains more than 100 percent of the Recommended Dietary Allowance for adults. These foods are also high in beta carotene, which the body converts to vitamin A, another antioxidant that is instrumental in building immunity.

Try zinc lozenges. Several studies have demonstrated that zinc lozenges can shorten the duration and/or severity of a sore throat. A diet that provides adequate zinc strengthens the body's immune defenses. Good sources include yogurt and other dairy products, oysters and other seafood, lean meat, eggs, and grains. Taking zinc supplements for a cold or as a preventive measure is not a good idea since getting more than 40 mg per day for an extended period of time can weaken your immune system, making it less able to fight against disease.

Avoid alcohol. Alcohol, which reduces immunity and irritates inflamed mucous membranes, should be avoided until the sore throat clears up. It's also a good idea to cut down on, or eliminate, caffeine; its diuretic effect increases the loss of body fluids and results in a drying of the membranes and thickening of mucus. Make every effort to stop smoking, and avoid secondhand smoke.

EASING SYMPTOMS

Nonalcoholic fluids, whether hot or cold, can alleviate painful swallowing. Some doctors even advise temporarily switching to a liquid diet to maintain nutrition without exacerbating throat pain. Good choices include milk shakes, fruit juices, broths and soups, and semiliquid foods such as custards, puddings, and gelatin.

Home sore throat remedies abound, and many are useful in alleviating symptoms. The most time-honored favorite is to gargle with salty warm water; you can make an alternative gargle by adding 2 teaspoons of cider vinegar to a half cup of warm water. ❖

DO ONE SIMPLE THING

SOOTHE A SORE THROAT WITH LEMON TEA

Lemons are loaded with vitamin C and can make a soothing and beneficial drink for sore throats when made into a hot drink. Squeeze the juice of a lemon into a cup of boiling water and add a teaspoon of honey.

SOUPS

BENEFITS
- Can be highly nourishing.
- An ideal food for convalescents.
- Easy to make and economical.

DRAWBACKS
- Commercial soups are generally high in salt and fat.

THE SOUP SOLUTION. *Whether it's a pasta and vegetable minestrone, a creamy carrot, apple and tomato combination, or a Thai-inspired broth with shrimp, soup is easy to make and nutritious.*

Nourishing, comforting, and inexpensive, soup is a staple food worldwide. Broth-based soups may even facilitate weight loss. In one study, the more soup people ate, the fewer calories they took in overall and the more weight they lost. One likely reason is that soup is high in volume, so it helps you feel full on fewer calories. (That doesn't mean that the fad diet based on cabbage soup is an effective way to lose weight. Like any severely restrictive diet, you'll get tired of it in no time and go back to your old eating habits.)

HOMEMADE SOUPS

Even a novice cook can make a delicious soup with a few basic ingredients: diced carrots, potatoes, and other vegetables simmered in a broth with herbs. Leftover meat or seafood can be added for more flavor and nutrition. Cooks who have the inclination can simmer leftover bones with vegetables to make a soup stock; reduced-sodium canned broths are also acceptable. Bouillon cubes can be used, but they are high in monosodium glutamate (MSG), sodium, and other additives; always taste the soup before adding salt or seasonings.

Although some vitamins may be lost during the slow cooking of vegetables, soups made with fresh ingredients still provide an excellent variety of nutrients, including vitamins, minerals, and protein. Vitamin loss can be minimized by adding the vegetables toward the end of the cooking process, bringing the soup to a boil, and cooking only until the vegetables are barely tender.

Making your own soup allows you to control the salt content, an important consideration for people with high blood pressure or those who are on a sodium-restricted diet. Use herbs and natural vegetable flavors to replace salt.

Chilling the stock forces any fat to congeal on the surface and makes it easy to remove for fat-free soups. Another way to remove the fat is by pouring the stock through a defatting cup. Cream soups and New England-style chowders contain higher amounts of saturated fat, but this can be reduced without losing flavor or texture by substituting evaporated skim milk for cream and whole milk. "Cream" soups can also be made with pureed cooked potatoes and milk.

COMMERCIAL SOUPS

Canned and instant soups have varied quality and nutritional value. Choose soups low in fat and sodium. Although canned soups are not as nutritious as homemade, they are better than instant soups, which are so highly processed that some experts have described them as little more than a mix of MSG, artificial flavors, sodium, dyes, and additives.

TYPES OF SOUP

Soups fall into one of six types. Cooking methods and ingredients frequently overlap.

- Chowders, such as bouillabaisse, combine coarsely chopped vegetables and fish, shellfish, or meat with stock for a thick, stewlike consistency.
- Clear broths, such as consommé or bouillon, are strained concentrated stocks made from a mixture of aromatic vegetables, either cooked in water or beef or chicken broth. Noodles, vegetables, and diced meat may be added to the strained broth. Some broths are thickened with a beaten egg just before serving. When a concentrated beef or chicken consommé is chilled, its natural aspic forms a solid jelly, which is a digestible and nutritious food for convalescents.
- Cold soups, such as the Spanish gazpacho and Scandinavian-style fruit soups, are always served chilled. Others, such as the leek-and-potato vichyssoise, can also be served hot.
- Cream soups, based on vegetables, meat, or seafood, are often thickened either with the same roux that is used for sauces or with cream. The fat and calorie content of cream soups can be drastically reduced by it with evaporated skim milk or double-strength reconstituted skim milk. (Low-fat yogurt can be used instead of sour cream in some soups, but it will curdle if the soup is boiled.)
- Vegetable purees (potage) are smooth and made from vegetables simmered in stock or other liquid, then blended or sieved.
- Vegetable soups, including minestrone, are made with chopped vegetables that are boiled quickly in water or stock. They are thickened with rice or pasta. ❖

SOY

BENEFITS

- A vegetarian source of high-quality protein and iron.
- A good source of B vitamins, potassium, zinc, and other minerals.
- Low in calories and saturated fat.

DRAWBACKS

- Fermented soy products are high in sodium and may provoke allergies.
- Soy protein may hinder iron absorption.

For many years, soy foods in North America were enjoyed mainly by vegetarians as an alternative to meat products. But in recent years as more consumers have pursued healthier lifestyles, the consumption of soy foods has risen steadily, bolstered by growing evidence of the many health benefits of these versatile foods. Research continues, however, as some questions about soy and its health effects remain unanswered.

Soybeans are one of the most nutritious and versatile plant foods available. Volume for volume, soy contains more protein than beef, more calcium than milk, more lecithin than eggs, and more iron than beef.

Soybean protein contains all of the essential amino acids, making it the only plant protein that approaches or equals animal products in providing a complete source of protein. This makes it a terrific choice for those looking for alternatives to meat products. Soybeans are also good sources of B vitamins and potassium, zinc, and other minerals. And to top it off, soybean oil is low in saturated fat, unlike the fat from animal sources. Soy contains important phytochemicals, including isoflavones, saponins, lignans, and phytosterols, all of which have a variety of positive effects on the health.

DO ONE SIMPLE THING

ADD FOODS HIGH IN VITAMIN C TO YOUR MEAL TO IMPROVE IRON ABSORPTION

Although many soy products are high in iron, it is not well absorbed. Improve absorption by adding foods high in vitamin C to your meal, such as orange juice, tomatoes, peppers, strawberries, or melons.

HEALTH BENEFITS OF SOY

The beneficial effect of soy foods on heart disease, some cancers, osteoporosis, and menopausal symptoms is the focus of much research. There is great deal of epidemiological evidence (studies of populations) supporting the health-protective effects of soy. For example, populations that

THE MANY FACES OF SOY

Tofu. Comes in firm, soft, or silken textures. It's made from pureed soybeans and processed into a "cake." This versatile food can be stir-fried, grilled, added to soups, lasagna, cheesecake, or blended into dips or smoothies.

Soy beverages. Can be bought fresh or in tetra packs. They can be substituted for other beverages or for milk in recipes. Some products are fortified with calcium and vitamin D, and they come in many flavors such as vanilla, chocolate, and coffee.

Soybeans. Convenient to use, canned soybeans just need to be rinsed before being added to casseroles, soups, or chili, or being mashed and added to veggie burger recipes.

Green soybeans (*edamame*). Edamame are bought shelled or still in the pod and can be served as a snack or a vegetable dish.

Soy flour. Adds protein to recipes when substituted for all-purpose flour. It can also be found in cereals, pancake mixes, frozen desert, and other common foods.

Textured vegetable protein. It is made from defatted, dehydrated soy flour. Once rehydrated, it can be used as a meat substitute in a variety of dishes, including chili, meat loaf, pasta sauce, or lasagna.

Tempeh. Made from fermented soybeans and formed into a chewy cake, this meat substitute can be used in a variety of dishes.

Miso. It is a delicious fermented soybean paste, and can be used as a base for soups or as a seasoning.

Soy nuts. These tasty nuts have more fiber and less fat than other nuts. They can be enjoyed as a snack or sprinkled on salads or in stir-fries.

Soy protein powders. Made from isolated soy protein, these powders can be added to shakes or smoothies for a protein-powered breakfast.

include high amounts of soy in their diet have low rates of breast cancer, prostate cancer, and menopausal symptoms. However, the evidence is stronger for some health benefits than for others:

HEART HEALTH

This is where the research is conclusive. A large body of evidence indicates that replacing some animal products with soy protein can reduce the risk of heart disease. This is because soy lowers levels of the artery-clogging LDL (low-density lipoprotein) cholesterol without reducing levels of the beneficial HDL (high-density lipoprotein) cholesterol. The evidence is so convincing that the U.S. Food and Drug Administration recently gave food manufacturers permission to put labels on products that are high in soy protein indicating that these foods may help lower the risk of heart disease.

CANCER

Throughout Asia, where soy has long been a dietary staple, the rates of breast and prostate cancer are much lower than in Western countries. Epidemiological studies of Asians show that it is soy intake early in life that is protective. Soy foods contain compounds called isoflavones, which are a subclass of a much larger group of food components called flavonoids. Genistein and daidzein are the two main types of isoflavones found in soy. Some researchers attribute the low incidence of these cancers to these isoflavones, which reduce the effects of estrogen on breast and prostate tissue. Estrogen is thought to stimulate tumor growth in genetically susceptible people. However, the evidence regarding soy and its effect on cancer rates is still inconclusive, and much more research needs to be done. While there is evidence that soy plays a role in preventing breast cancer, the jury is out on its effect in women who have the disease. The prudent recommendation is that they should consume soy in moderation and not increase their intake in response to a diagnosis of breast cancer.

OSTEOPOROSIS

Recent research has indicated that soy isoflavones may delay bone loss and might even build bone density. Not all research is consistent in this finding, however, with some studies showing no effect of soy on bone loss.

MENOPAUSAL SYMPTOMS

For some women, diets rich in soy foods can reduce menopausal symptoms, particularly the frequency and severity of hot flashes. The extent of improvement, however, varies from woman to woman.

SOME AREAS OF CAUTION

While there is agreement that soy foods offer distinct health benefits, some researchers have cautioned that there may be some health risks as well, particularly for those who consume large amounts of these foods, or who take soy supplements. Concerns have been raised about the effects of soy on the following:

- Cancer. We still have a lot to learn about isoflavones and how they work. Some recent findings have suggested that high isoflavone levels might actually increase the risk of certain cancers, particularly breast cancer. The concerns have mostly been raised with regard to isolated isoflavones in supplement form, not in whole soy foods. However, until further research helps clarify the role of isoflavones in human health, it is wise to avoid isoflavone supplements in general. People who are being treated, or who have been treated, for breast or prostate cancer should speak to their physician and/or exercise caution before adding soy to their diet.
- Dementia. Results of a recent study suggested that consuming tofu two or more times a week might increase the risk of dementia. At this point, this study raises more questions than it answers, and these results have not been supported by any other studies to date. In addition, this effect has not been seen in population studies looking at those who consume high amounts of soy foods.
- Thyroid function. Some studies have linked soy consumption to suppressed thyroid function. It appears that the risk is linked only to taking soy supplements or eating huge amounts of soy foods, but more research is needed to clarify this relationship.
- Infant formula. The National Institutes of Health is sponsoring a long-term study on the safety of soy infant formula. The study will compare young adults who consumed soy formula as infants with young adults who consumed milk-based formulas as infants. This study is a follow-up of earlier research findings that show high levels of isoflavones in the blood of infants who were consuming soy formula.

THE BOTTOM LINE

Overall, soy is a nutritious, beneficial food, and a welcome addition to a healthy diet. But it should be regarded as a food, not as a medication. It is a terrific protein substitute and can be used as an alternative to animal proteins. It can help protect us from coronary heart disease, and may help relieve menopausal symptoms for some women. It may also protect us from hormonally driven cancers and offer some protection from osteoporosis.

However, all foods, including soy, are complex mixtures of substances that researchers are only just beginning to understand. Many components are proving beneficial, but there is the risk with any food or component of food that they can also be harmful in certain amounts and for certain people. Don't overdo it and don't take soy or isoflavone supplements. Once again, there's no substitute for a balanced diet that includes a wide variety of wholesome foods in moderate amounts. ❖

ASIAN FLAVOR. *Triangles of tofu stir-fried with thin slices of meat and vegetables is a delicious way to include soy in your diet.*

SPICES

BENEFITS

- Add a variety of flavors to foods.
- Can act as an appetite stimulant.

Centuries ago, the taste for spices kindled international trade and sparked voyages of discovery. Today, spices are still prized for the variety they lend to the diet.

For thousands of years, spices have been used as flavorings, medicines, perfumes, dyes, and even as weapons of war. They can stimulate the appetite and add flavor and interest to humdrum dishes. Characterized by pungent aromas and flavor, spices are the fruits, flowerbuds, roots, or bark of plants. While they are rich in minerals, spices are used in minute amounts, so they provide little nutritional value. Because spices lose their pungency on exposure to light, heat, and air, store them in a dark, dry cupboard and replace them annually.

SPICY REMEDIES

Through the ages, spices have been used as remedies for almost every ailment. Although most specific health claims have not been borne out by scientific studies, several of the most popular traditional uses do seem to be grounded in fact.

Allspice gets its name from its flavor, which seems to blend the aromas of cinnamon, nutmeg, and cloves. It is believed to aid digestion.

Black pepper, like white pepper, is the fruit of a tropical vine; it accounts for 25 percent of the world's spice trade. Sniffing ground pepper may help prevent fainting attacks.

Caraway is a member of the carrot family. Caraway seeds are especially popular as a flavoring for breads, cakes, cheese, and red cabbage and other vegetable dishes. Drinking an infusion of caraway may stimulate milk flow in nursing mothers. The chemical called limonene in caraway may reduce cancer risk.

Cardamom is used to flavor coffee in Arab countries, sweet breads in Scandinavia, and to enhance the flavor of cooked fruit. Cardamon is also recommended to relieve indigestion.

Cayenne (also called chili pepper) and related spices are used to flavor the hot dishes of Mexico and many other countries. Capsaicin, a volatile oil, gives chilies their "bite" and is used as a topical painkiller. Consumption of cayenne and other fiery substances is thought to stimulate the production of endorphins, the brain's natural mood enhancers, which may explain the euphoria people feel after eating spicy food. Cayenne may help reduce the discomfort from allergies, colds, and flu.

Cinnamon, an ancient spice obtained from the dried bark of two Asian evergreens, is a highly versatile flavoring as well as a carminative that relieves bloating and gas. Cinnamon may have antibacterial and antimicrobial properties and may also reduce discomfort from heartburn.

Clove oil, long used as a home remedy for toothaches, is no longer recommended for this purpose because it can burn mucous membranes. However, eugenol, a mild derivative, is a popular flavoring ingredient in some brands of mouthwash and toothpaste. Eugenol may prevent heart disease by preventing blood clots from forming.

Coriander has been used as a digestive tonic since ancient times. The freshly chopped greens in large amounts are a good source of vitamin C. Coriander seed is thought to be helpful in relieving stomach cramps and may have the ability to kill bacteria and fungus. It contains limonene, which is a flavonoid thought to help fight cancer.

Cumin, a hot spice, blends well in chili, curries, and such Middle Eastern specialties as hummus. It is being investigated for potential antioxidant and anticancer effects.

Ginger, popular in Asian dishes as well as in desserts and soft drinks, is a common motion sickness remedy; sipping flat ginger ale may help to ease nausea. Substances in ginger—gingerol, shogaol, and zingiberene—have antioxidant capabilities that may help prevent heart disease and cancer. Also an anti-inflammatory, ginger may help against arthritis.

Juniper berries are used in pâtés and sauerkraut; the pungent berries also give gin its flavor. In large doses, juniper acts as a diuretic that may also cause uterine contractions.

Mustard has been used in poultices and smelling salts to relieve pain and congestion since Roman times. Mustard seeds contain allyl isothiocyanates, which studies suggest inhibit the growth of cancer cells.

Nutmeg and mace come from the same plant; nutmeg is the shelled seed, mace its hull. Very high doses of myristicin, a component of nutmeg oil, cause hallucinations. Eugenol, a monoterpene in nutmeg, is thought to help prevent heart disease by preventing blood cells from forming clots. Nutmeg may also have antibacterial properties that may destroy the foodborne bacteria *E.coli*.

Saffron, the most expensive of all spices, is obtained from the stamens of a single variety of crocus. It is used to flavor vegetable soups, rice dishes, fish, and sweet rolls. It is sometimes touted as an aphrodisiac.

Star anise gets its licorice flavor from an oil containing anethole. Anethole-based flavorings have long been used in cough syrups and digestive preparations, as well as in ouzo, arak, and anisette liquors. Star anise teas should not be given to children with colic. Doctors have reported a number of adverse reactions.

Turmeric is an essential ingredient of Indian curries and gives mustard its yellow color. Turmeric is a natural antibiotic that Ayurvedic practitioners use to treat inflammation and digestive disorders. ❖

SPINACH

BENEFITS

- A rich source of vitamin A (as beta carotene), vitamin K, folate, and potassium.
- Contains vitamins C and B$_6$ and riboflavin.

DRAWBACKS

- Oxalic acid reduces iron and calcium absorption, and can accelerate the formation of kidney and bladder stones.

Contrary to popular belief, spinach is not an especially good source of iron. The myth about its high iron content arose from an analysis in which a decimal point was erroneously dis-

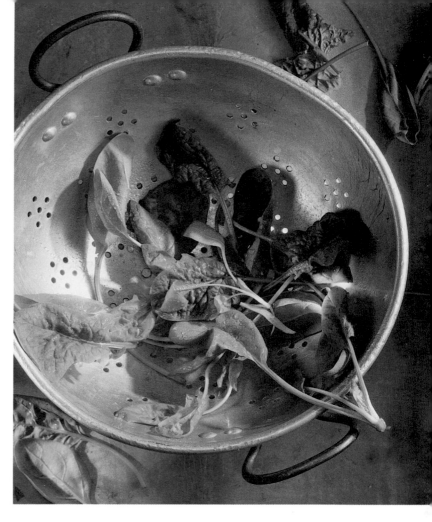

placed. But the vegetable's dark green leaves do contain many other valuable nutrients, especially the antioxidants and bioflavonoids that help block cancer-causing substances and processes. For example, spinach is rich in carotenoids, plant pigments that are responsible for its dark green color. Among these carotenoids are lutein and zeaxanthin, which help prevent macular degeneration, the leading cause of blindness in older adults. Cooking spinach helps to convert lutein into more bioavailable forms. To enhance the carotenoid absorption, eat spinach with some heart-healthy fat.

A half cup of cooked spinach provides a full day's supply of vitamin A and 105 mcg (micrograms) of folate, more than 25 percent of the Recommended Dietary Allowance (RDA). Folate is especially important for women who are pregnant or who may be planning a pregnancy, because it helps prevent congenital neurological defects. Folate deficiency can also cause a severe type of anemia. This half-cup serving of spinach also contains 419 mg of potassium, as well as vitamin C, riboflavin, and vitamin B$_6$.

VERSATILE VEGETABLE. *Young spinach leaves are delicious raw or lightly cooked. Either way, you should wash them thoroughly and discard damaged leaves and tough stalks.*

CAUTION

Excess vitamin K can counteract the effects of blood-thinning medication such as heparin and warfarin (Coumadin). If you are on these medications, it is wise to moderate your intake of vitamin K-rich foods, such as spinach.

On the negative side, the nutritional benefits of spinach are somewhat offset by its high concentration of oxalic acid. Spinach does contain iron, calcium, and other minerals, but their absorption is hindered by oxalic acid. Absorption can be increased by consuming spinach with other foods that are rich in vitamin C. Oxalic acid can also pose a problem for people susceptible to kidney and bladder stones that form from oxalates.

Phylloquinone is the most common form of vitamin K found in dark greens such as spinach. Vitamin K is needed for proper blood clotting and it may play a role in preserving bone health. Some research suggests that it may increase bone density and reduce fracture rates. Both the Nurses' Health Study and the Framingham Heart Study found that people who consume the most vitamin K have a lower risk of hip fractures than those who consume less.

SERVING SPINACH

Spinach can be served either raw or cooked. To avoid overcooking, try steaming or stir-frying it. These cooking methods preserve texture and flavor, and they minimize the loss of many water-soluble vitamins. Although some of these nutrients are lost in cooking, a ½-cup serving of the cooked vegetable actually provides more nutrition than 1 cup served raw because it takes a full 2 cups of leaves to cook down into a ½-cup serving. In addition, heating makes the protein in spinach easier to break down. The value of raw spinach can be enhanced by serving it with citrus slices for added vitamin C.

Before serving spinach, be careful to remove all the sand and dirt. One effective method is to submerge the spinach in a bowl of cold water and let the sand fall to the bottom, then remove and rinse the leaves. Dry them if making a salad. If you are cooking the spinach, the water left on the leaves may be just about the right amount with which to steam it. ❖

POPEYE'S SECRET WEAPON

Spinach's biggest fan may be Popeye the Sailorman. He first appeared on the scene with his trusty can of spinach at the ready in a 1929 comic strip. He jumped to the silver screen in 1933 and went on to star in nearly 600 Popeye cartoons. And it was always spinach that gave the indomitable sailor the strength to triumph over adversity.

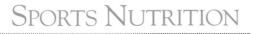

SPORTS NUTRITION

See Food and Fitness

SQUASH

BENEFITS

- Summer varieties provide some folate and vitamins A and C.
- Winter varieties are extremely rich in beta carotene and are a good source of potassium and fiber.

Members of the same family as melons and cucumbers, all types of squash are gourds—fleshy fruits protected by a rind. Squash is divided into two categories. The summer squashes include the chayote, patty pan, yellow crooknecks and straightnecks, and zucchini varieties. Acorn, banana, buttercup, delicata, dumpling, hubbard, spaghetti, and turban varieties make up the group called winter squashes. The flowers, immature and mature fruits, and seeds are all edible.

SUMMER SQUASH

Eaten while immature, summer squash has a soft rind and tender flesh. Because it has a high water content, it is low in calories (20 per cup, raw). A one-cup serving of raw summer squash provides about 15 percent of the Recommended Dietary Allowance (RDA) of vitamin C, 25 mcg (micrograms) of folate, and small amounts of beta carotene, which the body converts to vitamin A. Intensely colored squashes have more beta carotene than paler ones.

Summer squash can be eaten raw. If it is cooked, stir-frying or steaming minimizes nutrient loss and keeps the vegetable from becoming too mushy. The mild flavor complements stews, soups, and mixed vegetables, but squash can make some dishes watery. To avoid this problem, lightly salt the squash slices or pieces and place them on absorbent paper towels; rinse the pieces before adding them to the recipe.

WINTER SQUASH

Harvested when fully mature, winter squash has a hard shell and large seeds. It is larger, darker in coloring, and richer in nutrients than summer squash. Winter squashes such as acorn and butternut are rich in beta carotene, but the amount varies with the color of the flesh. Half a cup of acorn squash contains enough beta carotene to fulfill almost 100 percent of the RDA for vitamin A; 1 cup of light spaghetti squash provides less. A ½-cup serving of baked winter squash has at least 10 percent of the RDA of vitamin C, 450 mg of potassium, and 40 calories. Winter squash also has more fiber, more than 3 g per ½-cup serving. The strings and seeds are high in insoluble fiber, which helps prevent constipation; the flesh contains soluble fiber, which lowers cholesterol.

Winter squash can be stored for several months in a cool, dark place. Do not refrigerate it, because temperatures below 40°F (4°C) speed its deterioration.

Bake or steam winter squash; boiling is not recommended, because it destroys vitamin C and other nutrients. You can serve it with herbs and a little butter or margarine, stuffed and baked, or add it to breads, soups, and stews. It can be substituted for pumpkin in pies.

The seeds can be dried or baked for a snack; they are an excellent source of iron, potassium, zinc, and other minerals. They also provide some protein, beta carotene, and B vitamins. ❖

STRAWBERRIES

BENEFITS

- An excellent source of vitamin C.
- Contain folate and potassium.
- Low in calories and high in fiber.
- Provide anticancer bioflavonoids.

DRAWBACKS

- Provoke allergies in many people.
- Contain oxalic acid, which reduces mineral absorption and may aggravate kidney and bladder stones.

Strawberries are delicious, low in calories (about 40 per cup), and very high in vitamin C.

In fact, weight for weight, they are a better source of this vitamin than oranges. One cup contains about 90 mg, or 100 percent of the Recommended Dietary Allowance (RDA) for adults. Strawberries are also a good source of folate; 1 cup provides about 30 mcg (micrograms), or roughly 7 percent of the RDA, as well as 250 mg of potassium, 3 g of fiber, and useful amounts of riboflavin and iron.

The seeds in strawberries provide insoluble fiber, which helps prevent constipation; however, they can be irritating to people with such intestinal disorders as inflammatory bowel disease, or diverticulosis, a condition in which small pouches bulge outward along the intestinal wall.

Strawberries are a good source of pectin and other soluble fibers that help lower cholesterol.

They contain bioflavonoids, including red anthocyanin and ellagic acid, substances that may help prevent some cancers. Cooking does not destroy ellagic acid, so even strawberry pie and jam may be beneficial. Remember, though, that these usually have a very high sugar content.

Strawberries can be stored whole in the refrigerator for a few days (if sliced, the berries will gradually lose their vitamin C). Wash them well; unwashed strawberries have been linked to outbreaks of infectious diarrhea. To avoid molding, wash the fruit just before serving it.

Because strawberries contain a common allergen as well as a natural salicylate, an aspirin-like compound, many people are allergic to them. They also contain oxalic acid, which can aggravate kidney and bladder stones in susceptible people, and reduce the body's ability to absorb iron and calcium. Strawberries may contain relatively high levels of pesticide residues, so consider buying organic varieties. ❖

DID YOU KNOW?

FOLK REMEDIES FEATURE STRAWBERRIES

Aside from being delicious, people in many cultures have found strawberries useful for certain conditions. The Chinese, for instance, claim that a handful of the red berries is a cure for a hangover. They are also said to whiten teeth and are used to get rid of garlic breath.

STRESS
■ STRATEGIES FOR COPING ■

When people talk about stress, they are usually referring to tension or emotional distress. Medically, however, stress is defined as any condition or situation that places undue strain on the body. The sources can be a physical illness or injury, as well as numerous psychological factors—including fear, feelings of anger or frustration, and even unusual happiness. What constitutes almost unbearable stress to one person may be the spice of life to someone else. In either case, a stressor (a stimulus that causes stress) can trigger the body's automatic stress-response system. This sets the stage for decreased immunity and increased vulnerability to illnesses, ranging from the common cold to heart attacks and cancer.

Are you stressed?

Because stress can cause many different symptoms, both physical and mental, it's often difficult to determine the true source of many problems. A doctor may order medical tests, even if he suspects that stress is the real cause. The following are common manifestations of stress:

Physical symptoms
■ Palpitations, shortness of breath, chest pain, and other signs of heart disease (which must be ruled out).
■ Unusual rapid breathing, dizziness, or light-headedness.
■ Tingling sensations in the hands and/or feet.
■ Chronic or recurring backache and neck pain.
■ Frequent headaches.
■ Diarrhea or constipation.
■ Heartburn and other types of digestive problems.

Psychological symptoms
■ Difficulty in concentrating and in making decisions.
■ Sleep problems.
■ Chronic fatigue, even after adequate rest.
■ Prolonged anxiety.
■ Changes in appetite and an increased reliance on alcohol, nicotine, or other drugs.
■ Difficulty coping with what normally would be minor setbacks.
■ Decreased enjoyment of pleasurable activities and events.

Our natural fight-or-flight response

While physical stress is often episodic, emotional stress is part of daily life. This is not a modern phenomenon. Our early ancestors experienced much more stress than we do—from the constant quest for food to dangers from hostile neighbors and wild animals. While we don't usually encounter such situations, our bodies will still respond to any stress much as they would have in prehistoric times. This stress-coping mechanism, called the fight-or-flight response, floods the body with adrenaline and other hormones that raise blood pressure, speed up the heartbeat, tense muscles, and put other systems on alert. Metabolism quickens to provide extra energy; digestion stops as blood is diverted from the intestines to the muscles.

Nutritional needs

Good nutrition is especially important during periods of stress. Prolonged stress, whether psychological or physical, plays havoc with digestion and nutritional needs. Food provides energy, vitamins, and minerals for dealing with stress and helps to counter the negative effects on the body's immune system. Citrus fruits, bell peppers, and baked potatoes are rich in vitamin C, which helps your body maintain resistance to infection under stress. Also, one study showed that stressed people who took 1,000 mg of vitamin C daily had milder increases in blood pressure and lower levels of stress hormones. Foods high in zinc such as seafood, meat, poultry, milk, eggs, whole grains, and nuts also help to keep your immune system healthy.

When under stress, some people are always hungry and binge on food; others have to force themselves to eat. Because stress interferes with digestion, it's better to eat four to six small meals spaced throughout the day instead of the traditional three large ones.

Carbohydrate-rich meals can increase levels of serotonin, a brain chemical that is known to induce a feeling of calm. Studies have shown that stress-prone individuals who eat a diet higher in carbohydrates and lower in protein had less stress-induced depression.

Tips for eating during stressful periods

No diet will make stress disappear. However, there are steps you can take to help your eating during stressful times:

■ **Eat breakfast.** If you are running on empty, stress can be more difficult to handle.

■ **Eat slowly.** Eating quickly is often associated with digestive upset and this—coupled with stress—can make your food difficult to digest.

■ **Don't diet.** Changing eating habits is stressful at the best of times.

■ **Limit your intake of caffeine and alcohol.** They can affect your mood and sleep patterns. Alcohol can also heighten feelings of depression.

■ **Listen to your body** and avoid foods that cause you discomfort or digestive upset.

Comfort foods

Almost everyone has a favorite food that provides comfort during stressful times; the choices vary from one person to the next. For some people, it's a food that harks back to childhood, such as milk. Others crave chocolate or sweets, which increase the production of serotonin, a brain chemical that has a calming effect. Soups are also favorite choices, as are bland, easy-to-digest foods like rice pudding, custards, yogurt, and omelets. Experiment and go with whatever works best for you.

Better off without

Because stress can play havoc with normal digestion, foods that normally are well tolerated may trigger indigestion and heartburn when you are in a stressful period. Fatty foods, which are difficult to digest at any time, should be avoided as much as possible. Many people also find that hot or spicy foods cause them problems during times of stress.

Avoid caffeinated drinks, which can contribute to jittery feelings. Instead, try herbal teas such as chamomile and peppermint, which have a calming effect. Or substitute low-fat milk, fruit juice, or a noncaffeinated soft drink for caffeinated soft drinks. If you drink coffee, chose decaf.

Remember you can handle whatever life throws at you much better when you are eating and sleeping well, and by maintaining a positive outlook.

DO ONE SIMPLE THING

TAKE A MULTIVITAMIN PILL

Studies have shown that chronically stressed people have depressed levels of nutrients in their body, which can be corrected with a multivitamin and mineral supplement. So although there is no pill that will make stress go away or make it easier to cope, if you are not eating well during a difficult period, take a multivitamin and mineral supplement.

8 ways to relieve stress

1. Make sure you eat regular and healthful meals; several small meals may work best.
2. For a few minutes each day, sit quietly with your eyes closed.
3. Exercise regularly to increase the production of endorphins, brain chemicals that lift mood.
4. Listen to your favorite music; it, too, increases endorphin levels.
5. Learn a relaxation technique, such as yoga, meditation, or deep-breathing exercises.
6. Make a things-to-do list for the day; arrange the items by importance. Do an item at a time; move undone ones to the next day's list.
7. Consider having a pet; stroking an animal can help you relax.
8. Share your problems with a family member, friend, or counselor.

STROKE

MINISTROKES AREN'T SO MINI

So-called "ministrokes" are transient ischemic attacks, in which a part of the brain temporarily receives an insufficient amount of blood. A recent survey shows that 2.5 percent of all adults over the age of 18 have experienced these episodes, which are especially common in older adults. Although they usually only last from a few seconds to 24 hours and leave no permanent damage, ministrokes are a warning sign. It is estimated that up to 30 percent of people who have had these attacks will go on to have a full-blown stroke.

EAT PLENTY OF

- Fresh fruits and vegetables for vitamin C, potassium, and important antioxidants.
- Nuts, seeds, vegetable oils, wheat germ for vitamin E.
- Oily fish for omega-3 fatty acids.
- Oat bran, legumes, flax, psyllium, and fruits for soluble fibers.
- Onions and garlic, which may help to prevent blood clots.

LIMIT

- Animal and dairy products that are high in saturated fats and cholesterol.
- Salt, which may raise blood pressure.
- Alcohol use.

AVOID

- Smoking.
- Excessive weight gain.

On average, every 45 seconds, someone in North America has a stroke. Strokes are the third leading cause of death in the United States and the fourth in Canada, claiming over 283,000 American lives and 16,000 Canadians annually. African-Americans are 1.4 times more likely to die of a stroke than whites, and more than twice as likely as Hispanics and Native Americans, and at an earlier age, according to a recent study.

Approximately 88 percent of all strokes are ischemic, occurring when a clot blocks blood flow to a part of the brain. Most of these clots form in an artery that is already narrowed by atherosclerosis, either in the brain itself or, more commonly, in the carotid artery in the neck. Nine percent are hemorrhagic strokes, in which there is bleeding in the brain, such as from a burst blood vessel or severe head injury. Hemorrhagic strokes, which are more likely to be fatal than those caused by clots, are more common in people with high blood pressure.

The warning signs of a stroke include sudden weakness or numbness of the face, arm, and leg on one side of the body; difficulty speaking or understanding others; dimness or impaired vision in one eye; and unexplained dizziness, unsteadiness, or a sudden fall. Immediate treatment is critical, even if the symptoms disappear, as in the case of a ministroke (transient ischemic attack), a common prelude to a full-blown stroke. Prompt treatment may be lifesaving, and it may also minimize permanent damage, which can include impaired movement, speech, vision, and mental function.

REDUCING THE RISKS. *The key to avoiding stroke is a diet low in salt and saturated fat and high in fiber and the omega-3 fatty acids found in some oils and oily fish.*

PREVENTIVE MEASURES

Although the death rate from stroke decreased by 12.3 percent from 1990 to 2000, the actual number of stroke deaths rose by 10 percent. Despite the fact that we have a better understanding of the underlying causes, key risk factors, such as high blood pressure, heart disease, arteriosclerosis, and diabetes, many North Americans persist in a number of unhealthy lifestyle habits that increase the risk of a stroke; these include smoking, excessive use of alcohol, obesity, and a sedentary lifestyle.

Diet plays an important role in reducing or eliminating these risk factors. In fact, many of the same nutritional recommendations made for people who have heart disease, high blood pressure, and elevated blood cholesterol levels apply to people who are at risk for, or who have had, a stroke.

Adopt a diet that is low in fats. A good starting point is to reduce your consumption of fats, especially saturated animal fats, trans fats and tropical (palm and coconut) oils. Fruits, vegetables, lentils, legumes, and whole grains should be eaten for their vitamins, minerals, and flavonoids. Many of these foods, especially oats, lentils, and flax are high in the soluble fibers that help control cholesterol levels and reduce the risk of atherosclerosis, which narrows the arteries and sets the stage for developing the blood clots that block the flow of blood to the brain. Eating whole grains is important for stroke protection since data suggest a whole-grain based diet may reduce the risk for this condition. Preliminary evidence suggests that resveratrol, a phytochemical found in grapes, nuts, and red wine may inhibit blood clots and also help relax blood vessels. Population-based studies suggest that dietary flavonoids, particularly quercetin, found in apples and berries, may reduce fat deposits in arteries that can block blood flow to the brain.

Get lots of omega-3s. A number of other foods appear to lower the risk of a stroke. Some fish, for example, are rich in omega-3 fatty acids, which help to prevent blood clots by reducing the stickiness of blood platelets. Doctors recommend eating salmon, trout, mackerel, sardines, or other oily cold-water fish two or three times a week. Other good sources of omega-3 fatty acids include walnuts and walnut oil, canola (rapeseed) oil, flaxseed oil, soybeans, and leafy greens.

Eat plenty of garlic and onions. Garlic and onions appear to decrease the tendency of the

blood to clot, and they also boost the body's natural clot-dissolving mechanism.

Try Chinese tree ear mushrooms. A Chinese mushroom called the tree ear may have similar beneficial effects. This mushroom is available dried in Chinese markets and gourmet shops, and when rehydrated with a little boiling water, it makes a tasty addition to soups, stews, and casseroles. A recent study found that a tablespoon of the soaked mushroom consumed three or four times a week may be as effective in preventing strokes and heart attacks as a daily aspirin—but without the risk of gastrointestinal irritation that aspirin may cause.

Consume these foods for the right vitamins, minerals, and antioxidants. A growing body of scientific evidence shows that vitamin E, too, reduces the tendency to form blood clots. Foods high in this antioxidant include nuts, seeds, wheat germ, and green leafy vegetables. Other antioxidants include vitamin C, which strengthens blood vessel walls and thus may protect against brain hemorrhages; most fruits (especially citrus) and vegetables are good sources of vitamin C.

Fruits and vegetables are high in potassium, an electrolyte instrumental in maintaining normal blood pressure.

Anyone who has high blood pressure, or a family history of this disease or of strokes, should limit salt intake; excessive sodium—a main component of salt—increases the body's fluid volume and may raise blood pressure.

Limit alcohol. Numerous studies link excessive alcohol use, defined as more than two drinks a day for men and one for women, to an increased incidence of stroke; the risk is compounded if the person also smokes. The best approach is to abstain completely from smoking and to use alcohol in moderation.

Exercise. Regular exercise is helpful not only in reducing the risk of a stroke and heart attack by helping control weight and blood cholesterol levels, but also by promoting an enhanced sense of well-being. ❖

SUBMARINE SANDWICHES

See Fast Food

SUGAR AND OTHER SWEETENERS

BENEFITS
- Sugar satisfies an inborn taste for sweets.

DRAWBACKS
- High amounts may indirectly lead to obesity.
- Sugar fosters the growth of cavity-causing bacteria.

Refined sugar is a relatively new food in the human diet, becoming widely available only since the 1500s. It didn't take long for this sweetener to become a major commodity.

Sugars have been described as a "standard currency" for living organisms because all plants and animals store energy chemically as sugar. The sugars adapted for our diet are natural substances produced by photosynthesis in plants. Nutrition experts distinguish two main types of sugar: intrinsic sugar, which gives an appealing taste to such foods as fruits and sweet vegetables, and extrinsic sugar, which is added to food during preparation or processing or at the time of consumption.

Sugarcane and sugar beets are our main sources of sugar; some liquid sweeteners, such as molasses, are by-products of sugar refining. Manufacturers favor liquid sweeteners made from corn or potatoes because their sweetness and thickness can be regulated. They add a chewy texture to foods, and they prevent moisture loss and extend the shelf life of products.

> **KEY FINDING**
>
> A large study suggests that when it comes to diabetes, sugar is not a major factor. In the study, Harvard researchers looked at more than 38,000 healthy, middle-aged women enrolled in the Women's Health Study, an ongoing study of female health professionals. The women filled out food questionnaires and the researchers added up their total sugar intake, including table sugar (sucrose), fruit sugar (fructose), and milk sugar (lactose). Their analysis showed that women who consumed the most sugar were no more likely to develop diabetes than those who consumed the lowest amounts.

> **A UNIQUE SWEETENER**
>
> Artichokes contain cynarin, a unique organic acid that stimulates sweetness receptors in the taste buds. After eating artichokes, some people find that everything—including plain water—tastes sweet for a short time. However, efforts to convert this natural substance into a commercial sugar substitute have not yet been successful.

The main sugar in our diet is sucrose, familiar to us as white sugar.

FOOD VALUE

At 99.9 percent sucrose, white sugar is an extremely pure food. Sucrose is a disaccharide (double sugar) made up of two monosaccharides (single sugars): glucose (known as blood sugar, dextrose, or grape sugar) and fructose (the sugar in fruits and maple sap).

The intrinsic sugars in fruits, vegetables, and starches are bound up with essential vitamins, minerals, fiber, and oils. Extrinsic sugar, however, contains calories that supply energy but provide no valuable nutrients, although it satisfies our taste for sweetness and can enhance the flavor of many foods. And while many of the evils blamed on sugar—hyperactivity, acne, high blood pressure, obesity—have been found to be unrelated or only indirectly linked through overconsumption, it is true that sugar is a major cause of tooth decay and that people who turn to sugary fast foods for a quick energy boost may neglect less convenient but much more nutritious foods.

All forms of sugar provide about the same energy value: 4 calories per gram. In everyday terms, a cup of white sugar contains 770 calories, compared to 820 in a cup of densely packed brown sugar. A tablespoon of white sugar has 50 calories, and an individual serving packet, 25. Although sugar itself is not especially high in calories, many sweet foods, such as chocolates and pastries, are also high in fat, which contains 9 calories per gram.

Confectioners' sugar has about 385 calories in a cup. Although the sugar is pure sucrose, the product is packaged with cornstarch to prevent clumping. Because of this, people with allergies to corn may suffer adverse reactions from the powdered sugar in frostings and desserts. Raw sugar—the first crystals obtained during the refining process—is not sold in North America because it is contaminated with soil, plant refuse, and insect droppings and parts. Turbinado sugar, available in health-food stores, is raw sugar that has been purified.

Contrary to the claims of natural food enthusiasts, neither brown sugar nor honey is more nutritious than white sugar, but consumers who find the taste more appealing can substitute brown for white sugar in any recipe. Brown sugar is made by coating white sugar crystals with molasses. While molasses contains iron and other minerals, the amount in brown sugar is too small to be of nutritional value.

MAPLE SUGAR

Maple sugar and syrup are made by boiling down maple sap—a technique developed by North America's native people long before the arrival of white explorers. Pure maple products are expensive because production is limited. A tablespoon of maple syrup contains 50 calories, and 1 oz (30 g) of maple sugar has 100. Pure maple products contain traces of potassium, calcium, and other minerals, but not in amounts sufficient to be of much nutritional value.

DENTAL PROBLEMS

All types of sugar—white table sugar, brown sugar, honey, molasses—encourage the growth of the oral bacteria that are responsible for causing cavities. And when starchy foods are broken down by the enzymes in saliva, they, too, form cavity-causing sugars. More dangerous than the amount of sugar is the length of time the sugar remains in contact with the teeth. Thus, much of the damage can be prevented by brushing soon after eating a sweet.

Sugar alcohols, such as sorbitol, xylitol, maltitol, and lactitol, are used as sweeteners in chewing gums, candies, ice cream, and many baked goods. They provide fewer calories per gram than sucrose, do not promote tooth decay, and do not cause sudden jumps in blood glucose. In some people excessive consumption can cause bloating or diarrhea. If such problems do arise, start by adding a small amount of sugar alcohol in the diet and slowly increase it, allowing the body to grow accustomed to the substance. This usually overcomes the problem. Since sugar alcohols do not cause a sharp rise in insulin levels, they can be used by diabetics more readily than table sugar. Less than 10 g will cause no significant rise in blood glucose. ❖

HOW MUCH IS TOO MUCH?

A joint United States/Canada report from the Food and Nutrition Board, Institute of Medicine of the National Academies, released its recommendations for sugars in 2002. They concluded that based on the current scientific evidence, there is no level of total or added sugar intakes that increases the risk of adverse effects related to dental cavities, behavior, cancer, risk of obesity, and high cholesterol. Although no upper limit for sugar consumption was set, they suggest a maximum intake level of 25 percent or less of energy from added sugars for adults and children, which is considerably more than the current average intake.

However, an independent report from the World Health Organization (WHO) and the Food and Agriculture Organization of the United Nations (FAO) disagrees. It states that sugar leads to obesity when it displaces other nutrients in the diet. The WHO says that unless people limit their intake of added sugars, including sugar in soft drinks, to less than 10 percent of daily calories, they are looking at obesity and dental problems. For most people, that amount of sugar can be found in a single can of soda pop.

SUGAR BY ANY OTHER NAME. *Molasses, honey, and brown sugar all provide about 4 calories per gram.*

SUPPLEMENTS
■ WHO NEEDS THEM? ■

Millions of North Americans take dietary supplements. Some take them because they think they don't eat well enough for their diet to provide optimal levels of nutrients. Others take supplements because of a particular health problem they want to treat or try to prevent.

Nutritionists have always stressed that our diet is the best source of vitamins, minerals, fatty acids, amino acids, and fiber, and that food and nutrients in their natural form are best adapted to the human digestive system. In contrast, supplements contain only one isolated form of a nutrient, which lacks the energy, fiber, and other dietary components that provide proper nutritional balance.

In recent years, as we have shifted our focus from prevention of deficiency diseases to maximizing health and preventing chronic disease, interest in supplements has increased dramatically. However, it is not an easy task for researchers to prove the benefits of supplementation. Effects of supplements depend on the level of nutrients already being absorbed from the diet, as well as factors that influence nutrient absorption and metabolism. In addition, supplements may take years to have a significant beneficial effect, making their impact difficult to observe and measure. Despite these challenges, research is beginning to emerge supporting the benefits of certain supplements.

Multivitamins

The most common supplements are multivitamins. Few studies have looked at their effects, since most research addresses specific nutrients rather than groups of them. There is some evidence, however, that daily use of a multivitamin is associated with a lower risk of heart disease and stroke, and certain types of cancer, as well as illness from infection. Researchers recently concluded that most people could benefit from multivitamins. They are especially important for women of childbearing years, people who regularly consume one or two alcoholic drinks per day, those who do not eat enough fruits and vegetables, and the elderly. But popping a pill can't erase the effects of a poor diet, a sedentary lifestyle, smoking, or obesity, and a multivitamin can't replace healthy food; foods contain important components, such as fiber, plant chemicals, and essential fatty acids.

CAUTION

Beware of drug/nutrient interactions. Drugs and nutrients share the same route of absorption and metabolism in our bodies, which creates the potential for interactions. For example, calcium can bind to certain antibiotics, interfering with their absorption. So if you are taking, or planning to take, therapeutic doses of nutrients in supplement form, make sure you check for the possibility of these types of interactions. (See Medicine-Food Interactions: Hidden Dangers.)

Folic acid

There is now conclusive proof that folic acid can prevent neural tube birth defects such as spina bifida. This defect occurs when the neural tube of the fetus fails to close, which can result in death, or serious damage to the spinal cord. Folic acid can prevent half of these defects if women take it before conception. So it is wise for women who could become pregnant to take a supplement containing 400 mcg (micrograms) of folic acid daily.

There is also considerable evidence that folic acid can reduce the risk of heart disease. Research shows that people with higher levels of the amino acid homocysteine have a higher risk of heart disease; those who consume more folacin, or folic acid from a supplement, have lower homocysteine levels. Again, 400 mcg a day seems to do the job.

Vitamin B_{12}

Low blood levels of B_{12} are more common in older people because stomach acid, which often decreases with age, is needed for B_{12} absorption. Low levels of this nutrient are associated with higher homocysteine levels, which is a risk factor for heart disease. The type of B_{12} found in supplements does not require gastric acid for absorption, so taking a multivitamin or B-complex containing at least 25 mcg of B_{12} will ensure an adequate intake for most. Research suggests most seniors would benefit from a B_{12} supplement.

Vitamin D

Many people don't realize that vitamin D is just as important as calcium for healthy bones. Our two main sources are sun exposure and fortified milk. But people who live in northerly climates may not get sufficient sun exposure, and many adults do not drink milk. Also, as you age, your body becomes less efficient at producing the vitamin from sunlight. There is evidence that a significant number of people over 50 are vitamin D-deficient, which increases the risk of osteoporosis and fracture. Most people would benefit from taking a multivitamin that contained 400 IU of vitamin D; those over 70 who get little sunshine should take 600 IU daily. Because vitamin D is fat soluble, take it with the fattiest meal of the day (usually dinner) for best absorption.

Dangerous doses

The U.S. National Academy of Sciences and Health Canada have set Tolerable Upper Intake Levels (ULs) for many nutrients, including calcium (2,500 mg/day) and vitamin D (2,000 IU/day). The UL is defined as "the highest level of daily nutrient that is likely to pose no risk of adverse health effects for almost all individuals in the general population. As intake increases above the UL, the potential risk of adverse effects increases." Work continues in this area and tolerable upper limits will be identified for more nutrients in the future. In the meantime, common sense should prevail whether or not a tolerable upper limit has been set for a nutrient.

High doses of vitamin A can cause liver damage, skin problems, fatigue, and other symptoms. Taken before and during pregnancy, it can cause serious birth defects. High doses of vitamin D can result in calcium deposits in the heart and blood vessels, upset calcium metabolism, and lead to bone loss. Taken over an extended period, very large amounts of both vitamins can be fatal. Excessive zinc and several trace minerals have effects ranging from nausea and diarrhea to death if taken in doses that allow buildup in body tissues.

Remember . . .

■ Supplements won't make up for a bad diet. Eat a varied diet high in fruits and vegetables, whole grains, and quality protein foods every day.

■ Don't go overboard. While there's no need to worry about the amounts of nutrients in multivitamins, people planning to take therapeutic doses of single nutrients should consult a doctor, dietitian, pharmacist, or someone else knowledgeable in nutrition.

■ Beware of the latest cure-all product. Some supplements are heavily marketed without a whole lot of science to back up their claims. There are no magic bullets.

■ Anyone undergoing cancer treatment must discuss vitamin supplementation with their physician. In some cases, supplements may be contraindicated.

Sushi

BENEFITS

- Made from healthful ingredients, including seaweed, rice, vegetables, and fish.
- Low in fat

DRAWBACKS

- Many varieties made with raw fish, so should be avoided by pregnant women and those with immune disorders, because of the small risk of exposure to bacteria or parasites.

Once considered an esoteric dish, sushi has gone mainstream in North American restaurants and homes. And no wonder. This beautiful food is not just delicious and nutritious, it's also an art that has evolved over centuries.

Technically, the word sushi refers to vinegared rice, but the word is commonly used to describe a variety of finger-sized foods that include raw fish on a bed of rice (nigiri), or rice and seaweed rolls, both thin and larger sizes, with fish and/or vegetables (maki). These foods can be eaten as is, or dipped into shoyu (Japanese soy sauce) before eating. Much care and attention is put into the creation of these beautiful foods.

HEALTH BENEFITS

Sushi uses simple, healthful ingredients—rice, seaweed, fish, and vegetables, and it is low in fat and calories, so it's a great choice for those watching their weight or worried about their cholesterol. Those watching their salt intake should go easy on the seaweed (nori) wrapped varieties and the soy sauce.

The bite-sized pieces encourage the diner to eat slowly and savor the meal. A typical serving of sushi would consist of a variety of 10 pieces of nigiri and thin rolls, which would contain about 450 calories. As a general rule, nigiri ranges in calories from 40 to 100, with about 30 calories from the rice and the remaining from the various types fish or topping. Two pieces of thin roll are about equal to one piece of nigiri, and thick rolls vary considerably depending on their ingredients. One of the most popular, California roll, which contains fish and avocado, has about 40 calories per piece.

CAUTION

Although chefs trained in the art of preparing sushi usually maintain rigorous standards of freshness and cleanliness, eating raw fish carries certain risks. Both freshwater and saltwater fish can be intermediate hosts for parasitic worms. Many of the fish used to make sushi are chilled to a temperature that kills parasites; nonetheless, sushi-eaters should be aware that there is a risk of infection.

Because the fish used in sushi is uncooked, it should not be eaten by pregnant women or those with immune disorders, because of the small risk of exposure to bacteria such as *Listeria monocytogenes* and parasites. For most diners, however, these risks are considered minimal, as long as they eat in reputable restaurants. For anyone who prefers not to eat raw fish, there are many other options, including cooked crab, shrimp, egg, tofu, or vegetables. ❖

AN OLD ART FORM

Sushi had its beginnings in the 7th century when Southeast Asians introduced the technique of pickling. The Japanese adapted this method when packing rice and fish. As the fish fermented, the rice produced lactic acid, which in turn caused the fish to be pickled. After many improvements throughout the centuries, sushi has developed into a unique, healthful food, and its popularity continues to grow.

SUSHI SAVVY

California roll: Crab, smelt, or fish roe, and avocado rolled in rice.
Daikon: Long white radish, sweeter than red radish.
Ebi: Boiled shrimp.
Gari: Pickled ginger.
Gohan: Boiled rice.
Hashi: Chopsticks.
Make/norimake: Sushi roll made with nori seaweed on the outside, a layer of rice and vegetables or other fillings in the middle.
Makisu: Bamboo mat used to roll up sushi.
Nigiri: Fish, shellfish, or fish roe over rice.
Nori: Seaweed pressed into thin sheets, used to make norimake sushi.
Sashimi: Raw fish, chilled and sliced.
Shoyu: Soy sauce.
Wasabi: Japanese horseradish.

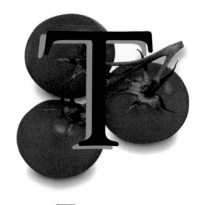

TACOS

See Fast Food

TANGERINES

BENEFITS
- A good source of vitamin C, beta carotene, and potassium.
- Contain pectin, a soluble fiber that helps control blood cholesterol.

DRAWBACKS
- Oils in peels may irritate the skin of some people.

We often use the terms tangerines and mandarins interchangeably, and indeed, tangerines, along with clementines and satsumas, are actually types of mandarin oranges. These sweet citrus fruits with loose-fitting skins originated in China, but they are now grown in many parts of the world. As they moved into other tropical and subtropical areas, the original mandarin oranges were crossed with other citrus fruits to produce a variety of hybrids, including tangelos and tangors.

Volume for volume, oranges have about twice as much vitamin C as tangerines, but even so, tangerines contribute a good amount of this antioxidant; a medium-size fruit fulfills about 30 percent of the adult Recommended

Dietary Allowance (RDA). In addition, tangerines are richer in vitamin A (in the form of beta carotene) than any other citrus fruit. A medium-size tangerine contains 775 IU (International Units) or 77 RE (Retinol Equivalents) of vitamin A, as well as 130 mg of potassium, and only about 35 calories. It is also high in pectin, a soluble fiber that helps lower blood cholesterol, and contains tangeretin, a flavonoid linked in experimental studies to reduced growth of tumor cells.

Like other citrus fruits, tangerine peels contain oils that can cause an itchy rash. Because tangerines are so easy to peel, this can usually be avoided.

TYPES OF TANGERINES
While most varieties are available from November to March, tangerines are especially popular at Christmas. The following are among the most common types sold in North America.

Clementine. This fruit is seedless, and smaller and sweeter than many of the other varieties. It is sometimes called an Algerian tangerine, but most clementines sold in North America are imported from Spain, Israel, and Morocco.

Honey tangerine. Also known as a murcott, this variety has a greener skin than other tangerines, but the flesh is more orange and the flavor is sweeter.

Satsuma. These are a little larger than clementines, nearly seedless, and very thin-skinned. Japan is the leading producer of satsumas.

Tangelo. A cross between a tangerine and a grapefruit, the tangelo looks like an orange, is tangier than a tangerine, and is sweeter than a grapefruit.

Tangor. This hybrid, also known as temple orange, looks like a tangerine but tastes like an orange; it is juicy and sweet, but contains many seeds. ❖

TEA MAY BE A POWERFUL INFECTION FIGHTER

Researchers report in the Proceedings of the National Academy of Sciences that they have found a chemical in tea that boosts the body's defense against disease fivefold.

They say they isolated from ordinary black tea a substance called L-theanine, also found in green and oolong tea. L-theanine is broken down in the liver to ethylamine, a molecule that primes the response of an immune blood cell called the gamma-delta T cell. Gamma-delta T cells in the blood are the first line of defense against many types of bacterial, viral, and parasitic infections. They might even have some antitumor activity. The T cells prompt the secretion of interferon, a key part of the body's chemical defense against infection.

TEA

BENEFITS

- A refreshing stimulant that is almost calorie-free if taken plain.
- Contains antioxidants and bioflavonoids, which may lower the risk of cancer, heart disease, and stroke.
- Contains tannins, which may provide protection against tooth decay.
- Herbal teas are caffeine-free.

DRAWBACKS

- Tannins decrease iron absorption if tea is consumed with meals.
- Has a diuretic effect that increases urination.
- May cause insomnia in caffeine-sensitive people.

Tea is the world's most popular nonalcoholic beverage. Most tea is grown in India, Sri Lanka, China, Japan, Taiwan, and Indonesia from a shrub in the camellia family. Like coffees, the best-quality teas are grown in the shade at high altitudes, and the finest leaves are plucked from the youngest shoots and unopened leaf buds, which also contain the highest levels of phenols, enzymes, and caffeine. Researchers are discovering evidence that tea may offer not only soothing warmth and mild stimulation, but also health benefits.

AN ANTIOXIDANT BREW

Tea contains hundreds of compounds, including various flavonoids, a class of chemical with powerful antioxidant properties. A subclass of flavonoids, the catechins, is responsible for the flavor as well as many of the beneficial health effects of tea.

The extent to which these compounds are present in the final beverage depends on how the leaves are processed. To make black tea, the dried leaves are crushed to liberate enzymes, which react with the catechins over a few hours to produce changes in color and flavor. This is often referred to as "fermentation." Green tea is not fermented, it is made by first steaming the leaves to halt any enzyme activity. Oolong tea is partially fermented. The highest concentration of catechins is found in green tea, although black tea is also a good source. Brand-name teas are mixtures of as many as 20 different varieties of leaves, blended to ensure a consistent flavor.

Researchers at Tufts University in Boston compared the ORAC capacity of tea with 22 vegetables. ORAC refers to the oxygen radical absorbance capacity, a measurement of the total antioxidant power of foods and other chemical substances. The higher the ORAC score, the greater its antioxidant capacity (see Antioxidants). Although there was variation among various teas, the highest scoring teas were green tea and black tea, brewed for 5 minutes—they outranked the best fruits and vegetables. While this doesn't suggest that tea should replace fruits and vegetables in daily consumption, it does underline the positive effects of this drink.

A cup of hot brewed tea has only 2 calories and—with one exception in green tea—no appreciable vitamins or minerals, except for fluoride. Green tea contains vitamin K, a nutrient needed for normal blood clotting.

TEA'S HEALTH BENEFITS

There are many positive studies regarding the health benefits of tea.

Heart disease. The antioxidants in tea may explain the fact that people who drink a lot of tea are much less likely to die from heart disease. Antioxidants prevent the oxidation of cholesterol, making it less likely to stick to artery walls.

Stroke. One study found that the risk of stroke was reduced by about 70 percent in men who drank five or more cups of black tea a day, and other studies showed that the risk of having a heart attack was reduced by more than 40 percent for men and women who consumed one or more cups of tea per day. Flavonoids may protect against stroke in two ways. They reduce the ability of blood platelets to form clots, the cause of most strokes. They also block some of the damage caused to arteries by free radicals, unstable molecules that are released when the body consumes oxygen.

Cancer. A number of studies have shown that tea offers protection against a variety of cancers. A type of catechin called EGCG (epigallocatechin gallate) is thought to be responsible for tea's anticancer properties. EGCG protects the DNA in cells from cancer-causing changes. It may also inhibit an enzyme that cancer cells need in order to replicate.

More benefits. The flavonoids in tea may suppress the growth of harmful bacteria, which helps prevent infections. Naturally occurring theophyllines in tea dilate the airways in the lungs and have been found to help some people with asthma and other respiratory disorders to breathe more freely. In fact, theophyllines have been developed as drugs to treat asthma and other constrictive lung disorders.

Tannins, which are found in wine as well as tea, are chemicals that bind surface proteins in the mouth, producing a tightening sensation together with giving the impression of a full-bodied liquid. They also bind and incapacitate plaque-forming bacteria in the mouth. The fluoride in tea—particularly green tea—also protects against tooth decay. Tea's binding action makes it useful against diarrhea.

OTHER EFFECTS

Tea leaves contain twice as much caffeine, weight for weight, as coffee beans do. But when measured by volume, tea has only half as much caffeine as coffee because tea is drunk weaker and coffee is more completely extracted from the grounds. A cup of black or green tea contains 35 to 45 mg of caffeine. Tea may trigger a migraine headache in hypersensitive people; for others, it may alleviate headaches when taken with aspirin or similar painkillers. Theobromine, which is also found in tea, has effects similar to those of caffeine but milder.

The tannins in tea can cut iron absorption by more than 80 percent when tea is drunk with an iron-rich meal. Tea-drinking vegetarians are especially susceptible. Individuals with a tendency to anemia can drink citrus juice at mealtimes to promote iron absorption; squeezing a wedge of lemon or adding milk to tea also binds the tannins and partly blocks their effect on iron. Tea drinking between meals does not affect iron absorption. Young children should not drink tea, which can increase their risk of iron-deficiency anemia. In addition, tannins can stain natural teeth and dental work, and some mouthwashes may intensify the staining.

Tea, like coffee, has a diuretic effect, which increases the kidneys' output of urine. Excessive urination can upset the body's fluid and chemical balance by washing potassium from the body.

HERBAL TEAS

Many plants, especially herbs, can be brewed into teas, also called infusions or tisanes. Because most of them do not contain caffeine, they offer a pleasant alternative for people who prefer to avoid this stimulant. Some herbal teas aid the digestion, and their soothing warmth can promote relaxation at bedtime.

Always choose herbs carefully. Although the herbs and spices used in herbal teas have been approved by government regulatory bodies for use as seasonings, a few herbs and spices are known to be unsafe when used medicinally. Nutmeg, for example, is harmless when used to flavor foods but can cause severe symptoms, including hallucinations, when brewed into a strong tea. Other herbs, such as oregano, have a stimulating effect and can cause wakefulness. Comfrey tea, if consumed regularly, is toxic to the liver.

Scientific information is inconclusive regarding the safety of various herbs and herbal products during pregnancy and while breast-feeding. The herbal teas considered safe if used in moderation include citrus peel, ginger, lemon balm, orange peel, and rose hip. It is wise for pregnant women to discuss use of these drinks with their health-care provider.

Folk healers have long used herbal teas for medicinal purposes, but few teas have been tested scientifically. Care is needed when self-treating with herbal teas, especially if the herbs have been gathered in the wild. Many plants are poisonous,

A CANCER CURE?

In test tubes, the catechins in tea are powerful inhibitors of cancer growth. And animal studies have suggested that tea can inhibit growth of tumor cells in lab animals. But it's unclear whether tea works the same way in the human body. Some population studies have found that heavy tea drinking appears to lower the rates of breast, skin, stomach, colorectal, and other cancers. Other studies have shown no link between cancer prevention and tea consumption. Ongoing research will shed more light on the subject. For example, scientists are studying the potential of green tea supplements and topical applications to slow or prevent skin cancer.

Cancer researchers in Arizona studied heavy smokers who were asked to drink four cups of decaffeinated green tea daily for 4 months. Test showed that DNA damage (which could lead to cancer) dropped 30 percent in that group, but not in control groups who drank decaffeinated black tea or water.

Other researchers, at the University of Rochester, found that two flavonoids in tea, EGCG and EGC, inhibit a molecule called the aryl hydrocarbon (AH) receptor. Tobacco smoke acts on this molecule and causes it to trigger potentially carcinogenic gene activity. By shutting down the AH receptor, green tea might help prevent smoking-related cancers.

ICED TEA

Iced tea becomes cloudy because caffeine and pigment molecules crystallize at low temperatures. Tea, made by steeping several tea bags in lukewarm water for several hours, is less likely to become cloudy than tea brewed with hot water.

Commercial iced teas, flavored with fruit syrups and sweetened with sugar, contain about as many calories as soft drinks.

and these may be mistaken for safe herbs. Among the more popular herbal teas are the following:

Chamomile. A mild sedative, chamomile tea is said to aid digestion and relieve menstrual cramps. Small amounts of pollen residue in chamomile tea may cause dermatitis or other allergic symptoms in people sensitive to ragweed, chrysanthemums, and members of the daisy family.

Dandelion. Tea made from this common weed is mildly diuretic. Some women use it to reduce problems of premenstrual bloating.

Elder flower. Extracts of elder are sometimes used in over-the-counter cold remedies, and elder-flower tea may alleviate cold and flu symptoms. The flowers and ripe berries of the elder are safe, but avoid the roots, stems, and leaves. The tea is a mild stimulant.

Fennel. With a flavor similar to licorice, fennel tea is used to soothe an upset stomach. Traditional herbalists often recommend it as an appetite suppressant and slimming aid.

Lavender flower. Tea brewed from dried lavender flowers is said to be mildly sedative.

Lemon balm. This minty tea may help soothe jittery nerves.

Nettle. Made from the same plant that causes stinging skin irritation, nettle tea is rich in vitamin C and several minerals. Herbalists recommend it to treat arthritis and gout and to increase milk production in nursing mothers.

Peppermint. Tea from this mint plant is refreshing and may stimulate digestion. It should be avoided by anyone with a hiatal hernia, because peppermint promotes reflux of the stomach contents into the esophagus.

Raspberry leaf. Herbalists recommend raspberry tea to ease menstrual cramps.

Rose hip. Rich in vitamin C, rose hip tea can substitute as an alternative to orange juice.

Rosemary. Tea from this popular garden herb is said to relieve gas and colic, but drinking more than two or three cups a day may irritate the stomach.

Thyme. Herbalists recommend thyme tea for gastrointestinal complaints and to alleviate lung congestion.

INSTANT TEA

Instant tea is made by brewing strong tea, then evaporating the water to leave a powder. The tea is reconstituted by adding water. Fruit juice can be used instead of water to make flavored iced tea. ❖

THYROID DISORDERS

EAT PLENTY OF
- Seafood, dark green leafy vegetables, and dairy products for iodine.

LIMIT
- Alcohol and caffeine, if the thyroid gland is overactive.
- Raw vegetables in the cabbage family, if the thyroid gland is underactive.

AVOID
- Smoking.
- High-dose kelp supplements.

The thyroid, a butterfly-shaped gland that lies over the windpipe (trachea) and just below the Adam's apple (larynx), produces triiodothyronine (T_3) and thyroxine (T_4), hormones that influence almost every function of the body. These hormones regulate metabolism, physical and mental development, nerve and muscle function, and circulation. Thyroid hormones also affect the actions of other hormones; for example, they intensify the action of insulin and the body's response to the adrenal hormones (catecholamines) that are instrumental in reacting to stress.

Unlike other hormone-producing glands, the thyroid needs a specific nutrient—iodine—to produce its hormones. Both too much and too little iodine can cause the thyroid to malfunction. Goiter, an overgrown thyroid that is marked by a swelling in the lower neck, usually signals a thyroid disorder. It is common in regions where crops are raised in iodine-poor soil and people do not receive iodine supplements in the diet. Goiter is also common among Japanese people, who often consume very large amounts of iodine-rich seaweed.

People who lack iodine appear to be more susceptible to the toxic effects of radioactive iodine, a contaminant released into the atmosphere during testing of nuclear weapons. That's why potassium iodide tablets may be distributed in case of an accident at a nuclear power plant. The iodide saturates the thyroid and blocks radioactive iodide from being taken up.

Iodine deficiency, although still a common cause of thyroid disorders in developing nations, has been almost wiped out in North America by the introduction of iodized salt. Because seawater contains high levels of iodine, food crops grown on coastal farmlands generally have sufficient levels of the mineral. Iodine deficiency more commonly occurs in mountainous regions, or in inland areas.

Although they affect both sexes, thyroid disorders tend to occur more frequently in women. Cretinism, a type of mental retardation and growth deficiency, is a birth defect caused by a lack of iodine in the mother during pregnancy. Cretinism still prevails in parts of China but is very rare in the United States and Canada, where babies are routinely tested at birth for thyroid deficiency.

Thyroid problems usually involve either overactivity or underactivity of the gland. Although there is some overlap, the symptoms of one disorder present almost a mirror image of the other. The usual causes of thyroid problems are an infection, autoimmune disorder, hormonal imbalance, tumor, exposure to high levels of ionizing radiation, or congenital or hereditary problems.

HYPERTHYROIDISM

People with overactive thyroids (hyperthyroidism, or Graves' disease) tend to be nervous and jittery. Their metabolism speeds up, and they experience unusual hunger, weight loss, muscle weakness, and rapid heartbeat, among other symptoms. They find heat hard to bear and sweat excessively. Whether or not a goiter distorts the neck, a person with an overactive thyroid develops protuberant eyes.

Treatment is aimed at the cause and involves reducing hormone production either by giving radioactive iodine or antithyroid drugs or by surgery to remove all or parts of the thyroid.

HYPOTHYROIDISM

An underactive thyroid, or hypothyroidism, slows down metabolism, causing weight gain and lethargy. Early symptoms are easily overlooked: progressive fatigue, sleepiness, and muscle weakness. People with hypothyroidism often complain of memory and concentration problems. They feel cold, even on hot days, and develop dry skin and thinning hair. Nails grow slowly and become brittle. Because metabolism slows down, weight gain is common, even though the person may be eating less than normal. Women often develop menstrual irregularities; constipation is another common problem.

Hypothyroidism is frequently caused by chronic inflammation due to an autoimmune disorder. Treatment usually requires lifelong hormone replacement with thyroxine pills.

DIETARY APPROACHES

The Recommended Dietary Allowance (RDA) for iodine is 150 mcg (micrograms) per day for adolescents and adults. Pregnant women need 220 mcg per day, nursing mothers 290 mcg. The use of iodized salt in the typical North American diet, which provides 2 to 6 g of salt each day, easily supplies more than these recommended amounts of iodine. However, iodine intake of up to 1,000 mcg a day has no adverse effects on the thyroid. Even people on low-salt diets get plenty of iodine from seafood, green leafy vegetables, and dairy products. Certain vegetables, mainly cabbage, broccoli, and other cruciferous vegetables, contain substances known as goitrogens, which block the effects of thyroid hormones and may lead to goiter. Cooking these foods inactivates the goitrogens; consumption of sufficient iodine also prevents adverse effects.

If you have a thyroid disorder, use small amounts of iodized salt and eat plenty of seafood, dairy products, spinach, and other vegetables for iodine. Fish, dairy products, eggs, as well as deep yellow or orange fruits and vegetables, and dark green vegetables provide vitamin A. The conversion of beta carotene (provitamin A) to two molecules of vitamin A (retinol) is accelerated by thyroxine. People with hypothyroidism may need a higher intake of beta carotene to meet vitamin A needs.

Stay away from caffeine. Caffeine may worsen the jittery feeling in someone with an overactive thyroid. Decaffeinated coffee, tea, and soda pop may refresh without adding to nervousness. The nicotine in tobacco also adds to feelings of nervousness. Alcohol may

CAUTION

Some people, usually women who are overly weight-conscious, take thyroid hormones as a diet aid. This can have dangerous results, including drug-induced hyperthyroidism, metabolic abnormalities, and irregular heartbeats. Thyroid pills should be taken only under careful medical supervision—never for weight control.

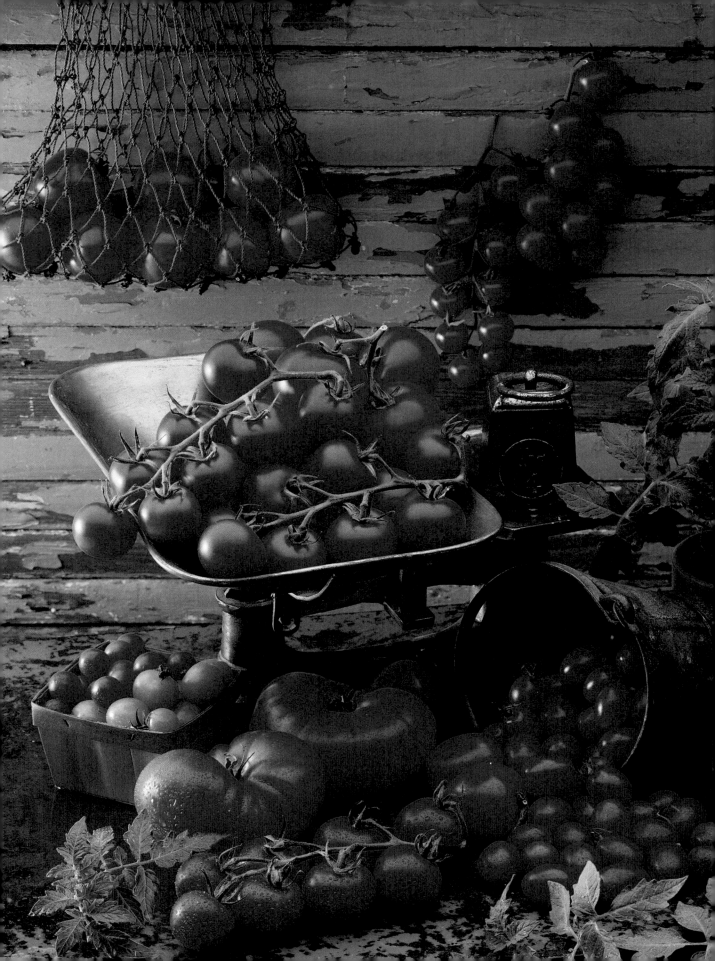

aggravate the sleepiness and fatigue in a person with an underactive thyroid gland. ❖

TOFU

See Soy

TOMATOES

BENEFITS

- A useful source of vitamin C, beta carotene, folate, and potassium.
- A good source of lycopene, an antioxidant that protects against some cancers.

DRAWBACKS

- Raw or cooked, may cause indigestion and heartburn.
- A possible cause of allergies.

Equally delicious raw or cooked, tomatoes are low in calories and rich in vitamins and other healthful substances. Tomatoes, like potatoes, sweet peppers, and eggplants, belong to the nightshade family. Brought to Europe from Central America by the Spanish during the 16th century, tomatoes were grown as decorative plants in northern Europe, where it was feared that the poisons in the leaves might be present in the fruit as well. Colonists emigrating from this area imported this misconception to the New World. Meanwhile, the Spanish and Italians discovered that tomatoes were indeed edible, and as they immigrated to North America, they brought their taste for tomatoes with them. Today, the tomato is one of the world's leading vegetable crops (though technically the tomato is a fruit).

SPECIAL BENEFITS

A well-known Harvard study showed that men who regularly ate tomato-based foods had lower rates of prostate cancer. Other studies continue to support this observation. The researchers theorize that lycopene—a powerful antioxi-

TOMATOES ARE ACTUALLY A TYPE OF BERRY, AND WERE CALLED "LOVE APPLES" IN THE 16TH CENTURY. *Tomato's flavor depends more on the variety and how ripe it is than on where it has ripened. Varieties include baby plum, beefsteak, cherry, plum, vine, and yellow cherry.*

dant—is the natural cancer-fighting agent in tomatoes. Other studies show that lycopene provides defense against a number of other conditions, including other cancers and heart disease. It is known to slow down damage to human cells caused by aging and disease. The best way to get lycopene is through tomatoes in their processed form—tomato sauce, tomato paste, tomato juice, and even ketchup. Lycopene is also found in pink grapefruits and watermelons, but it is most concentrated in tomato paste.

Although no single food can prevent cancer altogether, nutrition experts advise us to hedge our bets by consuming plenty of fruits and vegetables, such as tomatoes, that are rich in antioxidant nutrients, which protect against the cancer-causing cell damage that occurs when the body uses oxygen.

NUTRITIONAL VALUE

One medium-size ripe tomato contains only 26 calories, together with about 23 mg of vitamin C and 20 mcg of folate. Most of the vitamin C is concentrated in the jellylike substance that encases the seeds. Many recipes advise removing the seeds to prevent the development of a bitter taste during cooking; cooks who prefer to conserve all possible nutrients may use plum tomatoes, which have smaller seeds that impart less bitterness than larger ones. The jellylike substance around the seeds is actually high in salicylates, which have an anticlotting effect on the blood. This may be partially responsible for tomatoes' protection against heart disease.

Commercially prepared tomato sauces vary in calorie content, depending on added ingredients. Some tomato products may have high levels of added salt; people on low-sodium diets should look for those with no extra salt. On average, a half cup of canned tomato sauce contains about 40 calories, which may increase substantially with the addition of oil. A half cup of canned tomatoes contains only 25 calories. Tomato paste is a concentrated source of nutrients—a 3½-oz (100-ml) can contains

DID YOU KNOW?

WHEN IT COMES TO TOMATOES, REDDER IS BETTER

Tomatoes that have a crimson gene—making them a deep red color—contain more lycopene than paler tomatoes. A crimson tomato is said to have up to 50 percent more lycopene than a regular tomato. Vine-ripened tomatoes have more lycopene than those that are picked early and allowed to ripen off the vine.

DO ONE SIMPLE THING

LEAVE THE SKIN ON AND ADD A LITTLE OLIVE OIL

Lycopene is in the skin of tomatoes, so if you are making tomato sauce, leave the skin on. Also, lycopene is fat soluble, so cooking tomatoes with a little oil increases absorption.

about 90 calories, 50 mg of vitamin C, together with good amounts of beta carotene, the B-group vitamins, and 1,100 mg of potassium. Canned tomato juice, like fresh tomatoes, is a good source of vitamin C. Some vitamin C is lost in the processing, but some brands are fortified to raise the vitamin C content to the same level as found in fresh tomatoes.

Ripe tomatoes should be stored at room temperature; at 40°F (4°C) or below, the flesh becomes mealy. The green tomatoes left on the vine at the end of the season should be harvested and cooked, frozen, or pickled. Sun-dried tomatoes are a flavorful addition to dishes, but those packed in oil are high in calories.

DRAWBACKS

Solanines are toxic substances present in minute quantities in all members of the nightshade family; they may trigger headaches in susceptible people. Tomatoes are also a relatively common cause of allergies. An unidentified substance in tomatoes and tomato-based products can cause acid reflux, leading to indigestion and heartburn. People who often have digestive upsets should try eliminating tomatoes for 2 or 3 weeks to see if there is any improvement.

TOMATO CONDIMENTS

Many commercially prepared pickles and other condiments are based on tomatoes, including ketchup and chili sauce, pasta sauces, chutneys, and salsa, North America's most popular condiment. While these preparations certainly add zest to food, they contribute little nutrition in the quantities used. In addition, their calorie content is often boosted because of the generous quantities of sugar and oil with which they are made. And because many are high in salt, they should not be eaten by people who need to restrict their sodium intake. The healthiest tomato condiment choice would probably be a homemade salsa. ❖

TRANS FATS

See Fats

TUBERCULOSIS

CONSUME PLENTY OF
- Lean meat, poultry, eggs, and fish for high-quality protein.
- Fresh fruits and vegetables for vitamin C and beta carotene.
- Fortified milk, soy or rice beverages, and fatty fish for vitamin D.
- Lean meat, shellfish, milk, beans, and nuts for zinc.

AVOID
- Alcohol, smoking, and exposure to secondhand smoke.
- Sharing eating utensils and other personal objects.

With about 17,000 new cases a year, tuberculosis (TB) is relatively uncommon in North America, but worldwide it's a leading cause of death, claiming 3 million lives annually. Further, it is estimated that one-third of the world's population is infected with one of several strains of *Mycobacterium*, the bacillus that causes TB. Although the disease is inactive in most of these people, at any given time there are some 30 million active cases of TB.

The TB bacillus is spread when an infected person coughs or sneezes, releasing the microorganism into the air. Infection occurs when the bacillus is inhaled and enters the lungs, where it can silently multiply. The immune system usually eradicates the infection at this early stage, but in some people the bacillus remains dormant in the body. Even so, most infected people never develop symptoms, although they will still have a positive TB skin test, indicating the presence of antibodies against the disease-causing organism.

A latent infection can develop into full-blown TB if the immune system becomes weakened by malnutrition, age, or a serious disease, such as AIDS or cancer. The initial symptoms—loss of appetite and weight, night sweats, fever and chills, and general malaise—may resemble a lingering bout of flu. But as the disease progresses, more severe manifestations appear: typically, a chronic cough, profuse sputum that may be blood-tinged and malodorous, increasing weakness, and eventually, muscle wasting. Although the lungs are TB's most common target organ, the disease can attack almost any part of the body, including the brain, kidneys, spine, bones, and skin.

Throughout the 20th century, the number of TB cases in North America declined steadily. By the mid-1980s, however, a sharp increase was reported, mostly among AIDS patients and the homeless. In addition, some people who had been treated for (and presumably cured of) TB decades previous suffered recurrences.

ROLE OF DIET

The typical TB treatment regimen calls for long-term daily administration of several powerful antibiotics: usually isoniazid, rifampin, pyrazinamide, and either ethambutol or streptomycin. While undergoing treatment, patients must abstain from alcohol, which interacts with the drugs and also increases the risk of liver and nerve damage—common side effects of the TB regimen. Both the disease and the medications cause loss of appetite, but it is critical to maintain good nutrition to minimize weight loss, bolster immunity, and rebuild damaged tissue.

TB diet composition. The diet should provide high-quality protein, preferably from lean meat, poultry, fish, eggs, milk, and other animal products. (Although the results are inconclusive, some studies suggest that vegetarians are more vulnerable to TB and its complications than are people whose diets include some animal protein.) Citrus fruits and other fresh fruits and vegetables provide vitamin C and beta carotene, antioxidants that the body needs to boost immunity. Zinc is also important to foster healing and a strong immune system; good sources include oysters and other shellfish, lean meat, milk, beans, nuts, and whole grains.

Get lots of vitamin D. Researchers have found an explanation as to why TB patients who spend time in the sunshine and fresh air often improve faster. White blood cells that are armed with high concentrations of vitamin D appear to be more effective in destroying the bacillus. The body makes vitamin D when the skin is exposed to the sun; good dietary sources include fluid milk, fortified soy and rice beverages, margarine, eggs, and fatty fish.

Role of vitamin B$_6$. Isoniazid is especially destructive to the nerves. To counter this, some doctors prescribe B$_6$ supplements. Foods that are high in this nutrient include most animal products, grains, spinach, and potatoes.

Critical to maintain weight. It is critical to consume more calories than usual to counter the weight loss that is characteristic of TB. The diet should emphasize foods that are dense in calories and easy to digest. Good choices, in addition to the foods already mentioned, include legumes, pasta, grains, and other starchy foods; milk shakes or perhaps enriched milk-based drinks; and rich soups, custards, eggs, puddings, and ice cream.

OTHER MEASURES

Because tuberculosis usually damages the lungs, it's important to avoid exposure to tobacco smoke and other pollutants that are harmful to the lungs. It is imperative that smokers give up the habit; secondhand smoke should also be avoided as much as possible.

Although TB is highly contagious, the risk of spreading it can be minimized by practicing good hygiene and by not sharing eating utensils and other personal items. When coughing or sneezing, a person with TB should always cover his mouth and nose with a tissue and then promptly dispose of it.

Because sun and fresh air help destroy airborne bacilli, the living quarters should be aired frequently and as much sunshine as possible allowed in. Anyone who lives in close contact with a tuberculosis patient should undergo testing for the disease; in some cases, preventive antibiotic treatment may be warranted. ❖

TURNIPS

BENEFITS
- A useful source of vitamin C, as well as some calcium and potassium.
- A low-calorie source of fiber.
- May protect against certain cancers.

DRAWBACKS
- May cause flatulence.
- Contain substances that interfere with the production of thyroid hormones.

Turnips (including the yellow rutabagas) are economical, healthful, and easy to prepare and cultivate (even in soil of poor quality), and surprisingly full of vitamin C and some essential amino acids. One cup of boiled turnips yields only 35 calories while providing 18 mg of vitamin C, 35 mg of calcium, and 210 mg of potassium. They are also a useful source of fiber, including soluble dietary fibers that help soak

FACTS ABOUT TURNIPS
- Native to Europe and central Asia, turnips were first cultivated in the Middle East 4,000 years ago.
- Turnips are used as both table and hog food in eastern Europe.
- The rutabaga evolved from a cross between the turnip and cabbage, and thus it has more vitamin C than turnips do.

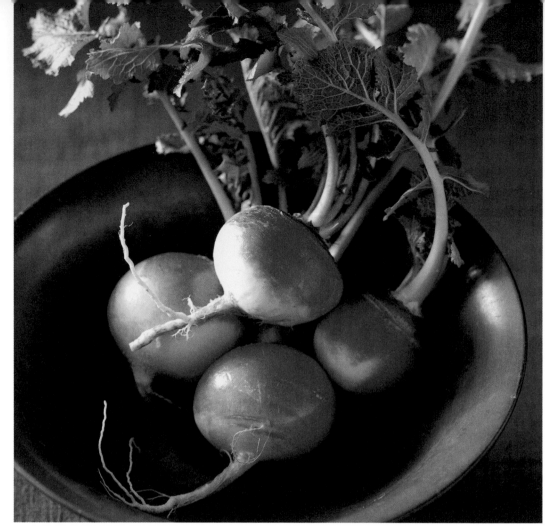

VERSATILE AND TASTY COMPLEX CARBOHYDRATES. *Turnips have been cultivated for 4,000 years and for good reason. They grow in poor soil, are low in calories, and high in nutrients, especially the greens.*

up LDL ("bad") cholesterol. They also contain lysine, an amino acid that may help to prevent and manage cold sores.

The turnip tops, or greens, which many cooks discard, are even more nutritious than the roots themselves. One cup of boiled greens provides 40 mg of vitamin C, about 200 mg of calcium, and nearly 300 mg of potassium. In addition, unlike the roots, the greens are an excellent source of beta carotene, an important antioxidant nutrient that the body converts to vitamin A. The same cup of boiled greens yields nearly 7,500 IU of vitamin A and 5 g of fiber.

As a member of the cruciferous family, which includes cabbage, broccoli, and radishes, turnips contain sulfurous compounds that may protect against certain forms of cancer. However, like other cruciferous vegetables, turnips can cause bloating and gas.

Turnips contain two goitrogenic substances, progoitrin and gluconasturtin, which can interfere with the thyroid gland's ability to make its hormones. These compounds do not pose a risk for healthy people who eat moderate amounts of turnips, but anyone with hypothyroidism should cook this vegetable since cooking appears to deactivate goitrogens.

Most people serve boiled turnips, but they can also be baked, braised, or steamed. They make a tasty addition to salads, stews, soups, or vegetable dishes.

Some herbal practitioners use turnips to treat bronchitis and sore throats. These benefits have not been proven. ❖

DID YOU KNOW?

TURNIPS CAN BE PINK

White turnips are given star billing in the Middle East. In fact, there is even a Lebanese saying that is paid as a compliment: "Her face is whiter than the inside of a turnip." In Middle Eastern cuisine, turnips are often pickled with beets to give them a pink color. Small white turnips are sliced or chunked and placed in a glass jar with pieces of beets, garlic cloves, and celery leaves. Salt (4 to 5 tablespoons) is dissolved in 1 cup of vinegar and 3 cups of water and then poured over the vegetables. The jar is sealed and left in a warm place for about 10 days.

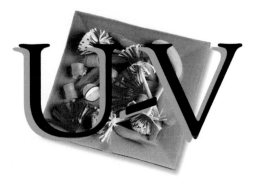

ULCERS

CONSUME

- A balanced, varied diet to promote healing.
- Lean meat, poultry, enriched or fortified breads and cereals, legumes, and dried fruits for iron lost through bleeding.

AVOID

- Coffee, including decaffeinated, and other sources of caffeine.
- Spices such as pepper, chili peppers, cloves, and garlic, which trigger acid secretion.
- Alcohol.
- Smoking.
- Fatty foods.
- Late-night snacks.

All sores that erode mucous membranes or the skin and penetrate the underlying muscle are referred to as ulcers. Those that occur in the lower part of the esophagus, the stomach, or the duodenum are known more specifically as "peptic ulcers," because they form in areas exposed to stomach acids and the digestive enzyme, pepsin. Peptic ulcer disease is one of the most common disorders diagnosed in North America today, and men and women are equally affected. When the erosion occurs in the duodenum, the upper part of the small intestine, the term duodenal ulcer is used to describe the lesion; an ulcer in the stomach is called a gastric ulcer.

A person with an ulcer may describe the pain as gnawing or burning and can often pinpoint the exact spot. The pain usually occurs 2 to 3 hours after eating, is worse when the stomach is empty, and can be relieved by eating a small amount of food or taking an antacid. Some people never have ulcer pain; however, they may develop intestinal bleeding, heartburn, bloating, and gas, as well as nausea and vomiting.

CAUSES OF ULCERS

The antacid industry is based on the notion that oversecretion of stomach acid causes ulcers as well as indigestion and heartburn. Although excess acid secretion plays a role, most ulcers develop when a common bacterium, called *Helicobacter pylori*, infects the intestinal tract. Smoking, emotional stress, and heavy drinking can also contribute to a person's risk of ulcers, and some people may have a hereditary predisposition. Ulcers frequently occur in people subjected to extreme physical stress, such as serious burns or surgery.

The other major cause of ulcers is the heavy use of drugs like aspirin, ibuprofen, naproxen, and other nonsteroidal anti-inflammatory drugs (NSAIDs), which erode the mucous membranes. Aspirin's effects are particularly serious, because it also inhibits blood clotting and promotes bleeding.

MEDICAL TREATMENT

Better understanding of the causes of ulcers has enabled doctors to devise new treatments. If tests confirm the presence of *H. pylori*, the treatment includes antibiotics to eradicate the bacteria and an acid secretion inhibitor to prevent secretion of acids by the cells of the stomach. The bacteria are usually eradicated in a week, but a significant percentage of patients experience side effects such as nausea, diarrhea, or a metallic taste. A daily yogurt supplement with live lactobacilli and bifidobacteria during treatment can reduce these symptoms.

Stop smoking. Smoking is one factor closely linked to poor healing and ulcer recurrence. Cigarette smokers often continue to suffer from ulcers until they quit.

Stop harmful medications. People with ulcers caused by NSAID use must discontinue the offending drug. People who need ongoing pain relief for a condition such as arthritis should ask their doctor to prescribe a gentler alternative.

Exercise to raise your endorphin level. Mindful that "it's not what you're eating, it's what's eating you," people with ulcers may benefit from relaxation techniques and biofeedback to cope with stress. Regular exercise promotes the release of endorphins, brain chemicals that dull pain and elevate mood.

DID YOU KNOW?

THE PRESENCE OF *H. PYLORI* BACTERIA INCREASES YOUR RISK OF STOMACH CANCER

H. pylori, the bacterium that causes peptic ulcers weakens the mucous coating that protects the stomach lining, allowing acid to do damage. Infection by the bacteria increases stomach cancer risk two- to sixfold, whether or not you develop an ulcer.

EAT MODERATE-SIZE MEALS AT REGULAR INTERVALS

When and how people eat may be more important than what they eat. Doctors no longer recommend frequent small meals, which can provoke rebound symptoms. Rather, they suggest several moderate-size meals spaced at regular intervals. Late-evening snacks should be avoided, because they stimulate acid secretion during sleep. It is also wise to avoid eating large quantities of food at one time.

HOME REMEDIES

Many people self-treat ulcer pain with over-the-counter drugs or with home remedies concocted from baking soda (sodium bicarbonate) to neutralize stomach acid. But long-term use of antacids containing aluminum hydroxide can prevent the body from absorbing phosphorus and result in the loss of bone minerals. Prolonged ingestion of baking soda or antacids containing calcium carbonate may lead to a buildup of calcium and alkali, resulting in nausea, headache, and weakness, with a risk of kidney damage. Check with a doctor before using acid-suppressant drugs.

One home remedy that seems to work well is a form of licorice called deglycyrrhizinated licorice (DGL). DGL is sold in wafer form at health-food stores. Follow the dosage instructions on the package. Another home remedy to try is aloe vera juice. Drink a half cup three times a day.

DIET AND ULCERS

A bland diet was once the mainstay of treatment, but it is no longer recommended as there is no evidence that it speeds the rate of healing. The main goal of diet is to avoid extreme elevations in gastric acid secretion and irritation of the gastrointestinal lining.

Avoid trigger foods. Triggers vary from person to person, but common offenders are coffee (including decaffeinated), caffeine in beverages and chocolate, alcohol, peppermint, and tomatoes and tomato-based products. Peppermint and chocolate can also interfere with the closing of the valve that connects the esophagus to the stomach, allowing acidic juices to "reflux" up the esophagus. This can cause heartburn. Fatty foods can slow down stomach emptying and stimulate acid release. Milk and dairy products temporarily relieve pain but can cause a rebound increase in acid secretion. Foods and seasonings that stimulate gastric acid secretion such as black pepper, garlic, cloves, and chili powder should be limited or avoided by people for whom they cause problems. Citrus juices may cause discomfort for some people.

Eat iron-rich foods. Bleeding from untreated ulcers can lead to iron-deficiency anemia. People with anemia should eat iron-rich foods, including lean meat, poultry, enriched or fortified breads and cereals, dried fruit, and dried beans and other legumes. ❖

UNDERWEIGHT

EAT PLENTY OF
- Larger portions and high-calorie choices.
- Nutritious between-meal snacks.

LIMIT
- Alcohol and caffeine, which can suppress the appetite.

In a society that prizes leanness and spends billions on weight-loss products, people find it hard to accept that excessive thinness (unrelated to anorexia nervosa) is unhealthy. But while obesity is dangerous, surveys show that people who are of average weight at age 50 live longer than those who are markedly underweight.

There's no such thing as a perfect weight; however, for every height and build there is a desirable range in which the rates of disease and death are lowest. Underweight is defined as 15 percent or more under the low end of the range (your doctor can advise you what your range should be). Mild underweight is not associated with serious health hazards, but people who are very thin lack energy reserves, are vulnerable to infections, and often feel the cold because they lack insulating fat. Patients weighing less than 80 percent of their desirable weight on admission to a hospital are at high risk for complications. Severely underweight people who are confined to bed rest easily develop pressure sores over bony areas.

WHEN THINNESS IS A PROBLEM

Thinness is a problem if it is a result of poor nutrition, such as chronic dieting, which can lead to infertility in women. For those who conceive, being underweight during pregnancy may cause anemia, heart and lung complications, and a high risk of toxemia. Their babies are often premature, have a low birth weight, and may experience slow growth and development.

TEN WAYS TO INCREASE CALORIES

1. Eat at least three well-balanced meals, including a hearty breakfast, and snacks throughout the day. For some people, it might be easier to eat smaller, more frequent meals than three large meals.

2. Eat hearty soups such as lentil, minestrone, split pea, or cream soups rather than broth. Make your canned soup with regular milk or evaporated milk instead of water and top it with Parmesan cheese and croutons.

3. Eat cereals with added fruit or nuts instead of the puffed varieties. Make cooked cereal with milk instead of water.

4. Add powdered milk to puddings, baked goods, milk shakes, and mashed potatoes.

5. To boost the calories and protein of a glass of milk, add a bit of milk powder to your regular milk.

6. Dried fruits such as raisins, dates, prunes, or dried apricots are high in calories and can be eaten as a snack or added to cereal or in baking.

7. Salads are low in calories but can be made more substantial by adding cheese or chickpeas or even sunflower seeds or raisins.

8. Nuts are high in fat and calories and make a good snack.

9. Choose desserts that have nutritional value but also are high in calories. Puddings, sweet breads such as banana bread or carrot muffins, ice cream, oatmeal cookies all make the grade.

10. Don't let anyone talk you into taking any supplements that are "guaranteed to put on weight." Be patient, try to keep a positive attitude about food, eat lots of healthy food, exercise regularly, and you will gradually start to see results.

Adolescents with erratic schedules are prone to slip below their ideal weight—especially if they exercise a lot. Overly thin teenagers and adults alike sometimes feel too busy to eat.

A CORRECTIVE DIET

Gaining 1 lb (0.45 kg) a week can require 500 to 750 extra calories a day. For some, dietary adjustments can be as taxing as a weight-loss regimen. The aim should be to build up muscle tissue and increase the level of energy to sustain the weight gain. Unless extremely weak, underweight people should exercise regularly to help build lean tissue as well as store some fat.

Extremely important to increase dietary calories from fat. A plan for increasing weight focuses, first, on increasing food intake and, second, on consuming foods that provide lots of calories in a compact volume. Raw vegetables, for example, are nutritious but satisfy hunger long before they've provided significant calories. And although a low-fat diet is important, an underweight person may need to relax the rules about fat consumption until the desired weight goal has been reached. Increasing dietary fat can rapidly make a difference, because fat contains more than twice as many calories (9 per gram) as protein and carbohydrates do (4 per gram).

Increase your portions of calorie-dense foods. Nutrition experts advise adhering to your food guide recommendations, but gradually increasing portions and choosing the more nutrient and calorie-dense foods within each group: peanut butter or cheese instead of lean meat, avocados instead of cucumbers, pancakes instead of toast, a milk shake instead of skim milk. Because caffeine suppresses the urge to eat, replace tea or coffee with juices and milk.

Augment your diet with liquid supplements. People who have lost weight due to illness may benefit from a concentrated liquid formula, which is easy to swallow. Doctors and dietitians can recommend liquid supplements.

Many underweight people feel uncomfortably full when they begin eating larger, more frequent portions to gain weight. This feeling eventually passes. People trying to gain weight, like those trying to lose it, occasionally reach a plateau. Increasing calorie intake is necessary to restart the process. ❖

URINARY TRACT INFECTIONS

CONSUME PLENTY OF
- Nonalcoholic and caffeine-free fluids to flush out the urinary system.
- Cranberry juice and blueberries.
- Citrus fruits and fresh fruits and vegetables for vitamin C.

AVOID
- Bladder irritants, such as coffee, tea, and alcoholic beverages.

Also known as cystitis, most urinary tract infections (UTIs) affect the bladder, but some may involve the kidneys, the ureters (the tubes that carry urine to the bladder), and the urethra (the tube through which urine exits the body). The

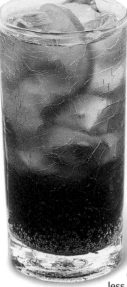

DO ONE SIMPLE THING

DRINK BERRY JUICE

A Finnish study followed 150 women who had a urinary tract infection but were not taking antibiotics. They found that giving women one glass of cranberry-lingonberry juice daily for 6 months significantly reduced recurrences of UTIs compared to women who received a placebo. Another study, published in the *American Journal of Clinical Nutrition,* showed that consumption of berry juices, particularly raspberry, cranberry, strawberry, and currant juices, one to three times per week was associated with a lower risk of UTI recurrence compared with drinking berry juice less than once a week. This same study showed that women who consumed fermented dairy products, which contained probiotic bacteria (such as yogurt with *Lactobacillus acidophilus*), also had a decreased risk.

most common symptom is an urgent need to urinate, even when the bladder is not full. Urination may be accompanied by pain or burning and, in severe cases, small amounts of blood. There may also be a low-grade fever and an ache in the lower back.

Most urinary infections are caused by *E. coli* bacteria, organisms that live in the intestinal tract but that can travel to the bladder. Chlamydia, a sexually transmitted organism, is another cause of UTIs. Women are more vulnerable to urinary infections because the female urethra is shorter than that of males, and its location provides a convenient entryway for bacteria. Many women develop so-called honeymoon cystitis, inflammation caused by sexual activity or an oversize diaphragm.

ROLE OF DIET

Antibiotics are needed to cure bacterial urinary infections, but dietary approaches can speed healing and help prevent recurrences.

- Doctors advise drinking at least 8 to 10 glasses a day of fluids to increase the flow of urine and to flush out infectious material.
- Avoid coffee, tea, colas, and alcoholic drinks, since these increase bladder irritation. Some people find that spicy foods also aggravate the urinary tract.
- Cranberry juice is a favorite home remedy, and one that is supported by research. Cran-

berries and blueberries contain substances that speed the elimination of bacteria by preventing them from sticking to the bladder wall.
- Vitamin C helps strengthen the immune system, fight infection, and acidify the urine. And calcium may help reduce bladder irritability.
- Consuming probiotics may be helpful since they are thought to inhibit the growth of microorganisms that cause UTIs. These beneficial bacteria, found in some yogurts, are also thought to foster the growth of friendly flora in the body, which may be reduced by antibiotic therapy.

ADDITIONAL PREVENTIVE TACTICS

Hygiene measures can help women avoid recurrent UTIs; many doctors recommend the following tactics.

- Wear loose-fitting white cotton underwear and panty hose that have cotton crotches.
- Avoid douching and using vaginal deodorants, which can cause bladder irritation.
- If you use a diaphragm, ask your doctor to check the size; one that is even slightly too large can irritate the urethra and bladder.
- Urinate and drink a glass of water before sexual intercourse and urinate within an hour afterward to flush out the urinary tract.
- After a bowel movement, wipe from the front to the back to reduce the risk of carrying intestinal bacteria to the urethra. ❖

VEGETABLES

BENEFITS

- Many are rich in vitamins A, C, and E, folate and other B vitamins, potassium and other minerals.
- High fiber content promotes regular bowel function.
- Rich in bioflavonoids and other compounds that help prevent disease.

DRAWBACKS

- Some are allergens.

Plants combine water, carbon dioxide from the air, and nutrients from the soil to synthesize all the compounds necessary for animal life. We live on vegetables whether we eat them directly or through animal intermediaries.

Root vegetables, such as beets, carrots, parsnips, and turnips, are food storage organs and valuable sources of carbohydrates. Stems, such as celery and fennel, conduct nutrients between roots and leaves, and in some plants, such as potatoes and water chestnuts, underground stems have evolved into storehouses for starch. Vegetables with dark green leaves, including members of the cabbage family (such as broccoli, cauliflower, collard greens, kale, and mustard greens) and spinach, are rich in antioxidants, bioflavonoids, and the B vitamins. The leaves of all vegetables are factories for the production of high-energy sugars through photosynthesis. They are the most fragile parts of the plant, which is the reason they shrink more than other parts when cooked. The leaves of plants in the onion family have grown into fleshy bulbs that store carbohydrates and water to nourish the plant during its next year of growth. The flowers of some plants are also eaten; broccoli stems are eaten with their unopened flower buds and the flowers of zucchini are a delicacy.

HOW MUCH IS ENOUGH?

It is highly recommended that we eat 5 to 10 servings of fruits and vegetables daily. A serving is a half cup of raw or cooked vegetables, a cup of leafy salad vegetables, or a half cup of juice. Nutritionists recommend choosing a variety of vegetables, both raw and cooked, including richly colored orange, red, dark green, and yellow vegetables, vegetables from the cruciferous family, and allium vegetables such as onion and garlic. In addition to antioxidants, vitamins, and minerals, these plants are teeming with the disease-fighting compounds known as phytochemicals.

NUTRITIONAL VALUE

Most vegetables are excellent sources of vitamins, fiber, folate, potassium, as well as some other minerals. They are also rich in various phytochemicals that provide protection from disease. Vegetables are low in fat and usually low in calories.

Green vegetables get their bright color from chlorophyll, the pigment that traps the energy from sunlight and makes it available for the production of sugars from water and carbon dioxide. Although chlorophyll is soluble only in fats, cooking vegetables in water liberates the enzyme chlorophyllase, which breaks chlorophyll down into water-soluble components. This has no nutritional consequence, but the green color of the vegetable is diminished. Some vitamins are also water-soluble, and are leached out into the cooking water. That's one reason nutritionists recommend using the water vegetables are cooked in as a basis for stock.

Color is a useful guide to the vitamin content of vegetables. Plants produce vitamin C from sugars formed by photosynthesis in their leaves. The larger and darker the leaves are, the more vitamin C and beta carotene they contain; the pale inner leaves of lettuce and cabbage, for instance, have only about 3 percent of the carotene found in the dark outer leaves. Unfortunately, outer leaves are often discarded because they are damaged or have been exposed to pollutants and pesticides.

Deep yellow, orange, or dark green vegetables derive their color from carotenoid pigments; these include beta carotene, an antioxidant that is converted to vitamin A in the intestinal wall. Because these pigments are stable in cooking and soluble in fat, the nutritional content is well preserved during baking or boiling.

Soluble and insoluble fiber in vegetables keeps bowel function regular and thereby reduces the colon's exposure to potentially toxic by-products of digestion. In some people, however, fiber can cause gas and bloating.

ANTICANCER FOODS

Cancer develops when mutant cells escape the body's immune system. Plants are also susceptible to cellular damage and have developed their own protective mechanisms. Beta carotene and vitamins C and E are natural antioxidants that hinder cell damage by scavenging and inactivating free radicals, the unstable molecules that are released when the body uses oxygen.

Some phytochemicals in vegetables block the growth of blood vessels that feed tumors, others inactivate the enzyme systems that allow cancer cells to spread, and still others suppress the hormones that promote cancer growth.

Indoles, found in cruciferous vegetables such as broccoli, cauliflower, turnip, and cabbage, appear to stimulate enzymes that offer some cancer protection. Lutein, found in corn, dark leafy greens, and peppers, is an antioxidant that helps prevent the age-related eye disease called macular degeneration. Lycopene, found in tomato products, watermelon, and pink grapefruit, has been shown to lower the risk of prostate cancer

MYTH BUSTER

Myth: Add a pinch of baking soda during cooking to produce a bright green color in the vegetable.

Reality: Although baking soda does keep the vegetables green, it also breaks down the plant tissues, making the texture mushy and destroying many of the vitamins.

as well as provide protection from heart disease. Onions and garlic contain sulfur compounds, many of which also offer disease protection. For example, in Vidalia, Georgia, where large amounts of onions are consumed, the death rate from stomach cancer is significantly reduced.

Studies have found that people who eat ample vegetables and fruits enjoy a reduced incidence of many cancers. By contrast, researchers have found that people who eat few vegetables are more prone to develop colon cancer.

Vegetables have a protective effect that goes far beyond what vitamin pills can offer. Most vegetables have more than one benefit. Broccoli, for example, contains beta carotene, vitamin C, fiber, folic acid, and the phytochemical sulforaphane. It is this variety of protective nutrients, plant chemicals, and as-yet-unidentified compounds in vegetables that helps keep cancer at bay.

PRESERVING NUTRIENTS

While vegetables provide starches, sugars, and proteins, their main contributions are vitamins, minerals, fiber, and protective phytochemicals. Their nutrient content, color, and texture are affected by the method of preparation, the length of cooking time, and the volume of water used.

The yellow carotene pigments are not water soluble and are well preserved in cooking, but vitamin C and the B vitamins leach into the cooking liquid. Vitamin C is also destroyed on exposure to oxygen. In addition, up to 20 percent of the vitamin C in a vegetable may be lost during each minute that it takes the water to heat from cold to boiling. This is because an enzyme that destroys vitamin C becomes more active as temperature rises; however, it stops its destructive action at the boiling point. For this reason, vegetables should be added to water that is already boiling. Steaming or cooking in a small amount of water retains more than twice as much vitamin C as boiling does.

The yellow and orange carotenoid pigments are changed only by the high temperatures reached with pressure cooking. The attractive brilliant green of chlorophyll in plant tissues is dulled, however, when heat causes chemical changes. This does not matter as chlorophyll cannot affect the human body internally since it is not absorbed.

Some cooks blanch vegetables such as beans and broccoli in boiling water for a minute or two, then plunge them into cold water to hold the color. This is satisfactory for vegetables that are served cold, but if they are served hot, they require rapid reheating, with further loss of nutrients.

To preserve the betacyanin in beets, avoid boiling them in water—it's best to roast, bake, or microwave whole beets in their skins. Peeled or cut-up beets leach the vegetable's pigments (and thus the betacyanin is lost). In addition, boiling in water depletes beets of their folate, which is water soluble.

STORAGE

Because harvested vegetables lose flavor, sweetness, and texture as they use up their own food stores, the least amount of time stored, the better. Corn and peas can lose up to 40 percent of their sugar if kept at room temperature for just 6 hours after picking. Beans and stem vegetables, such as broccoli and asparagus, are known to become tough.

Vegetables that originated in warm climates (including beans, eggplants, peppers, okra, squash, and tomatoes) keep best at 50°F (10°C). Potatoes convert their starch to sugar below 40°F (4°C); keep them cool and out of the light to prevent the formation of poisonous

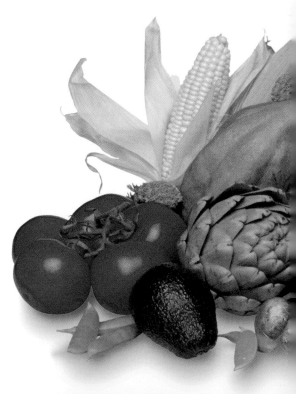

alkaloids. Most other vegetables keep best at 32°F (0°C). The salts and sugars in their sap prevent them from freezing until several degrees colder. Tomatoes should not be refrigerated: the cold temperature ruins the flavor. They are best stored on the kitchen counter and used within a few days. Potatoes, squash, and sweet potatoes are best stored in a cool, dark place, not in the fridge. Greens should be washed, drained, wrapped in paper or cloth towels, and stored in a tightly sealed container in the fridge. If bought in airtight packaging, store as is. Peppers should be stored in the refrigerator, away from the fruits.

POSSIBLE HAZARDS

Most vegetables are safe to eat either raw or cooked. The exceptions are lima and kidney beans and other legumes, which contain toxic substances that are inactivated through cooking. Broccoli, kale, and other cruciferous vegetables harbor goitrogenic compounds that can interfere with iodine metabolism. Cooking inactivates these compounds, but eating large amounts of these vegetables raw may worsen a pre-existing thyroid condition.

Most vegetables do not provoke allergies, but some people react to members of the nightshade family, which includes eggplants and tomatoes. Corn is another common allergen. ❖

EIGHT WAYS TO EAT MORE VEGGIES

1. When you make a sandwich or burger, load up on the veggies. Sliced tomatoes, shredded cabbage, peppers, cucumbers, onions, and dark greens are all perfect toppers.

2. Top homemade pizza with zucchini or squash slices, fresh spinach, mushrooms, onions, peppers, broccoli florets, shredded carrots, and fresh tomato slices.

3. Add extra fresh or frozen veggies to your favorite pasta sauce, chili, lasagna, casserole or stew.

4. Enjoy a bowl of minestrone or vegetable soup. In the summer, make gazpacho or cold cucumber soup.

5. Supplement take-out or frozen dinners with extra vegetables. When eating out, order extra vegetables as a side dish or a side salad or grilled vegetables as an appetizer.

6. Cut favorite vegetables into snack-size pieces. Store them in clear plastic containers and make sure they are the first thing you see when you open the fridge.

7. For convenience, shop for cut-up, cleaned, and ready-to-eat fresh vegetables.

8. For best value and top nutrition, buy in season. Get to know the produce manager at the store. He can tell you which is freshest and what to look for when choosing specific vegetables.

VEGETARIAN DIETS
■ HOW HEALTHFUL ARE THEY? ■

5 rules for healthy vegetarian eating

1. Choose a variety of foods, including whole grains, vegetables, fruits, legumes, nuts, seeds and, if desired, dairy products and eggs.
2. Choose whole, unrefined foods often and limit highly sweetened, fatty, and heavily refined foods.
3. Choose a variety of fruits and vegetables.
4. If dairy products and eggs are included, choose lower-fat dairy products and use both eggs and dairy products in moderation.
5. Use a regular source of vitamin B_{12} and, if sunlight exposure is limited, vitamin D.

It used to be that scientific research on vegetarian diets questioned their nutritional adequacy, particularly with regard to their protein content. But as most of these concerns have faded in recent years, researchers have begun studying vegetarian diets with respect to their role in both the prevention and treatment of disease.

As a result, there has been a growing appreciation for the benefits of vegetarian diets or those that include generous amounts of plant foods and limited amounts of animal foods. The American Institute for Cancer Research, the American Cancer Society, and the National Institutes of Health are some of the many health organizations now recommending these types of diets. Both the American Dietetic Association and Dietitians of Canada support appropriately planned vegetarian diets as "healthful, nutritionally adequate, and providing health benefits in the prevention and treatment of certain diseases." Vegetarianism has come a long way!

Technically, a vegetarian is defined as a person who does not eat meat, fish or fowl or products that contain them. However, in reality, the eating patterns of vegetarians can vary considerably, from strict vegetarians (vegans), to those who include dairy and/or fish in their diet. Some self-described vegetarians may even include occasional fish, chicken, and meat in their diet (see "Vegetarian Variations," next page).

Health benefits

Much of what we know about the health benefits of vegetarian diets comes from studies of Seventh-day Adventists. A high percentage of vegetarians is found among the adherents of this religious group. Many Seventh-day Adventists are strict vegans, others merely avoid meat. However, Seventh-day Adventists, as well as other vegetarians, often have healthier lifestyles in general, so it's difficult to link the health benefits of their lifestyle to any single dietary factor, such as the absence of animal foods.

■ **Obesity.** Plant-based diets have long been associated with decreased obesity, which is a risk factor for many chronic diseases, including heart disease, high blood pressure, diabetes, and some cancers. Some factors that may help explain lower body weight in vegetarians include lower fat intake, higher fiber consumption, and greater consumption of vegetables.

■ **Cardiovascular disease.** Numerous studies have shown a decreased incidence of heart disease among vegetarians compared with nonvegetarians. This may be explained in part by lower blood cholesterol levels in vegetarians. Compared to nonvegetarians, lacto-ovo-vegetarians and vegans have blood cholesterol levels 14 percent and 35 percent lower, respectively. Although most vegetarians don't eat low-fat diets, their saturated fat intake is considerably lower than that of nonvegetarians. They also consume between 50 to 100 percent more fiber, which helps reduce blood cholesterol levels. In addition, a vegetarian diet has the benefit of the many phytochemicals found in plant foods that have antioxidant properties, and antioxidants make blood cholesterol less likely to stick to artery walls.

■ **Hypertension.** In addition to having lower blood pressure in general, vegetarians also have lower rates of hypertension (high blood pressure) than nonvegetarians. Researchers have looked at possible explanations for this difference, including lower body weight, decreased dietary fat, absence of meat or milk protein, or differences in potassium, magnesium, or calcium intakes, but so far they have not been able to draw any conclusions.

■ **Cancer.** Vegetarians in general have a lower cancer rate compared to the general population. This difference is most significant for prostate cancer and colorectal cancer. A number of factors in vegetarian diets may affect cancer risk, such as lower fat consumption, more fiber, more fruits and vegetables, lower levels of heme iron (from animal sources) and higher intake of phytochemicals like isoflavones, hormonelike plant compounds found in soy and other plant foods.

■ **Diabetes.** There is some evidence that vegetarians have lower rates of diabetes. This protective effect may be the result of lower body weight among vegetarians, as well as a higher fiber intake, which can both improve blood sugar control.

Ensuring adequate nutrient intake

The nutritional needs of vegetarians are the same as those of nonvegetarians and can mostly be met by following general dietary recommendations. However, adjustments need to be made in a few areas to make up for the lack of animal sources of several nutrients, including protein, vitamins D and B_{12}, calcium, zinc, and iron.

Diets that include animal foods

Lacto-vegetarians and lacto-ovo-vegetarians can adequately meet their nutritional needs by following a balanced diet. A variety of foods should be included, with an emphasis on complex carbohydrates and lower-fat choices, including grains, legumes, fruits and vegetables, and lower-fat dairy products, as well as eggs, nuts, and seeds in moderation. This will ensure sufficient energy and protein, and provide good sources of all key nutrients.

Vegetarian variations

The reasons for being vegetarian are varied, including health concerns, ethics, religion, economics, as well as taste. Here are a few of the varieties:

■ **Semi-vegetarians.** Predominantly practice a vegetarian diet, but may include occasional animal foods in their diet.

■ **Lacto-ovo-vegetarians.** Include milk and products made from milk, as well as eggs, but avoid meat, fish, and poultry.

■ **Lacto-vegetarians.** Include milk and products made from milk.

■ **Vegans.** Consume no meat, poultry, fish, dairy, or eggs, and may also exclude honey.

DO ONE SIMPLE THING

EAT COMPLEMENTARY PROTEINS

Although plant foods contain various proteins, they are of an "incomplete" variety. This means they do not contain all the essential amino acids that the body needs. But combining plant foods to make a complete protein can be as simple as eating a legume (peanut butter) with a grain (whole-wheat bread). Alternatively, nuts and seeds can be combined with grains. Examples of complementary plant-protein combinations are:

- Rice and beans.
- Bean-vegetable chili served with tortillas.
- Baked beans and corn bread.
- Hummus (made with chickpeas and sesame seeds).
- Breadsticks with sesame seeds.
- Multigrain bread made with sunflower seeds.
- Split-pea soup served with a whole-wheat roll.

Vegan diets

Vegans need to plan their diets more carefully to make sure that their energy and nutrient needs are being met, particularly for children, adolescents, pregnant and breast-feeding women, and older adults.

Protein. Vegans can meet their protein needs by combining complementary plant protein sources to make complete proteins (see "Eat Complementary Proteins," at left). Adults don't need to eat complementary plant proteins at each meal as long as they are eaten in the same day, and as long as a balanced and varied diet provides enough protein on a regular basis. For growing children, whose protein needs are higher, complete protein sources at each meal, such as bread with peanut butter, or beans and rice, are recommended.

Calories. Because plant-based diets are high in fiber and lower in calorie-dense foods, care needs to be taken to make sure there is adequate energy in the diet, especially for children. Foods with higher caloric density, such as nuts and dried fruits, should be included often in meals and snacks.

Vitamin B_{12}. Because plant foods don't contain B_{12}, vegans need to include a reliable source in their diet daily, such as nutritionally enriched yeast, or a B_{12} supplement.

Vitamin D. Our two best sources of vitamin D are sun exposure and foods fortified with vitamin D, such as cow's milk, margarine, and fortified soy and rice beverages. If sun exposure and intake of fortified foods are not adequate, then vitamin D supplements are recommended.

Trace minerals. Iron, calcium, zinc, and other trace minerals are not as readily available from plant sources, so vegans need to develop strategies to make sure they're getting adequate amounts, such as: eating iron-enriched cereals, including sources of vitamin C at meals to help absorption of iron from plant foods, and eating dark green vegetables, tofu, legumes, almonds, and sesame seeds to ensure adequate calcium intake.

Children's needs

Children have high nutrient requirements, but they have small stomachs, so a strict vegetarian diet, containing mainly fruits and vegetables, whole grains, and a lot of bulky fiber, may be too low in calories and nutrients to meet a child's needs. But with some careful planning, a balanced vegan diet with good sources of protein and some concentrated sources of energy can adequately support growth and nutrition.

The daily diet should include: three meals plus plenty of appealing snacks like trail mix, muffins, and whole-grain cookies; sources of fat, such as nuts, seeds, avocados, and nut-butters; and plenty of protein-rich foods like tofu, nut-butters, soy cheese, and yogurt.

Vegetarians may need more iron and zinc

Phytates, compounds found mostly in cereal grains, legumes, and nuts, bind with iron and prevent the body from using it. Vegetarians should increase their intake of plant foods that are rich in iron, or should discuss the use of an iron supplement with their doctor. The Recommended Dietary Allowance (RDA) of iron for vegetarians who eat no animal products is 1.8 times greater than the RDA for nonvegetarians. For example, a 30-year-old vegetarian woman will need 32 mg instead of 18 mg daily. Vitamin C can help reduce the effects of phytates, and cooking or baking vegetables also releases some of the iron that is bound to the phytates.

VINEGAR

BENEFITS
- Basis for a low-calorie salad dressing.
- Can be used to preserve other foods.

DRAWBACKS
- May trigger an allergic reaction in people sensitive to molds.

For centuries, vinegar was a by-product of wine and beer making; in fact, the name comes from the French word *vinaigre*, which means sour wine. Apple cider and wine remain the most popular basic ingredients, but almost any product that produces alcoholic fermentation can be used to make vinegar, as evidenced by the dozens of varieties available today.

Although many people have accorded various healing powers to vinegar over the years, it lacks medicinal properties. It does, however, provide a low-sodium, low-calorie flavoring.

All vinegars are 4 to 14 percent acetic acid. They are made in two stages. First, yeasts or other molds are added to turn the natural sugars in the basic ingredient into alcohol. Then, bacteria are introduced to convert the alcohol into acetic acid.

VARIETIES OF VINEGAR
Plain white (clear) distilled vinegar is the type used for making pickles and other condiments. It can be transformed into a flavored or gourmet vinegar simply by adding various herbs, spices, or fruits—for example, dill, tarragon, lemon balm, mint, garlic, green peppercorns, chilies, citrus, or raspberries. These and many other varieties are widely available, or you can make your own by adding fresh herbs or fruit to distilled, cider, or wine vinegars. Cover tightly and store in a dark cupboard. The acetic acid keeps the herbs or fruits from spoiling.

DID YOU KNOW?

WHY BALSAMIC VINEGAR IS SO EXPENSIVE

It's the aging process. Rich, dark, and mild-flavored balsamic vinegar originated in Modena, Italy. It is considered by many to be the best-quality vinegar available. It is produced from a type of red wine, and the most-prized—and expensive—varieties are aged 15 to 50 years.

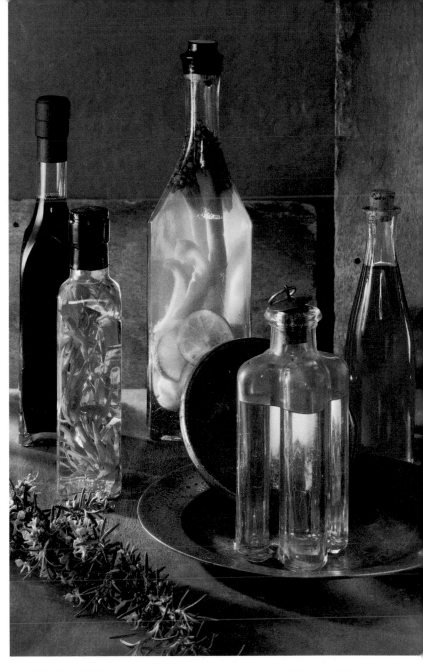

HEALTH BENEFITS
Various vinegars have often been recommended as a treatment for arthritis, indigestion, and other ailments. Such claims have never been proved scientifically, but some arthritis sufferers insist that a tonic of cider vinegar and honey alleviates joint pain.

Vinegar is virtually devoid of calories, so it's an ideal alternative to fatty salad dressings. To reduce its acid bite, the vinegar can be mixed with orange juice or fruit syrup and a little oil.

A note of caution: People who are allergic to molds may react to vinegar as well as to foods preserved with it. Symptoms include a tingling or itching sensation around the mouth, and possibly hives. ❖

SHARP FLAVORS. *As a preserving liquid, vinegar has no equal—once sealed, it can last indefinitely. Enliven salads with (from left to right) balsamic, tarragon, citrus, wine, and sherry vinegars.*

VITAMINS
■ ESSENTIAL NUTRIENTS ■

For more than 2,000 years folk healers and physicians have known that eating certain foods prevents or cures diseases. As far back as 400 B.C., Hippocrates found that eating liver cured night blindness. In another well-known example in 1747, James Lind, a British naval surgeon, carried out experiments and discovered the link between diet and scurvy. He advocated eating lemons and limes to prevent the dreadful disease that was common in sailors who lived on biscuits and salt pork on long voyages.

To date, 13 vitamins essential to health have been discovered. Other vitaminlike substances, such as bioflavonoids, have also been identified. Some appear to be essential to health, but Recommended Dietary Allowances (RDAs) for them have not yet been established. Researchers believe there are probably many more substances that may optimize health and may fall into the vitamin category. That is why they recommend eating a wide variety of foods for complete nutrition.

Only very small amounts—typically a few milligrams or even fractions of milligrams—of vitamins are needed to maintain good health.

Classification

Vitamins are classified according to how they are absorbed and stored in the body. Vitamins A, D, E, and K are soluble only in fats, whereas vitamin C and the B vitamins are soluble in water. The body can store fat-soluble vitamins in the liver and fatty tissue. Since most excess water-soluble vitamins are excreted in the urine, they need to be consumed more often.

Provitamins are substances that the body can convert into vitamins. Examples include beta carotene, a precursor of vitamin A, as well as a type of steroid in the skin that, after exposure to the sun's ultraviolet rays, is used by the body to make vitamin D.

Fat-soluble vitamins

These vitamins need fat in order to be absorbed into the bloodstream from the intestinal tract. Thus, people who have fat-malabsorption disorders can develop deficiency symptoms even though their diet supplies adequate amounts of a vitamin. On the other hand, toxic amounts may build up if a person takes high-dose supplements.

Vitamin A: There are several forms of this vitamin. The preformed, or active, ones are retinol, retinoic acid, and retinyl esters. Beta carotene is a precursor form. Vitamin A is essential to normal vision and to prevent night blindness. But it is also necessary for normal cell division and growth, the development of bones and teeth, and for the health of skin, mucous membranes, and the epithelial tissue that lines the intestines, airways, and other organs. Its antioxidant properties help prevent the cancer-causing cell damage inflicted by free radicals, unstable molecules that are released when the body uses oxygen. The body also needs vitamin A to synthesize amino acids as well as thyroxine and other hormones.

In general, vitamin A supplementation is not recommended. Excessive vitamin A can cause toxicity, which can lead to death in extreme cases. A woman contemplating pregnancy should never take high-dose vitamin A supplements or isotretinoin (Accutane), a powerful acne drug derived from

Why are they called vitamins?

In 1912 Dr. Casimir Funk, a Polish biochemist, put forth the theory that foods contained essential chemical substances that were vital to life. He coined the term *vitamines* referring to them as "vital amines," or nitrogen compounds. In fact, his 1922 work was titled *The Vitamines*. It later turned out that some of these substances were not amines and the *e* was dropped. The term vitamin has been part of our nomenclature ever since.

vitamin A. Because vitamin A is stored in the body, these should be stopped at least 3 months before attempting to conceive. As little as 5,000 IU (International Units) of vitamin A a day has been linked with easier bone fractures in men.

The amount of vitamin A may be listed in International Units or Retinol Equivalents (RE). One RE is equal to 3.3 IU of the retinol form of vitamin A and about 10 IU of beta carotene. One RE is also equal to 1 mcg (microgram) of retinol, or 6 mcg of beta carotene.

Vitamin D: There are two forms of this vitamin: D_2, which comes from plants, and D_3, which the body synthesizes when the skin is exposed to ultraviolet (UV) rays from the sun. In winter, in northern latitudes, when the angle of the sun's rays changes, you are unable to synthesize this vitamin by being outside, no matter how brilliant the sunshine.

The body must have vitamin D in order to absorb calcium. Vitamin D also promotes absorption of phosphorus and prevents the kidneys from excreting protein in the urine. Because of its role in mineral absorption, vitamin D promotes the growth of strong bones and teeth. A deficiency causes rickets in children and osteomalacia in adults (osteomalacia is the adult form of rickets; it is extremely rare in the industrialized world). Other deficiency symptoms include convulsions and muscle twitching.

Vitamin E: The tocopherols in vitamin E prevent oxidation, which results in the rancidity of fats and the destruction of vitamins A and D. They also help to maintain healthy red blood cells and muscle tissue, protect the lungs from pollutants, and regulate the synthesis of vitamin C and DNA. The value of vitamin E supplementation for heart disease prevention remains controversial. Although early studies involving people with cardiovascular disease have shown 20 to 40 percent reductions in coronary disease risk, findings in recent randomized trials with similar subjects have been less positive.

Researchers continue to explore this area in order to better understand the true potential of vitamin E. It may be that protection by vitamin E supplementation is afforded mainly to people without known coronary disease or a subset of heart disease patients, but this has yet to be determined.

Unlike other fat-soluble vitamins, tocopherols do not accumulate to toxic levels in the body. Any excess is excreted in the stools. People taking a blood-thinning medication, such as warfarin, should not take vitamin E without their doctor's approval, as it has anticlotting properties.

Vitamin K: The liver requires vitamin K to manufacture blood proteins that are essential for blood clotting. Intestinal bacteria make half the needed vitamin K; the rest comes from the diet. New research suggests that vitamin K might play a role in maintaining strong bones in adults. Studies suggest that it may increase bone density and also reduce fracture rates. Both the Nurses' Health Study and the Framingham Heart Study found that people who consume the most vitamin K have a lower risk of hip fractures than

(continued on page 380)

ALL ABOUT VITAMINS

VITAMIN	BEST FOOD SOURCES	ROLE IN HEALTH
FAT-SOLUBLE VITAMINS		
Vitamin A (from retinols in animal products or beta carotene in plant foods)	**Retinols:** Liver; salmon and other cold-water fish; egg yolks; fortified milk and dairy products. **Beta carotene:** Orange and yellow fruits and vegetables, such as carrots, squash, and cantaloupes; leafy green vegetables.	Prevents night blindness; needed for growth and cell development; maintains healthy skin, hair, and nails, as well as gums, glands, bones, and teeth; may help prevent lung cancer.
Vitamin D (calciferol)	Fortified milk and butter; egg yolks; fatty fish; fish-liver oils. (Also made by the body when exposed to the sun.)	Necessary for calcium absorption; hepls build and maintain strong bones and teeth.
Vitamin E (tocopherols)	Eggs, vegetable oils, margarine, and mayonnaise; nuts and seeds; fortified cereals.	Protects fatty acids; maintains muscles and red blood cells; important antioxidant.
Vitamin K	Spinach, cabbage, and other green leafy vegetables; pork, liver; and green tea.	Essential for proper blood clotting.
WATER-SOLUBLE VITAMINS		
Biotin	Egg yolks, soybeans, cereals, and yeast.	Energy metabolism.
Folate (folic acid, folacin)	Liver; yeast; broccoli and other cruciferous vegetables; avocados; legumes; many raw vegetables.	Needed to make DNA, RNA, and red blood cells, and to synthesize certain amino acids.
Niacin (vitamin B_3, nicotinic acid, nicotinamide)	Lean meats, poultry, and seafood; milk; eggs; legumes; fortified breads and cereals.	Needed to metabolize energy; promotes normal growth. Large doses lower cholesterol.
Pantothenic acid (vitamin B_5)	Almost all foods.	Aids in energy metabolism; normalizing blood sugar levels; and synthesizing antibodies, cholesterol, hemoglobin, and some hormones.
Riboflavin (vitamin B_2)	Fortified cereals and grains; lean meat and poultry; milk and other dairy products; raw mushrooms.	Essential for energy metabolism; aids adrenal function.
Thiamine (vitamin B_1)	Pork; legumes; nuts and seeds; fortified cereals; and grains.	Energy metabolism; helps maintain normal digestion, appetite, and proper nerve function.
Vitamin B_6 (pyridoxine, pyridoxamine, pyridoxal)	Meat, fish, and poultry; grains and cereals; green leafy vegetables, potatoes, and soybeans.	Promotes protein metabolism; metabolism of carbohydrates and release of energy; proper nerve function; synthesis of red blood cells.
Vitamin B_{12} (cobalamins)	All animal products.	Needed to make red blood cells, DNA, RNA, and myelin (for nerve fibers).
Vitamin C (ascorbic acid)	Citrus fruits and juices; melons, berries, and other fruits; peppers, broccoli, potatoes; and many other fruits and vegetables.	Strengthens blood vessel walls; promotes wound healing; promotes iron absorption; helps prevent atherosclerosis.

RECOMMENDED DIETARY ALLOWANCES
FOR ADULTS OVER 19

MALES	FEMALES	SYMPTOMS OF DEFICIENCY	SYMPTOMS OF EXCESS
900 mcg	700 mcg	Night blindness; stunted growth in children; dry skin and eyes; increased susceptibility to infection.	Headaches and blurred vision; fatigue; bone and joint pain; appetite loss and diarrhea; dry, cracked skin, rashes, and itchiness; hair loss. Can cause birth defects if taken in high doses before and during early pregnancy.
5 mcg[a]*	5 mcg[a]*	Weak bones, leading to rickets in children and osteomalacia in adults.	Headaches, loss of appetite, diarrhea, and possible calcium deposits in heart, blood vessels, and kidneys.
15 mg	15 mg	Unknown in humans.	Excessive bleeding, especially when taken with aspirin and other anticlotting drugs.
120 mcg*	90 mcg*	Excessive bleeding; easy bruising.	May interfere with anticlotting drugs; possible jaundice.
30 mcg*	30 mcg*	Scaly skin; hair loss; depression; elevated blood cholesterol levels.	Apparently none.
400 mcg	400 mcg	Abnormal red blood cells and impaired cell division; anemia; weight loss and intestinal upsets; deficiency may cause birth defects.	May inhibit absorption of phenytoin, causing seizures in epileptics taking this drug; large doses may inhibit zinc absorption.
16 mg	14 mg	Diarrhea and mouth sores; pellagra (in extreme cases).	Hot flashes; liver damage; elevated blood sugar and uric acid.
5 mg*	5 mg*	Unknown in humans.	Very high doses may cause diarrhea and edema.
1.3 mg	1.1 mg	Vision problems and light sensitivity; mouth and nose sores; swallowing problems.	Generally none, but may interfere with cancer chemotherapy.
1.2 mg	1.1 mg	Depression and mood swings; loss of appetite and nausea; muscle cramps. In extreme cases, muscle wasting and beriberi.	Deficiency of other B vitamins.
1.3 mg[b]	1.3 mg[b]	Depression and confusion; itchy, scaling skin; smooth, red tongue; weight loss.	Sensory nerve deterioration.
2.4 mcg	2.4 mcg	Pernicious anemia; nerve problems and weakness; smooth or sore tongue.	Apparently none.
90 mg	75 mg	Loose teeth; bleeding gums; bruises; loss of appetite; dry skin; poor healing. In extreme cases, scurvy and internal hemorrhages.	Diarrhea; kidney stones; urinary-tract irritation; iron buildup; bone loss.

This table presents daily Recommanded Dietary Allowances (RDAs), except where there is an asterisk. The values with an asterisk (*) represent daily Adequate Intakes (AIs). The RDAs are set to meet the known needs of practically all healthy people. Adequate Intakes are used rather than RDA when scientific evidence is insufficient to estimate an average requirement.

Source: Institute of Medicine, Food and Nutrition Board. National Academy Press, Washington, D.C.

[a] 10 mcg for males and females 51 to 70 and 15 mcg over 70

[b] 1.7 mg for males over 50 and 1.5 mg for females over 50

those who consume less. Deficiency is characterized by excessive bleeding from even minor cuts. Some newborn infants are especially vulnerable to vitamin K deficiency, because they lack the intestinal bacteria needed to make it.

Water-soluble vitamins

As water-soluble vitamins, the B vitamins and vitamin C are more easily absorbed than fat-soluble vitamins because there is always fluid in the intestines. At the same time, deficiencies may develop more quickly because the body stores water-soluble vitamins in only small amounts.

Biotin: Closely related to folate, pantothenic acid, and vitamin B_{12}, biotin is essential for the proper metabolism of carbohydrates, especially glucose, as well as proteins and fats. Some biotin is made by intestinal bacteria; it is also found in many foods. Deficiency occurs mostly in infants. In adults, it can be induced by eating lots of raw egg whites, which contain avidin, a substance that binds with biotin.

Folate: Also referred to as folic acid or folacin, this B vitamin is converted into enzymes that the body needs to make DNA, RNA, and red blood cells, and to carry out other important metabolic functions. During pregnancy, folate helps prevent neurological defects, particularly a malformed spinal column, in the developing fetus. Recent research indicates that mild folate deficiency is common, especially among infants, adolescents, and pregnant women. Alcohol and oral contraceptives interfere with absorption, increasing the risk of deficiency.

Niacin: Also known as vitamin B_3, nicotinic acid, and nicotinamide, niacin is important in energy metabolism, normal growth, and the synthesis of fatty acids, DNA, and protein. Mild niacin deficiency causes mouth sores and diarrhea. If unchecked, it can lead to pellagra, a disease characterized by chronic diarrhea, dermatitis, dementia, and if untreated, death.

When consumed in high doses, niacin may lower blood cholesterol levels. But such high doses should be taken only under careful medical supervision, with frequent blood checks for liver damage and high blood sugar. High doses can also cause flushing of the face, neck, and arms.

Pantothenic acid: As implied by its name, which comes from the Greek term for widespread, pantothenic acid is found in almost all plant and animal foods. It is also manufactured by intestinal bacteria. Pantothenic acid is required for the metabolism of carbohydrates, proteins, and fats and is used to make hormones, red blood cells, and fats. Deficiency is unknown, except in medical experiments.

Riboflavin: Essential for the release of energy, riboflavin is needed to metabolize carbohydrates, proteins, and fats. It is also necessary to utilize niacin and vitamin B_6, and it may play a role in the production of corticosteroid hormones. Riboflavin deficiency does not cause any specific diseases, but it can contribute to other B vitamin deficiency disorders. Riboflavin is responsible for the bright yellow color of the urine noted by supplement takers.

Thiamine: Also known as vitamin B_1, thiamine is instrumental in turning carbohydrates, proteins, and fats into energy. It is also needed to convert glucose into fatty acids. Still other important functions include promotion of normal nerve function, muscle tone, appetite, and digestion. A mild deficiency causes fatigue, listlessness, irritability, mood swings, numbness in the legs, digestive problems, and retarded growth in children. Severe deficiency leads to beriberi, a disease that now occurs mostly in alcoholics.

Vitamin B₆: Made up of three interchangeable and related compounds (pyridoxine, pyridoxamine, and pyridoxal), vitamin B_6 is a coenzyme that is essential for protein metabolism. It is needed to release energy in forms that the cells can use, and it is instrumental in the functioning of the nervous and immune systems and the manufacture of red blood cells. Deficiency is noted by oily, scaling skin, especially around the eyes, nose, and mouth; weight loss; muscle weakness; a smooth, red tongue; irritability; and depression. High-dose supplements can cause nerve damage.

Vitamin B₁₂: Like other B vitamins, B_{12} functions as a coenzyme, an organic molecule that helps the enzymes function. It is essential for the growth and division of cells, as well as for making red blood cells, genetic material, and myelin, the fatty sheath that surrounds nerve fibers. A deficiency can cause pernicious anemia, neurologic symptoms, and weakness.

The majority of cases of vitamin B_{12} deficiency in North America are not due to a poor diet; instead, it is almost always caused by an inability to absorb the vitamin from the intestinal tract due to a lack of intrinsic factor. The stomach's production of intrinsic factor declines with age. Many intestinal disorders also result in inadequate intrinsic factor. In these cases, B_{12} must be supplemented.

Vitamin C: Also called ascorbic acid, vitamin C is necessary to make and maintain collagen, the connective tissue that holds body cells together. It is an important antioxidant, associated with lowering risk of heart disease, certain cancers, and even some of the health concerns of aging. Vitamin C promotes healing of wounds and burns, helps to build teeth and bones, and strengthens the walls of capillaries and other blood vessels. In addition, it increases iron absorption.

A popular treatment for the common cold, most studies suggest that while it probably won't prevent your cold, it may lessen its severity and shorten its duration.

Deficiency symptoms are fatigue, joint pain, sore and bleeding gums, easy bruising, weakened bones that fracture easily, and the slow healing of wounds. With severe deficiency, these symptoms worsen into scurvy, gum ulcers form, the teeth loosen, and hemorrhages can develop.

A word about choline

Although not strictly speaking a vitamin, choline was classified in 1998 as an essential nutrient by the National Academy of Sciences. It was previously thought that our bodies made adequate amounts of this nutrient, but it is now recognized that we need to obtain choline from our diets. It is available in eggs, legumes, nuts, meats, and dairy products. Choline is an important nutrient in fat metabolism, and is needed to maintain healthy nerve function. It is also a precursor to acetylcholine, a brain neurotransmitter that is involved in memory.

WATER
■ VITAL FOR LIFE ■

Two parts hydrogen and one part oxygen (H_2O), water is the most abundant substance in the human body, accounting for up to 60 percent of our body weight. Even though water has no calories or other nutrients, we can go for only a few days without it. In contrast, a healthy person can survive for 6 to 8 weeks without food. A loss of only 5 to 10 percent of body water results in serious dehydration, while a 15 to 20 percent loss is usually fatal.

Vital functions

Water is essential to virtually every body function, including digestion, absorption, and transport of nutrients, elimination of body waste, and regulation of body temperature, as well as many other chemical processes. It provides a protective cushion for body cells, and in the form of amniotic fluid protects a developing fetus. Water is needed to build all body tissues and is the base of all blood and fluid secretions such as tears, saliva, and gastric juices, as well as the fluids that lubricate our organs and joints. It also keeps our skin soft and smooth.

As our body ages, it becomes dryer. The body of a newborn infant is 75 to 80 percent water, compared to 50 percent after age 65 or 70. This drying out is reflected in the wrinkled skin, reduced saliva flow, and stiffened joints that occur naturally with aging.

How much do we need?

The human body needs enough water to ensure that the urine is pale, not dark or bright yellow. For the average adult this may translate to six to eight glasses of water a day. Most of this comes from drinks—plain water, coffee, tea, juices, soft drinks—but surprisingly there's a substantial amount in foods as well. Fruits and vegetables, for example, are 70 to 95 percent water, compared to 75 percent of an egg, 40 to 60 percent of meat, poultry, and fish, and 35 percent of bread.

Our daily needs vary a lot. We need more water in hot weather, during exercise, or when we have a fever, cold, or other illness. We also need more during pregnancy to provide for the amniotic fluid and the expanded blood volume, as well as to meet the needs of the developing fetus. Nursing mothers need to increase their fluid intake to produce milk, which is 87 percent water.

As a general rule, the amount of water we take in should be equal to what is excreted. Many factors can affect this balance. For example, taking diuretics or other drugs that increase urination increases our needs for fluids. Drinking large amounts of tea or coffee has a similar diuretic effect, which can offset the fluid intake from these drinks. And eating salty foods also increases our need for extra water to maintain proper fluid balance.

Thirst decreases with age, so older people should drink water often even if they don't feel thirsty. As well, thirst may lag behind the body's need for water during intense exercise or when it's extremely hot and humid. By the time you feel thirsty, you may already be dehydrated. If you drink more fluid than you need, the kidneys excrete the excess by increasing the volume of urine. If you drink more water than the kidneys can handle, excess is absorbed by your cells.

Is our drinking water safe?

North Americans generally enjoy some of the world's safest and most reliable water supplies. However, especially in recent years, there have been significant episodes of serious waterborne illnesses, which have eroded the public's confidence in the water supply. In addition, a growing number of public health officials are warning that surface water supplies are becoming increasingly polluted by industrial waters, fertilizer runoff, pesticides, and chemical and nuclear wastes.

So just how safe is our water? The following are the most common or serious contaminants that may be affecting water safety:

Chlorine: Adding chlorine to our drinking water to destroy disease-causing bacteria has been a major public health success. But that success comes at a price. Chlorine can combine with other components of organic matter to form chlorinated disinfection by-products (CDBPs). Long-term exposure to one of the most common by-products, trihalomethanes, has been linked to increased cancer risk, specifically bladder and colon cancer.

Lead: Although most municipal drinking water contains little if any lead at its source, water can pick up this toxic metal in its journey to your home through various holding tanks and pipes, including the ones in your house. Lead can build up in the body over time and can be damaging to organs and blood cells. A common source of contamination is corrosion of old pipes and plumbing. To minimize your exposure, use only water from the cold water tap for drinking and cooking. Hot water is likely to contain more lead. And when you turn the tap on, run the water until it is cold to flush out any lead that may have accumulated. If you have concerns, have your water tested.

Turbidity: Turbidity results when matter like clay, decaying plants, and parasites become suspended in water. Disease-causing microorganisms can cling to these particles and escape disinfection. There have been instances where increased turbidity, while still well below regulated limits, has caused outbreaks of gastrointestinal illnesses.

Parasites: The parasites *Cryptosporidium parvum* and *Giardia lamblia,* which live in the intestines of humans and animals, can get into the water supply through sewage or animal waste. *G. lamblia* can cause diarrhea, loss of appetite, dehydration, and vomiting. It takes only very small amounts of this parasite to make some people ill. Campers and others who drink untreated water are most at risk, but there have been instances where people have been diagnosed with giardiasis from municipal drinking water. *C. parvum* infections are usually more serious—fever, diarrhea, stomach cramps, and even death can result. Both these parasites are hard to kill because their hard outer shells protect them from disinfection. And because they are very tiny, they can pass through most filters.

So, do you need to worry about these contaminants in your drinking water? Generally, our water supplies have a good safety record. But you can contact your local public health utility and ask for reports or other information on contaminant levels. You can also choose to use a water filter system, or switch to bottled water, but there is no guarantee that these options will totally eliminate contaminants from your drinking water. Different filter systems will remove different contaminants as well as varying levels of these contaminants. If you have concerns, have your water tested.

Home filter systems

There's a wide variety of filter systems available, ranging broadly in both cost and effectiveness in removing contaminants. You can choose an inexpensive counter-top pitcher or you can decide on an under-the-sink unit that can cost you more than $1,000. As with bottled waters, the only way to make an informed decision is to do a little detective work.

A good place to start is with NSF International in Ann Arbor, Michigan (www.nsf.org), an independent, nonprofit agency that works closely with the federal government in both the United States and Canada in setting standards in many areas, including water filters. They encourage consumers to educate themselves about the quality of their drinking water supply so they can determine whether or not they need a filter system, and which contaminants are cause for concern. Then you can select a filter system that can effectively remove those specific contaminants. If a product has been tested by NSF, there will be a statement on the packaging that will list which contaminants the filter is certified to remove.

6 interesting facts about bottled water

1. An estimated 25 percent of bottled water is actually filtered tap water.
2. Mineral water is often high in sodium.
3. Unlike municipal water supplies, bottled water may not contain enough fluoride to protect against cavities.
4. It's not a good idea to reuse plastic water bottles. Washing and reusing them over and over may accelerate the break-down of the plastic, increasing your exposure to potentially harmful chemicals.
5. Check the bottling date and best-before date to find out how fresh the water is. Bottled water normally contains low numbers of harmless bacteria, but if the water is stored for long periods at room temperatures, these bacteria can multiply rapidly. It's best to store the water in a cool place.
6. Opened containers of bottled water should be refrigerated in case potentially harmful bacteria have been introduced.

Arsenic in drinking water

Arsenic gets into our ground water supply when mineral deposits or rocks containing arsenic dissolve. Also, through the discharge of industrial wastes, and as fallout from the burning of fossil fuels—especially coal. Although the United States and Canadian governments have set strict standards that allow only minute trace amounts of arsenic in our drinking water, the International Agency for Research on Cancer considers arsenic a human carcinogen, and years of consumption of drinking water containing arsenic at levels close to, or higher than the guideline values have been found to increase the risk of skin cancer, as well as tumors of the bladder, kidney, liver, and lung. Long-term exposure to higher levels of arsenic in drinking water may also cause abnormal heart rhythm and blood vessel damage, decreased production of red blood cells, and thickening and discoloration of the skin. Again, if you have concerns, have your water tested, and consider investing in an in-home water treatment device to reduce the arsenic level in your water supply.

Bottled water

You might think that all bottled water is pretty much the same, but think again. Bottled water just means water that is packaged in a sealed container and offered for sale. The array of choice on the store shelves includes everything from imported mountain spring water to plain old municipal tap water in a bottle. Make sure you read the fine print so you're getting what you're looking for in terms of source, content, and taste. Here's the range of what you'll find:

Spring water. Flows from a natural underground spring source. Once the water is collected and bottled, it must have the same properties as it did underground. In theory at least, this water is better protected from pollution than river and lake water.

Mineral water. This is spring water that contains at least 500 mg of minerals per quart (or per liter). Some mineral waters are naturally carbonated because they contain carbon dioxide, while it is added to other types.

Drinking water. Bottled water can come from a spring or a municipal water supply. It is treated by distillation, deionization, or reverse osmosis. Other terms for water treated by one of these processes include "distilled water," "deionized water," and "reverse osmosis water."

Carbonated water. Bottled water that contains natural or added carbonation. Soda water and tonic water are considered soft drinks, not bottled water.

Is bottled water safer than tap water?

There's no easy answer to this question because there are so many variables affecting different municipal water sources, as well as the different sources and treatments of bottled water. Your best bet is to get more information on your tap water from your local water utility or to check out different bottled water brands. For more information on bottled water, contact the International Bottled Water Association (www.bottledwater.org, or 1-800-WATER-11) in the United States, or the Canadian Bottled Water Association (www.cbwa-bottledwater.org, or 905-886-6928) in Canada.

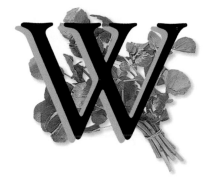

WATERCRESS

BENEFITS

- A good source of beta carotene and vitamin C.
- A useful source of calcium and potassium.
- Rich in antioxidants, which help prevent cancer and other diseases.

DRAWBACKS

- May be contaminated by parasites and bacteria, depending on where it's grown.

Whether it's eaten raw, used as a garnish, or added to salads, sandwiches, and soups, the dark green, peppery leaves of watercress are among the more nutritious salad greens.

Watercress is a cruciferous vegetable that is rich in antioxidants, bioflavonoids, and other substances that may protect against certain types of cancer, particularly those of the digestive system. It also has been found to contain a phytochemical called phenylethyl isothiocyanate (PEITC), which may detoxify the carcinogens that are linked to lung cancer. Watercress is also a good source of vitamins A (in the form of beta carotene, its precursor) and C, antioxidants that protect against cell damage by free radicals, unstable molecules that are produced when the body uses oxygen. A single cup of chopped watercress provides 1,600 IU of vitamin A, approximately 15 mg of vitamin C, and useful amounts of calcium and potassium, yet it contains less than 5 calories.

Many alternative practitioners suggest that watercress can alleviate gastrointestinal upsets and help to treat respiratory problems and urinary tract infections. Some claim that it also can be useful as a mild antidepressant, an appetite stimulant, and a diuretic. Application of its juice is recommended to clear up acne. These health benefits have not yet been verified, however.

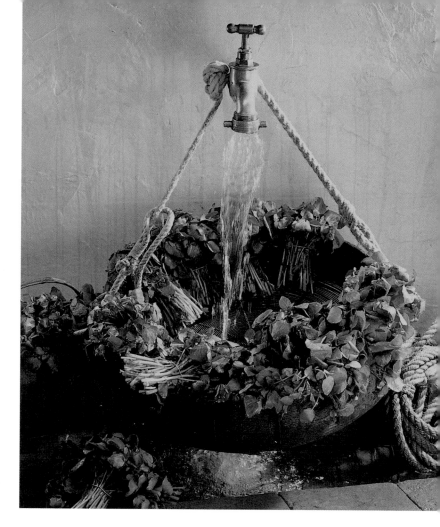

COOL AND FRESH. *Watercress, which grows in streambeds, is at its best in the early spring. It should be well washed to remove microorganisms.*

BUYING AND SERVING WATERCRESS

Watercress is only available fresh and is usually sold in bunches. When purchasing the vegetable, look for crisp leaves and a bright green color; bypass any with yellow or wilted leaves. Although watercress may be found in small streambeds, it's not a good idea to pick it in the wild. Streams often contain parasites and bacteria that may cause intestinal infections. Even watercress from a supermarket, which has usually been grown in a controlled environment, should be washed thoroughly before it is served.

The pungency of watercress is complemented by citrus. Use a light citrus dressing on a watercress salad, or toss orange or grapefruit slices with watercress for a refreshing fruit salad. Watercress can also be added to a variety of cooked dishes. However, to preserve its vitamins and to prevent the leaves from turning brown, it should be cooked rapidly (microwaving works well) and served right away. ❖

WHEAT GERM

BENEFITS

- A good source of vitamin E, zinc, and thiamine.
- Also contains folate, magnesium, and fiber.

Wheat germ is the nutritional heart of the wheat kernel. This germ is removed during the milling of white flour, and when this happens the resulting flour loses a significant amount of nutrition. Although it's the smallest part of the grain, the germ is packed with nutrients, including vitamin E, thiamine, folate, magnesium, and zinc. Two tablespoons of toasted wheat germ contain 55 calories, with more than 15 percent of the Recommended Dietary Allowance (RDA) of vitamin E, thiamine, zinc, and phosphorus, as well as 10 percent of the RDA for folate and magnesium and useful amounts of other B vitamins, iron, copper, potassium, and manganese. It also contains 4 g of protein and almost 2 g of fiber.

HEALTH BENEFITS OF WHEAT GERM

Wheat germ offers several heart benefits. The vitamin E it contains is a powerful antioxidant that is linked to heart health as well as a strong immune system. The fat in wheat germ (1.5 g in 2 tablespoons) is predominantly polyunsaturated fat, which can help lower LDL cholesterol levels when it replaces saturated fat in the diet. Wheat germ is also a source of plant sterols that help lower cholesterol levels.

Wheat germ is sold in both toasted and natural forms and it is often used to add extra nutrition to a variety of foods. It can be used in baking cookies, cakes, muffins, breads, and pancakes, sprinkled over cereals or on top of salads, mixed into meat loaf, burgers, or veggie burgers, or used as a substitute for bread crumbs when coating fish, chicken, or vegetables. Once it has been opened, keep the wheat germ jar tightly sealed and refrigerated to prevent it from going rancid. Defatted wheat germ contains much less vitamin E and does not need refrigeration. It can be kept in the cupboard. ❖

DO ONE SIMPLE THING

THROW A LITTLE WHEAT GERM INTO JUST ABOUT EVERYTHING YOU BAKE

Wheat germ is an exceptionally concentrated source of vitamin E, and this antioxidant may help to prevent cancer, heart disease, and vision loss. Always take every opportunity to include a little of this delicious whole grain in all sorts of baked goods, like banana or zucchini bread, rice puddings, coffee cake, apple crisp, pizza dough, bread and savory pie doughs, and even homemade cookies.

WINE

BENEFITS

- Moderate consumption may decrease the risk of heart disease and certain cancers.
- Contains bioflavonoids, phenols, and tannins, which have health benefits.
- Promotes relaxation.

DRAWBACKS

- May trigger allergies and migraine headaches in some people and increase the risk of a rare type of stroke.
- Excessive consumption can cause liver disease, cancer, and birth defects.

Although the art of wine making is some 7,000 years old, the process of fermentation was not understood until the discoveries of Louis Pasteur in the 19th century. Wine is palatable and resistant to deterioration only after it has undergone fermentation, which is a type of controlled spoilage. Alcohol, a waste product of fermentation, is toxic to all living beings; even the yeasts that excrete it cannot tolerate an environment of more than 15 percent alcohol, which is why fermentation stops at about this concentration. Most French wines are about 12 percent alcohol, and North American wines, 13 to 14 percent. Extra alcohol is added to fortified wines, such as sherry and port.

THE COMPONENTS OF WINE

Red wine is made from purple grapes, but white wine is not necessarily made from white grapes. Many white wines are made from purple grapes, but the skins are removed before they color the fermenting juice, called must. The skins contain most of the bioflavonoids, phenols, tannins, and other compounds that give wine its flavor and healthful properties. The longer the must stays in contact with the skins, the deeper the color will be. Some dessert wines are made with specially overripened grapes to achieve a prized sweetness and a rich consistency.

Four ounces (120 ml) of red wine contain about 80 to 90 calories, compared to 75 to 85 in the same amount of white wine and 175 in dessert wine. Many wines have trivial amounts of minerals; red wine has a trace of iron.

WINE AND THE HEART

Numerous studies show that moderate consumption of alcohol—one to two 4-oz (120-ml) glasses of wine a day, preferably with a meal—is associated with a lower risk of heart disease. According to a 1991 report, the French had a heart attack rate only one-third as high as that of North Americans, despite consuming as much or more fat as North Americans. Wine consumption may be at least partly responsible for this phenomenon, known as the "French paradox." Annual wine consumption in North America is between 2 to 3 gal (8–11 liters) per person, compared to about 15 gal (57 liters) per person in France.

Researchers have not determined what it is in wine that may prevent heart attacks, but some theorize that compounds such as quercetin and resveratrol in grape skins, as well as other bioflavonoids, may be responsible. These compounds tend to make the blood less sticky and less likely to form clots. It is thought that the French habit of drinking wine with meals may provide the small but regular intake of alcohol needed to reduce clot formation, a cause of most heart attacks. The bioflavonoids also have antioxidant properties and may help prevent damage to the artery wall and help keep the arteries dilated. Still other research suggests that moderate amounts of wine may raise the levels of the protective HDL (high-density lipoprotein) cholesterol.

OTHER HEALTH BENEFITS

Studies are under way looking at other benefits from the resveratrol found in wine. It is believed that it has a preventative effect on several types of cancer, including colon and prostate cancer. Laboratory studies indicate that the anthocyanin pigments and tannins in wine can fight viruses, but this effect has not been proved in humans. Tannins can inhibit the growth of plaque-forming bacteria on the teeth and may protect against cavity formation. Other studies are exploring the link between wine consumption and lowered risk of dementia.

Wine appears to contain substances (still to be identified) that slow the rate of alcohol absorption; studies show that a moderate amount of wine has a less intoxicating effect than the same volume of distilled liquor. Still, some claim that wine makes them more sleepy than other alcoholic beverages do; this effect may be due to ingredients other than alcohol.

NEGATIVE EFFECTS

The benefits of moderate wine drinking, which may extend to reducing the risk of some cancers, are lost when consumption exceeds 8 oz (240 ml) a day. Overconsumption can increase the risk of obesity, stroke, breast cancer, high blood pressure, as well as alcoholism, and cirrhosis and other liver disorders. Even moderate alcohol consumption may raise the risk of hemorrhagic stroke (involving a burst blood vessel). In addition, heavy use of alcohol in early pregnancy can cause birth defects.

Most wines contain sulfites and preservatives that can trigger allergic reactions in susceptible people. Wine, especially red, is a common trigger of migraines. ❖

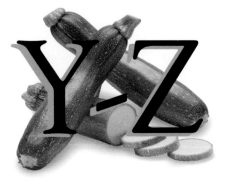

YAMS AND
SWEET POTATOES

BENEFITS

- A rich source of beta carotene.
- A good source of vitamins C and B$_6$, folate, and potassium.
- Naturally sweet and high in fiber.

SWEET POTATOES

Although the two vegetables are unrelated, sweet potatoes are often called yams in the United States and Canada. Sweet potatoes are also not related to the common white potato. In their own right, however, these sweet tubers are highly nutritious, and their rich, sweet flavor belies their humble origins as a New World plant that was introduced to Europeans by Columbus and other explorers.

Sweet potatoes derive their flavor from an enzyme that converts starches to sugar. As the tuber matures and is cooked, it becomes sweeter. Immediately after harvesting, sweet potatoes are cured—stored at about 85°F (30°C) for 4 to 6 days—to increase their sweetness and decrease the danger of spoiling.

A NUTRIENT-DENSE VEGETABLE

Like other brightly colored orange-yellow vegetables, sweet potatoes are an excellent source of beta carotene, an antioxidant precursor to vitamin A. On average, one medium sweet potato provides more than 100 percent of the Recommended Dietary Allowance (RDA) for vitamin A, about 33 percent of the RDA for vitamin C, 20 percent of the RDA for B$_6$, 400 mg of potassium, along with folate and some iron. Sweet potatoes also contain plant

BAKING OR BROILING SWEET POTATOES
enhances their beta carotene content and sweetens them as their starches turn to sugar.

sterols, which are cholesterol-lowering compounds. When eaten with its skin, a sweet potato is an excellent source of insoluble fiber, which may help prevent constipation and diverticulosis. It also contains the soluble fiber pectin, which may help control cholesterol. Beta carotene, the carotenoid that gives color to sweet potatoes, is a powerful antioxidant linked to lowered risk of heart disease and certain cancers.

Sweet potatoes spoil quickly, and any that have moldy spots or are shriveled should be thrown away. Cutting away the bad spots does not always help, because an unpleasant flavor may have already spread to the rest of the potato. Store sweet potatoes in a cool place but not in the refrigerator; temperatures below 50°F (10°C) gives them a hard core and an off taste.

Since their skins are very thin, sweet potatoes should be treated gently. If peeling is necessary, it is easily done after they are cooked.

Traditional recipes for candied sweet potatoes, a Thanksgiving basic, often call for a lot of sugar and fat. A lighter alternative is to use thickened apple juice as a glaze and to substitute pineapples for marshmallows. Sweet potatoes can replace white potatoes and pumpkins

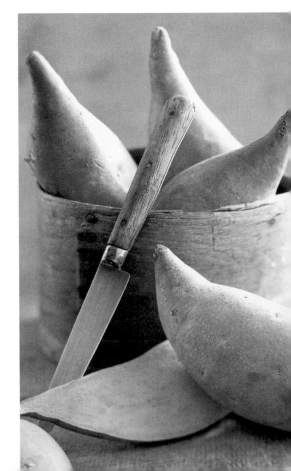

in a number of recipes, and mashed sweet potatoes with defatted broth or grated orange peel is a vitamin-packed side dish.

YAMS

Deriving their name from the Senegalese word *ñam* ("to eat"), yams are often confused with the sweet potato. Although many varieties of sweet potato are marketed as yams in North America, true yams are native to Africa and are seldom seen in the United States or Canada. Growing up to 100 lb (45 kg), they are much larger than sweet potatoes and not as rich in vitamins. They are, however, a good source of potassium and starch and are a carbohydrate staple in parts of Africa and Asia. ❖

YOGURT

BENEFITS

- An excellent source of calcium and phosphorus.
- Provides useful amounts of vitamin A, several B vitamins, and zinc.
- More digestible than milk for people with lactose intolerance.

DRAWBACKS

- Flavored, sweetened commercial yogurt may be high in calories.

To make yogurt, pure cultures of bacteria are added to pasteurized milk. Fermentation is allowed to proceed until the desired acidity is reached, then it is stopped by cooling the yogurt to refrigerator temperature. A mixed culture of *Lactobacillus bulgaricus* and *Streptococcus thermophilus* consumes the milk sugar, or lactose, for energy and excretes lactic acid, which curdles the milk. (This is similar to the acid that builds up in muscles during intense exercise and blocks energy production, making the limbs feel heavy.) Dried milk solids, gelatin, or other ingredients may be added for body.

The finished product reflects the fat, mineral, and vitamin content of the raw material, whether it be whole or skim milk. Following fermentation, yogurt has only one-third to two-thirds the amount of lactose found in milk, and therefore is more easily digested by people with intolerance to milk.

YOGURT AND HEALTH

Yogurt is a healthful food and a useful source of minerals and vitamins. What's more, yogurts

---

YOGURT GOES WITH EVERYTHING

- **Fruit smoothie:** Combine ½ cup plain yogurt with ½ cup diced ripe fruit, add one or two ice cubes, and puree in a blender.

- **Yogurt shake:** Blend ½ cup fruit-flavored, frozen nonfat yogurt with ½ cup low-fat milk until creamy.

- **Cucumber dip:** Peel, seed, and dice a large cucumber and combine with 1 cup plain yogurt, salt, pepper, and chopped fresh herbs. Serve as a dip for vegetables, a dressing for salad, or a sauce for fish.

- **Mild salsa:** Mix ½ cup plain yogurt with 1 mashed ripe avocado, 1 diced tomato, and chili powder to taste. Serve as a dip with tortilla chips or a sauce for enchiladas or hamburgers.

- **Vegetable sauce:** Mix plain yogurt with minced fresh dill and chopped cashews.

- **Garnish:** Top cold cucumber soup or vichyssoise with plain yogurt and minced chives.

---

that contain live or "active" bacteria cultures may help suppress the growth of harmful microorganisms in the body. (See Probiotics.) Some scientists question the health benefits of yogurt, in part because some studies indicate that *L. bulgaricus* does not survive human digestion. But more recent research disputes these findings and backs the age-old observation that yogurt is useful in restoring normal intestinal flora, the beneficial organisms that inhabit the intestinal tract. Regardless of who's right, eating yogurt when taking antibiotics (which can upset intestinal flora) does no harm and may well be helpful.

Yogurt or any fermented milk product must contain 100 million bacteria per dose to be effective. It should be absolutely fresh and contain live cultures of acidophilus or bifidobacteria, preferably both. Products that are heavily pasteurized or have been in the refrigerator for a long time will have very few active bacteria.

An excellent quick snack and a versatile dessert, yogurt can be served chilled or frozen, plain or flavored. Low-fat frozen yogurt contains only 110 calories in a ½-cup serving and gives almost the same pleasure as ice cream, with fewer calories and without the harmful saturated fats.

Because yogurt contains the same amount of fat as the milk it was made with, low-fat yogurt is the best choice for people on a low-fat diet. An 8-oz (240-ml) serving of plain yogurt made with whole milk contains 140 calories, compared to

150 calories for the same-size glass of whole milk. An 8-oz (240-ml) serving of plain yogurt contains 415 mg of calcium, about 530 mg of potassium, and 2 mg of zinc, with 24 mg of cholesterol. Vitamins include 1.2 mcg (micrograms) of vitamin B_{12}, 30 mcg of folate, and 0.5 mg of riboflavin.

Calorie content rises considerably with the addition of sweeteners and fruit purees: 8 oz (240 ml) of low-fat yogurt flavored with fruit and sugar contain about 230 calories, and whole-milk yogurt flavored with coffee, vanilla, or lemon essence and sugar contains 270 calories. Nonfat yogurt sweetened with aspartame is the least calorie-laden, but this sweetener is not recommended for children and is unsafe for people with phenylketonuria (PKU).

Custard-type yogurts are thickened with pectin, gelatin, cornstarch, or alginate (seaweed) thickeners. These ingredients do not make a substantial difference to the nutritional content, but people hypersensitive to corn and other additives should check labels carefully.

Goat's milk yogurts are made with whole goat's milk, which adds a sharp flavor. These yogurts are lower in saturated fat and somewhat lower in calories than cow's milk products.

Yogurt can be made at home by mixing a few spoonfuls of commercial yogurt that is made with live cultures into low-fat milk and leaving the covered mixture overnight at lukewarm or room temperature. ❖

ZUCCHINI

BENEFITS

- Low in calories.
- A good source of vitamins A, C, and folate.

ZUCCHINI FACTS

• Zucchini, like other varieties of squash, are New World plants that were cultivated by North America's Native people long before the arrival of European explorers and settlers.

• A single plant can produce more than 1 bushel (35 liters) of zucchini.

Elongated, dark green zucchini are sometimes mistaken for cucumbers. (There is also a golden variety of zucchini, as well as some that have dark green stripes.) Although both zucchini and cucumbers are members of the gourd family, zucchini are closer cousins to pumpkins than to cucumbers. Zucchini are by far the most popular summer squash in North America. Picked and eaten while still immature, zucchini have a soft shell and tender light-colored flesh that has a delicate, crisp, fresh flavor.

Zucchini, like other summer squash, are about 94 percent water, making them one of the lowest-calorie vegetables. One cup of raw sliced zucchini has less than 20 calories and provides 28 mcg (micrograms) of folate, about 7 percent of the adult Recommended Dietary Allowance

DO ONE SIMPLE THING

BAKE A CAKE WITH ZUCCHINI

You can eat cake, as well as a small serving of vegetables, by baking this delicious chocolate-zucchini cake. Cream 1/2 cup butter and 1 cup superfine sugar until fluffy and light. Slowly beat in 2 eggs. Sift 1 1/4 cups self-raising flour, 1/4 cup cocoa and 1/2 teaspoon cinnamon. Add flour into butter mixture with 1/4 cup milk, 1 cup grated zucchini and 1/2 cup chopped walnuts. Spread into greased and paper-lined loaf tin, and bake at 350°F (180°C) for 40 minutes.

(RDA), as well as 12 mg of vitamin C and 250 mg of potassium. Although zucchini is not as high in beta carotene as winter squash, it is still a source of this important antioxidant. The beta carotene is lost, however, if the skin is discarded.

VERSATILE VEGETABLE

The unobtrusive flavor of zucchini complements other ingredients in a variety of dishes. They are an especially suitable companion to tomatoes and are a splendid addition to vegetable lasagna, marinara sauce, and ratatouille. They are also delicious when grated and made into cakes and other baked goods.

Squash is an adaptation from several Native American words meaning "something eaten raw"; in fact, all summer squash are tender enough to eat uncooked. Raw zucchini is a pleasant addition to a vegetable platter or salad, and dieters sometimes keep bags of sliced zucchini in the refrigerator for easy snacking.

Orange-colored squash blossoms are edible and contain some of the same nutrients that are present in the squash. Of these, zucchini blossoms are the most often consumed and are considered a delicacy. However, the blossoms are often served battered and deep-fried—try sautéing or steaming them instead.

Zucchini can grow very large, and summer gardeners will often find them in gigantic proportions. However, zucchini taste best when eaten small—ideally, 6 to 9 in. (15–23 cm) long. As they grow larger, they are less flavorful, and become primarily ornamental. When buying zucchini, look for specimens that feel firm and heavy when you pick them up. Although they can be refrigerated for a few days, zucchini tend to spoil quickly. ❖

A DIFFERENCE OF COLOR. *Yellow and green varieties of zucchini are equally nutritious; the flowers are edible too.*

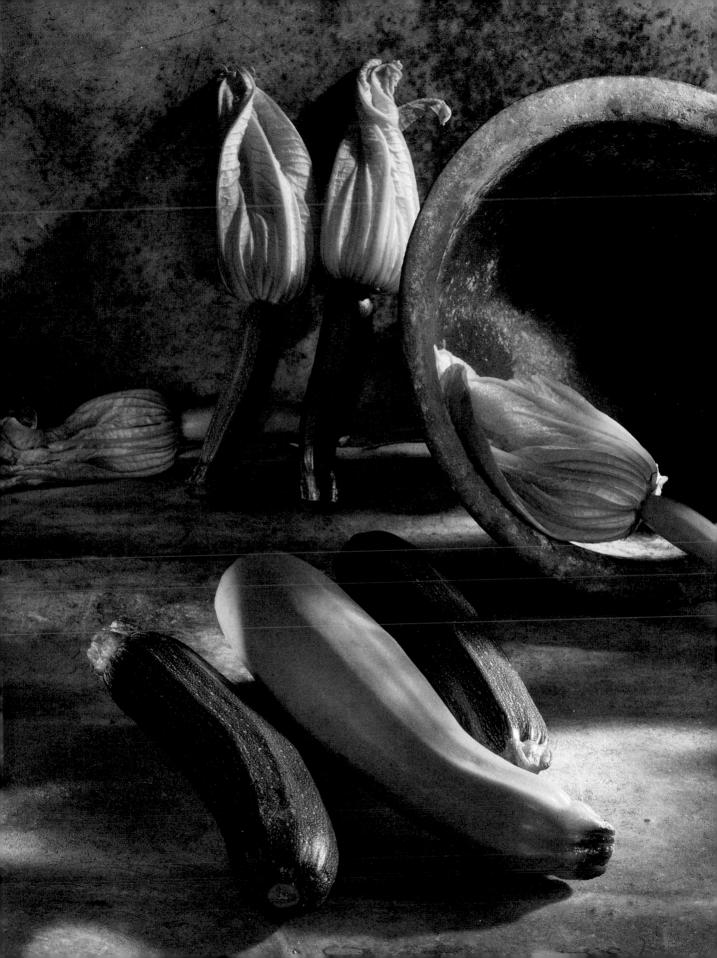

GLOSSARY

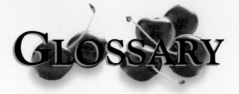

ADIPOCYTE A fat cell.

AFLATOXIN A toxin produced by molds that grow mainly on peanuts, cottonseed, and corn.

AJOENES Phytochemicals, found in garlic, that reduce LDL ("bad") cholesterol and possess anticlotting, anticancer, and antifungal activity, according to some studies.

ALBUMIN A protein found in most animal and many plant tissues that coagulates on heating.

ALLICIN A chemical that forms when garlic is crushed or cut and helps reduce LDL cholesterol levels. Responsible for garlic's pungent smell, allicin produces numerous sulfur compounds, possibly with antibacterial properties.

ALLYL SULFIDES Sulfur compounds, found in garlic, onions, leeks, scallions, and other members of the onion family, that help lower the risk of heart disease, stimulate the immune system, and are under review for their potential to fight cancer.

ALPHA-CAROTENE Like beta carotene, alpha-carotene is an antioxidant carotenoid and a precursor to vitamin A. It is found in apricots, carrots, pumpkins, and sweet potatoes.

ALPHA-LINOLENIC ACID An essential fatty acid linked to a wide range of health benefits. It cannot be made in the body and must therefore be obtained from foods. ALA is important for the maintenance of cell membranes and for creating substances in the body that protect against inflammatory conditions. ALA converts in the human body into two omega-3 fatty acids: EPA (eicosapentaenoic acid) and DHA (docosahexaenoic acid) and is found in canola oil, soybean oil, flaxseed, and walnuts. Smaller amounts are also found in dark green leafy vegetables.

AMINO ACIDS The building blocks of protein. Twenty amino acids are necessary for proper human growth and function. Nine amino acids are termed essential, because they must be provided in the diet; the body produces the remaining 11 as they are needed.

ANTHOCYANINS Responsible for the red and blue pigments found in certain fruits and vegetables, anthocyanins are flavonoids with the potential to suppress tumor cell growth, to lower LDL ("bad") cholesterol levels, and to prevent blood from forming clots. They are found in apples, berries, cherries, cranberries, black currants, red and purple grapes, plums, and pomegranates.

ANTIGEN A foreign substance that stimulates the body to defend itself with an immune response.

ARTERIOSCLEROSIS The stiffening and hardening of the arterial walls.

BACTERIA Single-celled microorganisms that are found in air, food, water, soil, and in other living creatures, including humans. "Friendly" bacteria prevent infections and synthesize certain vitamins; others cause disease.

BASAL METABOLIC RATE The energy required by the human body to maintain vital processes during a 24-hour period.

BETA CAROTENE One of the most studied of the carotenoids, beta carotene is a potent antioxidant plentiful in red, orange, and yellow plant foods (as well as in dark green vegetables where the orange color is masked by chlorophyll). It is converted by the body into vitamin A. Food sources include: apricots, carrots, brussels sprouts, dark leafy greens, pumpkin, spinach, sweet potatoes, and winter squash.

BETA-GLUCAN A type of soluble dietary fiber that helps to lower serum cholesterol levels. It is found in oats, oat bran, barley, brown rice bran, and shiitake mushrooms.

BETA-SITOSTEROL A plant sterol similar in structure to cholesterol, beta-sitosterol may help to manage benign prostatic hyperplasia (BPH), as well as protect against high cholesterol and cancer. It is found in avocados, corn oil, rice bran, seeds, soy foods, and wheat germ.

B-GROUP VITAMINS Although not chemically related to one another, many of the B vitamins occur in the same foods, and most perform closely linked tasks within the body, mostly by helping enzymes carry out their work. B vitamins are known either by numbers or names, or both: B_1, thiamine; B_2, riboflavin; B_3, niacin; B_5, pantothenic acid; B_6, pyridoxine; B_{12}, cobalamin; biotin; and folate.

BORON This bone-nourishing mineral is thought to enhance the body's ability to use calcium, magnesium, and vitamin D. It is found in beans and nuts.

BROMELAIN An enzyme derived from pineapples, bromelain is believed to have anti-inflammatory and pain-reducing properties.

CALORIE The basic unit of measurement for the energy value of food and the energy needs of the body. It is defined as the energy needed to raise the temperature of 1 g of water by 1 degree Celsius. Because 1 calorie is minuscule, values are usually expressed as units of 1,000 calories, properly written as kilocalories (kcal). One kilocalorie is what we commonly refer to as a food calorie.

CAROTENOIDS Pigments that give certain produce their characteristic orange, yellow, and red colors. They may possess potent antioxidant properties to fight heart disease, certain types of cancer, as well as degenerative eye diseases such as cataracts and macular degeneration. To date, more than 600 carotenoids have been identified, including alpha-carotene, beta carotene, beta-cryptoxanthin, lutein, lycopene, and zeaxanthin.

CELLULOSE One of the main ingredients of plant cell walls, this indigestible carbohydrate is an important source of insoluble fiber.

CHLOROPHYLL The green pigment of leaves and plants, chlorophyll not only helps to freshen breath but it may also help to prevent DNA damage to cells. Sources include dark leafy greens, kiwifruit, parsley, peas, and peppers.

COENZYMES Compounds that work with enzymes to promote biological processes. A coenzyme may be a vitamin, contain a vitamin, or be manufactured in the body from a vitamin.

COLLAGEN Fibrous protein that helps hold cells and tissue together.

COMPLEMENTARY PROTEINS Proteins that lack one or more of the essential amino acids but which when paired can supply a complete protein. For example, grains are high in the essential amino acid methionine, but they lack lysine. This essential amino acid is plentiful in dried beans, peanuts, and other legumes, which are deficient in methionine. So by combining a grain food with a legume, a complete range of amino acids can be obtained.

COMPLETE PROTEIN Contains all the essential amino acids. It is found in single animal foods; it can also be constructed by combining two or more complementary plant foods.

COMPLEX CARBOHYDRATES Fiber and starch in legumes, vegetables, and grains are complex carbohydrates. A diet that emphasizes complex carbohydrates can help protect against cardiovascular disease, improve blood sugar levels, relieve diarrhea, and ease insomnia. Sources include fruits, grains, legumes, potatoes, and rice.

CRUCIFEROUS VEGETABLES A family of phytochemical-rich vegetables named for their cross-shaped flowers, cruciferous vegetables are touted for their compounds that exhibit cancer-fighting activity in laboratory studies. Cruciferous vegetables include bok choy, broccoli, brussels sprouts, cabbage, cauliflower, kale, mustard greens, radishes, rutabaga, turnips, and watercress.

DEOXYRIBONUCLEIC ACID (DNA) The basic genetic material of all cells, DNA is the "genetic blueprint" that causes characteristics to be passed on from one generation to the next.

DHA An omega-3 fatty acid, DHA (docosahexaenoic acid) is important for all phases of the human life cycle. A major building block of human brain tissue and the primary structural fatty acid in the gray matter of the brain and the retina, DHA is vital for brain and eye health. Studies indicate that DHA may have cardiovascular benefits as well as neurological benefits. Although the body has enzymes that convert alpha-linolenic acid to DHA, you get it more efficiently by eating oily fatty fish such as herring, mackerel, salmon, sardines, and trout.

ELECTROLYTES Substances that separate into ions that conduct electricity when fused or dissolved in fluids. In the human body, sodium, potassium, and chloride are electrolytes essential for nerve and muscle function and for maintaining the fluid balance as well as the acid-alkali balance of cells and tissues.

ELLAGIC ACID A phenolic compound with potent antioxidant capabilities, ellagic acid is thought to fight cancer by inducing cancer cell death as well as by neutralizing carcinogens such as tobacco smoke or air pollution. Sources include apples, apricots, berries, grapes, pomegranates, and walnuts.

ENDORPHINS Natural painkillers made by the brain, with effects similar to those of opium-based drugs, such as morphine.

ENZYMES Protein molecules that are catalysts for many of the chemical reactions that take place in the body.

EPA An omega-3 fatty acid, eicosapentaenoic acid (EPA) is linked to cardiovascular and anticancer benefits, and may help improve inflammatory conditions such as rheumatoid arthritis. Although the body has enzymes that convert alpha-linolenic acid to EPA, you get it much more directly and more efficiently by eating oily fatty fish.

EPINEPHRINE Also called adrenaline, this is an adrenal hormone that prepares the body to react to stressful situations.

ESSENTIAL FATTY ACIDS (EFAS) The building blocks of necessary fats, EFAs must be obtained through foods. They help form cell membranes, aid in immune function, and produce important hormones. Food sources include canola oil, fatty fish (such as herring, mackerel, salmon, sardines, and trout), flaxseed oil, sunflower seeds, walnuts, and wheat germ.

FIBER, INSOLUBLE Composed of the indigestible parts of plants, insoluble fiber adds bulk to stools, which eases elimination. Insoluble fiber may promote satiety as well. Sources include fruits and vegetables, wheat bran, and whole grains.

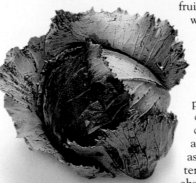

FIBER, SOLUBLE Soluble fiber forms a gel-like mass around food particles, slowing down the rate of digestion and absorption as well as preventing cholesterol from being absorbed. Pectin and beta-glucan are two types of soluble fiber that are particularly beneficial for lowering cholesterol levels. Soluble fiber also helps to manage diarrhea and may regulate levels of blood glucose as well. Sources include apples, barley, beans and lentils, citrus fruits, dried peas, flax, oats, and psyllium.

FLAVONOIDS Powerful antioxidants, flavonoids are phytochemicals linked to a reduced risk of cardiovascular disease and may impede the development of cancer. The free-radical scavenging properties of flavonoids are thought to inhibit clot formation, act as natural antibiotics, slow age-related decline in memory function, bolster blood vessels, and improve the potency of immune cells. Some important flavonoid compounds include anthocyanins, hesperidin, isoflavones, quercetin, and resveratrol. They are found in fruits, grains, tea, vegetables, and wine.

FREE RADICALS Unstable, highly reactive molecules that are the products of metabolism and also form as a result of environmental pollution such as cigarette smoke. Free radicals contribute to "oxidative stress," which is implicated in premature aging as well as the onset of many diseases.

FRUCTOOLIGOSACCHARIDES (FOS) Indigestible carbohydrate compounds, fructooligosaccharides are thought to encourage the growth of friendly bacteria in the body and may reduce the amount of toxins produced by unfriendly flora in the colon. They are found in asparagus, bananas, garlic, Jerusalem artichokes, and onions.

GENISTEIN A potent isoflavone with estrogenlike activity, genistein may help balance hormones and might reduce the risk for hormone-related cancer, such as prostate cancer, as well as help prevent fibrocystic breasts and premenstrual syndrome. It is found primarily in soy products.

GLUCOSE A simple sugar (monosaccharide) that is the body's prime energy source. Blood levels of glucose are regulated by several hormones, including insulin.

GLUTEN A protein in barley, buckwheat, oats, rye, and wheat. Certain people, particularly those with celiac disease, have an intolerance to it and experience an adverse gastrointestinal reaction necessitating the avoidance of foods made with these grains.

GLYCOGEN A form of glucose stored in the liver and muscles, which is converted back into glucose when needed.

GOITROGENS When eaten in large quantities, goitrogens in uncooked foods have the potential to interfere with the absorption of iodine and slow thyroid function. Goitrogens are primarily found in cabbage, turnips, mustard greens, and radishes, but in relatively small quantities.

HEME IRON Found in animal foods such as red meat, pork, and eggs; the body absorbs about four times as much heme iron as nonheme iron, which is found in plants.

HEMOGLOBIN The iron-containing pigment in our red blood cells that carries oxygen.

HESPERIDIN A flavonoid found in citrus fruits and juices, hesperidin may improve the integrity of capillary linings.

HIGH-DENSITY LIPOPROTEINS (HDLS) The smallest and "heaviest" lipoproteins, they retrieve cholesterol from the tissues and transport it to the liver to be removed from the body; called "good cholesterol," because high blood levels of HDLs are considered desirable in lowering heart disease risk.

HISTAMINE A chemical in the body's immune defense, it is released during allergic reactions to cause swelling, itching, rash, and sneezing.

HOMOCYSTEINE A compound that results from the breakdown of methionine, an essential amino acid, homocysteine, at high levels in the blood, increases the risk for atherosclerosis, and possibly other conditions. An estimated 20 to 40 percent of people with clogged arteries, or those who have suffered strokes or heart attacks, have abnormally high levels of homocysteine. The good news is that researchers have discovered that several B vitamins, folate, vitamin B_6, and B_{12}, can help lower homocysteine levels.

HORMONES Chemicals secreted by the endocrine glands that serve as molecular messengers triggering a host of body activities, including growth, development, and reproduction.

HYDROGENATION A process used by many manufacturers to make liquid oil more solid (as in the manufacturing of spreads). This process lengthens shelf life and provides the stability of many baked goods and processed foods. However, the process of hydrogenation creates trans fatty acids, which raise LDL cholesterol (the "bad" cholesterol) and also lower HDL cholesterol (the "good" cholesterol), increasing the risk of heart disease.

INCOMPLETE PROTEINS Proteins, usually from plant sources, that lack one or more essential amino acids.

INDOLES Partially responsible for the strong taste of broccoli and brussels sprouts, indoles are a class of glucosinolate phytochemicals present in cruciferous vegetables and may stimulate cancer-fighting enzymes.

INDOLE-3 CARBINOL A well-studied compound and a member of the glucosinolate phytochemical family, indole-3-carbinol is particularly abundant in broccoli and other cruciferous vegetables. It may offer protection against hormone-dependent cancers, such as breast cancer.

INSULIN A hormone that regulates carbohydrate metabolism.

ISOFLAVONES Found primarily in soy foods, isoflavones are a major class of phytoestrogens, plant chemicals with mild estrogen activity. Genistein and daidzein are the most prominent isoflavones. Soy isoflavones are under investigation for their potential to ease menopause symptoms and to protect against osteoporosis-related fractures, Alzheimer's disease, high cholesterol, and hormone-dependent cancers, such as breast and prostate cancer.

KETONES Potentially toxic waste products produced from the body's partial burning of fatty acids for fuel.

LECITHIN A phospholipid constituent of cell membranes and lipoproteins, lecithin is a natural emulsifier that helps stabilize cholesterol in the bile. Lecithin is not an essential nutrient, because it is synthesized by the liver.

LENTINAN A polysaccharide (carbohydrate compound) extracted from shiitake mushrooms, lentinan may have the potential to enhance immunity, as well as to protect against cancer, high blood pressure, and high cholesterol.

LIGNANS Phytoestrogens with mild estrogenlike activity. They may have antitumor effects, antimicrobial benefits, and provide relief from PMS and protection against osteoporosis. Food sources include flaxseeds (ground up), flaxseed oil, soy foods, and grains.

LIMONENE A phytochemical found in lemons, limes, and oranges. Now under review for its ability to inhibit tumors and protect the lungs from disease.

LINOLEIC ACID One of the omega-6 essential fatty acids.

LINOLENIC ACID One of the omega-3 essential fatty acids.

LIPID A fatty compound made of hydrogen, carbon, and oxygen, lipids are insoluble in water. The chemical family includes fats, fatty acids, cholesterol, oils, and waxes.

LIPOPROTEIN A combination of a lipid and a protein that can transport cholesterol in the bloodstream. The main types are high density (HDL), low density (LDL), and very low density (VLDL).

LOW-DENSITY LIPOPROTEINS (LDLs) These abundant, so-called "bad" lipoproteins carry most of the circulating cholesterol; high levels are associated with atherosclerosis and heart disease since this form of cholesterol builds up on artery walls.

LUTEIN AND ZEAXANTHIN Found in foods that are bright yellow, orange, and green, lutein and zeaxanthin are pigments in the carotenoid family that are linked to a reduced risk for macular degeneration and cataracts. Lutein is found in green leafy vegetables such as collard greens, kale, spinach, and watercress, as well as corn and egg yolks. Zeaxanthin is found in greens, red peppers, and corn.

LYCOPENE A powerful antioxidant that lends red color to numerous foods, lycopene is particularly abundant in tomatoes and tomato products. Studies have shown lycopene to be protective against prostate cancer, lung cancer, and heart disease.

MACRONUTRIENTS The food we eat provides two types of essential building blocks, or nutrients, known as macronutrients and micronutrients. Most food is primarily made up of water, a macronutrient. The remaining macronutrients—carbohydrate, protein, and fat—are vital energy-yielding nutrients that work in harmony with micronutrients to keep the body fit and functioning well.

METABOLISM The collective term for the body's physical and chemical processes that are needed to maintain life, including derivation of energy from food.

MICRONUTRIENTS Required in small amounts from the diet, vitamins and minerals are non-caloric essential nutrients known as micro-nutrients. They are critical for normal growth, development, and good health. Micronutrients promote and regulate chemical reactions vital for life and participate in all body processes, such as deriving energy from macronutrients, transmit-ting nerve impulses, and battling infections.

MONOTERPENES A family of phytochemicals that includes limonene, monoterpenes are under review for their ability to detoxify carcinogens, hinder cancer cell growth, and improve choles-terol levels. Food sources include cherries, citrus fruits, caraway, dill, and spearmint.

MONOUNSATURATED FAT Found in olive oil, canola oil, peanut oil, some margarine, avocado, nuts, and seeds, heart-healthy monounsaturated fat is not easily damaged by oxidation, so is less likely than saturated fat and trans fats to clog arteries. When consumed in place of saturated and trans fats, monounsaturated fats help lower LDL cholesterol levels. These fats are part of the Mediterranean diet, associated with lower rates of heart disease and cancer.

NEUROTRANSMITTERS Chemicals released from nerve endings that relay messages from one cell to another.

NITRATES Nitrogen-containing compounds that occur naturally in certain foods, nitrates are used as preservatives in some meat products, as fertiliz-ers, and in vasodilator drugs.

NITRITES Compounds that are produced in the body by the action of bacteria on nitrates, nitrites are also used as meat preservatives.

NITROSAMINES Compounds that are formed in food or in the body through the reaction of nitrites with amines. They are regarded as carcinogens, although no definite link has been established between nitrosamines and cancer in humans.

OLEIC ACID When consumed in place of saturated fat, this monounsaturated fat is linked to healthier cholesterol levels. Food sources include avocados, canola oil, and olive oil.

OXALATES Found in the greatest quantities in green vegetables, oxalates are compounds that

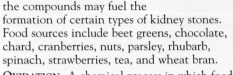

bind calcium, iron, and zinc, blocking their absorption in the body. In addition, people prone to kidney stones should avoid foods high in oxalates since the compounds may fuel the formation of certain types of kidney stones. Food sources include beet greens, chocolate, chard, cranberries, nuts, parsley, rhubarb, spinach, strawberries, tea, and wheat bran.

OXIDATION A chemical process in which food is burned with oxygen to release energy.

PASTEURIZATION The process of heating milk or other fluids to destroy microorganisms that might cause disease.

PECTIN A soluble fiber that helps to lower artery-damaging LDL cholesterol. Pectin may also be useful for managing diarrhea and diabetes. Sources include apples, apricots, bananas, carrots, figs, kiwifruits, and sweet potatoes.

PERISTALSIS Wavelike muscle contractions that help food and fluids move along through the digestive tract.

PHENYLKETONURIA (PKU) A condition caused by a genetic defect that prevents metabolism of the amino acid phenylalanine. People with PKU must follow a phenylalanine-free diet and avoid the artificial sweetener aspartame.

PHYTOCHEMICALS Naturally occurring plant chemicals that offer protection against a variety of diseases.

PHYTOESTROGENS Compounds found in plants that exhibit estrogenlike activity and may lower the risk of hormone-related cancers, as well as relieve fibrocystic breasts, osteoarthritis, and symptoms of perimenopause and menopause. The two major classes of phytoestrogens are isoflavones and lignans. Food sources include beans and soy.

PLASMA The clear yellow fluid that makes up about 55 percent of the blood and carries cells, platelets, and vital nutrients throughout the body.

PLATELETS Disc-shaped cells, manu-factured in the bone marrow, that are needed for blood coagulation.

POLYPHENOLS A class of antioxidants, polyphenol phytochemicals are under review for their potential to suppress tumor growth, detoxify carcinogens, interfere with the damaging effects of high estrogen levels, lower the risk of stroke, and prevent plaque buildup in the arteries. Sources include fruits, vegetables, tea, and red wine.

POLYUNSATURATED FATS Fats containing a high percentage of fatty acids that lack hydrogen atoms and have extra carbon bonds. They are liquid at room temperature (corn and sunflower oils, for instance) unless hydrogen is added. When hydrogen is added, these fats become more like saturated fats and have an adverse effect on blood cholesterol.

PROSTAGLANDINS Hormonelike chemicals involved in many body processes, including hypersensitivity (allergy) reactions, platelet aggregation (blood clotting), inflammation, pain sensitivity, and smooth muscle contraction.

PURINES Compounds that form uric acid when metabolized, purines are found in a number of foods, particularly high-protein foods, such as organ meats. Caffeine (in coffee and tea), theobromine (in chocolate), and theophylline (in tea) are related compounds. People prone to gout or kidney stones should avoid purines.

PYRIDOXINE One of the B vitamins, more commonly called B_6, this vitamin is essential for protein metabolism and the production of red blood cells. It is important for a healthy nervous and immune system. Food sources include meat, fish, whole grains, avocado, banana, and potatoes.

QUERCETIN Red onions, apples, grapes, red wine, and berries are rich source of quercetin, a potent flavonoid linked to a reduced risk of cancer, cardiovascular disease, and cataracts.

RESVERATROL A phytochemical particularly abundant in the skin of red grapes, resveratrol is under review for its potential to improve cholesterol levels, prevent atherosclerosis, and reduce the risks for stroke and cancer. Sources include red and purple grape juice, and red wine.

RIBONUCLEIC ACID (RNA) A substance present in every cell that translates the information contained in DNA into instructions telling the cell which proteins to synthesize.

SALICYLATES Compounds related to salicylic acid that are used for making aspirin and other painkillers and as a preservative. Naturally occurring salicylates in fruits or vegetables may produce allergic reactions in people who are sensitive to aspirin.

SALMONELLA A bacterium that is a frequent cause of food poisoning.

SATURATED FAT Fat found in animal products such as meat, poultry, and full-fat dairy products, as well as tropical oils such as palm and coconut. They are linked to an increased risk of heart disease, certain cancers, and other diseases.

SEROTONIN A neurotransmitter that helps promote sleep and regulates many body processes, including pain perception and the secretion of pituitary hormones.

SUCROSE Better known as table sugar, sucrose is composed of glucose and fructose. It is obtained from sugar cane and sugar beets; it's also present in honey, fruits, and vegetables.

SULFORAPHANE A notable sulfur compound, sulforaphane may increase the activity of cancer-fighting enzymes in the body, reduce tumor growth, block carcinogens from initiating cancer, and fight hormone-related cancer. Best food sources include broccoli and cabbage.

SULFUR COMPOUNDS Sulfur-containing phytochemicals abundant in garlic and the onion family are collectively called sulfur compounds and include allyl sulfide and ajoenes. Certain sulfur compounds are thought to stimulate cancer-fighting enzymes.

TANNINS Also called proanthocyanidins, tannins may detoxify carcinogens and scavenge harmful free radicals. Tannins in cranberries may protect against urinary tract infections. Note also that tannins reduce iron bioavailability. Sources include blackberries, blueberries, cranberries, grapes, lentils, tea, and wine.

TOXIN Any substance that when introduced into the body is capable of causing an adverse effect.

TRANS FATTY ACIDS Fats that are formed when vegetable oils are processed (hydrogenated) to improve their stability and to make them more solid. A food that lists "hydrogenated vegetable oil" on its ingredient list contains trans fatty acids. Growing concern about these acids is based on research that suggests high intakes of trans fatty acids may contribute to heart disease by elevating LDL ("bad") cholesterol and reducing HDL ("good") cholesterol. Some margarines (especially stick margarines), solid shortenings, snack foods, commercial frying fats (used in many fast-food establishments), and commercial baked goods are the major sources of trans fats.

TRIGLYCERIDES The most common form of dietary and body fat; high blood triglyceride levels have been linked to heart disease.

TRYPTOPHAN An essential amino acid, tryptophan is converted by the body into the B vitamin niacin. Tryptophan stimulates production of serotonin, a neurotransmitter that supports mental health. Complex carbohydrates enhance the absorption and use of tryptophan in the brain.

URIC ACID A nitrogen-containing waste product of protein metabolism, uric acid causes gout when it builds up.

ZEAXANTHIN See *Lutein and zeaxanthin*.

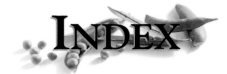

INDEX

*Note: Page numbers in **bold** are main discussions; illustrations are in italics.*
(Abbreviations: RDA is Recommended Dietary Allowance; UTIs are urinary tract infections.)

B

Photo Credits
Cover David Bishop, **31** Leland Bobbé/Corbis, **45** Alan Richardson, **49** Stockbyte, **52** Creatas, **79** Jay Hostetler/Still Life Stock,
80 Nicolas Eveleigh, **103** Douglas Kirkland/Corbis, **109** H. Amiard, **138** Corbis, **169** Julia Bigg,
171 Bob Winsell/Index Stock, **190** Todd Gipstein/Corbis, **238** Charles Gold/Corbis, **284** Corbis,
296–297 Annie Griffiths Belt/Corbis, **298** Corbis, **333** F. Vasseur/Visa, **374** Corbis, **384** Corbis.
Additional photo acknowledgments: Digital Vision, Digital Stock, Index Stock, Photodisc, PictureQuest,
and The Reader's Digest Association, Inc./GID.